P9-ELS-144

Vertebrate Endocrinology

Vertebrate Endocrinology

David O. Norris, Ph.D.
Professor of Biology, Department of Environmental, Population and Organismic Biology
University of Colorado, Boulder, Colorado

SECOND EDITION

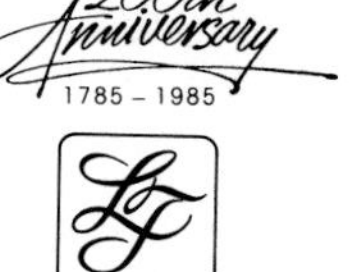

LEA & FEBIGER · 1985 · PHILADELPHIA

Lea & Febiger
600 Washington Square
Philadelphia, Pa. 19106
U.S.A.
(215) 922-1330

Library of Congress Cataloging in Publication Data

Norris, David O.
Vertebrate endocrinology.

Bibliography: p.
Includes index.
1. Endocrinology. 2. Vertebrates—Physiology.
I. Title.
QP187.N67 1985 596′.0142 84-19425
ISBN 0-8121-0967-8

PRINTED IN THE UNITED STATES OF AMERICA

Print Number 3 2 1

To Professor DONALD S. DEAN
inspiring teacher

Preface

This textbook is directed toward the advanced undergraduate zoology student who has some background in physiology as well as toward the graduate student seeking an introduction to the field. Because various disciplines encompassed by the field of endocrinology are changing so rapidly, it is difficult to keep any textbook on this subject current. *Vertebrate Endocrinology* has been extensively revised and updated in keeping with this need. New figures, tables, chemical regulators, sections dealing with clinical syndromes, and a glossary of endocrine abbreviations have been added. The organization of the book has been altered to provide a more logical sequence of topics.

The second edition is organized into four sections. Part One (Chapters 1–3) deals with introductory and background material on endocrinology including a general overview of endocrine systems and the mechanisms of action of hormones. A discussion of homeostatic mechanisms and phylogeny of vertebrates is provided for students who need this background. Part Two deals with the brain-pituitary system (Chapters 4–7) and the endocrine glands under its control (Chapters 8–11). Part Three includes all of the endocrine glands not regulated through the pituitary (Chapters 12–14) and many miscellaneous chemical regulators (Chapter 15). Part Four examines some major aspects of vertebrate biology and how they are regulated in particular vertebrate groups (Chapters 16–19). These chapters deal with osmoregulation (teleosts), metamorphosis (amphibians), migration (fish, amphibians, birds) and metabolism (mammals). Reproduction is treated comprehensively in Chapter 11. The purpose of Part Four is to remind us that although we may learn about endocrine systems "gland by gland", reality is a complex blending of the interactions of many different environmental factors and a variety of hormones. No hormone works in a "biological vacuum", and every internal adjustment influences many other processes. The Appendices are designed to supplement the text with background information (Appendices I and II), additional readings (Appendix III) and a glossary of abbreviations for quick reference (Appendix IV). The index is detailed and sufficiently cross-referenced to be a valuable aid in locating definitions of terms, functions, interactions with other hormones, etc.

There is considerable flexibility built into the text. It can be adapted to a number of approaches at the discretion of the instructor. Each chapter in Parts Two and Three is organized so that first mammals are discussed and then the nonmammalian groups. One approach would be to follow this sequence gland by gland. Alternatively, the mammalian portion of several chapters could be covered first or exclusively. The order of many chapters may be altered once the basics of the hypothalamo-hypophysial system have been completed (Chapters 4 and 5). Chapters from Part Four can be interspersed among those of Parts Two and Three where appropriate. For example, metamorphosis (Chapter 17) can follow thyroid (Chapter 8).

I have retained the practice of placing many references at the end of each chapter to direct the student to the voluminous literature on these subjects. Some references from the first edition have been replaced by more current ones, and many new references have been added. I have continued to cite references that should be available in most college and university libraries.

I would like to express my deepest appreciation to the many people who have contributed to the preparation of this edition. Particularly, I want to acknowledge the direct contributions of David Duvall, William A. Gern, Louis J. Guillette, Jr., Frank L. Moore, Richard Tokarz and Eugene Spaziani. My colleague and friend, Richard E. Jones, and my students, Mark Norman and Martha Pancak, provided thoughtful discussions and encouragement. I am indebted to my own students, numerous instructors and their students and many colleagues who have used the first edition for their critical comments. The contributions of the many scientists who are responsible for the rapid growth in our knowledge of comparative endocrinology are in evidence throughout the text.

The second edition of *Vertebrate Endocrinology* was completed during a sabbatical leave from the University of Colorado. I must also acknowledge the Department of Zoology at Oregon State University for providing use of university facilities during my sabbatical leave. Finally and most importantly, I am grateful to my wife, Kay, for providing editorial and secretarial skills. Without her support, encouragement and hard work, this edition would still be in progress!

DAVID O. NORRIS, PH.D.
Boulder, Colorado

Contents

PART I

1·An Introduction to Vertebrate Endocrinology

Endocrinology-Neuroendocrinology

Endocrinology is the study of certain glands known as endocrine glands and how these glands regulate the physiology and behavior of individual animals and populations. The endocrine system is basic to the abilities of an organism to adapt to its environment in both an ecological and an evolutionary sense. It is a chemical link between the environment and the organism.

At one time physiologists viewed the nervous and endocrine systems as discrete regulatory units each with their own brand of chemical messenger. The neurotransmitter released from neurons was easily distinguished from a hormone secreted into the blood (Table 1-1). This view began to change when it was discovered that neural activity could influence release of hormones from endocrine glands such as the pituitary and that hormones could in turn alter activity in the nervous system. Soon it was shown that some classic neurotransmitters could be released into the blood and function as hormones. Similarly, we learned that classic hormones were being used as neurotransmitters in the nervous system. Modified neurons were observed to produce special hormones that were released directly into the blood. Hypotheses appeared suggesting that many endocrine cells and neural tissues were derived embryonically from the same tissue. These observations gave birth to the field of *neuroendocrinology* which has become a dominant research area in the field of chemical regulation. This development has prompted some investigators to propose that endocrinology should be considered as a branch of neuroendocrinology.[32]

The endocrine system may be conceptualized as a series of reflexes much like the more familiar neural reflexes. The most simple reflexive unit in the endocrine system is the *endocrine reflex*. It is similar to the familiar neural reflex involving a stimulus, an integrating unit and an effector. A change in the amount of some substance circulating in the blood causes an endocrine cell to release a hormone into the blood that ultimately brings about a return of the circulating substance to "normal" levels. The *neurohormonal reflex* involves modified neurons within the central nervous system that secrete special hormones into the blood in response to information collected by neural receptors. This reflex may deal not only with information obtained from internal receptors but also information obtained from the external environment. The *neuroendocrine reflex* is the most complex of these reflexes involving neurohormonal control over activities of specific endocrine glands. It integrates external and internal information into precise regulatory control over major physiological processes such as reproduction, growth and metabolism. These reflexes are described in more detail in Chapter 2, but some general aspects of endocrinology must be considered before these reflexes are discussed.

TABLE 1-1. *Comparison of Chemical Regulators*

AGENT	DESCRIPTION	EXAMPLE
Neurotransmitter	Produced by neurons; secreted into extracellular synaptic spaces; travels short distances; local regulator	Acetylcholine
Hormone	Secreted by specialized endocrine cells into the blood; travels relatively long distances to targets	Thyroxine
Neurohormone	Hormone produced by a neuron (neurosecretory neuron)	Oxytocin
Paracrines	Produced by paraneurons; secreted into extracellular spaces; diffuse short distances	Somatostatin
Parahormone	Substance of general origins that produces generalized effects	Histamine
Semiochemical	Specific substance secreted into the environment that modify physiology and behavior of other organisms	Pheromone
Intracellular endocrine mediator	Intermediate in the cellular action of hormones that do not penetrate the cell but bind to receptors on the plasmalemma	cAMP

Glands and Glandular Secretion

There are many different kinds of glands in vertebrates that are highly specialized for secretion (Fig. 1-1; Table 1-2). Classically, they have been segregated into two kinds: endocrine and exocrine. The vertebrate endocrine system includes a variety of endocrine glands that secrete (synthesize and release) into the blood specific chemical messengers known as *hormones.* These chemical messengers travel via the blood to specific target tissues where they cause changes in the activities of the target tissue cells. Glands that secrete their products directly into the blood are termed *endocrine glands.* In recent years, this definition has been expanded to include the observation that some hormones are secreted into the cerebrospinal fluid. The pituitary gland, thyroid gland and the adrenal cortex are examples. *Exocrine glands* secrete their products into ducts through which the secretions pass to an internal or external surface. Salivary glands, sebaceous glands, sweat glands and mammary glands are all examples of exocrine glands.

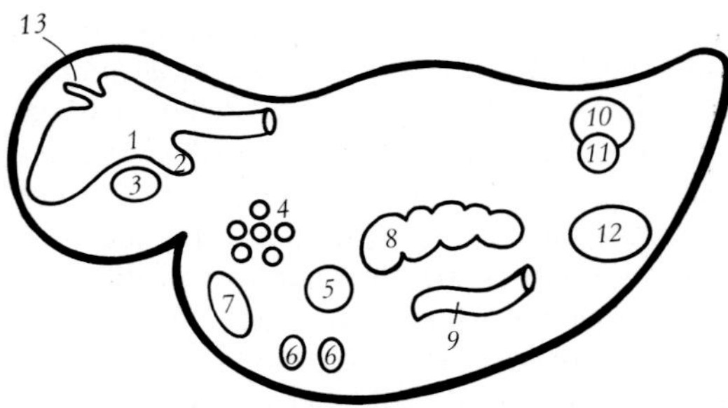

FIG. 1-1. Generalized endocrine structures in vertebrates. *1,* hypothalamus; *2,* pars nervosa (neurohypophysis); *3,* adenohypophysis; *4,* thyroid; *5,* ultimobranchial body; *6,* parathyroid glands; *7,* thymus; *8,* endocrine pancreas; *9,* stomach and duodenum (gastrointestinal tract); *10,* adrenal cortex; *11,* adrenal medulla; *12,* gonad; *13,* pineal gland. (Modified from Gorbman and Bern.[10])

Frequently glands are characterized according to the manner by which their secretory products are liberated. *Merocrine* secretion involves the process of *exocytosis,* which is essentially a reverse of pinocytosis or phagocytosis. The membrane-bound secretory granule or droplet containing the intracellular secretion product fuses with the cell membrane (plasmalemma), and the contents are dumped outside the secretory cell. Such a process causes no damage to the secretory cell and is typical of most endocrine cells as well as of certain exocrine cells (for example, the enzyme-secreting cells of the pancreas). Some exocrine cells slough the apical portion of the cell (that portion nearest the duct) containing the secretory products. This type of secretion is termed *apocrine* and is characteristic of cells

TABLE 1-2. *Cellular Patterns of Secretion*

SECRETORY PATTERN	DESCRIPTION	EXAMPLE
Endocrine	Product secreted into the blood for transport internally to target tissues	Hormones
Exocrine	Product secreted into a duct that opens onto an external or internal surface	Sweat
Exocytosis	Product released from secretory cell via a process essentially the reverse of pinocytosis	Peptide hormone release
Merocrine	Product secreted without visible damage to the secretory cell (involves exocytosis)	Thyroxine secretion
Apocrine	Product released by sloughing of "outer" or apical portion of secretory cell	Sebaceous gland secretion
Holocrine	Product released through cell death and lysis	
Cytogenous	Release of whole, viable cells	Spermatozoa

of the mammary gland. Still other glandular cells may die and undergo lysis upon releasing their stored products. Sebaceous gland cells exhibit this type of secretory pattern, which is termed *holocrine*. Finally the term *cytogenous* has been proposed for situations in which live, viable cells are "secreted" by organs such as the testes and ovaries, which release spermatozoa and ova respectively.

Neurosecretion: Neurohormones

The nervous system is usually viewed as a complex of neurons, most of which secrete specific chemicals, *neurotransmitters,* from their axonal endings. Such a neuron secretes neurotransmitter substance into an extracellular space (the synaptic cleft) through which it diffuses to bind with specific receptors in the postsynaptic cell (which may be another neuron, a muscle cell or a gland cell). Many different kinds of neurons have been identified in the central and peripheral nervous systems, each secreting its particular neurotransmitter. These neurons are frequently designated according to the chemical nature of their neurotransmitter such as cholinergic neurons (acetylcholine), adrenergic (norepinephrine), aminergic (amines such as dopamine), peptidergic (peptides), serotonergic (serotonin) and purinergic (purines). The pharmacological investigation of vertebrate nervous systems largely deals with the specific roles for these various neuronal types and the actions of drugs as they influence one or another type of neuron.

The neurotransmitter substance produced by a specific neuronal type can be partially identified by means of the electron microscope. Each neurotransmitter is stored prior to release within small membrane-bound droplets (synaptic vesicles) located in the expanded axonal tips (Fig. 1-2). Cholinergic synaptic vesicles have a diameter of 30–45 nm and are not electron dense, whereas adrenergic synaptic vesicles are larger (approximately 70 nm diameter) and exhibit electron-dense cores.

A number of years ago it was discovered that another type of axonal secretory product associated with certain highly specialized neurons could be identified at the light-microscope level by selective staining techniques (such as paraldehyde fuchsin, pseudoisocyanin and the Gomori chrome-alum hematoxylin procedure). Later, with the electron microscope, these secretory products were identified as large electron-dense granules (100–300 nm diameter). Anatomical studies suggested that these neurons release their secretory products directly into the blood vascular system. These neurons are termed *neurosecretory neurons,* and the dyes that they selectively accumulate are termed *neurosecretory stains.* Their secretory products are peptidergic substances (small peptides) or amines termed *neurohormones.* The process of secreting neurohormones is termed *neurosecretion.* A large num-

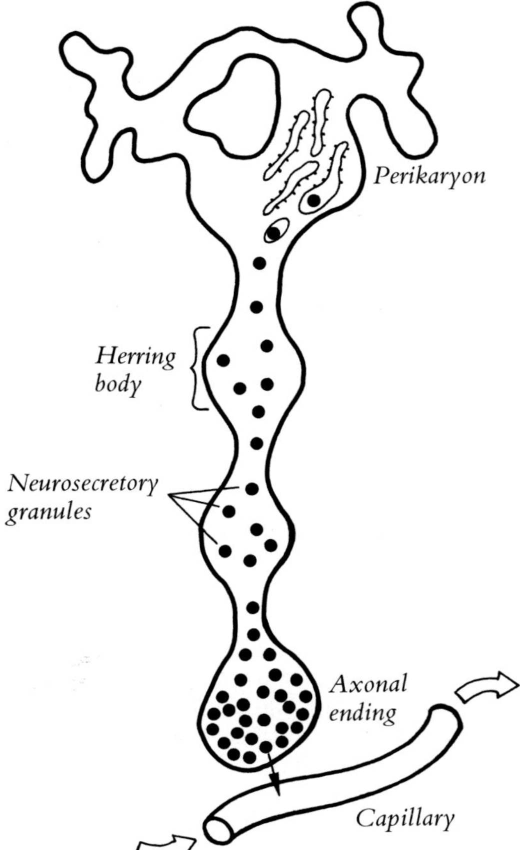

FIG. 1-2. Generalized neurosecretory cell. Neurosecretory granules containing neurohormones plus "carrier" protein are synthesized in the rough endoplasmic reticulum and migrate through the axon. Neurosecretory granules may accumulate in enlargements of the axon (Herring bodies) but eventually reach the tip of the axon where they may be stored until released by exocytosis into nearby capillaries. When many neurosecretory axons terminate in a highly vascularized structure the latter is termed a neurohemal organ.

ber of neurohormones have been chemically characterized and others have been proposed. Phylogenetically neurohormones constitute the first type of endocrine system to appear in animals and the only endocrine-secreting mechanism in many invertebrate groups.

The neurosecretory (NS) neuron is capable of conducting an action potential, although duration of action potentials measured from NS neurons is longer than that of "ordinary" neurons. The secretory granule of the NS neuron consists primarily of the neurohormones plus a "carrier" protein (Fig. 1-2), called a *neurophysin.* Although several neurophysins have been identified, their role in neurohormonal secretion is not clear. They may be related to the process of synthesizing the neurohormones.

An aggregation of perikarya (neuronal cell bodies) within the central nervous system is known as a *nucleus.* Perikarya of NS neurons typically occur in groupings called *neurosecretory nuclei.* Such nuclei are demonstrated easily with the use of NS stains. Generally NS neurons secreting a particular neurohormone occur in the same NS nucleus.

The classical NS neuron described above must now be modified somewhat. In the vertebrate brain at least two types of NS elements have been described on the basis of cytological details. The classical NS neurons are characterized by large cytoplasmic granules (100–300 nm diameter) in the axon terminals. The secretion products of these neurons are peptide neurohormones. Other NS neurons typically exhibit smaller granules (about 70 nm diameter). At least some of these NS neurons secrete amines such as dopamine (hence termed *aminergic*), but others secrete specific peptides (termed *peptidergic* neurons).

Neurosecretory tracts consisting of bundles of NS cell axons also can be stained within the central nervous system by NS stains. The endings of NS axons may accumulate in a highly vascularized area known as a *neurohemal organ.* Neurohormones are stored in these neurohemal organs prior to release. These organs usually stain intensely with NS dyes because of dense accumulations of NS material.

Neurosecretory dyes appear to stain the carrier proteins (neurophysins) in the secretory granules but will also stain other cellular inclusions and organelles such as other protein granules, mitochondria and endoplasmic reticulum. Consequently one cannot be sure that these dyes are staining only NS material by using this approach. A further caution in the use of NS staining procedures is related to the occasional observation that "stainability" of NS material does not always parallel neurohormonal content as determined by biological tests. High stainability may be correlated with high levels of the neurohormone on one occasion but with low levels on another.

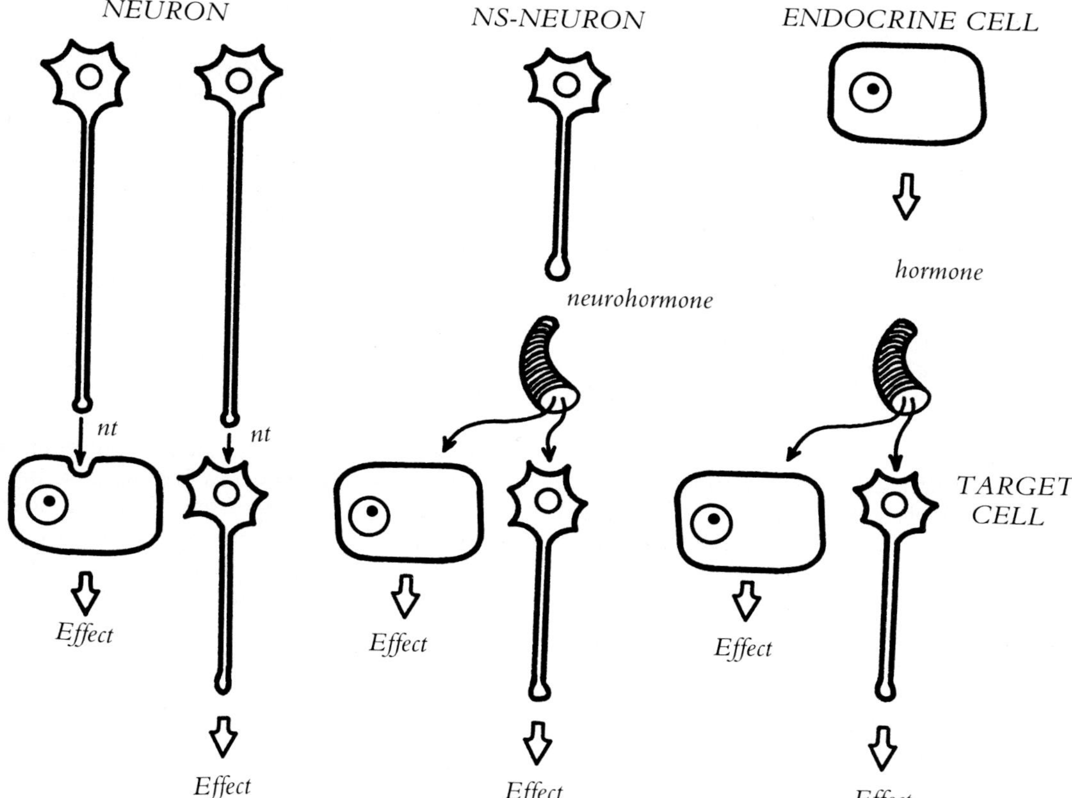

FIG. 1-3. General patterns of chemical regulation by neurons, NS neurons and endocrine cells. Paracrine secretion would be like the action of a neuron. See text for explanation. nt, neurotransmitter.

Many neurosecretory neurons release more than just their reputed neurohormone. Secretory granules in these cells may contain other peptides, enzymes and amines which are released along with the hormones.

Neuroendocrine Responses

The cells of endocrine glands may be influenced by neurohormones circulating via the blood vascular system. Scharrer has emphasized that in addition to direct innervation of endocrine cells by neurons forming the typical secretomotor junctions associated with neurotransmitters, some NS neurons form "neurosecretomotor junctions" with endocrine cells.[38] These junctions are usually of the peptidergic type, although some are apparently aminergic. Scharrer has described another variation on the general theme of NS influences on endocrine cells in which NS neurons release their secretory products into an extracellular matrix, thereby relying on diffusion to accomplish the actual contact with an endocrine cell. Any of these variations involving NS neurons and endocrine cells constitutes a neuroendocrine control mechanism.

Types of Chemical Regulators

The knowledge that individual neurons can function like endocrine cells, that many known neurotransmitters are released into the blood where they function as classical hormones and that widely distributed cells release chemical regulators into extracellular fluids has altered the field of endocrinology. Chemical regulators of the latter type that diffuse short distances are designated as *paracrines.*[5] Internal chemical regulators occur as a continuum from classical neurotransmitters to paracrines to classical hormones. Attempts to provide rigid definitions for these various types of regulators may be counterproductive, for evolution has assured that we cannot provide discrete categories. These types are simply categories for convenience and are not meant to be mutually exclusive. Epinephrine, for example, is a neurotransmitter when released from a neuron into a synaptic extracellular space. It is a paracrine substance if released into a generalized extracellular space through which it diffuses to a nearby target cell. When released into the blood from the adrenal medulla, epinephrine is a hormone.

The situation is complicated further by the existence of other chemical messengers. *Parahormones* are one category of such compounds; they are specialized substances that may be produced by a variety of cellular types and often have rather generalized effects. Histamine and angiotensin II might be considered parahormones because of their widespread effects on smooth-muscle contractions. Carbon dioxide produced by all respiring cells has generalized effects on many tissues, including rather specific effects on the respiratory centers in the brain.

The so-called *semiochemicals* form another category of chemical messengers that cannot be classified strictly as hormones. They are often produced by specialized cells but are secreted outside the body and influence the physiology and behavior of other individuals. Some of these semiochemicals may be modified steroid hormones, which helps justify their inclusion under the umbrella of endocrinology. Semiochemicals are given special "endocrine" status in Chapter 15.

A variety of intracellular chemical messengers have also been identified. The prostaglandins and certain cyclic nucleotides are important intracellular messengers that are involved in the mechanisms of action for hormones that are bound to the plasmalemma and do not enter the cytoplasm of their target cells.

Chemical Nature of Hormones and Neurohormones

Vertebrate hormones and neurohormones may be proteins, polypeptides, derivatives of amino acids or lipids. Most of the lipid hormones are steroids derived from cholesterol (Chap. 9) or fatty acid derivatives such as the prostaglandins (Chap. 15). Steroid hormones differ further from polypeptide hormones and those derived from amino acids in that they are not generally stored in glandular cells but are released immediately after their synthesis. Secretion of the nonsteroidal hormones and the neurohormones can be readily separated into synthetic and release phases that may be regulated separately.

The mode of action of hormones is also different, correlated in part to their chemical and physical properties. Water-soluble hormones tend not to enter their target cells but bind to the plasmalemma, whereas steroids and thyroid hormones (derived from the amino acid tyrosine) are nonpolar molecules and readily move across cell membranes. Transport of steroids and thyroid hormones into cells may not be simple diffusion but may involve a membrane-mediated process. These latter hormones require binding proteins in the blood plasma to facilitate their transport and reduce their rate of removal from the blood, metabolism and excretion.

Cytological Features and Hormone Synthesis

Cells responsible for elaboration of peptide hormones possess a well-developed rough endoplasmic reticulum where hormone synthesis takes place. The hormonal products are stored in membrane-bound secretion granules in the cytoplasm. Peptide hormones are synthesized on ribosomes as part of a larger peptide called a *preprohormone.* A special terminal segment of the preprohormone is a short amino acid sequence called a *signal peptide.*[21] The presence of this segment allows the newly synthesized peptide to enter into the cisterna of the endoplasmic reticulum. In the process, the signal peptide is enzymatically removed leaving a large peptide called a *prohormone.* This peptide travels through the endoplasmic reticulum to the Golgi apparatus where it is packaged into secretory granules. Addition of carbohydrates may occur in the Golgi when the final products are glycoproteins. Enzymatic cleavage of the prohormone occurs within the secretory granules. This cleavage produces the specific hormone and a separate peptide fragment. The neurophysins may be produced as the non-hormonal fragment of a prohormone.

Synthesis of proteins and peptides is controlled by the activity of nuclear genes or, in certain cases, mitochondrial genes. A given gene determines the sequence of messenger RNA that will be transcribed. Messenger RNA leaves the nucleus and travels to the ribosome where it directs the specific sequence by which amino acids are linked to construct a particular polypeptide. By identifying the sequence of amino acids in the hormone as well as in its preprohormone and prohormone fragments, it has been possible to construct artificial genes which can be inserted into cultured cells or cells of intact animals. Once incorporated into their genome, these cells can synthesize large quantities of specific hormones. Already, the synthesis of genes for producing growth hormone, insulin and many others has been achieved. Such genetic engineering offers the promise that some day similar gene insertions may alleviate clinical problems associated with underproduction of a peptide or protein hormone.

It is the storage granules in endocrine cells that are responsible for their unique affinities for various dyes and their identification at the light microscope level. Furthermore, depending upon their size, shape, or both, these storage granules may provide cytological markers for particular cellular types at the ultrastructural level.

Steroid-secreting cells are characterized by abundant smooth endoplasmic reticulum for steroidogenesis and a well-developed Golgi apparatus for packaging lipid droplets. Steroidogenic cells can be identified histochemically by localization of specific enzymes involved in steroid hormone synthesis (for example, Δ^5, 3β-hydroxysteroid dehydrogenase). Quiescent steroidogenic cells may contain large cholesterol-positive droplets in their cytoplasm, but as a rule most of the steroid hormones synthesized from cholesterol are released into the blood as they are produced and are not stored. Enzymatic activity or cholesterol content is an index of hormone synthesis.

Histological Organization of Endocrine Cells

Endocrine cells are grouped or clumped in characteristic arrangements, although in certain instances isolated cells may be diffusely distributed among other cellular types such as occurs in the gastrointestinal tract. A common arrangement for endocrine cells is in folded sheets or *cords* of cells as found in the pituitary (Chap. 4) or the adrenal cortex (Chap. 10). In some cases separate clumps of endocrine cells or *islets* may be found embedded within another tissue. The endocrine pancreas consists of islets of cells dispersed among the exocrine-secreting tissue of the pancreas (Chap. 13). Other endocrine cells are arranged in hollow balls of cells or *follicles.* In this arrangement there is only a single layer of endocrine cells in each follicle surrounding a central space filled with fluid or colloidal material secreted primarily by the endocrine cells themselves. Such a follicular organization is characteristic of thyroid glands (Chap. 8).

Internal Rhythms in Endocrine Secretion

Hormones are released episodically or in bursts (phasic secretion) rather than at a constant rate (tonic secretion). Many of these bursts show a decisive diurnal, monthly or seasonal cyclicity or rhythm. Diurnal fluctuations are being observed commonly in all kinds of animals as a consequence of the development of precise techniques for monitoring blood levels of hormones. The daily to seasonal variations in reproductive hormones during the menstrual cycles of higher primates and the estrous cycles of other mammals are well known to students of zoology. Not only do hormone levels vary, but the sensitivities of target tissues to the same hormone dose may also exhibit diurnal or seasonal fluctuations.[4,20]

The establishment of variations in secretory patterns of endocrine glands on a daily or seasonal basis or both, as well as rhythmic variations in sensitivities of target tissues, means that additional caution is required in interpreting experimental results, especially when no effects of a given treatment are observed or when two investigators obtain opposite results in the same system. Indeed the response observed to one hormone may depend upon the rhythm of another hormone.

The relationship of cyclical exogenous (external or environmental) rhythms to migration, reproduction and other phenomena is of great interest to all types of zoologists. Endocrine glands are proving to be important mediators of cyclic environmental phenomena that program physiological events in other endocrine glands. Many studies, for example, have shown that alterations in photoperiod can influence endogenous (internal) endocrine rhythms dramatically. The discovery of these endogenous hormonal rhythms and the involvement of exogenous or external factors (Zeitgebers) to set internal timers has opened research into one of the most exciting areas of endocrinology and will alter the direction of future endocrine research.

Hormones and Age

Throughout the life of any vertebrate, developmental changes are occurring with respect to maturation of hormonal secretory patterns and to the responsiveness of particular target tissues. Many of the changes associated with development and aging may be caused by hormones themselves.[7] Fetal tissues may respond differently than neonatal tissues to the same hormone. Young animals may respond differently than neonates. The secretory patterns for certain hormones may be altered by the attainment of sexual maturity, and they may be altered again after the animal ceases to be reproductively active (a rare event in nature but common in humans and some domesticated animals). The role of growth hormone is very different in a growing animal and an adult animal, for example. The action of growth hormone on certain growing tissues can be altered markedly by the secretion of gonadal steroids at puberty. Consequently it is important to consider developmental ages of animals when interpreting endocrine data.

Mammalian Hormones: An Overview

The major hormones and glands of the mammalian endocrine system are listed below. All of these hormones and certain others will be considered in greater detail in later chapters.

The central figure of the mammalian endocrine system is the *hypothalamo-hypophysial axis.* The *hypothalamus* is the ventral portion of the brain immediately beneath the thalamus and above the *pituitary gland* or *hypophysis.* Neurosecretory centers in the hypothalamus produce neurohormones that independently control release of several different hormones from the pituitary. These hypothalamic NS centers are in turn influenced by neurons from higher neural centers in the brain. The hypothalamic neurohormones are termed releasing hormone(s) (RH) or release-inhibiting hormone(s) (RIH). They are sometimes designated as the *hypothalamo-hypophysiotropic hormones.*

The pituitary hormones include *prolactin* (PRL); *growth hormone* (GH); *thyrotropin,* or thyroid-stimulating hormone (TSH); *luteinizing hormone* (LH); *follicle-stimulating hormone* (FSH); *corticotropin,* or adrenocorticotropic hormone (ACTH); *melanophore-stimulating hormone* (MSH); and *lipotropin,* or lipotropic hormone (LPH). These hormones are termed collectively the *tropic hormones* since several of them influence the activities of other endocrine glands. Thyrotropin controls the synthesis of thyroid hormones *triiodothyronine* (T_3) and *thyroxine* (T_4) by the thyroid gland. Corticotropin regulates synthesis and release of corticosteroids such as *cortisol* and *corticosterone* by adrenal cortical cells. Luteinizing hormone and FSH influence the gonads (testes, ovaries) by stimulating gametogenesis (gamete production) and synthesis and release of male sex hormones or *androgens* (for example, *testosterone*) and female sex hormones or *estrogens* (for example, *estradiol-17β*) and *progestogens* (*progesterone*). The other tropic hormones do not have endocrine targets. Prolactin influences lactation by the mammary gland. Growth hormone has metabolic effects on muscle, adipose cells and other tissues. Pigment cells in the skin are targets for MSH, and LPH produces metabolic effects on adipose cells.

Two neurohormones produced by hypothalamic centers are stored in a special region of the pituitary, the *pars nervosa.* When released, *oxytocin* stimulates contraction of uterine smooth muscle and initiates labor. Oxytocin also causes contraction of modified cells in the mammary gland that cause milk ejection following suckling by the young. The *vasopressins* are similar molecules to oxytocin that enhance water reabsorption in the kidney and have been termed antidiuretic hormones.

In addition to the hypothalamo-hypophysial hormones there are a number of important endocrine glands that are not influenced by neurohormones although they may be influenced by direct innervation with sympathetic or parasympathetic fibers. Parathyroid glands produce *parathyroid hormone* (PHT) which, together with *calcitonin* (CT) from the thyroid, regulates calcium balance. The *endocrine pancreas* produces at least two hormones that control intermediary metabolism, *insulin* and *glucagon.* A variety of cellular types distributed in particular regions of the digestive tract produce a series of *gastrointestinal hormones* including *gastrin, secretin* and *pancreozymin-cholecystokinin* (PZCCK). In recent years the secretions of the *thymus gland* have achieved recognition as hormones in controlling differentiation of immunologically responsive tissues.

Two organs derived from neural tissue are well-known hormone sources. The *adrenal medulla* releases both *epinephrine* (adrenaline) and *norepinephrine* (noradrenaline) into the circulation. Norepinephrine binds primarily to target tissues with alpha-type receptors on the cell surface (plasmalemma). Epinephrine may bind to either alpha-type or beta-type receptors and consequently may influence different targets than norepinephrine. (See Appendix II for a discussion of alpha and beta receptors.) The *pineal gland* produces *melatonin* as well as several peptides that appear to deserve hormonal status. These substances may influence thyroid and reproductive functions in mammals, and the pineal gland may be an endocrine transducer that mediates the effects of photoperiod on reproductive cycles (see Chap. 11).

Three hormones are made by the kidney. Renin is secreted by the kidney and influences secretion of *aldosterone,* a hormone involved with regulation of sodium and potassium balance, by the adrenal cortical cells. The second involves production of *erythropoietin,* a hormone controlling formation of red blood cells (erythropoiesis) in the bone marrow. The kidney converts a derivative of vitamin D to the third hormone, *1,25-dihydroxycholecalciferol.* This hormone is responsible for stimulating calcium uptake in the small intestine.

Inactivation and excretion of hormones occur in many target tissue cells. In addition, the liver, primarily, and the kidney, to a lesser extent, also metabolize and excrete hormones via the bile or urine respectively.

Origin of Endocrine Cells

Endocrinologists have recognized four separate embryonic origins for hormone-secreting cells exclusive of the NS cells that are derived from neural ectoderm. Cells of the pituitary gland that secrete peptide and protein tropic hormones, such as thyrotropin and corticotropin, classically have been believed to develop from oral (non-neural) ectoderm (see Chap. 4). The steroid-synthesizing cells of the gonads and adrenal glands are mesodermal in origin. Each adrenal medulla is a modified sympathetic ganglion and is derived from neural ectoderm. Finally the majority of endocrine glands appear to have their origins from the endodermal primitive gut, and they all synthesize protein hormones, polypeptide hormones, or modified amino acids.

A considerable revision in thinking followed the discovery of a peculiar property of many hormone-secreting cells previously thought to characterize only cells that secrete biogenic amines such as epinephrine. This property is known as *amine content* and *amine precursor uptake and decarboxylation* or simply as APUD.[31] Cells possessing APUD characteristics were originally proposed by Pearse to originate from the *neural crest,* which is a series of small masses of neuroectodermal cells located adjacent to and distributed along the neural tube of very young vertebrate embryos. The neural crest gives rise to the sympathetic ganglia, the adrenal medulla, all of the melanin-producing pigment cells of vertebrates, the branchial skeleton of the head region and other structures. The discovery of APUD characteristics in many endocrine cells led to the elegant demonstration of a neural crest origin for the CT-producing cells that migrate to the ultimobranchial body, which eventually becomes incorporated into the thyroid gland of mammals[19] (see Chaps. 8 and 12). Parathyroid cells that secrete PTH arise from neural ectoderm in the frog *Rana temporaria,* and a similar origin may occur in birds and mammals.[7] Later, this definition was broadened to encompass cells originating from other neural and even non-neural tissue. For example, endocrine cells of the gut, pancreatic islets, adenohypophysis, hypothalamus, placenta, thymus and others were included. Although some of the pituitary cells lack the APUD characteristics, Pearse argues that because of their purported origin from neural ectoderm they should be included.

Although there is considerable debate concerning the common origins of all of these cellular types, it is agreed that almost all secrete regulatory peptides. Some consider that the possession of APUD characteristics and certain enzymes is probably related to similar metabolic requirements and not to common embryonic origins.[1]

Fujita proposed the *paraneuron concept*[13] to recognize paracrine secreting cells that have properties in common with neural cells. The origins of paraneurons have not been established. They do have APUD characteristics, but it is not clear whether they are derived from ectoderm or endoderm. Their name was coined in the belief that, although they are not neurons, they do receive environmental input and release their secretory products into extracellular spaces. It has been hypothesized that paracrine hormones, neurohormones and hormones all had a common origin. This hypothesis is strengthened by the discovery that many vertebrate regulatory peptides are present in unicellular organisms and that many invertebrate regulatory peptides are present in the vertebrates.[17] Moreover, peptides that serve as neurotransmitters in the central and peripheral nervous systems may also function as neurohormones, paracrines and/or hormones in the same animal.

Regulatory peptides may have been basic to the first living cells. During evolution, they may have been adapted in various ways; first as paracrine secretions, later as neurotransmitters, neurohormones and finally as endocrine hormones.

Mechanisms of Hormone Action

This brief account of possible mechanisms of hormone action is designed only to introduce the topic so that these points may be considered in reference to hormones discussed in the following chapters. More will be said about how specific hormones produce their effects as actions of each hormone on its target cells are considered.

In order that a hormone produce any effect on a target cell it must be bound specifically by the target cell either intracellularly or at the cell surface. Those cells that respond to a given hormone synthesize *receptors* that selectively bind only the appropriate hormone. Nontarget cells lack these receptors. Steroid and thyroid hormone receptors are located intracellularly, and these hormones must pass through the plasmalemma before being bound. Polypeptide, protein and amine hormones bind to receptors in the plasmalemma and are believed not to enter the cell. Recent studies, however, have unequivocally demonstrated that polypeptide hormones attached to their receptors enter target cells. It appears that the entrance of the hormone-receptor complex is related to enzymatic degradation of the complex.[34,35] It is possible that "delayed" actions on enzyme synthesis that take place much later than the initial actions are related to internalization of the hormone-receptor complex.

Hormones may bring about their effects through a variety of mechanisms and may influence a variety of different cellular activities. Many hormones influence specific synthetic or catabolic enzymatic reactions. Certain hormones act to stimulate or inhibit release of other hormones. One hypothalamo-hypophysiotropic hormone is known to inhibit release of GH from the pituitary, whereas another is believed to stimulate its release. Epinephrine is a known inhibitor of insulin release from the endocrine pancreas, which is an action entirely separate from its effect of increasing blood glucose levels through alteration of liver metabolism. Permeability changes in membranes may occur as a consequence of binding of hormone molecules to receptor molecules embedded in the plasmalemma. The consequence of binding might alter the conformation of the membrane, allowing for ionic fluxes to occur across the membrane. Movements of ions may increase or decrease metabolic reactions in the cell, or they may alter the influx or efflux of some important nutrient. One hypothesis for explaining all of the many actions of insulin is based entirely upon changes induced in membrane structure and hence permeability following binding of insulin to the receptor molecule in the plasmalemma (see Chap. 13).

Hormones do not generally initiate reactions in target cells de novo but only influence the biochemical machinery already there. One of the first biochemical events measured in hormone target cells was an increase or decrease in activity of certain enzymes (Table 1-3). Other chemical substances are known to affect enzyme activity, but the mechanism by which hormones operate is different. For example, two known stimulators of the level of tryptophan pyrrolase (a liver enzyme) are found to increase the in-vivo activity in different ways.[33] Cortisone, a steroid hormone produced by the adrenal cortex, stimulates synthesis of this enzyme, but the amino acid tryptophan inhibits degradation of the enzyme, which also raises the effective level of enzyme in the liver cells.

The common biochemical target for many hormones is frequently some *rate-limiting step* in a biochemical pathway. Generally, complex enzyme systems possess at least one rate-limiting step; that is, one enzyme-activated transformation that can operate as a valve or control step. Once activated, this rate-limiting reaction occurs and allows the synthesis of some substrate that starts a sequence of transformations. Hormones alter the rate of reaction by influencing availability of the enzyme responsible for catalyzing that rate-limited step. This action of a hormone on the rate-limiting step may be due to an increase in the synthesis of an enzyme or an effect on the activity of enzymes already present. In the latter case the hormone might activate or inactivate an enzyme already present or simply alter the permeability of the plasmalemma such that additional substrate becomes available, which in turn stimulates enzyme activity. Research on the mechanisms of hormonal action on enzyme systems has centered around these three basic phenomena: transport of substrates, new enzyme synthesis and activation of inactive enzymes.

Membrane Transport and Enzyme Activity

In some cases the action of the hormone may be simply an effect on transport. Some effects of hormones on transport of materials both through the cell membrane (plasmalemma) and across intracellular membranes are summarized in Table 1-4. Transport regulation would determine the availability of certain substrates, cofactors, etc., essential for activity of specific enzymes. Thus hormones might increase or decrease the activity of specific enzyme systems via the availability of some essential substrate or cofactor. Insulin, for example, accelerates lipogenesis in adipose cells in part by facilitating entrance of glucose into the adipose cells. Intracellular glucose is metabolized to glycerol and other substances necessary for the synthesis of triglycerides

TABLE 1-3. *Effects of Some Hormones on Enzyme Activity*

HORMONE	SOURCE	ENZYME	% CHANGE	HR[a]
Cortisone	Adrenal cortex	Arginase	(+) 400	5
Testosterone	Testis	Salivary gland esteropeptidase	(+) 300–500	48
Glucagon	Endocrine pancreas	Serine dehydratase	(+) 2000	6
Growth hormone	Pituitary	Tyrosine aminotransferase	(−) 80–100	4

SOURCE: Modified from Pitot, H.C. and M.B. Yatvin (1973). Interrelationships of mammalian hormones and enzyme levels *in vitro*. Physiol. Rev. 53:228–325.
[a]Time in hrs required to observe maximum response.

Table 1-4. *Actions of Selected Hormones on Transport across Cellular Membranes*

HORMONE	SOURCE	ACTION
Aldosterone	Adrenal cortex	Stimulates Na^+ reabsorption in nephron
Estradiol	Ovary	Stimulates H_2O, Na^+ and K^+ uptake by uterus
Glucagon	Endocrine pancreas	Stimulates glucose uptake by adipose cells
Growth hormone	Pituitary	Stimulates amino acid uptake by muscle, liver, adipose tissue
Insulin	Endocrine pancreas	Stimulates amino acid and glucose uptake by muscle cells
Parathyroid hormone	Parathyroid glands	Stimulates movement of Ca^{++} and phosphate ions from bone into the blood

(fats). In muscle cells, insulin stimulates uptake of both glucose and amino acids, which respectively increase glycogen synthesis and protein synthesis as a result of increased substrate availability.

Gene Action and Enzyme Activity

Following the lead of microbial investigations on the genetic apparatus and control of enzyme synthesis, a "repressor" or "inducer" role for hormones has been sought in eukaryotic cells.[32,46] Several workers studying the peculiar polytene salivary chromosomes of dipteran larvae observed that "puffs" appeared in particular regions of these chromosomes correlated with particular stages of development.[18] Ecdysone, the insect molting hormone, stimulated formation of a certain puffing pattern (that is, formation of puffs at specific loci along the chromosome), suggesting an action of ecdysone on chromosomal events. These puffs were shown to be active sites of DNA-dependent RNA synthesis. Analogous experiments were performed with chromosomes of newt oocytes. These cells exhibit attenuated chromosomes with peculiar loops consisting of single DNA strands extending outward from the body of the chromosome. These chromosomes are termed lampbrush chromosomes (after the brushes used for oil lamps that they supposedly resembled), and the loops have been shown to be sites of DNA-dependent RNA synthesis like the puffs of the dipteran polytene chromosomes. ^{3}H-estradiol-17β, a vertebrate steroid hormone similar in structure to ecdysone, binds specifically to some of the unwound loops of lampbrush chromosomes, and subsequently a number of steroids have been shown to bind to nuclei of their target cells.

The effect of cortisone on synthesis of the enzyme tryptophan pyrrolase is mediated via DNA-dependent RNA synthesis that is inhibited by actinomycin D.[12] Such stimulation of RNA synthesis has been shown by a variety of experiments to be an integral part of hormone-induced responses in target cells. Estradiol stimulates RNA and protein synthesis of a specific egg protein, ovalbumin, in chicken oviducts. Chick-oviduct RNA extracted following estradiol treatment can direct synthesis of ovalbumin in a cell-free system.[29] Some hormones that induce RNA synthesis in certain target tissues are listed in Table 1-5.

Once it was shown that steroid hormones affect nuclear RNA synthesis, investigations were launched to identify earlier events in hormone action, in other words, what happens during the interval between arrival at the cell and the stimulation of nuclear events. One of the central questions examined was whether hormones have a direct or an indirect action on RNA synthesis. These studies have not only elucidated some of the early events in the stimulation of enzyme synthesis by hormones but have also identified how activity of existing enzymes can be influenced by hormones. Most of the studies with steroid and thyroid hormones have centered around the binding of hormones to intracellular receptors, while the majority of studies with polypeptide and amine hormones have emphasized binding to receptors in the plasmalemma and activation of a plasmalemma-bound enzyme, *adenyl* (adenylyl, adenylate) *cyclase* (see p. 15).

TABLE 1-5. *Some Hormones That Stimulate RNA Synthesis in Target Tissues*

HORMONE	HORMONE SOURCE	TISSUE EXAMINED	TISSUE SOURCE
Growth hormone	Pituitary	Liver	Hypophysectomized rat
		Muscle	Hypophysectomized and castrated rat
Thyroxine	Thyroid gland	Liver	Thyroidectomized rat
Testosterone	Testis	Prostate	Castrated rat
		Muscle	Hypophysectomized and castrated rat
		Liver	Castrated rat
Estradiol	Ovary	Uterus	Ovariectomized rat
Cortisone	Adrenal cortex	Liver	Rat

SOURCE: Modified from Frieden and Lipner.[8]

Mechanism of Steroid Action on Protein Synthesis

Binding of steroid hormones to target tissues is essentially the study of protein receptor molecules and behavior of a hormone-receptor complex in activating enzyme synthesis.[28] Such receptor molecules have been found to be highly specific for a given hormone and are not present in significant amounts in nontarget cells. Receptor molecules for estradiol-17β extractable from known target tissues will not bind other steroid hormones appreciably, including the biologically inactive 17α-isomer of estradiol.

Jensen[14] proposed a model for the binding of estradiol-17β and the role of the hormone-receptor complex in stimulation of nuclear RNA synthesis in the uterus. This model has undergone several revisions and is outlined in Figure 1-4. Simply stated, estradiol (E) enters through the cell membrane and is bound to a *receptor molecule* to form a *hormone-receptor complex.* The complex migrates to and enters the nucleus where it binds to a nuclear *acceptor site.* This hormone-receptor complex has a molecular weight of approximately 70,000 daltons, but it may form a dimer (MW = 130,000) before being translocated to the nucleus. After binding of the hormone-receptor complex to the nuclear acceptor site the complex is believed to activate a specific gene, resulting eventually in new synthesis of hormone-specific enzyme. This action on enzyme synthesis may be achieved by blocking the synthesis of a specific repressor molecule or by inactivating the repressor itself. New messenger RNA (mRNA) and translation of messenger are enhanced, and an increase in enzyme synthesis occurs. After activating the synthesis of mRNA the hormone-receptor complex is degraded metabolically, and the gene may again be repressed. In addition to stimulating synthesis of enzymes associated with the overt actions of estradiol on uterine tissues, it appears that estradiol also stimulates synthesis of new receptors so that more estradiol may be bound by the cell.[3]

The actions of other steroid hormones (corticosteroids, progesterone and androgens) have not been studied as extensively, but their mechanisms of action appear to be very similar to estrogens. They may bind to cytoplasmic receptors prior to translocation and binding to nuclear chromatin. One difference has appeared in many androgen-sensitive tissues in that the major circulating androgen, testosterone, must be enzymatically converted to another androgen, 5α-dihydrotestosterone or DHT, before it can be bound to the receptor.[22] Androgens may also be converted to estrogens,[5] and this alteration may be important in the actions of androgens on the central nervous system (see also Chap. 9).

The Jensen hypothesis should be treated as a working hypothesis for steroid hormone action since many aspects of the model as presented here require experimental verification, and considerable revision may still take place.[11] For example, the observations that unoccupied estrogen receptors may occur in the nucleus of intact cells[24,47] suggests that the demonstration of receptors in the cytoplasm of cell homogenates (an integral part of

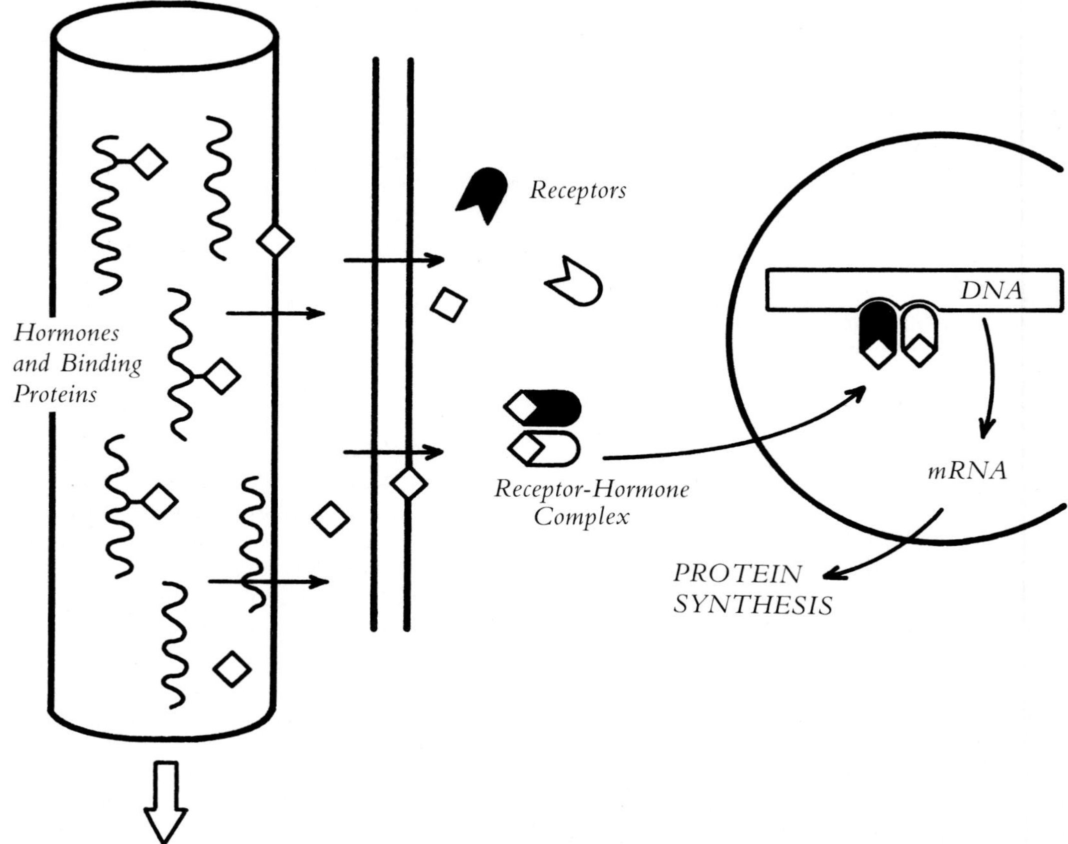

FIG. 1-4. Model of the proposed mechanism of action for steroid hormones. Steroids dissociate from plasma-binding proteins and enter the target cell where they bind to intracellular receptors or are enzymatically converted to another steroid which binds to the receptor. The hormone-receptor complex activates nuclear genes to stimulate synthesis of specific proteins which bring about effects specific for each target cell. The precise location of intracellular steroid receptors (cytoplasmic or nuclear) is not certain (see text). If the receptor is located in the cytoplasm, then the hormone-receptor complex must translocate to the nucleus before protein synthesis can be activated.

the Jensen hypothesis) could be artifactual. Nevertheless the Jensen hypothesis has been of immeasurable value in stimulating research and furthering understanding of steroid hormone actions.

Additional Mechanisms for Steroid Action

Estrogens not only stimulate growth of the uterine lining (endometrium) but also cause increased vascularity (hyperemia). A number of investigators believe that the hyperemic action of estrogens is mediated by an estrogen-dependent release of histamine, a potent local vasodilator.[23] A local action for estrogens possibly involving histamine has been reported also for the ovary of a lizard.[15,45]

Alterations of the properties of the plasmalemma by corticosteroids has been reported for cultured mammalian cells.[2] Corticosteroids stimulate new enzyme synthesis in these cells and also produce changes in cell adhesiveness and in electrophoretic and antigenic properties. The importance of these observations for in-vivo action of corticosteroids is not clear.

Thyroid Hormones and Gene Function

The mechanism of action for thyroid hormones appears to be analogous to the Jensen hypothesis for steroids, although some major differences are noted. Some evidence indicates that thyroid hormones are not bound to cytoplasmic receptors but bind directly to nuclear receptors.[30] Once bound to the nucleus, thyroid hormones stimulate DNA-dependent protein synthesis similar to that produced by steroid hormones in their target tissues. Others provide evidence for mitochondrial receptors for thyroid hormones.[43] Following binding of thyroid hormones to the mitochondrial receptors the synthesis of mitochondrial protein is stimulated. The possible significance of these divergent observations and their relationship to the functions of thyroid hormones are discussed in Chapter 8.

Enzyme Activation by Hormones: The "Second Messenger" Hypothesis

The discovery of the effect of epinephrine (the "emergency" hormone released from the adrenal medulla) on the formation of the cyclic nucleotide *cyclic adenosine 3′, 5′-monophosphate* (cAMP) and its subsequent role in cardiac muscle responses resulted in the awarding of a Nobel Prize to E.W. Sutherland in 1972. Studies by Sutherland and his coworkers showed that the first measurable effect of epinephrine was a fourfold increase in the level of cAMP *within 3 seconds* after the hormone was administered.[44] The formation of cAMP from ATP is catalyzed by the enzyme *adenyl cyclase* associated with the plasmalemma and a guanine-nucleotide-binding protein (see p. 16). Cyclic AMP activates an enzyme, *protein kinase,* in the cytosol. This protein kinase phosphorylates other enzymes, causing them to assume or lose catalytic activity. The changes in catalytic activity of these enzymes determines the cellular events that characterize the actions of the given hormone. Epinephrine, glucagon and FSH are among those hormones whose action is mediated via a cAMP-dependent mechanism. Other peptide and polypeptide hormones that stimulate cAMP are LH, TSH, GH, ACTH, MSH, some hypothalamic releasing hormones, vasopressin and gastrin. The hormone might be considered the first messenger, and cAMP produced following the binding of the hormone to the plasmalemma would be the *second messenger.* This scheme is outlined in Figure 1-5.

Another "Second Messenger". *Guanyl (guanylyl, guanylate)* cyclase converts guanosine triphosphate to a cyclic nucleotide, *cyclic guanosine 3′, 5′-monophosphate* (cGMP), and this enzyme is activated by acetylcholine (ACh) in heart muscle. Heart rate may be depressed by addition of ACh or cGMP, whereas cAMP or adrenergic substances accelerate heart rate (Table 1-6). The mechanism of GH release from the pituitary involves activation of cAMP by a specific GH-releasing hormone (GHRH). A second hypothalamic neurohormone (somatostatin or GH release-inhibiting hormone [GHRIH]) has been found to inhibit GH re-

Table 1-6. *Systems in Which Antagonists Have Been Demonstrated to Operate through Interaction of cAMP and cGMP Production*

Neural function: Cholinergic and adrenergic innervation of cardiac muscle		
Acetylcholine	Increases cGMP	Slows heart rate
Epinephrine	Increases cAMP	Accelerates heart rate
Liver and glycogen metabolism: Antagonism of glucagon and insulin		
Glucagon	Increases cAMP	Favors conversion of glycogen to glucose
Insulin	Increases cGMP	Favors conversion of glucose to glycogen
Pituitary gland: Hypothalamic control of growth hormone release		
Growth hormone–releasing hormone	Increases cAMP	Stimulates growth hormone release
Growth hormone release–inhibiting hormone	Increases cGMP	Inhibits growth hormone release

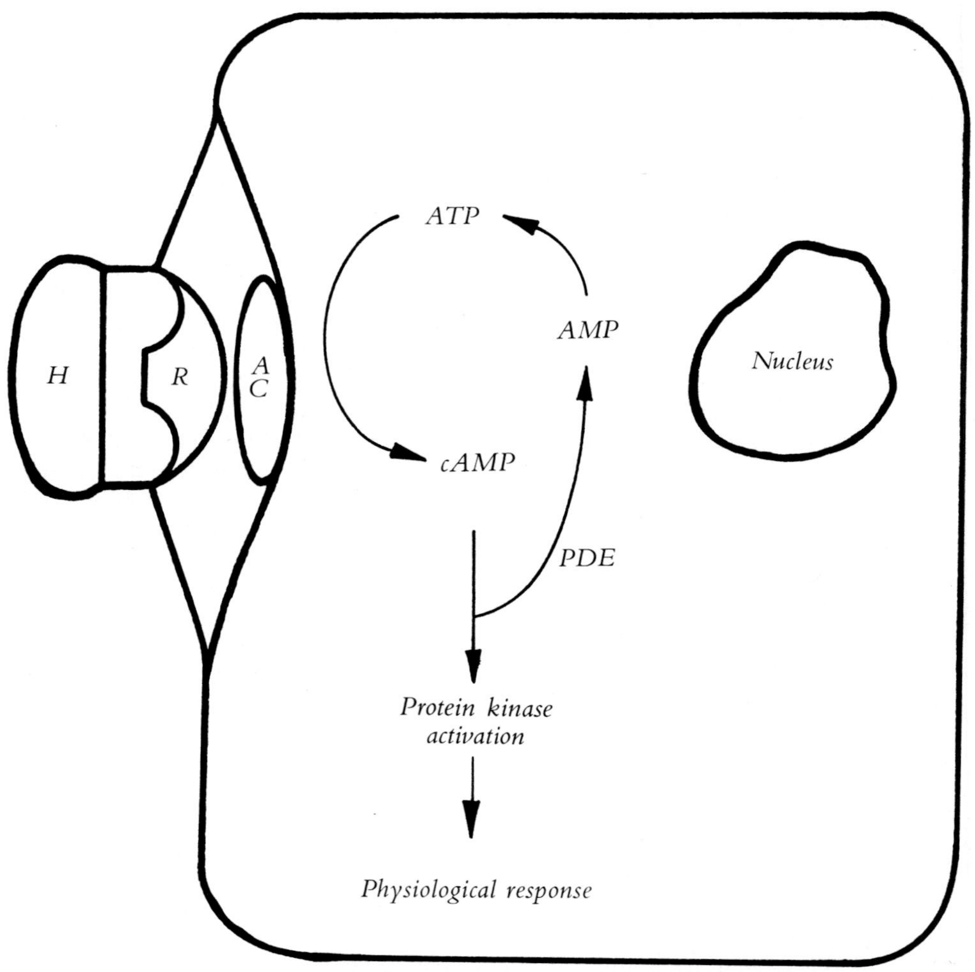

FIG. 1-5. Schematic representation of the role of cAMP in the mechanism of peptide and protein hormone action. *H,* hormone; *R,* receptor; *AC,* adenyl cyclase; *PDE,* phosphodiesterase. See text for explanation. Note: The plasmalemma has been enlarged on the left side to emphasize the relationship of both receptor and adenyl cyclase to the plasmalemma. It has not yet been determined whether the receptor is a separate protein from the enzyme.

lease. This GHRIH elevates cGMP levels and depresses cAMP levels.[16] Similar observations have been reported for liver, where both glucagon and epinephrine stimulate glycogen conversion to glucose via a cAMP-dependent mechanism. Insulin stimulates cGMP formation and depresses cAMP levels. One hypothesis[42] suggests that the hormone receptor is separate from the adenyl cyclase which occurs on the cytoplasmic side of the plasmalemma. A component of the enzyme is a guanine nucleotide-binding protein (GNBP). When guanine triphosphate (GTP) is bound, the GNBP interacts with the catalytic unit of adenyl cyclase and cAMP is formed from ATP. Hydrolysis of GTP to cGMP frees the GNBP and adenyl cyclase activity is reduced (Fig. 1-6). A hormone could also act by altering the ability of the GNBP to bind GTP.

There is reason to suspect that the cytoskeleton of the target cell may be involved in the mode of action of peptide hormones.[47] Microfilaments are associated with GNBP, adenyl cyclase, and the hormone-receptor complex. Any factors that might alter the cytoskeleton could influence hormone action.

PHOSPHODIESTERASE. Another enzyme complex, *phosphodiesterase* (PDE), is responsible

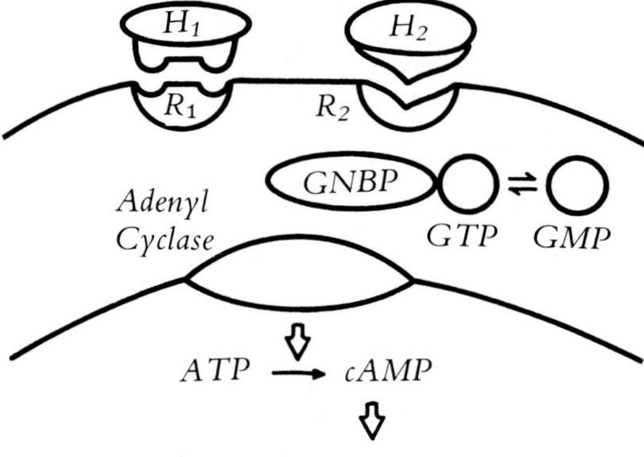

FIG. 1-6. Current hypotheses concerning the mechanism of action for protein and peptide hormones (H_1) suggest the interaction of the receptor (R_1) with a guanine nucleotide binding protein (GNBP) is necessary to activate the enzyme adenyl cyclase. Action of the first hormone can be inhibited by binding of a second hormone (H_2). Its receptor (R_2) causes release of guanosine triphosphate from GNBP, rendering it incapable of interacting with R_1.

for degradation of cAMP to 5′-AMP, which has no activity in this system but is used in the resynthesis of ATP. The activity of PDE is readily blocked by drugs known as methyl xanthines, such as caffeine and theophylline. Methyl xanthines potentiate the action of hormones by extending the biological life of cAMP, and they have proved useful for investigating the mechanism of action of many hormones in addition to epinephrine. Theophylline is used clinically to potentiate the actions of endogenous epinephrine. The discovery that there are at least three forms of the enzyme PDE in liver cells may provide clues to the interactions between these nucleotides. Only one of these PDEs is specific for cGMP, and the other two are specific for cAMP. Of the last two, one is activated by low levels of cGMP. Thus a hormone that elevates cGMP levels could reduce effective levels of cAMP and antagonize processes dependent on cAMP.

A "THIRD MESSENGER"? A number of small lipids known as prostaglandins (see Chap. 15) have been implicated as agents that influence cyclic nucleotides in hormone target tissues. Prostaglandins inhibit cAMP production in adipose (fat) cells, which can be stimulated by hormones like epinephrine. They also stimulate cAMP formation and progesterone synthesis in a manner similar to the effects of LH on the mouse ovary. One prostaglandin stimulates cAMP and causes venous vasodilation in the cow, whereas another one stimulates cGMP formation and brings about vasoconstriction. These compounds or related substances (see Chap. 15) may be confirmed as mediators in the mechanism of action for peptide hormones, but more research is needed.

Role of Calcium in the Action of Hormones

Calcium ions have been implicated in presynaptic and postsynaptic events associated with neural transmission and action potential generation; in regulation of glycogenolysis (hydrolysis of stored glycogen) within muscle cells; in synthesis of glucose from noncarbohydrate sources (amino acids, fats) in kidney and possibly in liver cells; in the action of MSH on pigment cells of the skin, of vasopressin on the toad bladder, of PTH on bone cells, and of hypothalamo-hypophysiotropic hormones, to name a few.[24,25,36,41]

The actions of calcium ions may be related to microtubular contractions involved with such processes as migration and exocytosis of secretion granules (for example, in stimulating hormone release) or intracellular movements of specialized organelles (for example, dispersal of pigmented organelles throughout the cytoplasm of melanophores). Activation of numerous enzymes caused by certain hormones and mediated via cAMP-protein kinase mechanisms may also be influenced by the availability of intracellular calcium ions. Binding of polypeptide hormones to the plasmalemma of a target cell apparently results in an increase of intracellular calcium that is essential for the general action of the hormone.

Techniques in Endocrinology

Numerous techniques developed in other areas of physiological and biochemical research have been applied to the study of endocrine systems (Table 1-7). The basic approach to determine if a suspected tissue may produce a hormone is extirpation and replacement. This classic approach is described here along

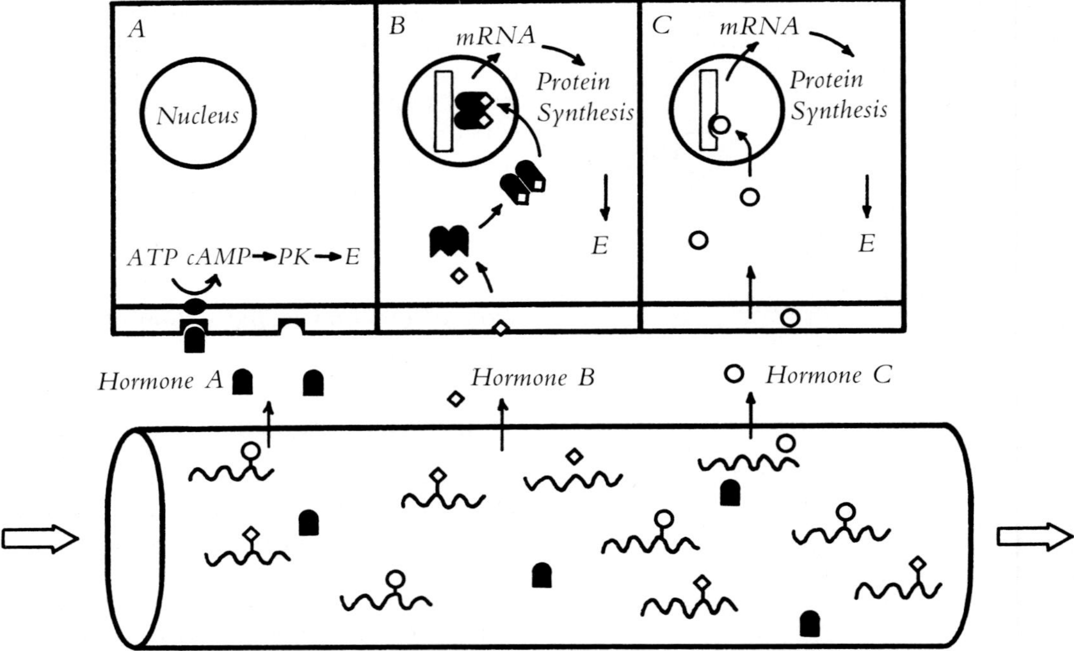

FIG. 1-7. Mechanisms of actions for peptide (A), steroid (B) and thyroid hormones (C) on target cells. Binding proteins are shown only for steroids and thyroid hormones but peptides may interact with plasma proteins, too. Peptides may produce secondary effects on protein synthesis but their first action is on cell membrane permeability and/or activation of protein kinases (PK) in target cells. E, effect of hormone action.

with two "borrowed" approaches: bioassay and radioimmunoassay. Bioassay is discussed in some detail here and elsewhere in the text because of its historical importance and because of its continued importance for validating other techniques such as radioimmunoassay. Bioassay techniques are the only approaches available for quantifying hormone levels in some systems. Radioimmunoassay is one of the most sensitive probes available to endocrine researchers for monitoring changes in hormone levels. Consequently it is essential to understand the theory of its use and its limitations.

The Classic Technique

Historically the technique for identifying an endocrine gland has involved (1) *extirpation* (removal) of the putative gland and (2) *observation* of the effects of removal; (3) *replacement* of the gland by implant or by injection of a homogenate or extract prepared from the putative gland or by injection of some purified chemical substance and (4) *observation* to see whether the consequences of extirpation are reversed to the "normal" or pre-extirpation condition. This procedure (extirpation-replacement) is often referred to as the classic technique of endocrinology although it is still in common use.

Bioassay

The next step following the classic procedure to establish the existence of a hormonal substance has been identification of the active chemical principle responsible for the effects of the gland. This procedure requires development of some suitable bioassay system so that the investigator has a simple, quantitative response system in which to test extracts and chemical fractions for biological activity. The bioassay need not be conducted in the same organisms in which the gland is found. For example, in the mature pigeon a structure termed the *crop sac* produces a cytogenous secretion called *crop milk* that is regurgitated

TABLE 1-7. *Some Techniques for Investigating Endocrine Systems*

Disruptive techniques
1. Severing of peripheral neural or vascular connections
2. Production of lesions in brain or spinal cord
3. Transplantation of a gland to another site in the organism where it may revascularize but no neural connections can recur

"Inject 'em, inspect 'em"
1. Inject a substance (hormone, inhibitor, precursor, etc.) and observe the effects

Radioisotopic techniques
1. Determine accumulation rates and/or sites for particular radioisotopes (e.g., radioiodine, ^{125}I and ^{131}I, and thyroid tissue)
2. Metabolism of radioactively labeled molecules (^{3}H or ^{14}C) to identify synthetic pathways or degradative pathways
3. Binding of radioactively labeled hormones to target tissues and cell organelles utilizing autoradiographic techniques

Fluorescence immunoassay
1. Identification of a peptide or protein hormone-secreting cell using the antibody specific for the hormone that has been combined with a fluorescing compound

and fed to the young birds while in the nest. This secretion is abolished in hypophysectomized animals (extirpation of the hypophysis or pituitary gland) but can be restored by subcutaneous injection of pituitary extract directly over the crop sac (replacement). Crop milk is secreted only in that portion of the crop sac directly beneath the injection site. This crop-milk material can be scraped from a given area around the injection site, dried, weighed and compared quantitatively to a similar site in the same crop sac beneath an injection of saline or of an extract prepared from some other tissue. (The pigeon crop sac is conveniently proportioned into two halves such that the test may be made on one side of the bird and the control injection given on the other hemi-crop sac of the same individual.) The amount of crop-sac secretion (dry weight of the unit area for comparison) increases proportionately to the amount of pituitary extract administered over a defined range. The crop-sac bioassay allowed endocrinologists to identify the pituitary crop-stimulating factor as the hormone prolactin. The pigeon crop sac also responds to prolactins or pituitary extracts from amphibians, reptiles and other birds and mammals but not to fish preparations.

Because biological systems are subject to fluctuations induced by environmental conditions such as temperature, it is essential that conditions for the bioassay be rigidly defined. For example, the crop sac bioassay may be done in 6-week-old inbred White King pigeons to reduce variability in the response due to genetic differences between individuals and other strains of pigeons and to insure that prepubertal pigeons are used.

An important feature of a good bioassay system is the dose-response relationship, that is, the relationship between amount injected and degree of response. Some bioassays are designed so that one identifies the minimal quantity of extract that will cause a response in the system. It is desirable, however, to have a bioassay in which there is a minimum dose that will produce a response with quantitatively dose-related increments in response up to some maximum. Frequently supramaximal doses will produce no additional response, and in some cases may reduce the response (toxicity effect). Some dose-response relationships derived from different types of bioassay are depicted in Figure 1-8.

One frequent error of researchers is failure to ascertain a dose-response relationship before deciding what dose of a hormone, inhibitor, etc., is to be used. Rather, they choose a dose arbitrarily or make a guess from published literature. Effective doses of hormones are generally in the microgram (μg, 10^{-6} g), nanogram (ng, 10^{-9} g) or picogram (pg, 10^{-12} g) range, and circulating hormone levels are expressed as a weight to volume of plasma or serum (0.1 μg/ml, 10 ng/dl). Hormone doses that approximate levels that can be experienced by the animal are often termed *physiological,* whereas excessive or supramaximal doses are referred to as *pharmacological.* Although pharmacological doses may produce marked effects, it is difficult to ascertain the biological significance of such data.

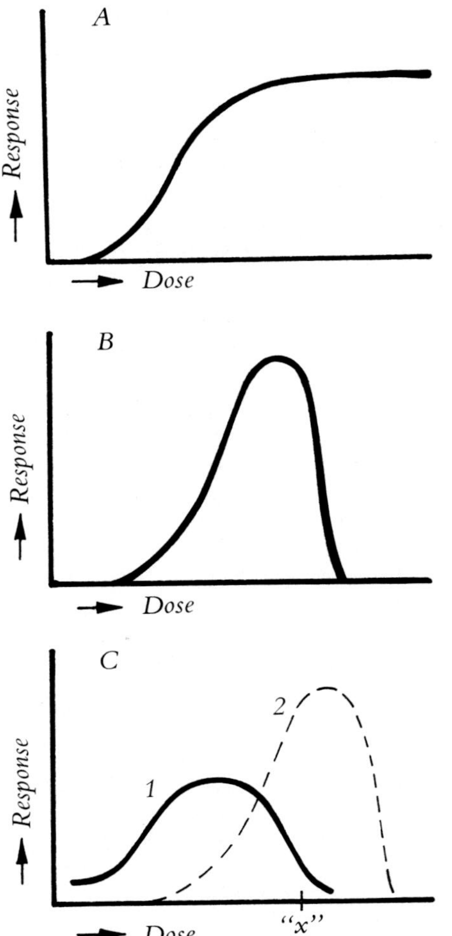

FIG. 1-8. Some examples of dose-response relationships.
A. Dose-response relationship in which additional increases beyond a maximum effective dose produce no increase in response.
B. Increasing dose above maximum effective dose causes inhibition of response. Eventually a suppressive dose is reached, probably because of toxicity of the substance used.
C. Different tissues (*1* and *2*) in a given animal may exhibit different dose-response relationships. A dose of "X" is inhibitory to tissue 1 but stimulatory to tissue 2. This could also represent different sensitivities of two species.

Knowledge concerning minimally effective doses of hormones is especially important when one is considering the effects of one hormone on another. A given hormone may produce a *priming effect* (increase in sensitivity of target tissue to another hormone), inhibit release or action of another hormone, increase release of another hormone or act cooperatively to produce an enhanced effect. This last action may involve either an *additive effect* or a *synergistic effect.* An additive effect occurs when the action of a particular dose of two hormones produces a response that is equal to the sum of the two hormones working alone ($1 + 1 = 2$). The term synergism is loosely applied to situations in which the combined effect is greater than additive, implying a different kind of cooperative effort ($1 + 1 = 3$).

Pharmacological doses of seemingly purified hormones may produce effects characteristic of the contaminants. For example, stimulation of the thyroid gland of the European crested newt following administration of massive doses of mammalian PRL is most likely due to contamination with TSH.[9] Similarly, induction of metamorphosis in tiger salamander larvae by injection of FSH is due to the presence of TSH as a contaminant.[27]

Radioimmunoassay

Radioimmunoassay (RIA) is being employed widely in comparative studies to measure blood levels of specific hormones. This technique allows direct and more accurate assessment of the endocrine state of the organism, whereas many other techniques such as histological examination or application of exogenous hormones tend to be indirect, inconclusive or both. RIA is essentially the same in principle and method as competitive protein-binding assays and the newer highly specific radioreceptor assays.

An antibody produced against any antigen (in this case a hormone) has a binding site on the antibody molecule that is specific for the antigen, much like the binding site of an enzyme for its substrate. A given amount of antibody (a given number of antibody molecules) quantitatively possesses a given number of binding sites for antigen. For purposes of this discussion, one antigen-binding site per molecule of antibody will be assumed. The antibody, however, cannot distinguish between an antigen that contains radioactive atoms (that is, labeled atoms) from one that does not. The assay technique is based upon the assumption that, at equilibrium, increasing quantities of cold hormone (unlabeled) will displace proportionately increasing amounts of hot hormone (radioactively labeled) from the antibody, because there will be competition for a limited number of binding sites. A standard curve can be prepared by placing increasing amounts of cold hormone in separate reaction tubes with a constant number of antibody molecules and constant quantity of labeled hormone. The quantity of labeled hormone bound to the antibody can be accurately determined by precipitating the antibody and measuring the amount of radioactivity bound to it. Unbound labeled hormone is discarded with the supernatant. The radioactivity measured in the precipitated antibody is inversely proportional to the amount of cold hormone added. These data may be plotted in various ways (ratio of bound to free label, percentage of total label added as measured in the antibody precipitate, the reciprocal of the radioactive counts per minute bound to the antibody, etc.) to yield a dose-response curve (Fig. 1-9). The hormone concentration of an unknown plasma or serum sample can be assayed in the same manner and the quantity of hormone extrapolated from the standard curve using the amount of label bound to the antibody.

RIAs require a pure source of hormone in order to prepare an antibody against it as well as a source of radioactively labeled pure hormone. Furthermore, the system must be tested rigorously for specificity to determine whether molecules closely related chemically but lacking the same biological activity of the hormone assayed might also displace hot hormone from the antibody. The problem of a purified source becomes particularly acute when one is investigating endocrine systems of nonmammalian vertebrates in which the chemical structures for most protein and polypeptide hormones are unknown and the hormones are not available in pure form. Frequently such hormones may have activity similar to mammalian hormones, but there are often important biological differences reflecting variations in the structure of the hormones themselves. The use of antibodies prepared against mammalian peptide and protein hormones to measure nonhomologous molecules in nonmammals results in uncertain interpretations. Immunological data may not parallel data obtained by biological assay,[26]

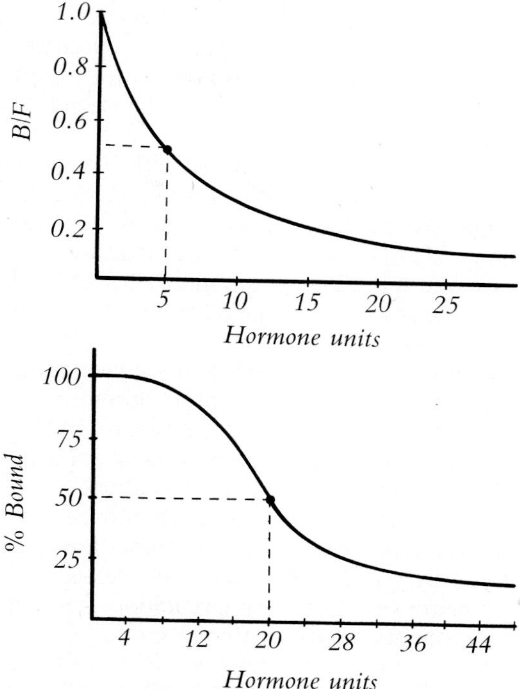

FIG. 1-9. Standardized curves for radioimmunoassay determination of hormone concentrations.
A. Calculated from the ratio of bound to free label *(B/F)* that is equal to the radioactivity (labeled hormone) bound to the antihormone antibody vs. the radioactivity displaced by cold or unlabeled hormone and hence "free" in the solution. An unknown sample resulting in a B/F ratio of 0.47 would be equal to 5 units of hormone activity.
B. Another form for a standard RIA curve is to plot the percent of the total labeled hormone added to the mixture vs. the amount of unlabeled hormone added. In this example an unknown sample exhibiting binding of 50% of the labeled hormone would contain 20 units of unlabeled hormone.

and the tendency should be to accept the bioassay data.

The determination of receptor levels is considered by many to be important in understanding the status of a given system. If receptor levels in the target tissue are low, there are fewer sites to bind hormone molecules and less effect is produced. In many systems, there is evidence that binding of the hormone to the target cells results in a reduction in the number of receptors. This "*down-regulation*" reduces the observable hormone effects on the target when circulating levels are constant or even increasing. Later, production of new receptor is initiated, and the target tissue becomes more responsive. Special biochemical procedures have been developed to measure the levels of specific receptors in target tissues using techniques similar to those described for RIA.

The difficulties encountered with the application of mammalian RIA techniques to nonmammals may be circumvented by development of radioreceptor assays that employ hormone-specific receptor molecules isolated from the animal's own target tissue in place of the antibody. The principle of the assay is still the same, but the problem of not knowing the structure of the animal's native hormone becomes irrelevant. Although this approach also has its technical difficulties, it is of value to investigations of a comparative nature.

Endocrine systems must constantly be considered as dynamic states. Hormones are continuously being synthesized and released and are being lost from the circulation through metabolic inactivation, excretion or both. The effectiveness of a hormone and its circulating levels will be determined not only by rates of synthesis and release but also by rates of inactivation and excretion. Consequently it is helpful to know *turnover rates* or the *biological half-life* (time for half of a given population of hormone molecules to be inactivated, excreted or both) in assessing endocrine states. Turnover rates for peptide hormones are very short and can be measured in minutes. Steroids have much longer half-lives in blood because they are bound to specific binding proteins and are not removed as rapidly. Their half-lives are usually measured in hours. Thyroid hormones are more tightly bound to binding proteins in the blood than are steroids. For example, the half-life of thyroxine in humans is about 7 days.

The presence of binding proteins adds another complication in measuring hormone levels. An equilibrium is established between bound hormone and unbound or free hormone. It is the free hormone that is considered by most researchers to be available for entering tissues and therefore the important parameter to measure. Not only is the rate of secretion of hormones important, but the circulating levels of binding protein may influence the availability of free hormone. Thus, the levels of binding protein may be important, too. Another hypothesis has been proposed[40] that suggests the binding protein actually facilitates entry of the hormone into target cells, and free hormone is destined for excretion. This hypothesis is based in part on the presence of binding protein within steroid target cells.

The limitation of using blood level data as a diagnostic tool may be illustrated further by considering attempts to localize the source of an abnormal endocrine state. The demonstration of unusually low or high circulating hormone levels does not distinguish between changes in secretion rates and excretion rates for the hormone, and additional tests are required. Similarly, are hormone levels higher in a fish adapted to 10°C than in one adapted to 20°C because the former fish is secreting more or because the rates of excretion are markedly reduced at lower temperatures?

In spite of the cautions listed above, RIA has provided the endocrinologist with a highly sensitive probe with which to investigate dynamic endocrine events. When used with appropriate methods and experimental designs, RIA techniques are providing considerable insight into the functioning of the vertebrate endocrine system, bringing about major revisions in some established concepts while strengthening or rejecting others.

High Performance Liquid Chromatography

One tool has facilitated greatly the purification of peptides: high performance liquid chromatography or HPLC. This method is capable of cleanly separating peptides differing by a single amino acid. Differences in small molecules like steroid hormones allow their separation by HPLC as well. By coupling HPLC with RIA, it is possible to separate potentially contaminating molecules from the fraction to be assayed. If suitable sensitivity can be achieved, HPLC validated with RIA and bioassay may someday be used for determination of circulating levels of hormones.

Man-made Hormones

Positive identification of a hormone with a physiological response involves the artificial synthesis of that hormone. Recent advances in biochemical techniques have made it possible to synthesize a new peptide shortly after verification of its structure. The final verification involves administration of the synthetic hormone and comparison of its actions to data obtained using the procedures discussed earlier. Once the true nature of the hormone is known, biochemists produce structurally altered forms called *analogues*. By comparing the actions and metabolism of these analogues they can better understand how the structure of the hormone relates to its effects. Some synthetic analogues are many times more potent than the naturally occurring hormone and prove very useful in both experimental and clinical work. Inhibitory analogues block actions of the natural hormone by binding to the same receptor but not effecting the anticipated actions.

Summary

The heterogenous nature of endocrinology should be evident from this brief introduction. The variety of chemical regulators defies attempts by scientists to erect exclusive or inclusive categories. The terms *neurohormone, neurotransmitter* and *semiochemical* can be limited more readily than *hormone. Paracrine* secretion is similar to both neurotransmitter and hormonal secretion. The structural and functional features of these regulators together with current concepts of cellular origins for their secretory cells serve to emphasize the closeness of neural and endocrine physiology.

Protein, peptide and amine hormones bind to receptors embedded in the plasmalemma of target cells and cause permeability changes in the plasmalemma and/or activation of intracellular enzymes. These intracellular events are mediated by cyclic nucleotides. Steroid and thyroid hormones enter target cells and bind to intracellular receptors. Intracellular conversion to other molecules may be prerequisite to binding for some (androgens, thyroxine). Following binding, the hormone-receptor complex activates nuclear transcription and protein synthesis in the target cell. Protein, peptide and amine regulators may produce delayed effects on protein synthesis. Stimulation of cellular division may be a delayed consequence of hormone action.

Endocrinology has its own approach to identification of chemical regulators which involves extirpation, replacement and bioassay. Validation of chemical procedures for quantifying hormone levels also employs bioassays. Endocrinologists make imaginative use of every biochemical, cytological and physiological technique available in their efforts to understand how life processes are regulated by chemical messengers.

References

1. Andrew, A. (1982). The APUD concept: where has it led us? Br. Med. Bull. 38:221–225.

2. Ballard, P.L. and G.M. Tomkins (1969). Hormone induced modification of the cell surface. Nature 224:344–345.

3. Barnea, A. and J. Gorski (1970). Estrogen-induced protein. Time course of synthesis. Biochemistry 9:1899–1904.

4. Burns, J.T. and A.H. Meier (1971). Daily variations in pigeon cropsac responses to prolactin. Experientia 27:572–574.

5. Callard, G.V. (1983). Androgen and estrogen actions in the vertebrate brain. Am. Zool. 23:607–620.

6. Epple, A. (1982). Functional principles of vertebrate endocrine systems. Verh. Dtsch. Zool. Ges. 1982, 117–126.

7. Finch, C.E. (1976). The regulation of physiological changes during mammalian aging. Q. Rev. Biol. 51:49–83.

8. Frieden, E. and H. Lipner (1971). Biochemical Endocrinology of the Vertebrates. Prentice-Hall, Englewood Cliffs, N.J.

9. Frye, B.E., P.S. Brown and B.W. Snyder (1972). Effects of prolactin and somatotropin on growth and metamorphosis of amphibians. Gen. Comp. Endocrinol. Suppl. 3:209–220.

10. Gorbman, A. and H.A. Bern (1962). A Textbook of Comparative Endocrinology. John Wiley and Sons, New York.

11. Gorski, J. and F. Gannon (1976). Current models of steroid hormone action: A critique. Ann. Rev. Physiol. 38:425–450.

12. Greengard, O., M.A. Smith and G. Acs (1963). Relation of cortisone and synthesis of ribonucleic acid to induced and developmental enzyme formation. J. Biol. Chem. 238:1548–1551.

13. Fujita, T., S. Kobayashi, R. Yui and T. Iwanaga (1980). Evolution of neurons and paraneurons. In S. Ishii, T. Hirano and M. Wada, eds., Hormones, Adaptation and Evolution. Japan Sci. Soc. Press, Tokyo and Springer-Verlag, Berlin, pp. 35–43.

14. Jensen, E.V. and E.R. DeSombre (1973). Estrogen-receptor interaction. Science 182:126–134.

15. Jones, R.E., R. Tokarz, J.J. Roth, J.E. Platt and A.C. Collins (1975). Mast cell histamine and ovarian follicular growth in the lizard, *Anolis carolinensis.* J. Exp. Zool. 193:343–352.

16. Kaneko, T., H. Oka, M. Manemura, S. Suzuki, H. Yasuda and T. Oda (1974). Stimulation of guanosine 3′5′ monophosphate accumulation in rat anterior pituitary gland *in vitro* by synthetic somatostatin. Biochem. Biophys. Res. Commun. 61:53–57.

17. Kreiger, D. (1983). Brain peptides: what, where and why? Science 222:975–985.

18. Laufer, H. (1968). Developmental interactions in the dipteran salivary gland. Amer. Zool. 8:257–272.

19. LeDouarin, N. and C. LeLievre (1971). Demonstration of the neural origin of the ultimobranchial body glandular cells in the avian embryo. In Proc. Third Int. Symp. Endocrinology, William Heinemann Medical Books, London, pp. 153–163.

20. Lee, R.W. and A.H. Meier (1967). Diurnal variations of the fattening response to prolactin in the golden topminnow, *Fundulus chrysotus.* J. Exp. Zool. 166:307–316.

21. Lingappa, V.R. and G. Blobel (1980). Early events in the biosynthesis of secretory and membrane proteins: the signal hypothesis. Rec. Pro Horm. Res. 36:451–476.

22. Mainwaring, W.I.P. (1977). The mechanism of action of androgens. Monog. Endocrinol. 10, Springer-Verlag, New York.

23. Maraspin, L.E. and W.J. Bo (1971). Effects of hormones, pregnancy and pseudopregnancy on the mast cell count in the rat uterus. Life Sci. 10:111–120.

24. Martin, P.M. and P.J. Sheridan (1982). Towards a new model for the mechanism of action of steroids. J. Steroid Biochem. 16:215–229.

25. Means, A. (1981). Calmodulin: properties, intracellular localization and multiple roles in cell regulation. Rec. Pro Horm. Res. 37:333–367.

26. Nicoll, C.S. (1975). Radioimmunoassay and the radioreceptor assays for prolactin and growth hormone: A critical appraisal. Am. Zool. 15:881–904.

27. Norris, D.O., R.E. Jones and D.C. Cohen (1973). Effects of mammalian gonadotropins (LH, FSH, HCG) and gonadal steroids on TSH-induced metamorphosis of *Ambystoma tigrinum* (Amphibia: Caudata). Gen. Comp. Endocrinol. 20:467–473.

28. O'Malley, B.W. and A.R. Means (1974). Female steroid hormones and target cell nuclei. Science 183:610–620.

29. O'Malley, B.W., S.L. Woo, S.E. Harris, J.M. Rosen, J.P. Comstock, L. Chan, C.B. Bordelon, J.W. Holder, P. Sperry and A.R. Means (1975). Steroid hormone action in animal cells. Am. Zool. 15, Suppl. 1:215–225.

30. Oppenheimer, J.H., H.L. Schwartz, M.I. Surks, D. Koerner and W.H. Dillmann (1976). Nuclear receptors and the initiation of thyroid hormone action. Recent Prog. Horm. Res. 32:529–566.

31. Pearse, A.G.E. (1968). Common cytochemical and ultra-structural characteristics of cells producing polypeptide hormones (the APUD series) and their relevance to thyroid and ultimobranchial C cells and calcitonin. Proc. R. Soc. Lond. 170:71–80.

32. Pearse, A.G.E. and T. Takor Takor (1976). Neuroendocrine embryology and the APUD concept. Clin. Endocrinol. 5, Suppl. 229s–244s.

33. Pitot, H.C. and M.B. Yatvin (1973). Interrelationships of mammalian hormones and enzyme levels *in vivo.* Physiol. Rev. 53:228–325.

34. Posner, B.I., M.N. Khan and J.J. Bergeron (1982). Endocytosis of peptide hormones and other ligands. Endo. Revs. 3:280–298.

35. Rao, G.S. (1981). Mode of entry of steroid and thyroid hormones into cells. Mol. Cell. Endocrinol. 21:97–108.

36. Rasmussen, H. (1970). Cell communication, calcium ion, and cyclic adenosine monophosphate. Science 170:404–412.

37. Scharrer, B. (1972). Comparative aspects of neuroendocrine communication. Gen. Comp. Endocrinol. Suppl. 3:515–517.

38. Scharrer, B. (1975). The role of neurons in endocrine regulation: A comparative overview. Am. Zool. 15, Suppl. 1:7–11.

39. Schrader, W.T., M.E. Birnbaumer, M.R. Hughes, N.L. Weigel, W.W. Grody and B.W. O'Malley (1981). Studies on the structure and function of the chicken progesterone receptor. Rec. Prog. Horm. Res. 37:583–633.

40. Siiteri, P.K., J.T. Murai, G.L. Mammond, J.A. Nisker, W.J. Raymoure and R.W. Kuhn (1982). The serum transport of steroid hormones. Rec. Prog. Horm. Res. 38:457–510.

41. Simkiss, K. (1974). Calcium translocation by cells. Endeavor 33:119–123.

42. Spiegel, A.M., R.W. Downs, Jr., M.A. Levine, M.J. Singer, Jr., W. Kraweietz, S.J. Marx, C.J. Woodard, S.A. Reen and G.D. Aurbach (1981). The role of gua-

nine nucleotides in regulation of adenylate cyclase activity. Rec. Prog. Horm. Res. 37:635–665.

43. Sterling, K. and J.H. Lazarus (1977). The thyroid and its control. Ann. Rev. Physiol. 39:349–372.

44. Sutherland, E.W. (1972). Studies on the mechanism of hormone action. Science 177:401–408.

45. Tchernitchin, A., X. Tchernitchin and P. Galand (1975). Correlation of estrogen-induced uterine eosinophilia with other parameters of estrogen stimulation, produced with estradiol-17β and estriol. Experientia 31:993–994.

46. Tomkins, G.M. and T.D. Gelehrter (1972). The present status of genetic regulation by hormones. In G. Litwack, ed., Biochemical Actions of Hormones. Academic Press, New York, Vol. 2, pp. 1–20.

47. Welshons, W.V., M.E. Lieberman and J. Gorski (1984). Nuclear localization of unoccupied estrogen receptors. Nature 307:747–749.

48. Zor, U. (1983). Role of cytoskeletal organization in the regulation of adenylate cyclase-cyclic adenosine monophosphate by hormones. Endocr. Rev. 4:1–21.

2·Homeostatic Model for Endocrine Systems

Homeostasis

Claude Bernard formulated the concept of homeostasis in the nineteenth century. However, it was the American physiologist Walter B. Cannon who in 1929 coined the term *homeostasis* to describe balanced physiological systems operating in the organism to maintain a dynamic equilibrium, that is, a relatively constant steady state maintained within certain tolerable limits.

> When we consider the extreme instability of our bodily structure, its readiness for disturbance by the slightest application of external forces and the rapid onset of its decomposition as soon as favoring circumstances are withdrawn, its persistence through many decades seems almost miraculous. The wonder increases when we realize that the system is open, engaging in free exchange with the outer world, and that the structure itself is not permanent but is being continuously broken down by the wear and tear of action, and as continuously built up again by processes of repair . . . .
>
> The constant conditions which are maintained in the body might be termed equilibria. That word, however, has come to have fairly exact meaning as applied to relatively simple physico-chemical states, in closed systems, where known forces are balanced. The coordinated physiological processes which maintain most of the steady states in the organism are so complex and so peculiar to living beings—involving, as they may, the brain and nerves, the heart, lungs, kidneys and spleen, all working cooperatively—that I have suggested a special designation for these states, homeostasis. The word does not imply something immobile, a stagnation. It means a condition—a condition which may vary, but which is relatively constant. (Walter B. Cannon, The Wisdom of the Body, 1929)

A Homeostatic Model

Cannon's original formulation of the homeostatic mechanism emphasized the maintenance of such parameters as blood levels of various chemical substances (for example, calcium, sodium, glucose), blood osmotic pressure, blood volume and blood pressure. Models that simulate homeostatic mechanisms emphasize the regulatory components that stabilize these dynamic equilibria as well as the flexibility in these components to alter "set" levels to meet temporary elevated or lowered demands on the system. The act of identifying or categorizing (or both) various components of a complex regulatory system in order to make it "conform" to a hypothetical model can be of considerable value to the student who is attempting to understand endocrine systems. The models that will be developed in this chapter and the basic terms applied to the models are borrowed from the field of cybernetics. Although cybernetics has more to do with control systems in engineering and computer science, these models can be developed and applied successfully to endocrine systems. There are many different formal models for describing physiological systems, some of which are highly sophisticated and complex.

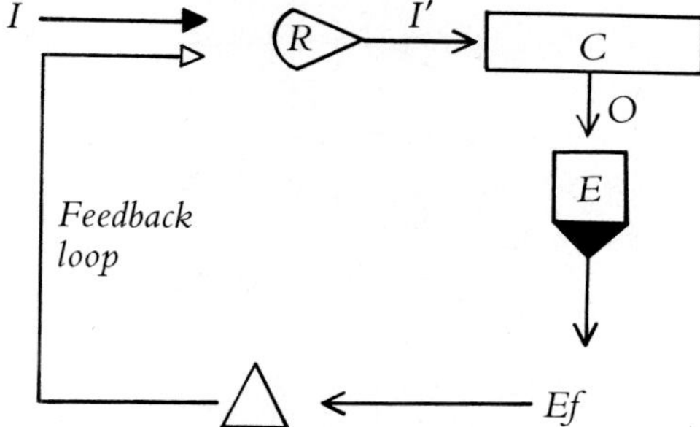

FIG. 2-1. A highly simplified homeostatic model. Information *(I)* is detected by a receptor *(R)*, transduced to input *(I′)* and relayed to the controller *(C)*. By making a comparison with programmed data (set point), the controller assesses whether a response is necessary. To initiate a response the controller sends a message (output [*O*]) to an effector *(E)*, which in turn responds in a predetermined manner (effect, [*Ef*]). The action of the effector produces a change in the system (Δ), which can then be detected by a receptor (i.e., feedback). Feedback loops are depicted here and in subsequent figures by open arrowheads.

The format used in this chapter is outlined in Figure 2-1 in its simplest form. The mathematical aspects have been eliminated, and the homeostatic models described are presented primarily to stress qualitative relationships.

In this model a change in the system (*information*) is detected by a *receptor* (*transducer*) that translates or converts (transduces) this information into the language of the control system. For example, blood pressure information can be translated to electrochemical neural impulses. The receptor relays this translated message, termed *input,* to the controlling center (*controller*), which compares the input with programmed data (sometimes called the *set point*) and determines, or rather computes, the appropriate adjustment (if any) necessary to preserve the homeostatic condition. It might also be considered that the controller functions as a *comparator* and *error detector* as well as a control center. If after comparing the input data to the set point the controller computes that a corrective response in the system is necessary, a new message (*output*) is relayed to one or more *effectors* which will perform some specific action (*effect*) that will bring about a corrective change in the system. The actions of the effectors will cause changes in the system that can be detected by receptors (the original receptor or others) and provide new input to the controller, which checks whether the response called for was adequate, appropriate, etc., and whether or not additional corrective changes will be necessary. The mechanism whereby the controller is apprised of the effectiveness of the corrective change is termed a *feedback loop.* If feedback indicates the response was inadequate to bring the system back into balance, additional effectors may be brought into operation. Similarly, if the response overcorrects the condition (termed an *overshoot*), other effectors can be activated to bring the system into balance. Overshoot as a result of corrective actions is a common biological phenomenon causing specific systems to oscillate in time around a mean, first exceeding the homeostatic mean, then falling below. Such an oscillation is depicted in Figure 2-2. The type of feedback loop operating to continually drive a homeostatic system toward the optimum mean conditions is termed *negative feedback.*

Positive feedback would identify a feedback loop that drove the system progressively away from the "optimum condition," that is, away from the present homeostatic mean determined by a given set point in the controller. Positive feedback for more than a short period may be detrimental to the organism and even result in death. It would appear that positive feedback might be invoked in an emergency type of response or an adaptive response necessary to complete some particular series of

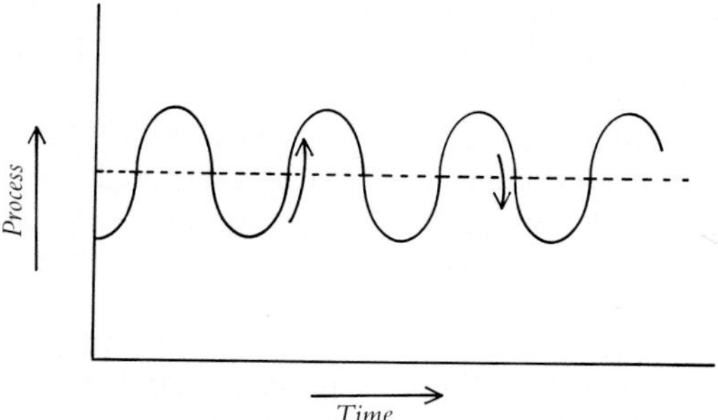

FIG. 2-2. A stable oscillation produced around a homeostatic mean and maintained by negative feedback. Arrows indicate overshoot. This idealized figure does not represent daily or hourly fluctuations necessarily, but probably minute-to-minute or short-term regulation. The limits of this oscillation are well defined, and the system's response time is due largely to the sensitivity of receptors.

physiological changes at some point in the life cycle such as sexual maturity.

A physical model of this simple type of control system might be a controlled temperature room that has a programmable thermostat (representing receptor and controller components), an air conditioner and a heater (effectors). The receptor that determines the air temperature is a bimetal strip that expands or contracts with changing air temperature. The mechanical deformations produced in the bimetal strip are transduced to electrical impulses (input). The controller component of the thermostat compares the air temperature to the programmed set point (where the thermostat is "set" manually) and accordingly turns on or off the appropriate effector or effectors to provide minimum fluctuations around the optimum temperature. The use of two opposing types of effectors (an air conditioner and a furnace) allows for more rapid responses and more precise control. The sensitivity of the receptor will also influence response time and precision of the system.

As an exercise, this physical temperature control system can be contrasted to that for regulating body temperature in mammals as described in an introductory physiology textbook. Where are the receptors located? The controller? What are the effectors? Via what route does feedback operate? In the same manner consider the control of breathing rate in humans and the roles of blood CO_2, lactate, pH and O_2 as information. If these nonendocrine systems can be fitted into the format of the basic model discussed here, one is ready to consider endocrine systems in a similar manner.

Four basic reflexes for controlling vertebrate physiology will now be examined: *neural, endocrine, neurohormonal* and *neuroendocrine*. The specific examples employed will be examined more fully in later chapters. The purpose of these examples is to illustrate the model rather than to provide detailed data about particular endocrine systems.

The Neural Reflex

The neural reflex as outlined in Figure 2-3 includes the classical conditioning reflexes and automatic reflexes such as the "cold-hand-on-the-hot-stove" phenomenon. In this simple example of a neural reflex, the information would be the temperature of the stove (heat). The temperature receptor in the skin relays this information as neural impulses (input) to nerve cell bodies of the spinal cord, which compute that an immediate response is required and send impulses (output) to appropriate muscles (effectors), causing them to relax or contract (effect). These events result in an immediate withdrawal of the hand from the stove (change in the system), even before higher control centers have received the input and computed "hot."

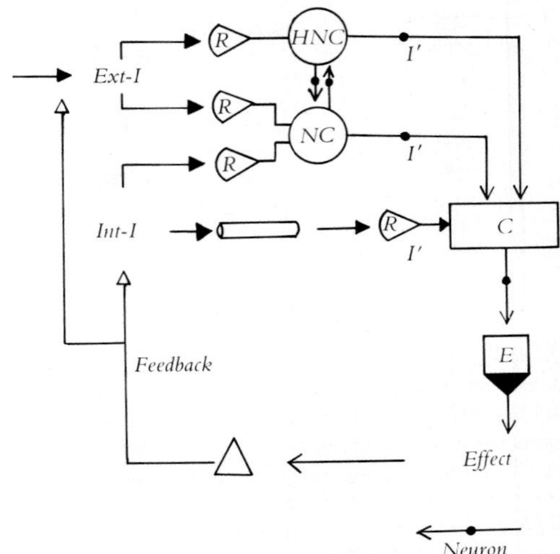

FIG. 2-3. The neural reflex. This diagram is somewhat more complicated than Fig. 2-1, but it contains the same basic elements. Input and output are in the form of neural impulses. Higher neural centers *(HNC)* may directly influence the controller *(C)* either by altering the set point or by influencing the response by the controller (i.e., altering output). The effect, change in the system and feedback loops may involve only the nervous system or may include other effectors such as muscles or exocrine glands. *NC,* neural center; *Ext-I,* external information; *Int-I,* internal information. For key to other abbreviations see Fig. 2-1.

The Endocrine Reflex

The endocrine reflex is involved primarily with internal (biochemical) information, such as blood levels of calcium or sodium (Fig. 2-4). For the most part these are substances whose levels in the blood must be precisely maintained to preserve normal functions of neurons, muscle cells, etc. Deviations from homeostatic means could yield serious pathological

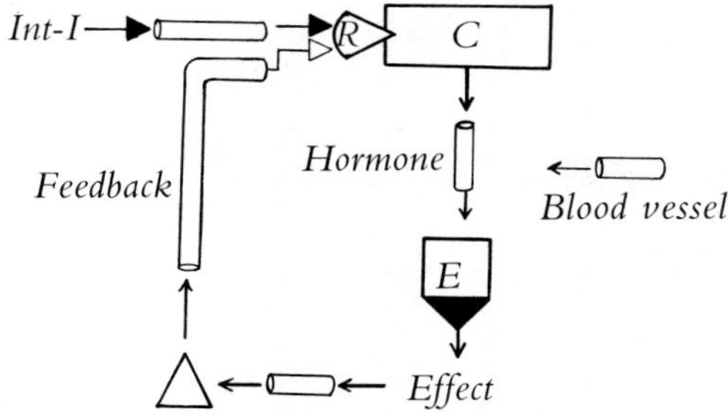

FIG. 2-4. The endocrine reflex. In this example the internal information *(Int-I)* is the level of some molecule in the blood. In general, the receptor *(R)* is a protein in the plasmalemma or the cytosol of the same endocrine cell that synthesizes and releases the specific hormone. Input might be in the form of an intracellular messenger such as cAMP or a steroid-receptor complex. The change produced in the system would be an alteration in circulating level of the same molecule responsible for initiating the reflex. For key to other abbreviations see Fig. 2-1.

conditions and possibly death for the organism, and variations in these internal parameters must be minimized. The response time for an endocrine reflex relying upon the blood for transport of hormones is much slower than for a neural reflex. The influence of parathyroid hormone (PTH) on blood calcium levels provides an excellent example of an endocrine reflex. Parathyroid cells are directly sensitive to (that is, have specific receptors for) circulating free calcium ions in the blood. If blood calcium levels decrease the parathyroid cells acting as both receptors and controllers release PTH (output), which travels via the blood to one of its effectors, bone tissue. Parathyroid hormone causes calcium to be released from bone into the blood (effect), resulting in an increase of blood calcium (change in system) proportional to the amount of PTH released. The new level of calcium feeds back on the parathyroid cells, which compare this new input to the established set point. As will be seen in Chapter 12, there is more to the regulation of blood calcium than is outlined here, but this example serves well as an illustration of a simple endocrine reflex.

The Neurohormonal Reflex

The neurohormonal reflex (Fig. 2-5) involves the neurosecretory (NS) neuron. The NS neuron is responsible for synthesis and release of specific neurohormones into the blood. Frequently the axonal endings of NS neurons accumulate in a highly vascularized structure, the neurohemal organ, in which the neurohormone may be stored until release is stimulated. This system involves both neural and endocrine components and is intermediate between them with respect to response time. Information may come to the system as external factors (for example, transduced via the visual system) or as blood-borne internal factors (ions, hormones, etc.)

The vertebrate hypothalamo-hypophysial system involving the octapeptide neurohormones stored in the pars nervosa (see Chap. 7) provides a good example of a neurohormonal reflex. The absorption of large volumes of water following the imbibition of a large quantity of liquid reduces the osmotic concentration of the blood and increases blood volume (and pressure). The hypothalamus (controller) located in the brain receives neural input from various osmoreceptors (osmotic concentration) and baroreceptors (hydrostatic pressure) indicating a change in the system has occurred. There follows a reduction in the amount of vasopressin (a neurohormone) released from the pars nervosa. Vasopressin would normally travel via the blood to the kidney (effector) where it brings about increased permeability of the collecting ducts to water. As a result of the action of vasopressin on the collecting ducts, reabsorption of water from the urine within the lumen of the collecting ducts is increased. (Hence vasopressin is sometimes called the mammalian antidiuretic hormone or ADH.) The reduction in circulating vasopressin as a consequence of the large volume of water absorbed through the gut results in reduced water reabsorption from the urine such that a larger volume of dilute urine is passed to the urinary bladder and eliminated. The increased blood pressure would have elevated the glomerular filtration rate (GFR) so that more urine would be formed per unit time (a nonendocrine homeostatic mechanism). These two factors (increased GFR and decreased circulating levels of vasopressin) would bring about a reduction in blood volume and an increase in blood osmotic pressure (changes in the system) that would feed back on the hypothalamic centers.

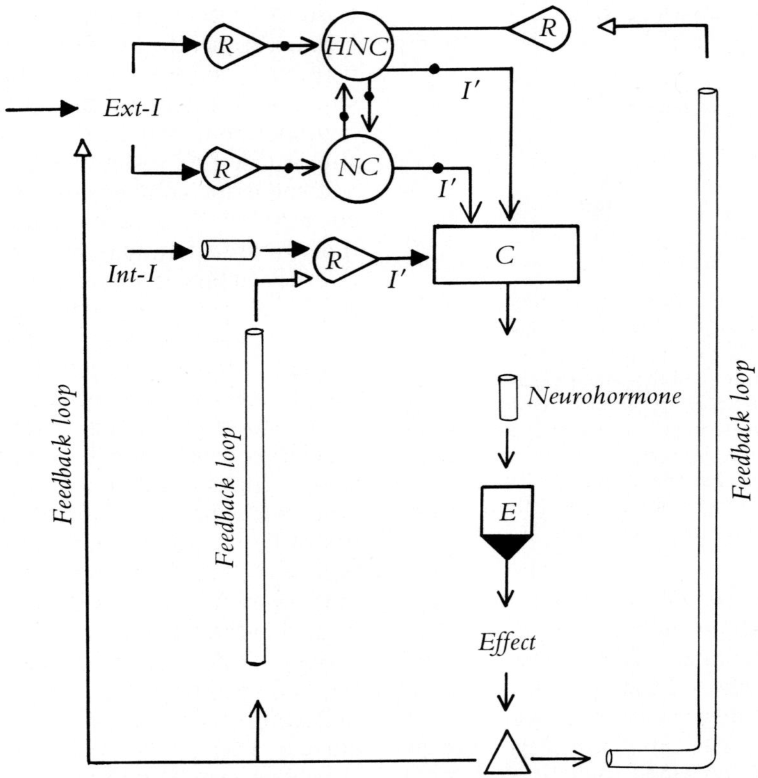

Fig. 2-5. The neurohormonal reflex. In this example, input *(I′)* may reach the controller *(C)* from several sources. See Figs. 2-1, 2-3 and text for explanation and Figs. 2-1 and 2-3 for key to other abbreviations.

The Neuroendocrine Reflex

The neuroendocrine reflex is depicted in Figure 2-6. It involves the superimposition of a neurohormonal reflex over an endocrine reflex. Such complication allows for more precise regulation of physiological patterns, as will become evident in later discussions. It also follows that the increased number of sites in the model allows for more points where modifications can occur and where imbalances could result in pathological states. The so-called *stress response* (see Chap. 10) provides an elegant and complicated example of a neuroendocrine reflex (see Fig. 2-7). There is also a reflex as part of the total stress response involving the adrenal medulla and epinephrine, but only the neuroendocrine reflex involving the pituitary gland and the adrenal cortex will be discussed here. Neural receptors perceive information (internal or external), translate it to neural input and relay the message to the central nervous system (CNS; brain). The controller for the stress response is located in the hypothalamus. Hypothalamic NS neurons secrete a specific neurohormone, corticotropin-releasing hormone (CRH), which travels via a special blood vascular link (called the hypothalamo-hypophysial portal system) to an endocrine gland, the adenohypophysis (the anterior portion of the pituitary gland). Release of the hormone corticotropin (ACTH), from certain adenohypophysial cells into the general circulation is stimulated by CRH. ACTH stimulates the adrenal cortex, another endocrine gland (effector 2), to synthesize and release a second hormone, corticosterone (effect 2). This second hormone travels via the blood to other effectors (effector 3) that produce specific effects that together enable the organism to respond to the stressful stimulus (change in the system). The blood levels of ACTH and corticosterone (and even possibly CRH) provide feedback loops. This specific neuroendocrine reflex is outlined in Figure 2-7.

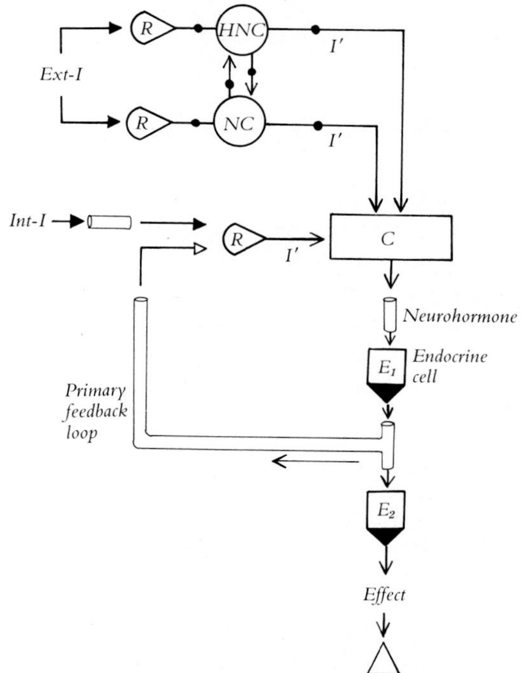

FIG. 2-6. A simplified neuroendocrine reflex. This scheme involves two effectors functioning in series. The first effector is an endocrine cell *(E_1)* that releases a hormone in response to the neurohormone *(O)* from the controller *(C)*. See Figs. 2-1, 2-3 and text for explanation and Figs. 2-1 and 2-3 for key to other abbreviations.

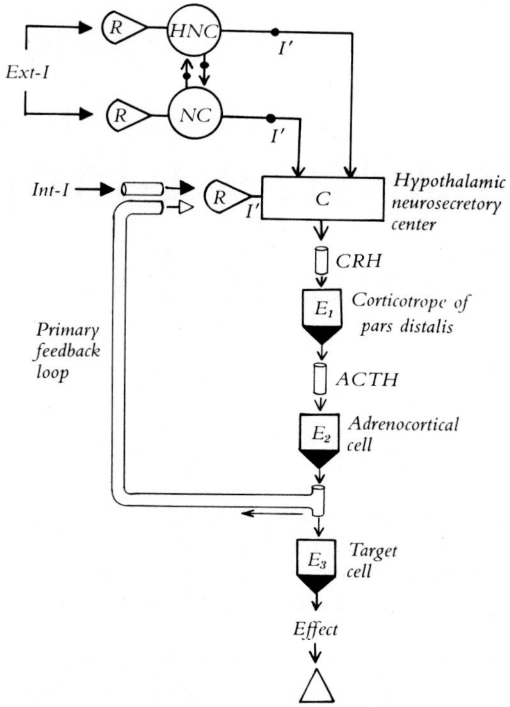

FIG. 2-7. Neuroendocrine reflex controlling adrenocorticoid secretion. This scheme involves three effectors in series. *CRH,* corticotropin-releasing hormone. See Figs. 2-1, 2-3, 2-6 and text for explanation and Figs. 2-1 and 2-3 for key to other abbreviations.

Summary

Endocrine systems can be categorized as endocrine, neurohormonal and neuroendocrine reflexes combined in complicated arrays to regulate physiological patterns of responses. No hormone-induced effect is without consequence on other homeostatic mechanisms, nor are many homeostatic mechanisms free from hormonal modification. There may be multiple receptors and a complex of external or internal factors or both providing relevant information to the controller of a specific physiological parameter. In order to comprehend these interrelationships it is essential to identify first the simple reflexes and their components (receptors, input, effectors, controller, output, feedback). Once the individual reflexes are identified and categorized it becomes possible to integrate several simple reflexes on a larger scale to gain an overview of more complex physiological and behavioral patterns such as those described in Chapters 16 to 19.

3·A Brief Glimpse of Chordate Evolution

A comparative study of vertebrate endocrine systems necessitates knowledge of the major vertebrate groups, their evolutionary history and relationships to one another. It is essential not only to be aware of the evolutionary position of each group but also to know something about the environments in which they arose. Each group of vertebrates, each species, in fact, is a product of individualistic evolutionary change and "progression" as well as a product of adaptations to similar environmental problems faced by unrelated groups. The comparative endocrinologist faces the task of sorting out similarities due to convergent evolution of structures and functions as opposed to similarities due to common ancestry. The purpose of this chapter is to provide a brief overview of the major evolutionary events in vertebrate phylogeny as a framework for later discussions.

Phylum Chordata

The basic features of the phylum Chordata are *pharyngeal gill slits,* a *dorsal, hollow nerve cord* (that is, a spinal cord) and a supportive endoskeletal element, the *notochord,* which lies beneath the dorsal nerve cord. Each of these features must be present at some stage in the life cycle to qualify for membership in the Chordata. In addition, most chordates possess a postanal tail. The aquatic tadpole-like larva is basic to the phylum. In many fishes and amphibians as well as in reptiles, birds and mammals, however, the larval stage per se no longer exists, having been reduced to a transitory embryonic sequence recapitulating many of the developmental features of the tadpole.

The phylum Chordata consists of three subphyla: *Urochordata* (tailed chordates or ascidians or tunicates), *Cephalochordata* (head chordates) and *Vertebrata* (vertebrates).

Subphylum Urochordata

The all-marine subphylum Urochordata is considered to be the most primitive chordate group. A free-swimming aquatic tadpole larva is characteristic. The larva possesses the three basic chordate features, but these are modified when the larva undergoes drastic structural modifications or metamorphosis to become a sessile aquatic adult (that is, attached firmly to some substrate). The dorsal, hollow nervous system degenerates to a single neural ganglion, the notochord is obliterated and the animal secretes an exoskeleton or *tunic* that completely encases the adult (Fig. 3-1).

The adult tunicate (sometimes called a sea squirt because of its habit of ejecting a fine stream of water when disturbed by an eager biologist) retains only one of the unique chordate characteristics: a gill structure called a *branchial basket.* This apparatus is covered with cilia and has a mucus-secreting structure, the *endostyle,* associated with it. Coordinated ciliary movements cause a current of water to flow into the branchial basket (via the

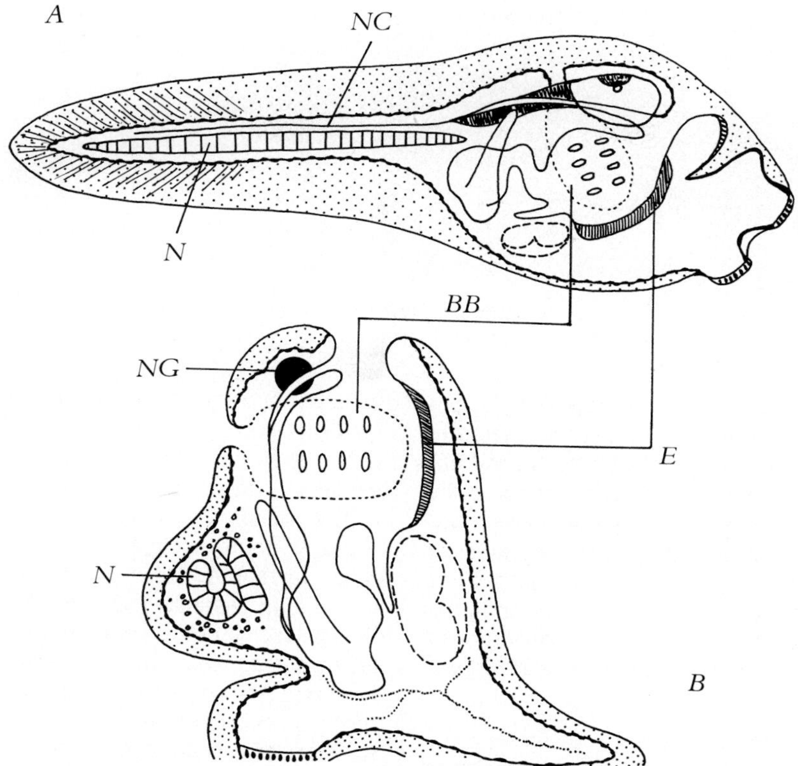

FIG. 3-1. Tunicata. A larval tunicate *(A)* attaches itself to the substrate and undergoes extensive metamorphosis to the sessile adult form *(B)*. *N*, notochord; *NC*, nerve cord; *E*, endostyle; *BB*, branchial basket with gill slits; *G*, gut; *NG*, neural ganglion. (Redrawn from Romer.[8])

mouth of the larva or the incurrent siphon of the adult) and out via the gill slits (the excurrent siphon of the adult). Mucus secreted by the endostyle traps minute food particles, and the mucus plus trapped food is moved by ciliary action into the gut, where both mucus and trapped food particles are digested. This method for obtaining food is common among the invertebrate groups believed to have given rise to the chordates, and organisms possessing such a mechanism are called *ciliary-mucus* or *pharyngeal-filtration feeders.*

Subphylum Cephalochordata

The sessile urochordate or tunicate is considered to be an evolutionary dead end, but some ancestral form similar to the larval tunicate may have given rise to the marine Cephalochordata. Certain living tunicates (for example, *Oikopleura*) never undergo metamorphosis to a sessile adult but remain free living and attain sexual maturity while retaining the larval body form. Prolongation of larval life or retention of larval characteristics in sexually mature animals often is termed *paedomorphosis.* If paedomorphosis is brought about by delayed development of nonreproductive tissues, it is called *neoteny.* In the most extreme form of neoteny the larva itself becomes sexually mature.

The cephalochordates (such as the living Amphioxus) have a body plan very similar to larval urochordates, including a branchial basket with mucus-secreting endostyle and a persistent notochord throughout their life (Fig. 3-2). Furthermore, cephalochordates anatomically resemble the larvae of the most primitive members of the Subphylum Vertebrata, the cyclostomes. Cephalochordate larvae are ciliary-mucus feeders like the urochordates. Similarities among cephalochordates, urochordates and vertebrates support a common

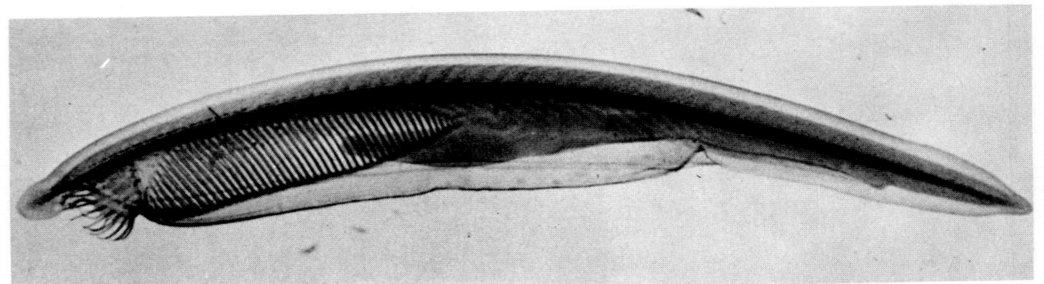

FIG. 3-2. Adult Amphioxus. Compare to the ammocetes vertebrate larva in Figure 3-3. (Courtesy Carolina Biological Supply Co.)

evolutionary origin for all three subphyla, but it is not certain how the groups are related to one another. The ancestral vertebrate may not have been a member of either invertebrate chordate group.[3] Vertebrates have many features not found in either urochordates or cephalochordates; for example, specializations of the head, anterior nervous system and pharyngeal breathing apparatus that are responsible for the active predaceous life of vertebrates.

Subphylum Vertebrata

Eight major groups (classes) comprise the subphylum Vertebrata of which only one is entirely extinct. In addition to possession of the three chordate characteristics the vertebrates all have special body structures, *vertebrae,* that surround and protect the spinal cord. Furthermore, there is a special bony case, the *cranium,* that protects the enlarged anterior portion of the nervous system, the brain. This latter feature is the basis for another name sometimes applied to these chordates, the subphylum Craniata.

Class Agnatha

The class Agnatha consists of primitive, jawless fishes (*a* without + *gnathos* jaws) believed to have evolved directly from cephalochordates or some cephalochordate-like ancestor. They are divided into an extinct subclass the Ostracodermi and the extant subclass Cyclostomata (*kyklos* round + *stoma* mouth).

The ostracoderms were all small fishes covered with bony plates (armor). They were limited to the ocean bottom where they existed as ciliary-mucus feeders. Although the ostracoderms were not sessile like the urochordates, they nevertheless lived a "sit-and-sift" existence close to the bottom sediments of the oceans.

Many adult cyclostomes are parasitic on other vertebrate fishes, but the larvae are ciliary-mucus feeders. There are two groups of living cyclostomes, the marine hagfishes, *Myxinoidea,* and the essentially freshwater lampreys (*Petromyzontidae*). The *ammocetes larva* of the lamprey has a branchial basket with an endostyle, and in general, the body form looks much like the cephalochordate, Amphioxus (Figs. 3-2, 3-3). Although some biologists suggest these structural similarities imply a close evolutionary relationship, others would argue against such an interpretation.[3]

When the ammocetes larva metamorphoses to the adult lamprey, the endostyle differentiates into the thyroid gland of the adult (see Chap. 8). The Myxinoidea do not have a larval form and are more primitive than lampreys in many features. However, modern hagfishes may not be like the first vertebrate, and their apparent simplicity may be a degenerate condition. Lampreys could be the best living example of a primitive vertebrate.[4] A comparison of lampreys and hagfishes is provided in Table 3-1.

Class Placodermi

The ostracoderm fishes were ancestral to the first jawed vertebrates, the class Placodermi, a heterogeneous collection of extinct, heavily armored fishes. Hinged jaws developed in the placoderm fishes from modifications of the first gill arch, and this same event

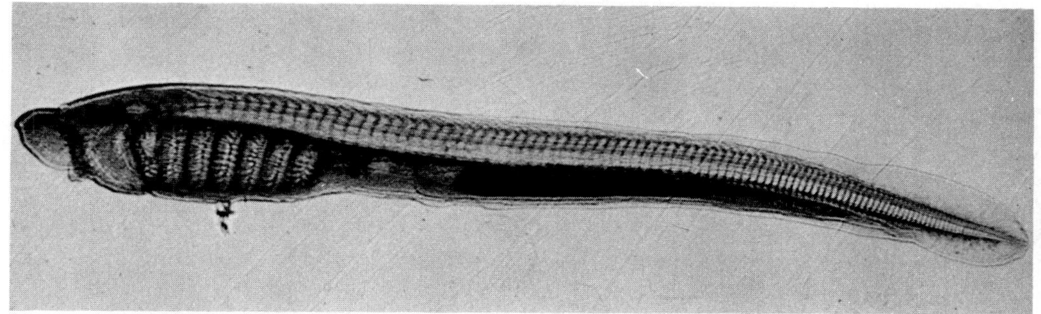

Fig. 3-3. Ammocetes larva. This larva of the lamprey, a living, jawless vertebrate (Agnatha: Cyclostomata), is structurally much like the cephalochordate in Figure 3-2. (Courtesy Carolina Biological Supply Co.)

can be observed early in embryonic development of all jawed vertebrates (Fig. 3-4). Many zoologists consider development of jaws to be the most significant single event in vertebrate evolution. Certainly it was a significant advancement enabling the placoderm fishes to abandon the bottom-dwelling existence of their ancestors. They could discard the ciliary-mucus feeding behavior for a pelagic, predatory behavior, so to speak, although some retained the ancestral filter feeding. The placoderms became abundant, attained great size and sported heavy armor. They were the dominant vertebrates of the Devonian period, but they suddenly declined and disappeared altogether. During the Devonian, the placoderms gave rise to two important piscine classes: the bony fishes, *class Osteichthyes,* and the cartilaginous fishes, *class Chondrichthyes* (Fig. 3-5). These descendants retained the jaws of their ancestors but shed the bony armor, emphasizing speed and agility.

Class Chondrichthyes

The class Chondrichthyes (*chondros* cartilage + *ichthy* fish) includes fishes whose skeletons are primarily composed of cartilage or calcified cartilage. True bone is not present in this group. Since cartilage forms prior to bone in the normal developmental sequence, some zoologists suggest that this group arose from the placoderms via neoteny. Included in the class Chondrichthyes are the sharks, rays and skates (*Selachii* or *Elasmobranchii*) and the ratfishes or chimaeras (*Holocephali*) (Fig. 3-6). The cartilaginous fishes flourished for a time but declined. Although in recent geological time they are increasing in abundance, they are believed to represent an evolutionary

Table 3-1. *Comparison of Some Features of Living Agnathan Fishes: Cyclostomata*

FEATURES	LAMPREY (PETROMYZONTIDAE)	HAGFISH (MYXINOIDEA)
Oral disc	Present	Absent
Teeth	On tongue and oral disc	On tongue plus "palate"
Eyes	Moderately developed	Degenerate
Buccal glands	Present	Absent
Barbels	Absent	Present
Gill pouches	Ectodermal origin	Endodermal origin
Kidney	Mesonephros	Pronephros anteriorly; Mesonephros posteriorly
Eggs	Small, unkeratinized and without hooks	Very large (about 2 cm), keratinized and with hooks
Spawning frequency	Die after first spawning	Apparently breed more than once
Larval stage	Ammocetes larva	No larval stage

Data from Jensen[5] and Hubbs and Potter.[6]

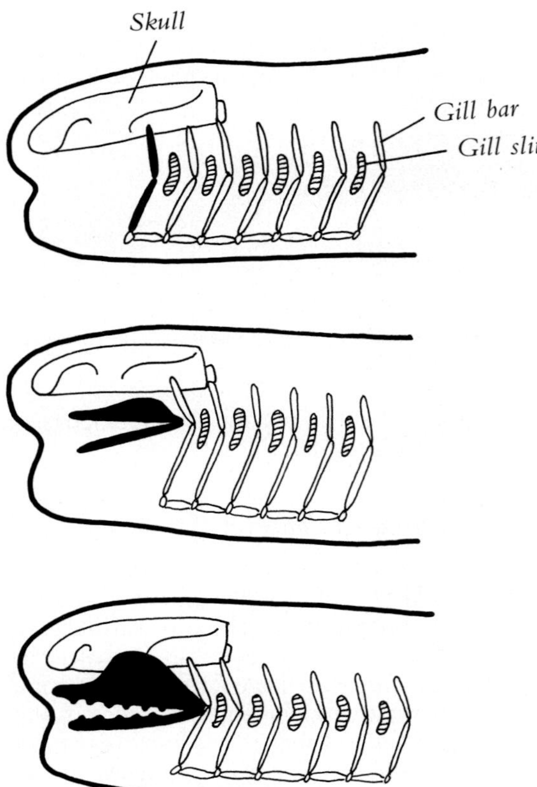

FIG. 3-4. Evolution of hinged jaws. The jaw arose through modification of the first set of gill-supporting bars, enlarged and eventually became endowed with teeth. (Redrawn from Keeton.[7])

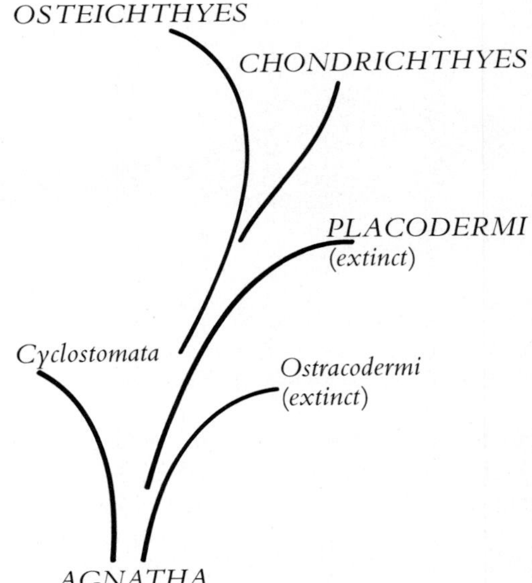

FIG. 3-5. Evolution of primitive fishes. (Redrawn from Colbert.[2])

dead end in not having given rise to any other vertebrate group. The cartilaginous fishes have not been as successful as the higher bony fishes (teleosts) in exploiting the aquatic environment (especially fresh water), and they represent a secondary fish fauna today (Fig. 3-7).

Class Osteichthyes

The class Osteichthyes (*osteon* bone) has excelled in exploitation of freshwater and marine habitats. The bony fishes had their origin in fresh water and secondarily invaded the marine habitat. Consequently the modern marine bony fishes are all derived from freshwater ancestors. It was the freshwater bony fishes that gave rise to the first terrestrial vertebrates, the amphibians. It is important to keep in mind the freshwater origins of modern fishes as well as the origin of amphibians from freshwater fish species when considering endocrine function and evolution.

The bony fishes can be readily separated into two subclasses: the *Actinopterygii* or ray-finned fishes, and the *Sarcopterygii* or lobe-fin fishes. The Actinopterygii (spiny wings or fins) have distinct rays that support the fins, whereas the Sarcopterygii (fleshy fins) have lobed fins with internal skeletal supports (bones) that are homologous to the limb bones of tetrapods.

Early in the evolution of the bony fishes (or possibly in the placoderm group that gave rise to the bony fishes) a pouch developed ventrally off the gut anterior to the stomach and remained connected to the gut by a duct. In the actinopterygian fishes this *air bladder* was used as a flotation device or swim bladder. Among the sarcopterygians the air bladder became modified as an accessory breathing device homologous to the lungs of tetrapods.

SUBCLASS ACTINOPTERYGII. The Actinopterygii includes most of the living bony fishes. There are four superorders, which are listed in order of evolutionary progression: *Polypteri, Chondrostei, Holostei,* and *Teleostei.*

The most primitive ray-finned fishes are found in the superorder Polypteri. Two living

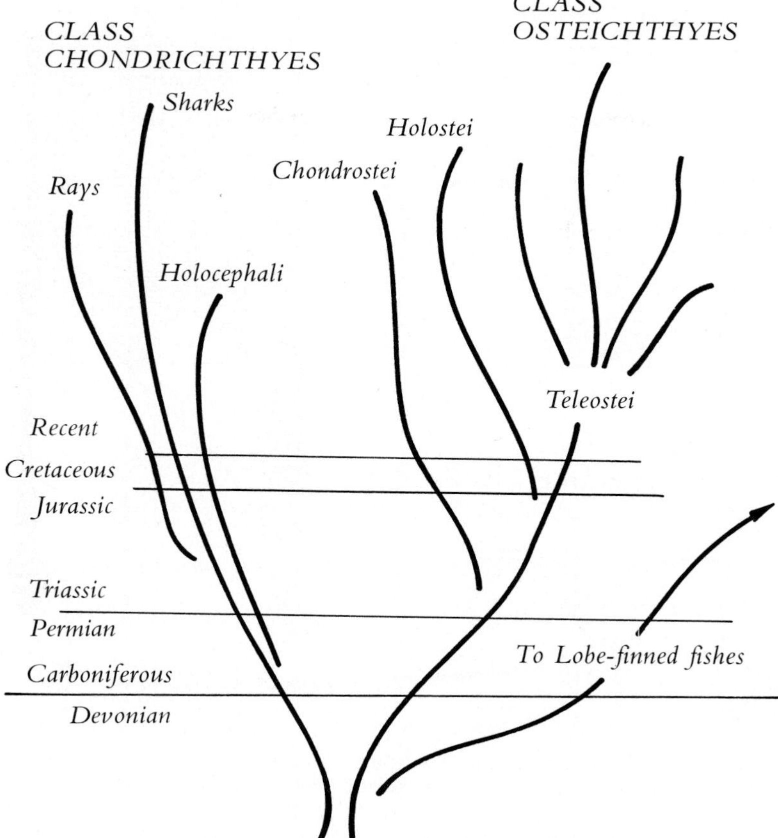

Fig. 3-6. Evolution of class Chondrichthyes and class Osteichthyes (Actinopterygii). A branch of the modern sarcopterygian bony fishes is indicated and an expansion of this line is shown in Figure 3-7. (Redrawn from Colbert.[2])

freshwater genera (*Polypterus,* the bichir, and *Erpetoichthyes*) are found in Africa. These fishes possess a number of very primitive features that make them especially interesting to the comparative endocrinologist.

The superorder Chondrostei includes sturgeons (for example, *Acipenser* spp.) and the spoonbills (*Polyodon*) of China and North America. Zoologists sometimes include the Polypteri as the most primitive members of this group. The chondrostean fishes are all freshwater fishes.

The superorder Holostei is restricted to North America, occurring only in the Mississippi drainage. This group consists of the bowfin, *Amia calva,* and several species of gar (*Lepisosteus*). The teleostean fishes, superorder Teleostei, are the most advanced Actinopterygii. The teleosts have produced a tremendous adaptive radiation in fresh water and have secondarily invaded the marine habitat where they are the most abundant and successful vertebrate group. The majority of extant fish species are teleosts. Sometimes the teleosts are divided into the so-called lower teleosts, exemplified by the salmonid fishes such as trout and salmon, and the higher teleosts, such as the centrarchids (large-mouth bass and bluegill sunfish, etc.). The higher teleosts can be recognized by the strong tendency for the pelvic (ventral) paired fins to move anteriorly to the vicinity of the pectoral (shoulder) fins.

Subclass Sarcopterygii. The ancestors of the first four-footed or *tetrapod* vertebrates were the Sarcopterygii. Two orders of sarcopterygian fishes are living today: *order Crossopterygii* (fringe fins) and *order Dipnoi* (*dipnoos* double breathing). Both of these groups

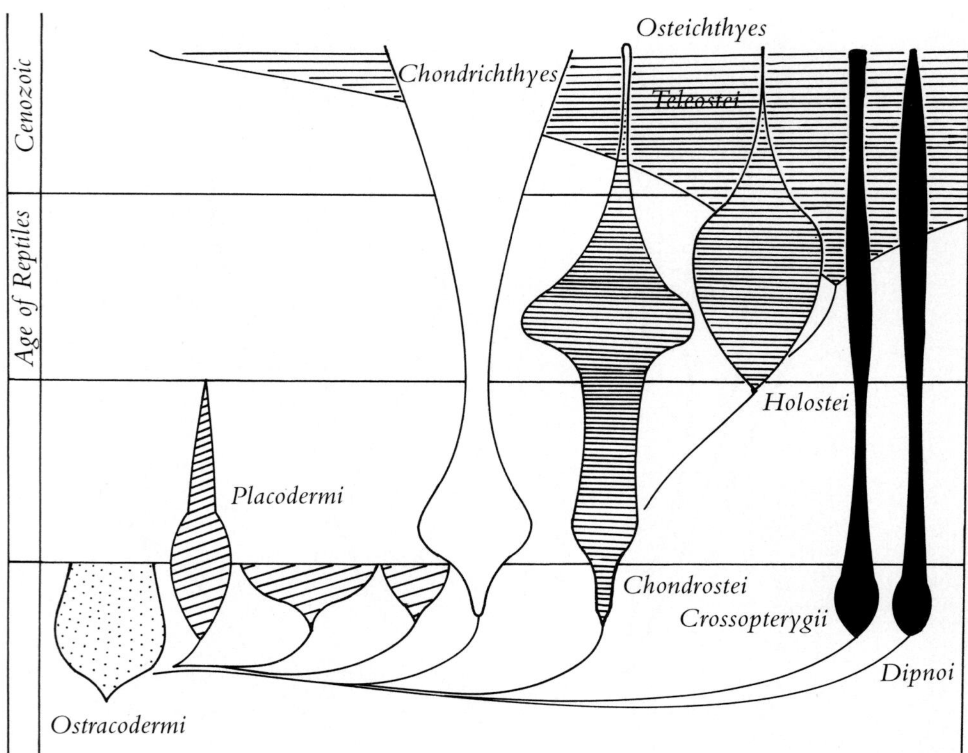

FIG. 3-7. Relative abundance of fish groups throughout geologic time. The relative abundance is proportional to the width of the bars. Note the sudden disappearance from the fossil record of two groups of placoderms at the end of the Devonian and the disappearance of the last placoderms (acanthodians) during the Permian. The teleosts appeared during the late Cretaceous and have become the dominant fishes of recent times. (Redrawn from Colbert.[2])

represent side ventures off the main line of evolution within the Sarcopterygii, which gave rise to the first semiterrestrial vertebrates, the class Amphibia (Figs. 3-8, 3-9).

Crossopterygian fishes were known only from their excellent fossil record until 1938 when a living crossopterygian, *Latimeria chalumnae* (Fig. 3-10), was caught by some fishermen off the coast of Madagascar. Since that time a number of these bizarre giants have been captured and their anatomy and physiology closely scrutinized by comparative zoologists. *Latimeria,* like other crossopterygian fishes, has internal nares and a lung-like air bladder. It may reach 5 to 6 feet in length and is viviparous (live bearing).

The order Dipnoi consists of three genera of lungfishes restricted to the tropical regions of three continents: *Protopterus* in Africa, *Lepidosiren* in South America and *Neoceratodus* in Australia. These fishes are gill breathers that use their lungs as accessory breathing structures. Only *Protopterus* survives breathing air alone. *Protopterus* can secrete a mucus-lined cocoon in which it resides and breathes air during periods of intense drought when its aquatic habitat may disappear altogether. The unusual distribution for these genera of lungfishes relates to the theory of formation of the present continents following the breakup of a "super continent" and a movement or drifting apart of the fragments (that is, continental drift).

Class Amphibia

Class Amphibia (*amphi* both + *bios* life) exhibits three living groups: *order Caudata* (*Urodela*), which includes salamanders and newts; *order Apoda* (without feet), the limbless caecilians, a tropical group about which little

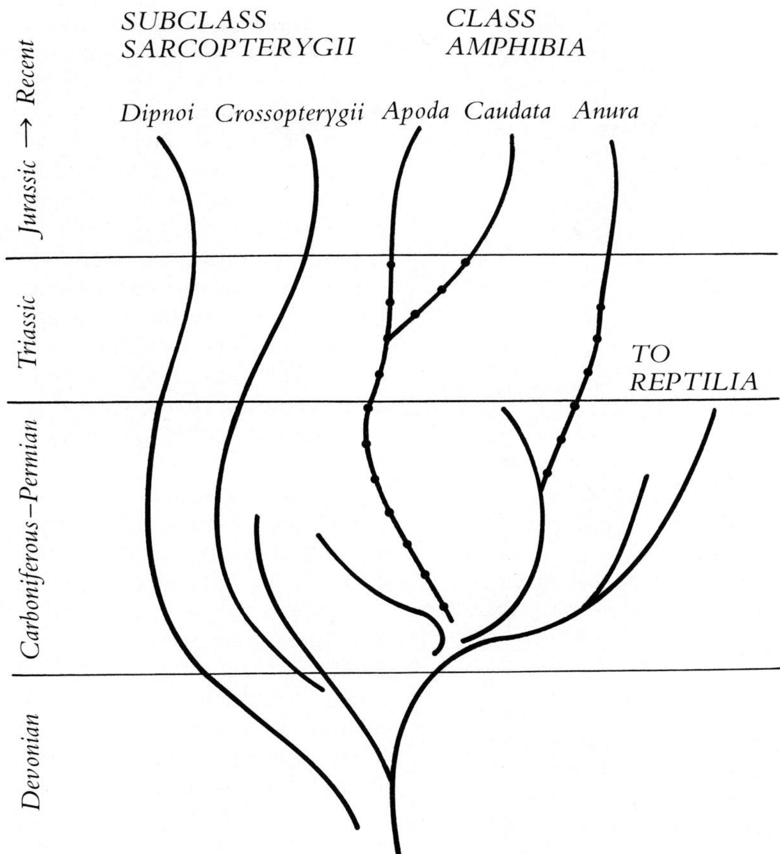

FIG. 3-8. Evolution of the Sarcopterygii and Amphibia. Note that the reptilian stock appeared early in the Carboniferous (see Fig. 3-9). (Redrawn from Colbert.[2])

is known; *order Anura* (without tail), the tailless frogs and toads.

The primitive amphibians (labyrinthodonts) had their origin from the crossopterygian fishes that had developed internal nares and lungs for air breathing and had supportive skeletal elements in their fleshy lobed fins. The labyrinthodonts were large-tailed amphibians that gave rise to the first reptiles. The modern amphibians arose from two or three separate lines of evolution (Fig. 3-8), depending upon where the Apoda are placed. Current thought suggests a common ancestral group for all three extant orders.

As the name of this class implies, some amphibians lead double lives: one as aquatic larvae and the second as terrestrial or semiterrestrial adults. This "typical" life history involves laying eggs in fresh water where they develop into tadpole-like larvae. The larvae remain in fresh water as did their ancestors for a period of growth followed by a remarkable metamorphosis involving drastic structural and biochemical alterations to attain the different adult body form and the physiology to survive in a desiccating environment. The process of metamorphosis will be discussed in more detail in Chapter 17.

Many amphibians, however, have abandoned the aquatic phase of their life cycle to varying degrees. A number of species lay their eggs on land in moist places where larval development is completed within the egg (for example, *Batrachoseps, Pseudotriton, Plethodon*). The so-called marsupial frogs of Ecuador, *Gastrotheca* spp., develop on the back a hormone-dependent pouch in which the eggs are placed. After hatching, the tad-

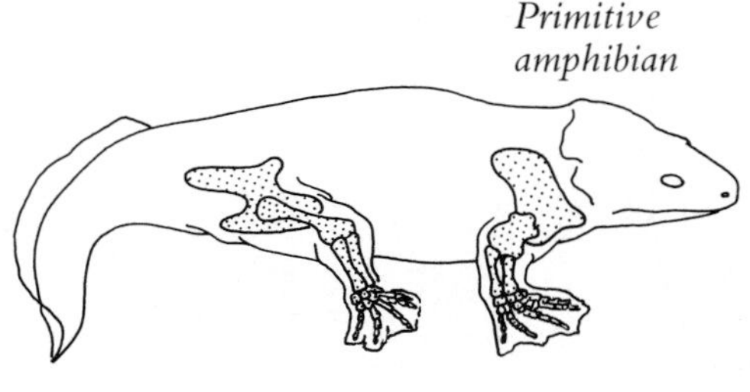

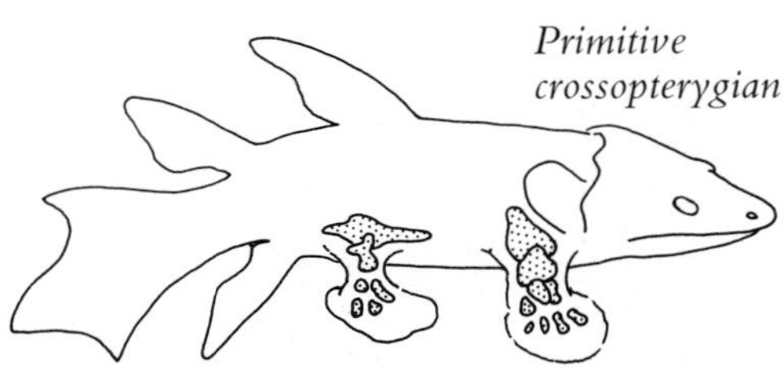

FIG. 3-9. Evolution of limbs in the Tetrapoda. The bones in the limbs and the pectoral and pelvic girdles of crossopterygian fishes are believed to be homologous. (Redrawn from Wilson et al.[9])

poles are placed in water to continue their larval development until metamorphosis occurs. The male midwife toad *Alytes obstetricans* "incubates" the eggs on land by wrapping around his legs the strings of eggs laid by the female. Periodically he travels to the water to moisten the eggs. *Salamander atra,* a European salamander, is viviparous and gives birth to two fully metamorphosed young. Many species of apodans and some anurans are viviparous.

Class Reptilia

In a sense it was a mistake for the amphibians to give rise to the reptiles, for the reptiles quickly replaced them as the dominant terrestrial organisms. Class Reptilia owed its success in exploiting the terrestrial environment in part to the development of a unique "land egg," which enclosed the aquatic environment for embryonic development within a membrane (the amnion). This amniote egg could be laid on land where it was safe from aquatic predators. The reptilian egg is much more resistant to desiccation than the "terrestrial" eggs of amphibians. Furthermore, the reptiles were no longer tied to water for reproduction, which placed fewer restrictions on their movements. The large eggs allow young to hatch at a size considerably greater than is possible from eggs of either oviparous fishes or amphibians.

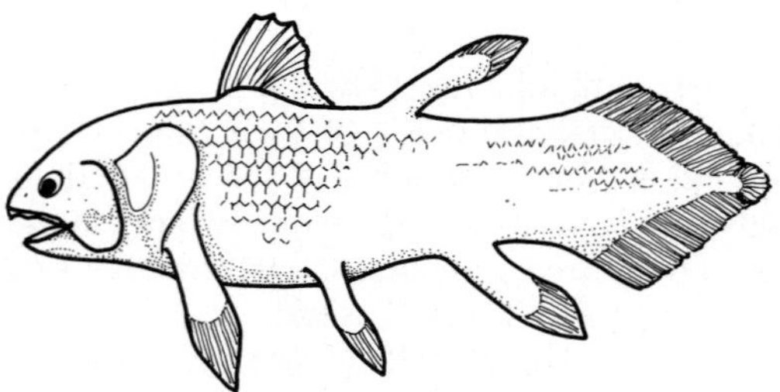

FIG. 3-10. The coelacanth. Adult specimens of this crossopterygian fish, *Latimeria chalumnae,* may exceed 6 feet (2 meters) in length. (Redrawn from Keeton.[7])

Birds and mammals have retained many of the features of the reptilian egg, including the amnion and other membranes (the chorion, allantois and in some cases the yolk sac). Bird eggs are little different from reptilian eggs, and embryonic development is very similar. Mammals have greatly modified the use of these membranes, especially the placental mammals. Reptiles, birds and mammals are often referred to collectively as the *amniote vertebrates* (that is, they all possess an amnion), whereas fishes and amphibians are termed *anamniotes* (without an amnion).

Primitive amphibians gave rise to the cotylosaurs or stem reptiles, which early in reptilian evolution diverged into several separate pathways (Fig. 3-11). Only four of these pathways have living representatives (as far as is known).

One pathway (the *subclass Anapsida*) separated early and gave rise to the heavily armored *order Chelonia,* the turtles, tortoises and terrapins. The chelonians are anatomically a conservative group, having changed little in appearance over several million years. However, it might be a mistake to assume that their physiology has also remained conservative.

A second pathway (*subclass Lepidosaura*) produced two important groups, the *order Squamata* (snakes and lizards) and the *order Rhynchocephalia,* which contains only the New Zealand tuatara, *Sphenodon.* The tuatara is of special interest because it is the only living representative of a very old reptilian group.

The *subclass Archosaura* represents a third

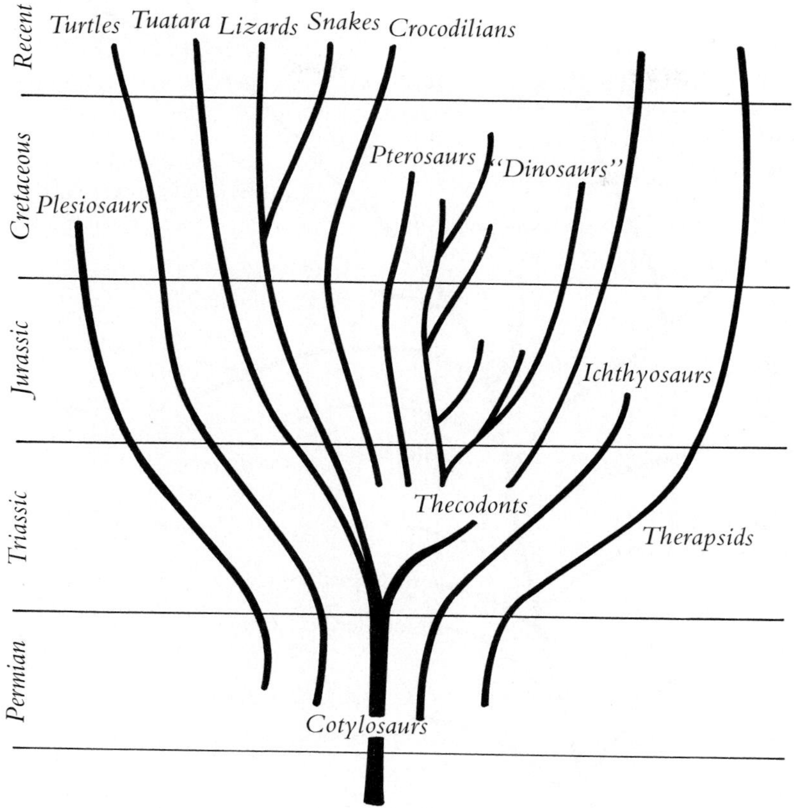

FIG. 3-11. Evolution of the Reptilia. The primitive reptiles (cotylosaurs) are closely related to several lines of extinct and extant reptilian groups as well as to the reptilian ancestors of both the birds and mammals. (Redrawn from Keeton.[7])

evolutionary line of which only the *order Crocodilia* (crocodiles and alligators) has living representatives. The extinct dinosaurs were part of this evolutionary line. In addition, the archosaurs (thecodonts) gave rise to birds (class Aves).

The final reptilian group that gave rise to extant organisms was the *subclass Synapsidia,* from which evolved the mammals (Fig. 3-11). This group separated early from the main line of reptilian evolution.

None of the reptilian ancestors of the mammals remains today. Apparently the ability to regulate a relatively constant body temperature developed in the synapsids (specifically in the therapsid reptiles) independently of its development in the thecodont reptiles, which gave rise to the birds.

Class Aves

Birds are characterized by having *feathers,* no teeth, a relatively constant body temperature (37°–43°C), a four-chambered heart analogous to that of mammals and numerous structural modifications for flight. Nevertheless, birds are not much more than glorified reptiles. Although viviparity has developed in all other tetrapod classes (as well as some fishes), all birds lay eggs. However, birds have been successful at exploiting the terrestrial habitat in such a way as to avoid undue competition with mammals and exhibit an impressive adaptive radiation. There are many diverse groups within the class Aves (Fig. 3-12), but a more detailed account is beyond the scope of this chapter. Primarily, studies of avian endo-

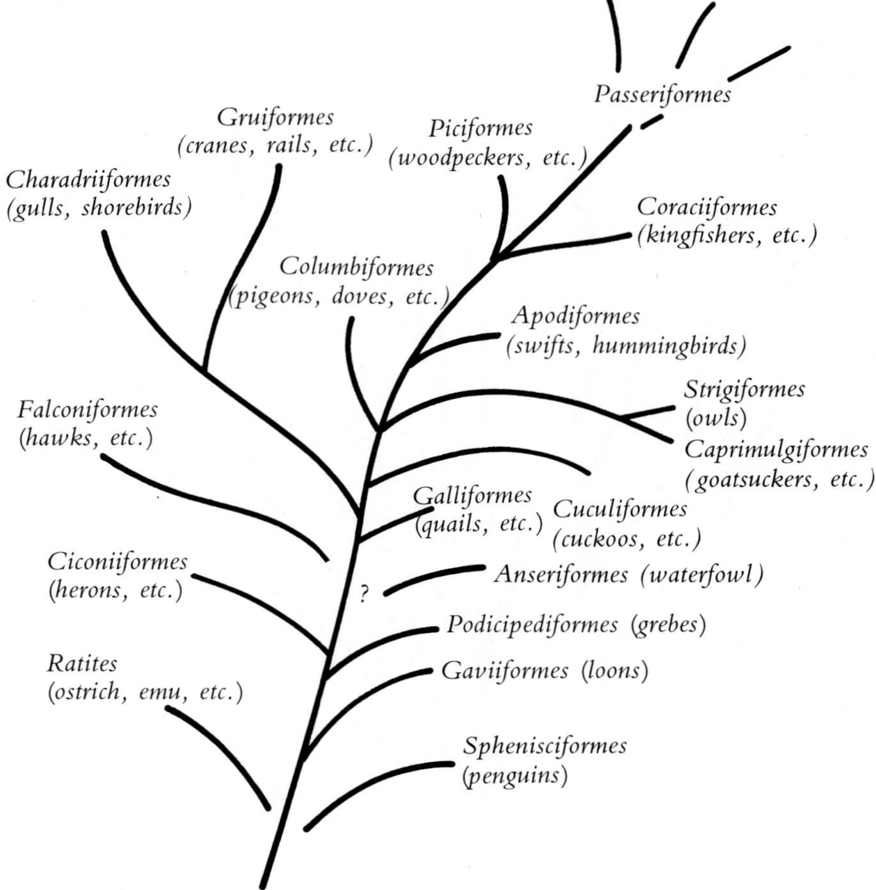

FIG. 3-12. Major orders of modern birds. (Based on Zim and Gabrielson.[10])

crinology have been limited to domestic species, and only a few wild species have been examined.

Class Mammalia

The most distinctive and uniform features of mammals are the possession of *hair* and *mammary glands,* for which the group is named. Class Mammalia may be separated into three subclasses: *subclass Prototheria* (*protos* first + *therion* animal), *subclass Metatheria* (*meta* middle) and *subclass Eutheria* (*eu* good).

The most primitive mammals are the *order Monotremata* in the subclass Prototheria. This group includes the duckbill platypus (*Ornithorhynchus anatinus*) and the spiny anteater, *Tachyglossus.* All members of this group lay eggs, and they are found only in Australia.

Subclass Metatheria consists of a single order, *Marsupialia,* the pouched mammals such as the kangaroos and wallabys of Australia and the opossum of North America. The fossil record indicates that the marsupials were just beginning their adaptive radiation when continental drift began to separate the continents. This explains in part their present skewed distribution, with the vast majority of extant species being found in Australia.

The subclass Eutheria consists of the placental mammals. From a primitive insectivore stock, 13 orders have evolved (Fig. 3-13 and Table 3-2). The *order Primates* is considered (by man, of course) to be the highest group of mammals, that group showing the most ad-

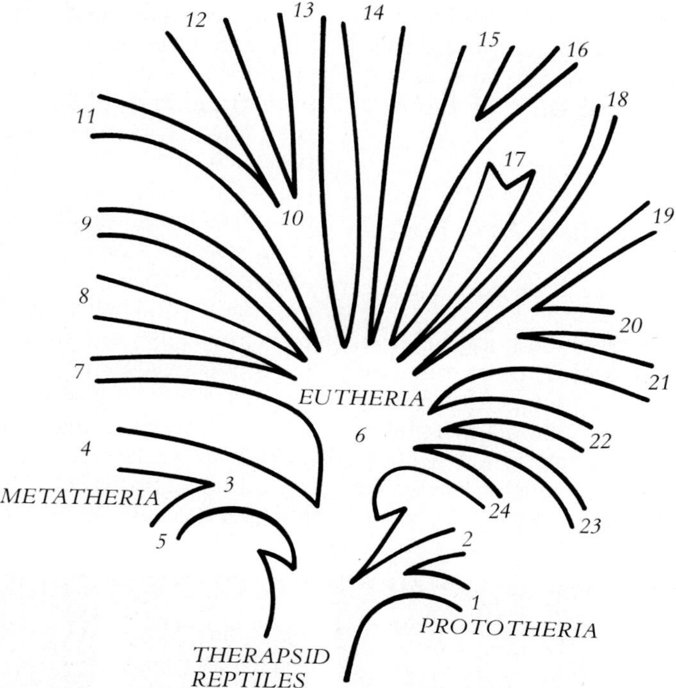

FIG. 3-13. Evolution of mammals. The three major divisions (Prototheria, Metatheria and Eutheria) are indicated along with the orders. (After Romer.[8])
1, echidna (spiny anteater); *2,* duckbill platypus; *3,* opossum; *4,* kangaroos and other herbivores; *5,* carnivores; *6,* insectivore stock of eutherian mammals; *7,* bats; *8,* primates; *9,* lagomorphs; *10,* primitive rodents; *11,* squirrel group; *12,* guinea pig group; *13,* mouse group; *14,* carnivores; *15,* toothed whales; *16,* whalebone whales; *17,* artiodactyls; *18,* perissodactyls; *19,* hydrax; *20,* elephants; *21,* sirenians; *22,* aardvark; *23,* pangolin; *24,* edentates (anteaters)

TABLE 3-2. *Thirteen Orders of Extant Mammals*

ORDER	COMMON REPRESENTATIVES
Insectivora	Shrews, hedgehogs, moles
Chiroptera	Bats
Dermoptera	Flying lemurs
Carnivora	
Suborder Fissipedia	Toed carnivores (dogs, cats, bears)
Suborder Pinnipedia	Limbs modified for aquatic life (seals)
Rodentia	Rodents (rats, squirrels, mice)
Lagomorpha	Rabbits, hares
Edentata	Toothless mammals (sloths, anteaters, armadillos)
Cetacea	Whales, dolphins, porpoises
Proboscidea	Elephants
Sirena	Manatees
Perissodactyla	Odd-toed mammals (horses, zebras, rhinoceroses)
Artiodactyla	Even-toed ungulates (swine, cattle, deer, goats, hippopotamuses, antelopes, sheep)
Primates	Lemurs, tarsiers, monkeys, apes, man

vanced evolutionary adaptations and success among the mammals. Eutherians invaded the western hemisphere from Asia and almost eliminated the marsupial fauna of the New World.

A Concluding Note about Vertebrate Evolution

It is tempting to think of the so-called lower groups of vertebrates as being more primitive than the so-called higher groups. However, it is important to remember that old in a phylogenetic sense does not imply primitive. Certainly the teleostean fishes, which have existed as a definitive group much longer than mammals, have had more time for evolutionary processes to operate upon the ancestral progenitors than mammals have had to diverge from therapsid reptiles (Fig. 3-14). Figure 3-15 is an attempt to summarize vertebrate evolution such that all living groups appear at the top of the phylogenetic scheme rather than the more traditional form that implies that once a group appears it no longer undergoes any evolutionary change. Of special interest to the evolutionist and hence also to the comparative endocrinologist are those forms that were transitional between extant classes. Zoologists become very excited when new species are discovered representing groups previously thought to be extinct. Sometimes the discovery of "living fossils" can be a disappointment, however, because the true missing links prob-

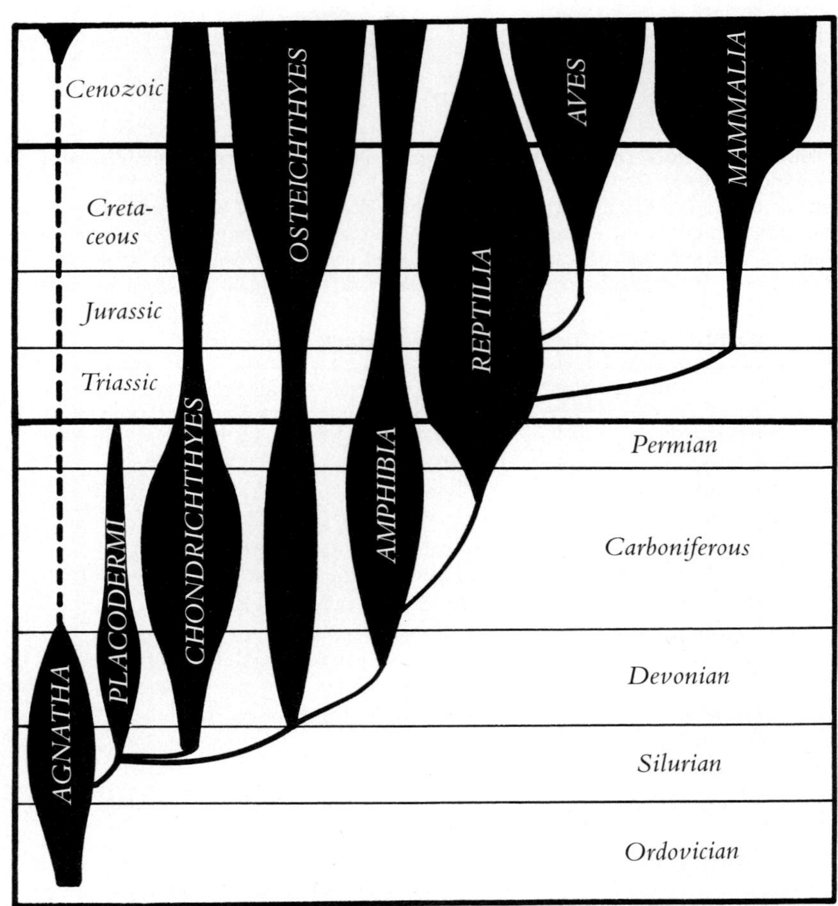

Fig. 3-14. Relative abundance of vertebrates in geologic time. All eight classes are indicated. The width of the bar is proportional to the relative abundance (species) based upon the fossil record and extant species. (Redrawn from Keeton.[7])

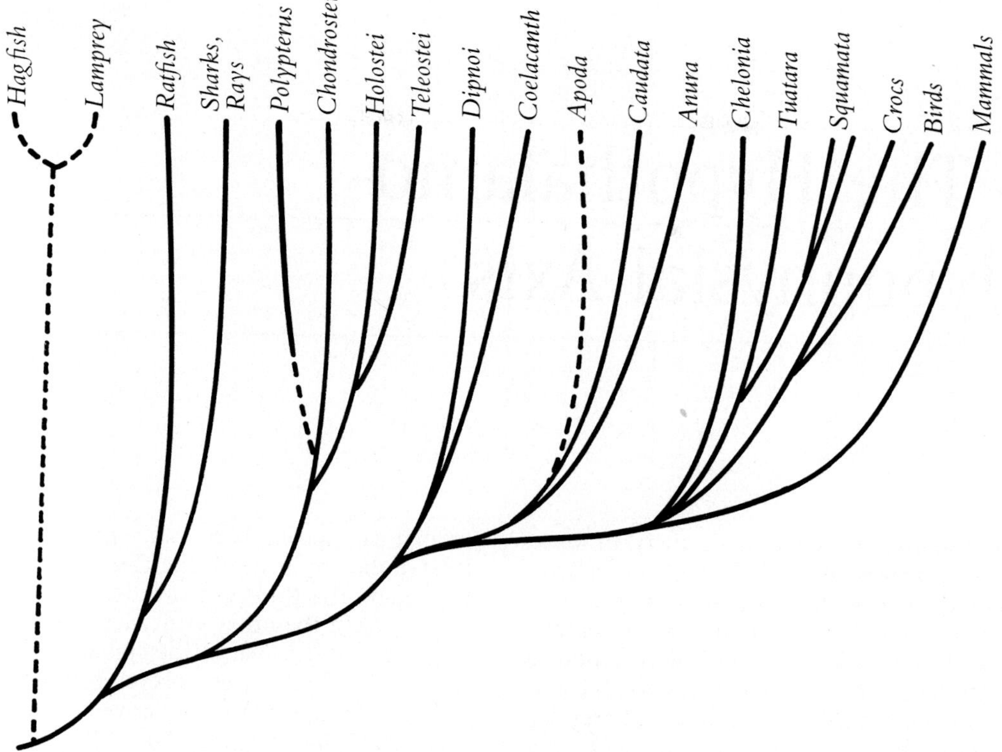

FIG. 3-15. Phylogenetic tree of extant vertebrates. This way of drawing phylogenetic relationships emphasizes that all living representatives are at the top of the diagram. Dotted lines indicate phylogenies that are not clearly established. (Redrawn from Bern.[1])

ably are all well fossilized by now. Such living fossils have not necessarily retained primitive features of their ancestors and may have diverged significantly.

References

1. Bern, H.A. (1972). Comparative endocrinology—The state of the field and the art. Gen. Comp. Endocrinol. Suppl. 3:751–761.
2. Colbert, E.H. (1955). Evolution of the Vertebrates. John Wiley and Sons, New York (Reprint).
3. Gans, C. and R.G. Northcutt (1983). Neural crest and the origin of vertebrates: a new head. Science 220:268–274.
4. Gorbman, A. (1980). Endocrine regulatory patterns in Agnatha: In S. Ishii, T. Hirano and M. Wada, eds., Hormones, Adaptation and Evolution, Japan. Sci. Soc. Press, Tokyo/Springer-Verlag, Berlin, pp. 81–92.
5. Hubbs, C.L. and I.C. Potter (1971). Distribution, phylogeny and taxonomy. In M.W. Hardisty and I.C. Potter, eds., The Biology of Lampreys. Academic Press, New York, Vol. 1, pp. 1–65.
6. Jensen, D. (1966). The Hagfish. Sci. Am., 214 (Feb):82–90.
7. Keeton, W.T. (1972). Biological Science, 2nd ed. W.W. Norton and Co., New York.
8. Romer, A.S. (1962). The Vertebrate Body, 3rd ed. W.B. Saunders Co., Philadelphia.
9. Wilson, E.O., T. Eisner, W.R. Briggs, R.E. Dickerson, R.L. Metzenberg, R.D. O'Brien, M. Susman, and W.E. Boggs (1973). Life on Earth. Sinauer Associates, Stamford, Conn.
10. Zim, H.S. and I.N. Gabrielson (1965). Birds. Golden Press, New York.

PART II

4·The Hypothalamo-Hypophysial Axis

The majority of endocrine activity in vertebrates is generated through the hypothalamo-hypophysial axis. Under neurohormonal directives from the hypothalamus, the hypophysis secretes hormones that control secretion by the thyroid gland, adrenal cortex and the gonads. In addition, the hypophysis secretes several other hormones. The structure and function of the vertebrate hypothalamus and hypophysis are discussed in this chapter, and the hormones of the hypophysis are the foci for Chapters 5, 6 and 7. The hypothalamo-hypophysial-thyroid axis is covered in Chapter 8, and the steroid-secreting glands are the subjects of Chapters 9 through 11.

The hypothalamo-hypophysial axis consists of the neurosecretory (NS) portions of the hypothalamic region of the brain and the hypophysis or pituitary gland (Figs. 4-1, 4-2). During development of the brain the diencephalon differentiates into three regions: Most of the diencephalon becomes the thalamus, a major relay station between higher and lower portions of the brain. The floor or ventral portion of the diencephalon becomes the hypothalamus, containing various NS nuclei, which are sources for neurohormones. The third portion, the epithalamus, is derived from the roof of the diencephalon and gives rise to the endocrine epiphysial complex that includes the pineal gland (see Chap. 15).

The pituitary gland or hypophysis develops through fusion of a ventral growth from the diencephalon, the *infundibulum,* with an ectodermal sac known as *Rathke's pouch,* and is located directly beneath the third ventricle of the brain. The third ventricle is a cavity continuous with the other ventricles of the brain and the central canal of the spinal cord. It is filled with a fluid known as cerebrospinal fluid.

The term hypophysis is derived from *hypo* under (the brain) + *physis* growth. Its alternate name, pituitary gland, is derived from *pituita* slime or phlegm. The pituitary was believed to be the source of phlegm, one of the four humors of the body proposed by Galen centuries ago. The other humors were blood, black bile and yellow bile.

The mammalian hypothalamo-hypophysial axis will be discussed first and followed by descriptions of nonmammalian vertebrates. Although in an evolutionary sense such a discussion should begin with agnathan fishes, the mammalian system is better understood and provides the nomenclature with respect to structures, hormones and functions that are applied to the nonmammalian systems. The entire field of endocrinology has branched in similar fashion from mammalian investigations to nonmammalian.

The Mammalian Hypophysis

The hypophysis of adult mammals is located ventral to the brain just posterior to the optic chiasma, and it remains attached to the hypothalamus by a stalk-like connection. Embryo-

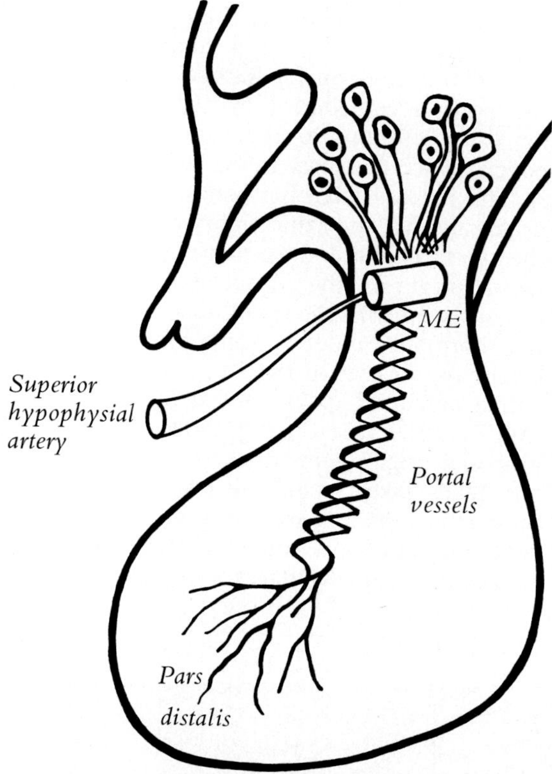

FIG. 4-1. The mammalian hypothalamo-adenohypophysial system. Hypothalamic neurosecretory neurons discharge hypophysiotropic factors into the vasculature of the median eminence *(ME)* from which they travel via the portal vessels to the tropic cells of the pars distalis. The superior hypophysial artery conducts blood to the median eminence. Tropic hormones enter the general venous drainage system.

logically the hypophysis has been described as having two separate origins: The *adenohypophysis* develops from Rathke's pouch, which has been thought to develop from oral (nonneural) ectoderm. The adenohypophysis is an epithelial structure (*adeno* gland) and can be subdivided into three regions: the *pars* (body) *distalis, pars tuberalis* and the *pars intermedia.* These regions are distinguished by their cytological features as well as their anatomical relationships to the remainder of the pituitary gland, the *neurohypophysis.* The infundibulum growing out ventrally from the floor of the diencephalon gives rise to the neurohypophysis, whose name reflects its neural origin. Two distinct subregions can be identified in the neurohypophysis: the *median eminence* and the *pars nervosa.* The median eminence consists mostly of aminergic axonal endings. The majority of axonal endings in the pars nervosa are peptidergic. An extensive vascular portal system, the *hypothalamo-hypophysial portal system,* develops between the median eminence of the neurohypophysis and the adenohypophysis. This portal system carries blood from the median eminence directly to the epithelial cells of the pars distalis.

The classic concept of the neurovascular link between the hypothalamus and the pituitary gland (the hypothalamohypophysial portal system) is based upon the pioneering anatomical studies of Wislocki. Presumably blood containing the hypophysiotropic regulating substances flows from the median eminence to the adenohypophysis, and the venous drainage

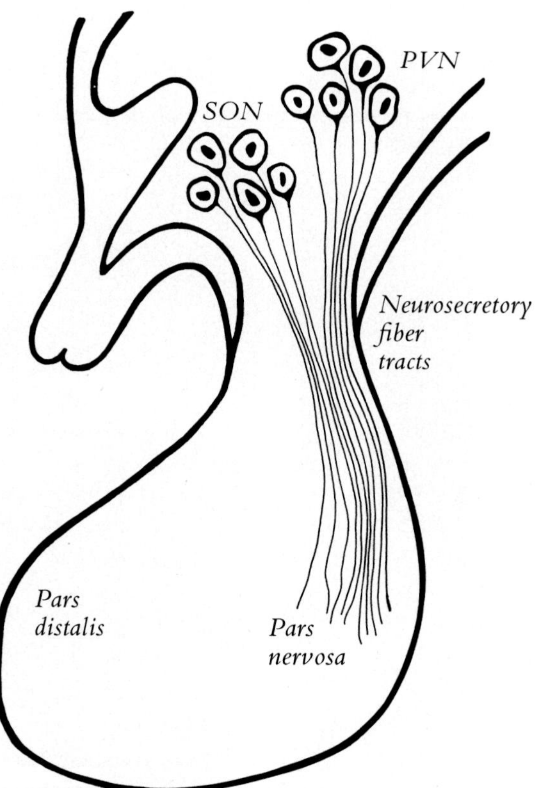

FIG. 4-2. The mammalian hypothalamo-pars nervosa system. Axonal fibers from the neurosecretory neurons of the supraoptic nucleus *(SON)* and paraventricular nucleus *(PVN)* travel through the infundibular stalk to the pars nervosa where their secretory products, the neurohypophysial octapeptide hormones, are stored.

from the latter carries pituitary hormones into the general circulation. Data gathered over the last several years, however, suggest that there may be significant blood flow from the adenohypophysis to the hypothalamus as well, and such a pathway may prove to be important in actions of pituitary hormones on the central nervous system.

Frequently in mammalian studies, the terms anterior lobe and posterior lobe are used to represent two divisions of the pituitary gland. These terms will not be used in this text since they do not refer to the same components of the gland as do adenohypophysis and neurohypophysis. Furthermore, the "posterior lobe" includes cells derived from both Rathke's pouch and the infundibulum, whereas the preferred terminology divides the pituitary according to its origin from Rathke's pouch and the infundibular process.

Recent reexamination of the hypothalamo-hypophysial axis supports a common origin from neuroectoderm for Rathke's pouch and the portion contributed by the diencephalon.[31,107] According to these studies, Rathke's pouch, which gives rise to the adenohypophysis and its associated hormones, is of neural origin and has the same embryonic origin as the hypothalamus and the neurohypophysis. A neural origin for the adenohypophysis would be consistent with the hypothesis that all peptide hormone-producing cells are of neural origin and belong to the amine content and amine precursor uptake and decarboxylation (APUD) series (see Chap. 1). Because of the proposed origin from neuroectoderm, Pearse and Takor Takor include all tropic hormone-producing cells as part of the general APUD series although no amines can be demonstrated in certain cellular types.[107] The neuro-

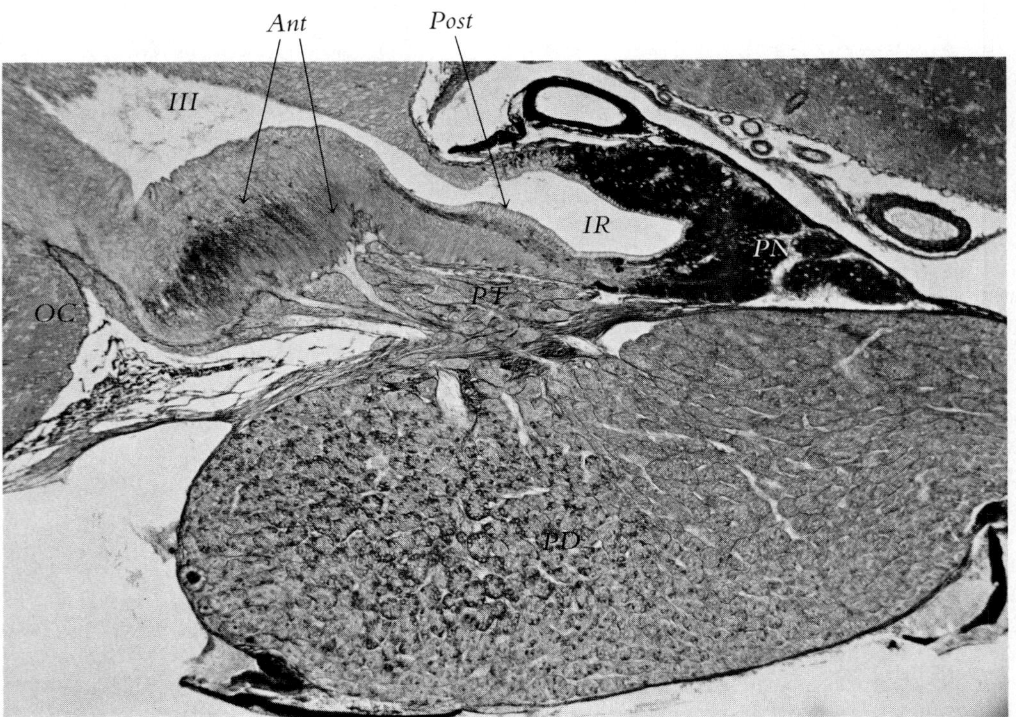

Fig. 4-3. Midsagittal section of the hypothalamo-hypophysial system of the white-crowned sparrow. Aldehyde fuchsin-positive neurosecretory fibers can be seen in the anterior median eminence and in the posterior median eminence *(arrows). III,* third ventricle; *IR,* infundibular recess extending from the third ventricle; *OC,* optic chiasm; *PT,* pars tuberalis; *PD,* pars distalis; *PN,* pars nervosa. The avian pituitary has no discrete pars intermedia. (Reprinted with permission from Bern, H.A., R.S. Nishioka, L.R. Mewaldt and D.S. Farner (1966). Photoperiodic and osmotic influences on the ultrastructure of the hypothalamic neurosecretory system of the white-crowned sparrow, *Zonotrichia leucophrys gambelii.* Z. Zellforsch. 69:198–227.)

ectodermal origin for adenohypophysial cells is further strengthened by the demonstration of pituitary hormones in the brain.[41,42]

The Adenohypophysis

Pars Tuberalis. The pars tuberalis consists of a thin layer of cells projecting rostrally (anteriorly and dorsally) from the adenohypophysis, and it is in contact with the median eminence of the neurohypophysis. The blood vessels of the hypothalamo-hypophysial portal system pass near or through the pars tuberalis en route to the pars distalis.

The pars tuberalis has long been termed a portion of the adenohypophysis of unknown function but characteristic of all tetrapod vertebrates. Recent evidence seems to imply that it is only an extension of the pars distalis related primarily to reproduction (see p. 55).

Structurally the cells of the pars tuberalis are connected to the cerebrospinal fluid of the third ventricle in the brain through cellular processes originating in modified ependymal cells known as *tanycytes* (Fig. 4-4). It has been suggested that tanycytes may selectively remove materials (neurohormones?) from cerebrospinal fluid and transfer them to cells of the pars tuberalis, causing the latter to release their stored products (?). Although this is a highly speculative idea, such an interesting anatomical relationship demands some imaginative research to provide a better understanding of both tanycytes and the cells of the pars tuberalis.

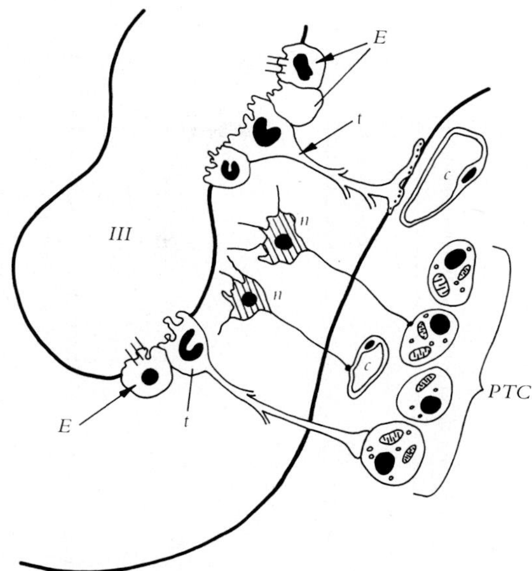

Fig. 4-4. Relationship of modified ependymal cells lining third ventricle to the pars tuberalis. Modified ependymal cells or tanycytes *(t)* provide connections between the third ventricle *(III)* and capillaries *(c)* and possibly pars tuberalis cells *(PTC)*. Similar connections by neurons *(n)* have also been observed. *E,* ciliated ependymal cells. (Modified from Holmes and Ball.[59])

Pars Intermedia. That portion of the adenohypophysis that makes contact with the pars nervosa of the neurohypophysis is defined as the pars intermedia. Indeed, formation of the pars intermedia occurs only if physical contact takes place with the infundibulum during development. In some species the pars intermedia becomes separated from the remainder of the adenohypophysis by a cavity or cleft. Only one cellular type appears in the mammalian pars intermedia as identified by selective staining procedures, and it is supposedly responsible for secretion of the peptide hormone *melanophore-stimulating hormone* or *melanotropin* (MSH). Cells associated with the skin and known as melanocytes in mammals synthesize a brown pigment, melanin, under the influence of MSH. This peptide hormone has also been identified in the hypothalamus,[14] although its importance there is not clear.

Pars Distalis. The major portion of the adenohypophysis is designated as the pars distalis. A variety of cellular types can be identified in the pars distalis by selective staining procedures. These various cellular types are responsible for secretion of seven pituitary hormones: *corticotropin,* or adrenocorticotropic hormone (ACTH); *thyrotropin,* or thyroid-stimulating hormone (TSH); *lipotropin,* or lipotropic hormone (LPH); *growth hormone* (GH); *prolactin* (PRL); and two *gonadotropins,* or gonadotropic hormones (GTHs). The two GTHs are *follicle-stimulating hormone* (FSH) and *luteinizing hormone* (LH), both of which are named for their effects in female mammals. All of these hormones are polypeptides or proteins. These seven hormones, together with MSH from the pars intermedia, are referred to as the *tropic hormones* of the adenohypophysis. The cells responsible for secreting tropic hormones are called *tropes.* Hence a corticotrope is a cell that produces ACTH. The

TABLE 4-1. *Synonyms, Abbreviations, Cellular Source, Targets and Actions for Mammalian Adenohypophysial Tropic Hormones*

NAME	ABBREVIATION[a]	SYNONYMS	OTHER ABBREVIATIONS	CELLULAR SOURCE	TARGET	ONE ACTION ON TARGET
Prolactin	PRL	Mammotropin, luteotropin, luteotropic hormone	LTH	Lactotrope	Mammary gland	Stimulates milk synthesis
Growth hormone	GH	Somatotropin, somatotropic hormone	STH	Somatotrope	Muscle	Stimulates incorporation of amino acids into protein
Corticotropin	ACTH	Adrenocorticotropic hormone, adrenocorticotropin		Corticotrope	Adrenal cortex	Stimulates synthesis and secretion of corticosteroids
Lipotropin	LPH	None		Corticotrope?	Adipose tissue?	Stimulates hydrolysis of fats to free fatty acids and glycerol
Melanotropin	MSH	Intermedin, melanocyte- or melanophore-stimulating hormone		Pars Intermedia	Melanocyte, etc.	Stimulates synthesis of melanin pigment
Thyrotropin	TSH	Thyroid-stimulating hormone		Thyrotrope	Thyroid gland	Stimulates synthesis of thyroid hormone
Follicle-stimulating hormone	FSH	Follitropin		Gonadotrope	Gonad	Stimulates follicular development in females and spermatogenesis in males
Luteinizing hormone	LH	Interstitial cell-stimulating hormone, lutropin	ICSH	Gonadotrope	Gonad	Stimulates estrogen and progesterone synthesis in females and androgen secretion in males

[a] The names in the first column and the abbreviations are used throughout the text.

functions of these hormones are discussed in the following chapter, and a listing of these hormones, alternate names for them, their targets and their general physiological roles are summarized in Table 4-1.

Cellular Types of the Adenohypophysis

Staining Procedures and Light Microscopy. A variety of cellular types can be distinguished in the pars distalis by utilizing special dyes in particular staining combinations. This differential uptake of dyes is due to the differential affinity of cytoplasmic granules for these dyes. Some cytoplasmic granules bind acidic dyes, and cells with these granules are termed *acidophilic cells* or *acidophils* (*philos* love). Other granules bind basic dyes and the cells containing these granules are termed *basophils*. Cells containing granules that may bind acidic and basic dyes are said to be *amphophilic*. A basophil in the pars distalis is defined as a cell that is stained by the aniline blue dye of the Mallory trichrome staining method. However, since aniline blue is in reality an acidic dye, some investigators have preferred to use the term *cyanophil* (*cyanos* blue) to designate these cells. The endocrine literature is filled with the term basophil, so use of this term continues, although it is recognized to be technically inappropriate. Cells that do not contain stainable cytoplasmic granules are called *chromophobes*. Various types of basophils or acidophils may be distinguished from one another in terms of their specific affinities for other dyes. Some cells contain granules that stain with the periodic acid-Schiff(PAS) method for staining glycoproteins and mucopolysaccharides. Such cells are termed PAS(+). A listing of dyes and associated terms is found in Table 4-2. A unified scheme for nomenclature of the hormone-secreting cells of the adenohypophysis is summarized in Table 4-3.

Cellular Types in the Pars Distalis. Generally speaking there is one cellular type responsible for synthesis and release of each tropic hormone. Only two strongly basophilic cells are found, however, and they are responsible for secretion of three glycoprotein hormones: TSH, LH and FSH. The traditional mammalian designation for these various cellular types is given with the corresponding generalized vertebrate cellular type indicated within the parentheses. The PAS(+) *beta basophil* (type 1 basophil) that secretes TSH can be distinguished from the gonadotropic PAS(+) *delta basophil* (type 2 basophil) by the affinity of the former for aldehyde fuchsin (AF[+]). It has not been possible to differentiate between LH- and FSH-secreting gonadotropes on the basis of stainability for light microscopy or with the aid of the electron microscope (Table 4-4). In the past, immunological tests have not been able to distinguish separate cellular types, and it may be that both mammalian GTHs are produced by the same cell. Recent studies employing sensitive microscopic and immunocytochemical procedures suggest there may be separate cellular sources for gonadotropins in tetrapods.[142] However, throughout this book the source for gonadotropic hor-

Table 4-2. *Some of the Dyes Used in Cytological Observation of Adenohypophysial Cells and Their Abbreviations*

Dye or staining procedure	Abbreviation	Chemical specificity (if known)
1. Aldehyde fuchsin	AF	—
2. Alcian blue	AB	Disulfide bonds, mucopolysaccharides
3. Periodic acid-schiff	PAS	Glycoproteins, mucopolysaccharides
4. Orange G	OG	—
5. Azocarmine	AZ	—
6. Lead hematoxylin	PbH	—
7. Iron hematoxylin	FeH	—

TABLE 4-3. *Simplified Scheme for Naming Certain Cellular Types in the Vertebrate Pars Distalis*

STAINABLE CELLULAR TYPE	STAINING CHARACTERISTICS	TROPIC HORMONE PRODUCED
Type 1 basophil	PAS[a](+) AB[b](+) AF[c](+)	Thyrotropin (TSH)
Type 2 basophil	PAS(+) AB(+); some OG[d](+) cytoplasmic granules	Gonadotropin (FSH, LH)
Type 3 basophil	May be basophilic or almost chromophobic; often PbH[e](+)	Corticotropin (ACTH)
Type 1 acidophil	Azocarmine (+), erythrosine (+)	Prolactin (PRL)
Type 2 acidophil	OG(+)	Growth hormone (GH)

[a] Periodic acid-Schiff.
[b] Alcian blue.
[c] Aldehyde fuchsin.
[d] Orange G.
[e] Lead hematoxylin.

mones will be referred to as the type 2 basophil.

Two cells staining with acidic dyes have been found to be sources for GH and PRL respectively (Fig. 4-5). The *alpha acidophil* stains with orange G (orangeophilic) and is the source of GH in mammals. The *epsilon acidophil* exhibits a strong affinity for azocarmine (carminophilic) and secretes PRL. The PRL-secreting epsilon acidophil (type 1 acidophil) is called a lactotrope. The alpha acidophil (type 2 acidophil) is known as a somatotrope.

Corticotropin-secreting cells have proved especially difficult to identify, partly because of their similarity to other cellular types and the chemical similarity of ACTH to other pituitary hormones, MSH and LPH (see Chap. 5). Corticotropes are considered to be intermediate between chromophobes and basophils for they stain very weakly PAS(+) and AF(+). Corticotropes may be termed *type 3 basophils*. They have been identified at the light microscope level by means of immunofluorescent techniques coupled with adrenalectomy and administration of corticosteroids. Corticotropes are polyhedral with occasional long cytoplasmic processes. In many cytological respects, corticotropes are like thyrotropes. Both cells are PAS(+) and AF(+) and frequently respond to the same experimental manipulations. Furthermore, TSH and ACTH activities have been associated with the same size of

TABLE 4-4. *Some Light and Electron Microscopic Features of Cellular Types in the Mammalian Par Distalis*

CELLULAR TYPE	TROPIC HORMONE SECRETED	STAINABILITY[a] FOR LIGHT MICROSCOPE	IN SITU GRANULE SIZE (nm)	ISOLATED GRANULE SIZE[b] (nm)
Beta basophil	TSH	PAS (+), AF(+)	150	140
Delta basophil	FSH, LH	PAS(+), AF(−)	200	200
Corticotrope	ACTH	weakly PAS(+), AF(+); maybe PbH(+)	200	35–150
Epsilon acidophil	PRL	azocarmine (+)	600–900	600
Alpha acidophil	GH	OG+	variable to 350	variable to 350

SOURCE: Data compiled from Baker,[2] Fawcett et al.,[29] Siperstein and Miller.[132]
[a] See Table 4-3 for explanation of abbreviations.
[b] Granules isolated from pituitary extracts with tropic hormone activity.

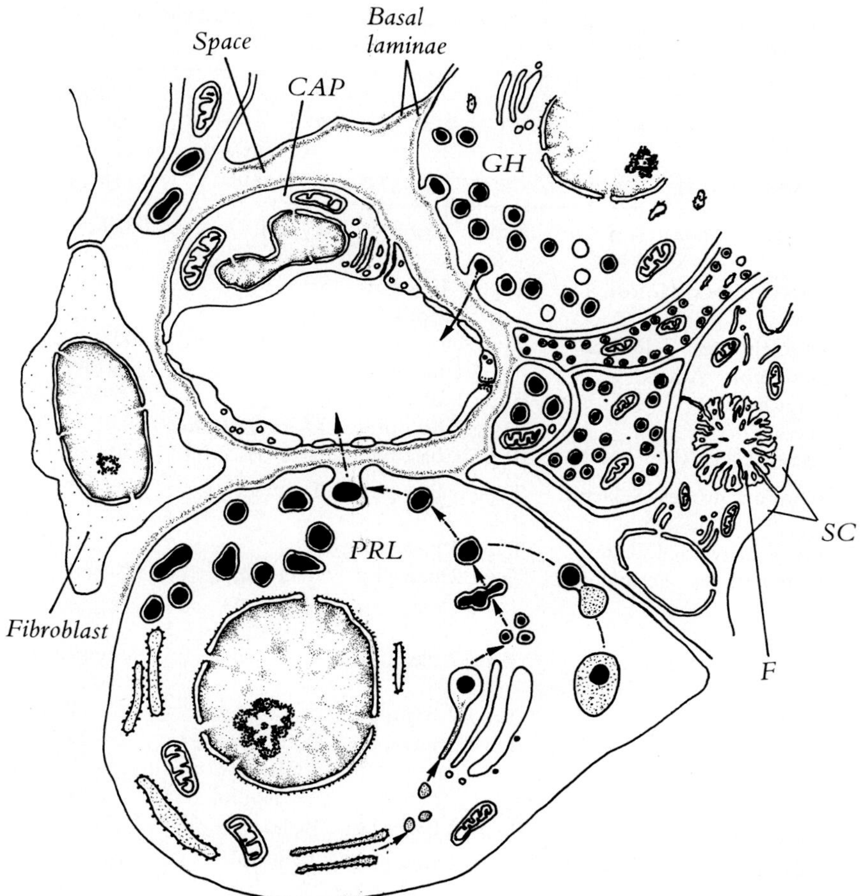

Fig. 4-5. Some cellular types characteristic of the mammalian adenohypophysis. Two tropic cells (growth hormone [*GH*] and prolactin [*PRL*]) border on a capillary *(CAP)*. Two follicular or stellate cells *(SC)* form an extracellular follicle *(F)* where they contact one another. Extensions of some other granular tropic cellular types are also shown. (After Baker.[4])

small granules (35–150 nm) extractable from the pars distalis. The type 3 basophil may also be the source of lipotropin.

The sixth cellular type in the mammalian pars distalis is the chromophobe. Chromophobes may represent inactive, depleted or undifferentiated cells, and they may differentiate into either basophils or acidophils, depending upon the experimental manipulations applied.[148] A special type of chromophobic cell, the *stellate* or *follicular* cell, has been observed in some mammals with the aid of the electron microscope. The processes of the stellate cell are very long and form a sort of network or reticulum between capillaries throughout the pars distalis. They are called follicular in some mammals because of the way these processes will sometimes surround or enclose small spaces or lumina (Fig. 4-5). These stellate cells may perform a supportive or nutritional function. They are probably not the source of any tropic hormones,[2] although some investigators have suggested them to be the source of ACTH. The term stellate cell, however, should not be applied to the ACTH-secreting cell.

The electron microscope has been used to characterize cellular types of the pars distalis on the basis of general cellular morphology and the size and shape of electron-dense cytoplasmic granules (Table 4-5). A combination of ultrastructural, tinctorial and immunofluores-

TABLE 4-5. *Comparative Cytology of the Pars Distalis from Representatives of Different Vertebrate Groups*

HORMONE[a]	VERTEBRATE GROUP	CELLULAR TYPE	ALTERNATE NAMES	ULTRASTRUCTURAL DETERMINATION OF CYTOPLASMIC GRANULE SIZE (nm)
TSH	Chondrichthyes: Selachii[b]	Type 1 basophil (?)	Type I	90–120
	Osteichthyes: Holostei[c]	Type 1 basophil (Amphophil)		–
	Osteichthyes: Teleostei[d]	Type 1 basophil	Delta basophil	400
	Amphibia: Anura[e]	Type 1 basophil		150–400
	Reptilia[f]	Type 1 basophil		300–400 × 200–250
	Aves[g]	Type 1 basophil	Delta basophil	50, 100, 200
	Mammalia[h]	Type 1 basophil	Beta basophil	150
GTH	Chondrichthyes: Selachii	Type 2 basophil (?)	Type V, VI	100–700
	Osteichthyes: Holostei	Type 2 basophil		
	Osteichthyes: Teleostei	Type 2 basophil	Beta and gamma basophils	60–160; 80–240
	Amphibia: Anura	Type 2 basophil		polymorphous to 900
	Reptilia	Type 2 basophil		150–270; 600–800
	Aves	Type 2 basophil	Beta basophil; Gamma basophil	120–200 120–400
	Mammalia	Type 2 basophil	Delta basophil	200
ACTH	Chondrichthyes: Selachii	Type 3 basophil (?)	Type II	140
	Osteichthyes: Holostei		Acidophil	–
	Osteichthyes: Teleostei	Type 3 basophil	Epsilon cell	110–250
	Amphibia: Anura	Type 3 basophil		100–200
	Reptilia	Type 3 basophil (Amphophil)		–
	Aves	Type 3 basophil	Epsilon cell	150–300
	Mammalia	Type 3 basophil		200
PRL	Chondrichthyes: Selachii	Type 1 acidophil (?)	Type IV	263
	Osteichthyes: Holostei	Type 1 acidophil		–
	Osteichthyes: Teleostei	Type 1 acidophil	Eta cell	polymorphic; 170–350
	Amphibia: Anura	Type 1 acidophil		180–500
	Reptilia	Type 1 acidophil		–
	Aves	Type 1 acidophil	Eta cell	polymorphic; 250–300
	Mammalia	Type 1 acidophil	Epsilon acidophil	polymorphic; 600–900

Table 4-5. *Comparative Cytology of the Pars Distalis from Representatives of Different Vertebrate Groups (Continued)*

HORMONE[a]	VERTEBRATE GROUP	CELLULAR TYPE	ALTERNATE NAMES	ULTRASTRUCTURAL DETERMINATION OF CYTOPLASMIC GRANULE SIZE (nm)
GH	Chondrichthyes: Selachii	Type 2 acidophil (?)	Type III (?)	200
	Osteichthyes: Holostei	Type 2 acidophil		–
	Osteichthyes: Teleostei	Type 2 acidophil	Alpha cell	–
	Amphibia: Anura	Type 2 acidophil		180–250
	Reptilia	Type 2 acidophil		310
	Aves	Type 2 acidophil	Alpha acidophil	250–300
	Mammalia	Type 2 acidophil	Alpha acidophil	350

[a] The cellular source for lipotropin is not known.
[b] *Sycliorhinus caniculus.*[69]
[c] *Amia calva.*[7]
[d] *Zoarces* sp.[103]
[e] *Rana temporaria.*[141]
[f] General summary from Holmes and Ball.[59]
[g] General summary based upon domestic duck and Japanese quail (Mikami et al.,[87] Tixier-Vidal and Follett.[136]).
[h] See Table 4-3.

cent techniques plus differential isolation and biological assay of granules leaves little doubt as to the origins of most of the tropic hormones. The source for LPH remains unresolved as well as whether one or two cellular types are responsible for production of GTHs (FSH and LH).

Cellular Types in the Pars Intermedia. One type of epithelial cell occurs in the pars intermedia. This MSH-secreting cell characteristically stains with the lead hematoxylin procedure (PbH). Corticotropin and LPH activities have been identified in the pars intermedia, but they appear to be present within the MSH-secreting cells.

Cellular Types in the Pars Tuberalis. Three cellular types have been identified in the primate pars tuberalis by means of light and electron microscopic techniques.[67] Type I stains with PAS and exhibits small cytoplasmic granules (170 nm diameter). Type II cells stain with the dye alcian blue (AB) and contain somewhat larger granules (350 nm). The remaining cellular type is described as having occasional granules. Cells reacting specifically to antibody to pituitary LH and FSH are believed to be gonadotropic cells and probably correspond to type I.[3] Thyroptropic cells that specifically bind antibody to TSH are thought to be the type II cells, although granule sizes are much larger than for pars distalis thyrotropes (Table 4-3). Occasionally, rare cells are observed that bind antibody to ACTH and GH, but PRL cells are absent. Gonadotropin-containing cells have also been found in the pars tuberalis of rats.[4] These data would suggest that the pars tuberalis may represent only a "fragment" of the pars distalis and that in some species it may function to secrete tropic hormones in response to either hypothalamic regulatory hormones or other substances in the portal blood or cerebrospinal fluid.[3,59]

The Neurohypophysis

The mammalian neurohypophysis consists of two distinct components. The *median eminence* is defined as the more anterior portion of the neurohypophysis that has a blood supply in common with the adenohypophysis, specifically the hypothalamo-hypophysial portal system. (Note that in some terminologies the median eminence is considered to be a subdivision of the hypothalamus.) An abundant but separate blood supply characterizes the *pars nervosa*, which is that portion of the neurohypophysis in contact with the pars intermedia. Both the median eminence and the pars nervosa are neurohemal structures composed of axonal tips of NS neurons originating in hypothalamic nuclei, capillaries and special cells known as *pituicytes*.

The function of pituicytes is unknown, but they could play a role as supportive elements or may be involved actively in storage and release of neurohormones from the neurohypophysis. Pituicytes are thought to be derived from ependymal or glial cells. Ependymal cells are specialized neural cells that line the ventricles of the brain and the central canal of the spinal cord as well as form an outer protective layer around the brain and spinal cord. Glial cells are sometimes called the connective tissue of the nervous system although they may play a nutritive or some other role with respect to the neurons. There is some evidence that might suggest an influence of ependymal cells on tropic hormone release,[59] but more work must be done in this area before a definitive role can be established.

The Mammalian Hypothalamus

The hypothalamus contains many NS nuclei that produce neurohormones. The neurohormones associated with the median eminence and adenohypophysis are termed *hypothalamic hypophysiotropic hormones* and are identified as either *releasing hormones*, or *release-inhibiting hormones*, depending on whether they stimulate or inhibit tropic hormone release from the adenohypophysis (Table 4-6). These regulating hormones are mostly small peptides, although at least one has been found to be an amine derived from an amino acid.

The neurohormones associated with the pars nervosa are all of very similar structure. Each is an *octapeptide neurohormone* consisting of nine amino acid residues. The use of "octa" has come about because the two cysteine residues form a disulfide bridge to become a single amino acid, cystine. Formation of the disulfide bond results in the characteristic five amino acid-ring structure with a side chain of three amino acids. The mammalian octapeptide hormones, oxytocin and vasopressin, are discussed in Chapter 7.

The region of the mammalian hypothalamus that controls hypophysial function consists primarily of the mediobasal hypothalamus containing a number of bilaterally paired NS nuclei, including the *anterior hypothalamic, suprachiasmatic, ventromedial, dorsomedial, posterior hypothalamic* and *arcuate* nuclei (Fig. 4-6). These nuclei are responsible for producing the hypothalamic hypophysiotropic neurohormones that regulate release of tropic hormones from the hypophysis. In addition there are two adjacent, bilaterally

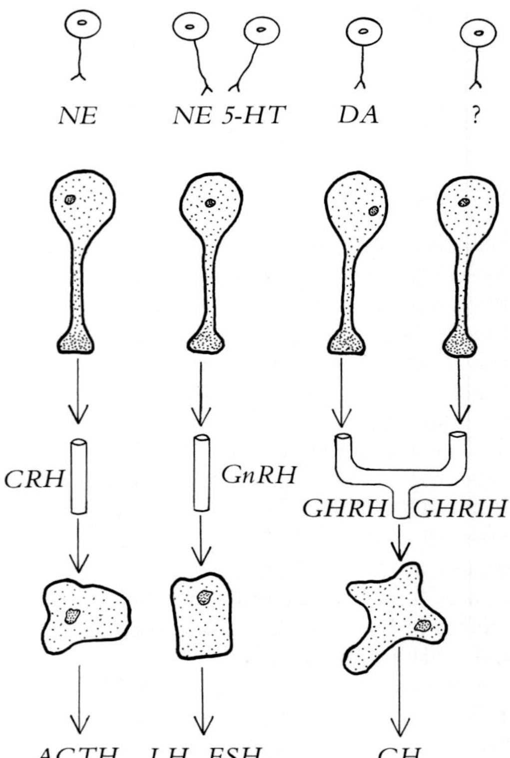

FIG. 4-6. Representation of relationships between the nervous system, hypothalamic neurosecretory neurons and release of tropic hormones. Ordinary neurons *(top row)* release neurotransmitters that influence release of hypophysiotropic hormones from the neurosecretory cells *(second row)* into the portal vessels. Arrival of the hypophysiotropic hormones at the secretory cells of pars distalis *(bottom row)* influences release of tropic hormones into the general circulation. *NE*, norepinephrine; *DA*, dopamine; *5-HT*, serotonin; See Table 4-6 for explanation of other abbreviations.

TABLE 4-6. *Confirmed and Proposed Mammalian Hypothalamic Hypophysiotropic Hormones*

NAME	ABBREVIATION	ALTERNATE ABBREVIATION	CHEMICAL STRUCTURE
Thyrotropin-releasing hormone	TRH	TSHRH, TRF	(Pyro)-Glu-His-Pro-NH_2
Gonadotropin-releasing hormone	GnRH	LRH, LHRH,	(Pyro)-Glu-His-Trp-Ser-Tyr-Gly-Leu-Arg-Pro-Gly-NH_2
Somatostatin	GHRIH	GRIH, STHRIH	Ala-Gly-Cys-Lys-Asn-Phe-Phe-Trp-Lys-Thr-Phe-Thr-Ser-Cys (S—S bridge between Cys residues)
Growth hormone-releasing hormone	GHRH	GRH, GRF	Peptide, possibly 40 amino acids
Prolactin release-inhibiting hormone (dopamine)	PRIH	PIF	Dopamine
Prolactin-releasing hormone	PRH	PRF	Same as TRH?
Corticotropin-releasing hormone	CRH	ACTHRH, CRF	Peptide, 41 amino acids
Melanotropin release-inhibiting hormone[a]	MSHRIH	MRIH, MIF	Cys-Tyr-Ile-Gln-Asn-Cys-OH (S—S bridge between Cys residues)
	MSHRIH	MRIH, MIF	Pro-Leu-Gly-NH_2
	MSHRIH	MRIH, MIF	Pro-His-Phe-Arg-Gly-NH_2
	MSHRIH	MRIH, MIF	Dopamine
	MSHRH	MRH, MRF	Cys-Tyr-Ile-Gln-Asn-OH (SH on Cys)

Data from Hadley and Hruby,[51] Saffran,[120] Schalley et al. [127], Rivier et al., [117] Vale et al.[138]
[a]Dopamine is most likely MSHRIH; others may be fragments of neurohypophysial octapeptides.

paired nuclei responsible for production of the octapeptide neurohormones of the pars nervosa. These are the *supraoptic* nuclei and, immediately posterior, the dorsoanteriorly located *paraventricular* nuclei.

Much of our knowledge about these hypothalamic centers has been accumulated from observing the effects of particular hypothalamic lesions or of localized electrical stimulation in the hypothalamus and adjacent regions or from studies involving implants of crystalline hormones into the hypothalamus (related to negative feedback effects). Some cautions of interpretation from such studies are in order, however. The use of disruptive lesions, for example, requires careful bilateral placement of comparable lesions and leaves some uncertainty as to exactly what was destroyed by the lesions. Alterations in pituitary function following placement of lesions might involve destruction of the NS neurons that elaborate a given hypothalamic hypophysiotropic hormone or may only disrupt a NS tract. The lesion might have damaged non-NS neurons that would normally modulate the activity of these NS neurons. Damage to vascular elements of the median eminence might also alter tropic hormone release patterns. Ideally, secretion of all tropic hormones should be monitored following placement of a particular lesion, yet, for practical reasons, this is rarely done. Usually only one or, at most, two tropic hormone systems are examined (such as, TSH or GTH), whereas others (PRL, ACTH and GH) are ignored.

In spite of such drawbacks the use of combinations of these approaches has helped establish the general localization of different NS centers.[59,91] The thyrotropic center appears to be located anteriorly behind and dorsal to the optic chiasma (anterior hypothalamic and suprachiasmatic nuclei). Gonadotropic centers are located more posteriorly (mediobasal hypothalamus), and, in particular, the ventromedial nuclei appear to be responsible for controlling ovulation in some species. Corticotropin release is influenced most strongly by experimental alterations associated with the ventroanterior and ventromedial portions of the hypothalamic hypophysiotropic area. Release of GH appears to be localized in the ventral hypothalamic hypophysiotropic area, and the hypothalamic center for regulating PRL release seems to be located somewhere posterior to the optic chiasma in the ventral portion of the hypothalamic hypophysiotropic area.

Hypothalamic Hypophysiotropic (Regulating) Hormones

Numerous studies have confirmed that the hypothalamus exerts a direct influence over functioning of the adenohypophysis. Observations indicate the absence of neural connections between the hypothalamus and the adenohypophysis but the presence of the hypothalamo-hypophysial portal system led to the establishment of what is now termed the *neurovascular hypothesis.* Severing the portal connections or transplanting the pituitary to some avascular site elsewhere in the body (an *ectopic* transplant) causes marked changes in the secretory pattern of the tropic hormones (Table 4-7). Generally such operations are followed by a marked reduction in circulating levels of TSH, FSH, LH, GH and ACTH,

TABLE 4-7. *Some Evidence for Negative Hypothalamic Control of MSH Release*

1. Removal of pituitary from hypothalamic control decreases MSH content of pituitary by
   a. transplanting gland to ectopic site
   b. section of the pituitary stalk
   c. producing appropriately placed lesions in the hypothalamus
2. Injection of hypothalamic extracts from frogs and several mammals results in increased pituitary MSH content.
3. Addition of rat hypothalamic extracts to pituitaries cultured in vitro reduces the MSH content of the tissue culture medium.
4. Injection of purified bovine hypothalamic extracts reduces plasma MSH levels.
5. Injection of hypothalamic extracts into frogs darkened as a result of hypothalectomy results in lightening of the frogs.
6. Weasels with pituitary autografts grow brown pelage under conditions in which only white pelage would normally be produced.

Modified from Kastin, A.J. et al.[65]

whereas PRL and MSH levels increase. These data led to the interpretation that release of the first group of tropic hormones is under stimulatory hypothalamic control (releasing hormones) and that MSH and PRL release is under inhibitory control. If the severed blood vessels of the hypothalamo-hypophysial portal system are allowed to regenerate so that blood may again flow from the median eminence to the adenohypophysis, the normal secretory patterns for the tropic hormones resume. These latter observations support strongly the neurovascular hypothesis of hypothalamic control over tropic hormone release.

In recent years as many as nine different hypothalamic regulatory hormones have been proposed. The chemical identities are established for most of these regulatory hormones. (Andrew Schally and Roger Guillemin shared a Nobel Prize for their initial isolation and characterization of TRH and GnRH, respectively.) The others are frequently referred to as factors rather than as hormones. In this text a unified terminology is used for simplicity. Each regulatory hormone is named for the tropic hormone it influences and is designated according to whether it causes release (R) or is release inhibiting (RI). Thus the neurohormone that stimulates release of thyrotropin is termed TRH (thyrotropin-releasing hormone). Similarly the single neurohormone believed to cause release of both FSH and LH is termed the gonadotropin-releasing hormone (GnRH). Prolactin release is inhibited by PRIH (prolactin release-inhibiting hormone).

Thyrotropin-releasing Hormone. The first hypothalamic regulatory hormone that was identified chemically was the tripeptide TRH. It is found in the hypothalamus, appears in the hypophysial blood following electrical stimulation of the hypothalamus and causes release of TSH in vivo and in vitro.[116] It appears that this tripeptide is the endogenous hypothalamic hypophysiotropic TRH in mammals.

Extrahypothalamic TRH is present in the brain as well as in the spinal cord, the pineal gland and the neurohypophysis (Table 4-8). The common occurrence of TRH outside the hypothalamus and its presence in extrahypothalamic regions of the nervous system of mammals, nonmammalian vertebrates and even invertebrates has led to the suggestion that TRH may also function as a neurotransmitter. It has been demonstrated that administration of synthetic TRH causes depression of firing in certain neurons.[147]

The biological half-life for TRH in peripheral blood is very short (for example, 2 minutes in mice[12]) apparently because peptidases in the blood rapidly inactivate TRH. Consequently it is very difficult to measure endogenous levels of circulating TRH in peripheral blood even with radioimmunoassay.

Gonadotropin-releasing Hormone. Endogenous GnRH is a decapeptide originating in the arcuate and ventromedial NS nuclei of the hypothalamus. Apparently GnRH causes release of both GTHs, FSH and LH, from the adenohypophysis, although a greater amount of LH release is always observed following

Table 4-8. *Concentrations of Gonadotropin-Releasing Hormone and Thyrotropin-Releasing Hormone in the Hypothalamus and Extrahypothalamic Tissues of Male and Female Rats*

	GnRH (ng/g wet weight)		TRH (ng/wet weight)	
LOCATION	MALE	FEMALE	MALE	FEMALE
Hypothalamus	205	112	116	63
Pituitary	167	178	16	20
Midbrain	84	11	9.5	4.2
Cerebellum	32	9	4.7	0.87
Brain stem	6.8	14.3	1.8	3.1
Cerebral cortex	6.4	2.7	2.9	1.2

Modified from Wilber et al.[147]

administration of synthetic GnRH. It is the marked effect of this regulatory hormone on LH release and subsequent induction of ovulation that accounts for its originally being named an LH-releasing hormone (LHRH or LRH). Although there is evidence for a separate FSHRH,[88,130] it is generally accepted that endogenous GnRH causes release of both gonadotropins. Since GnRH was first synthesized, approximately 1400 analogues have been created, ranging from stimulatory to inhibitory on gonadotropin release.

Like TRH, GnRH has been identified immunologically in extrahypothalamic nervous tissue and in the pineal gland of some species.[146] Similarly, GnRH, like TRH, can cause depression of neural function in the central nervous system.[147] Thus GnRH may have a role as a neurotransmitter in addition to its involvement with gonadotropin release.

Gonadotropin-releasing hormone is rapidly degraded in peripheral plasma, and the success of several potent synthetic analogues appears to be related to their relative resistance to degradation. One superreleaser has approximately 150 times the activity of the native GnRH.[49]

Growth Hormone-releasing and Release-inhibiting Hormones. The release of GH by the hypothalamus is under both inhibitory (GHRIH) and stimulatory (GHRH) control. Also known as *somatostatin,* GHRIH is a very strong inhibitor of GH release.[50] Somatostatin also blocks the action of synthetic TRH on TSH release from the adenohypophysis. It is a tetradecapeptide (Table 4-6).

Somatostatin occurs in extrahypothalamic nervous tissue (both brain and spinal cord), and a possible neurotransmitter function has been suggested similar to that for TRH and GnRH.[147] It is also present in the mucosa of the stomach and has been shown to inhibit release of the gastric hormone, gastrin (see Chap. 14). In addition, somatostatin is present in the pancreatic islets where it appears to be involved in the inhibition of both glucagon and insulin release (see Chap. 13).

The importance of stimulatory control over GH release is emphasized by the reduction in GH release following disruption of the portal vessels. There is evidence for the existence of hypothalamic GHRH associated with the ventromedial nucleus of the hypothalamus.[39] It is possible that direct neural control of GH release occurs and may account for the stimulatory actions of various physiological stresses on increasing GH release. A potent releaser of GH has been isolated from a human pancreatic tumor.[117] This peptide (40 amino acid residues) is related chemically to the glucagon family of peptides (see Chap. 14).

Prolactin-releasing and Release-inhibiting Hormones. The primary control over prolactin release, as mentioned earlier, is inhibitory in mammals. The mammalian PRIH appears to be dopamine released from hypothalamic neurons into the hypothalamo-hypophysial portal system. The inhibitory nature of hypothalamic control is evidenced by enhanced release of PRL following certain hypothalamic lesions, separation of the adenohypophysis from the hypothalamus by insertion of a physical barrier to blood flow or transplantation of the adenohypophysis to an ectopic site.

There is evidence for an endogenous factor that stimulates PRL release. This PRL-releasing hormone (PRH) may be the tripeptide already known as TRH since administration of synthetic TRH stimulates PRL release as well as TSH release.[116] This action of TRH on PRL secretion is not influenced by somatostatin.[49] It is not clear whether endogenous TRH has any physiologically important influence over PRL secretion since its effects would normally be counteracted by the presence of PRIH. Furthermore, the occurrence of enhanced PRL release in vitro in the absence of any hypothalamic factors tends to argue against any endogenous PRH. It remains to be demonstrated that factors which evoke TRH release with ensuing release of TSH are accompanied by increases in PRL release without a change in PRIH levels.

Corticotropin-releasing Hormone. The amino acid sequence of CRH has been determined, and synthetic CRH is now available.[137] It is a peptide of 41 amino acid residues and releases ACTH from the corticotrope. There is considerable homology (at 20 positions) to sauvagine, a 40-residue peptide isolated from skin of the frog, *Phylomedusa sauvagii.* There is also overlap with the structure of a hypotensive agent, urotensin I, isolated from teleosts (see Chap. 16).

Melanophore-stimulating Hormone Release-inhibiting Hormone. Experimental studies similar to those described for PRL established that hypothalamic control of MSH release from the pars intermedia was primarily inhibitory. It is not clear whether MSH release is controlled by a neurohormone or by direct innervation. Several peptides have been shown to possess intrinsic MSHRIH activity (Table 4-6), but the exact chemical identity of the endogenous neurohormone is not known. Extrahypothalamic MSHRIH activity has been demonstrated, and at least one of the synthetic releasers of MSH is an antidepressant when administered to humans.[116] Numerous investigators believe that dopamine released into blood traveling to the pars intermedia is MSHRIH.

Role of Cyclic Nucleotides

Hypothalamic hypophysiotropic hormones produce several initial changes in adenohypophysial cells prior to release of tropic hormones. One such effect is an increase in the permeability of the membrane to calcium ions, causing an influx of these ions. The role of calcium ions is essential to tropic hormone release, and release does not occur in calcium-free medium in vitro. The specific involvement of calcium has not been settled but it appears to be necessary for the action of cyclic adenosine 3′,5′-monophosphate (cAMP). Most of the hypothalamic regulating hormones have been shown to activate adenyl cyclase in the cell membrane, which causes an increase in cAMP production. Cyclic AMP operates through a cAMP-dependent protein kinase to effect hormone release. (The adenyl cyclase-protein kinase mechanism is described in Chapter 1.)

Control of Hypothalamic Hypophysiotropic Hormone Release

Release of hypothalamic regulatory hormones is influenced by neural activity.[21] A variety of neurotransmitters (for example, dopamine, norepinephrine, serotonin) and drugs that selectively block neuronal function (such as reserpine, which blocks adrenergic neurons by depleting them of neurotransmitters) affect tropic hormone release. The same agent may stimulate release of one tropic hormone and inhibit release of another. Presumably these neuronal agents influence release of the hypothalamic hypophysiotropic hormones (Fig. 4-7).

Many pharmacological studies of nervous regulation over hypothalamic NS centers have been conducted employing different neurotransmitters or drugs that either mimic or block the activity of various known neurotransmitters (Tables 4-9, 4-10). Studies of this type have led to identification of the kinds of neurons that regulate release of individual hypothalamo-hypophysiotropic hormones. For example, application of dopamine to cultured pituitary cells with and without cocultured hypothalamic tissue has made it possible to distinguish between the indirect stimulatory

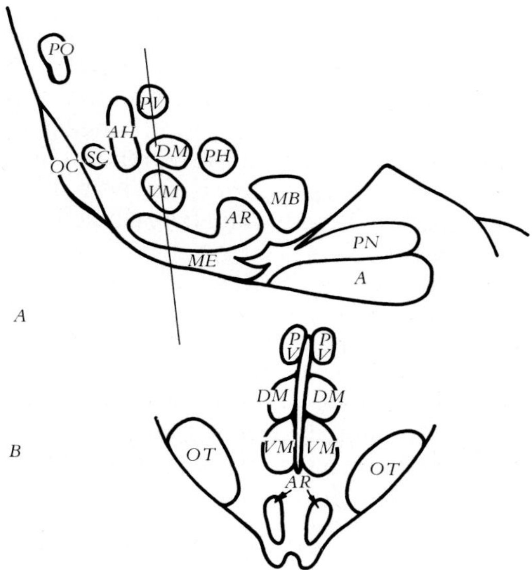

Fig. 4-7. The hypophysiotropic centers of the hypothalamus. (Modified from D'Angelo.)
A. Sagittal section of hypothalamus showing locations of various neurosecretory nuclei in relation to the anterior optic chiasm *(OC)* and the posteriorly located mammillary body *(MB)* and pituitary gland. *A,* adenohypophysis; *PN,* pars nervosa; *ME,* median eminence.
B. Cross-section of the hypothalamus at the level indicated by the line through *A.* The more lateral optic tracts *(OT)* are visible in cross-section.
Hypophysiotropic nuclei: *AH,* anterior hypothalamic nucleus; *AR,* arcuate nucleus; *DM,* dorsomedial nucleus; *PH,* posterior hypothalamic nucleus; *PO,* preoptic area; *PV,* paraventricular nucleus; *SC,* suprachiasmatic nucleus; *VM,* ventromedial nucleus.

TABLE 4-9. *Action of Some Neurotransmitters on Tropic Hormone Release Primarily through Effects on Release of Hypothalamic Neurohormones*

NEUROTRANSMITTER	STIMULATORY	INHIBITORY	NO EFFECT
Dopamine	TSH ?	MSH[a]	
		PRL[a]	
		TSH ?	
Serotonin	ACTH	TSH	
	LH		
	PRL		
	GH[b]		
Norepinephrine	GH	ACTH	
	LH		
	TSH		
Acetylcholine	ACTH		TSH
	LH		

[a] May be direct actions on pituitary cells.
[b] Sleep-induced increase in GH.

activity of dopamine on LH release and its inhibitory action on PRL release. Utilization of catecholamines and related drugs has also contributed much to the understanding of neuronal regulation of hormone release. Norepinephrine and epinephrine may both influence release of hypothalamo-hypophysiotropic hormones.

The response of NS cells to specific neurotransmitters is determined by the presence of receptors for these substances on the cell membranes of the NS neurons. The inhibitory action of dopamine on PRL release mentioned above is accomplished through the binding of dopamine to receptors in the plasmalemma of the PRL-secreting cells. The ergot alkaloids such as ergocornine and ergocryptine can mimic the action of dopamine by binding to another receptor on the PRL cell membrane termed an alpha receptor.[105] Stimulation of this receptor might ordinarily evoke PRL release, but the use of these alpha receptor-blocking drugs (alpha blockers) can completely inhibit hormone release. (A discussion of alpha and beta receptors and their relationships to norepinephrine, epinephrine and various pharmacological agents can be found in Appendix II.)

Oxytocin and vasopressin, two of the octapeptide neurohormones associated with the

TABLE 4-10. *Effects of Some Anesthetics on Tropic Hormone Release*

ANESTHETIC	STIMULATORY	INHIBITORY	NO EFFECT
Ether	LH		
	FSH		
	PRL		
Pentobarbitol		LH	
		PRL	
Pentobarbitone		PRL	
Urethane			PRL
Chloral hydrate		PRL	
Ketamine		PRL	

pars nervosa, as well as melatonin, a derivative of tryptophan secreted by the pineal gland, have been shown to alter tropic hormone release, probably at the hypothalamic level. These hormones may reach the hypothalamus either via the cerebrospinal fluid or through the general circulation following their release from the pars nervosa. It is also possible that neural fibers release octapeptide neurohormones in the vicinity of the median eminence and influence release of regulatory hormones into the portal vessels. Most of the supportive data for the action of octapeptide neurohormones and melatonin on tropic hormone release are based on studies applying large doses, and it may not be justified to extend such data to in-vivo control mechanisms. Another interesting observation is that two of the peptides indicated in Table 4-6 that have MSHRIH activities are fragments of one of the neurohypophysial octapeptides, oxytocin. Furthermore, melatonin is structurally very similar to the neurotransmitter serotonin, an intermediate in the synthesis of melatonin from tryptophan. This structural similarity may account in part for some of its purported activities on hypothalamic neurons.

Other peptides have been identified in hypothalamic neurons, and some of these may influence tropic hormone release, at least indirectly. Two peptides, known as *neurotensin* and *substance P*, are probably neurotransmitters and thus could indirectly affect release of the hypothalamo-hypophysiotropic hormones. A family of peptides that mimic morphine effects in the central nervous system are also present in the median eminence. They are known as the *endorphins* and *enkephalins* (see Chap. 5), and they appear to be capable of stimulating GH and PRL release due to presynaptic effects on dopaminergic neurons rather than direct actions on cells of the pars distalis. Enkephalins and endorphins are extractable from the adenohypophysis, too.

Feedback and Tropic Hormone Release

The release of adenohypophysial tropic hormones can be influenced through negative feedback at the hypothalamus or at the pituitary, as was discussed in Chapter 2. Thyroid hormones produced by the action of TSH on the thyroid gland can reduce circulating TSH by inhibiting release of either TRH or TSH or both through effects on the hypothalamus and the pituitary gland respectively (Fig. 4-8). Similarly, corticosteroids produced by the adrenal cortex and gonadal steroids from ovaries or testes inhibit release of ACTH and GTHs respectively through similar action. (Figs. 4-9, 4-10). Growth hormone release can be influenced by either circulating glucose or amino acid level in a similar negative feedback loop (Fig. 4-11). Circulating glucose and amino acid levels are in part determined by the actions of GH on its target cells. Negative feedback of PRL and MSH release does not seem to be necessary because of the strong inhibitory

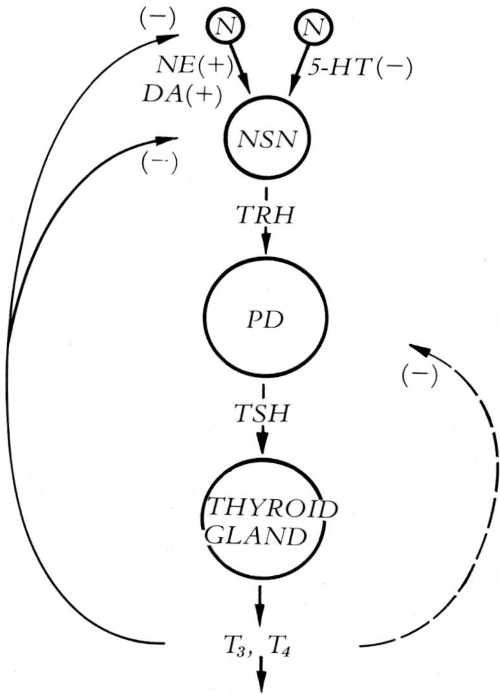

FIG. 4-8. The hypothalamo-hypophysial-thyroid axis. Ordinary neurons, *N;* neurosecretory neurons, *NSN;* pars distalis, *PD;* thyrotropin-releasing hormone, *TRH;* thyrotropin, *TSH;* thyroid hormones, T_3, T_4. For key to other abbreviations see Fig. 4-6. *Long arrows,* feedback loops. *Dotted arrows,* feedback directly on pituitary cells; (−) = inhibitory influences; (+) = stimulatory influences.

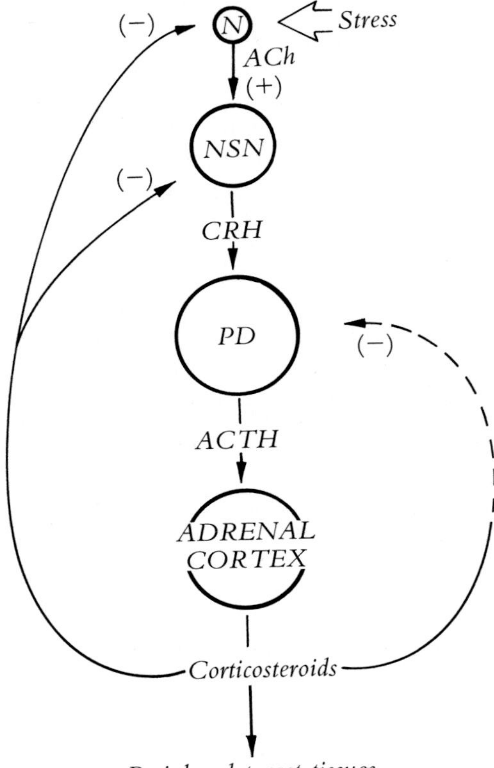

FIG. 4-9. The hypothalamo-hypophysial-adrenal axis. *ACh,* acetylcholine. For explanation and key to other abbreviations see Figs. 4-6, 4-7 and 4-8. See also Figs. 2-1, 2-3, 2-6 and 2-7.

influence of the hypothalamus over their release (Fig. 4-12).

In female mammals, gonadal steroids have differential effects on hypothalamic NS centers. There appears to be a "tonic center" for regulating gonadotropin release that is inhibited by either estrogens or progesterone and a "surge center" inhibited by progesterone but stimulated by estrogens (Fig. 4-9). Consequently the increase in estrogens produced by the growing follicles in the ovary causes a massive release (surge) of gonadotropin that triggers ovulation (see Chap. 11 for details). Estrogens have also been shown to stimulate release of PRL (Fig. 4-12), but it is not clear whether it inhibits dopamine release (PRIH) or whether it stimulates TRH release (PRH?).

The Hypothalamic Octapeptide Neurohormones

This second group of hypothalamic neurohormones, the so-called octapeptide hormones, are synthesized in the supraoptic and paraventricular hypothalamic nuclei. The octapeptides consist of nine amino acid residues, but two cysteine residues are joined by disulfide bonds, resulting in formation of cystine; hence, "octapeptide" rather than "nonapeptide." These hormones are stored in the pars nervosa until they are released into the general circulation. The targets for these hormones are located at considerable distances from the pars nervosa (for example, kidney, mammary gland, uterus).

Two neurohypophysial octapeptide hormones are present in the pars nervosa of most adult mammals. *Arginine vasopressin* (AVP) and *oxytocin* (OXY) are the common two octapeptide neurohormones. A variant of AVP

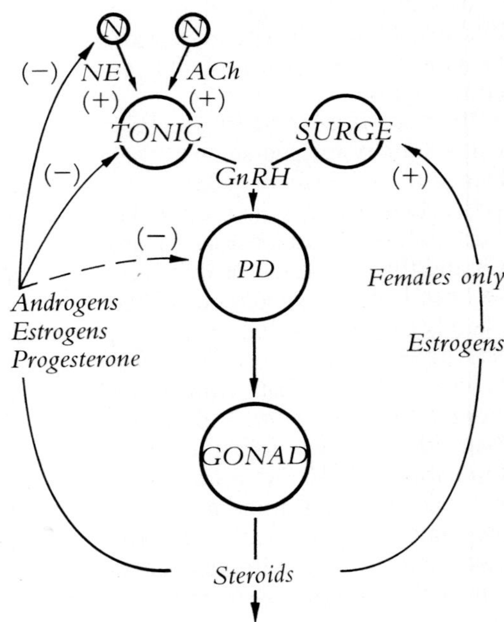

FIG. 4-10. The hypothalamo-hypophysial-gonadal axis. Both male and female mammals exhibit a tonic neurosecretory center controlling reproductive function, but females also exhibit a second neurosecretory center, the surge center, that is activated by estrogens. *ACh,* acetylcholine; *PD,* pars distalis. For explanation and key to other abbreviations see Figs. 4-6, 4-7 and 4-8.

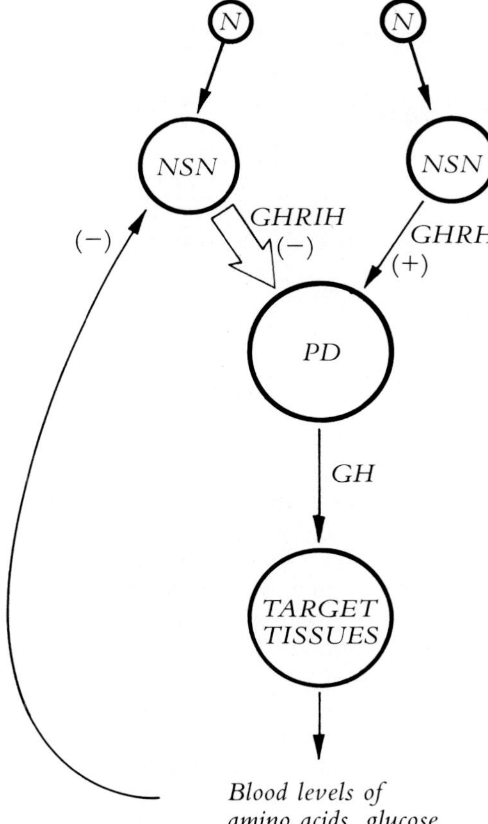

FIG. 4-11. Hypothalamic regulation of growth hormone secretion. The relative sizes of the two neurosecretory centers *(NSN)* reflect the relative importance of these dual control mechanisms. For explanation and key to other abbreviations see Figs. 4-6, 4-7 and 4-8.

known as *lysine vasopressin* (LVP) is produced by the Suina, which includes peccaries, domestic pigs and the hippopotamus. Most of the species in this group exhibit both AVP and LVP in addition to OXY (see Chap. 7 for details). A unique vasopressin-like molecule, *phenypressin,* has been isolated from the pars nervosa of marsupials.[20] Fetal mammals have been shown to produce what at first appears to be a hybrid of AVP and OXY, being composed of the side chain of AVP with the ring structure of OXY. This octapeptide is known as *arginine vasotocin* (AVT) and is characteristic of adult nonmammalian vertebrates (Table 4-11; see Chap. 7). The pineal gland of at least some adult mammals also contains AVT.

The vasopressins (AVP, LVP) function as antidiuretic agents affecting the ability of the kidneys to reabsorb water from the glomerular filtrate. At higher doses, vasopressins cause vasoconstriction and can elevate blood pressure (a pressor effect). This action may increase glomerular filtration and water excretion. Arginine vasotocin produces a similar type of action in nonmammals and has been suggested to play an osmoregulatory role in fetal mammals.[109]

Oxytocin stimulates contraction of uterine smooth muscle and contraction of the myoepithelial cells lining the ducts of the mammary glands. The action of OXY on the uterus is related to the induction of labor and the birth

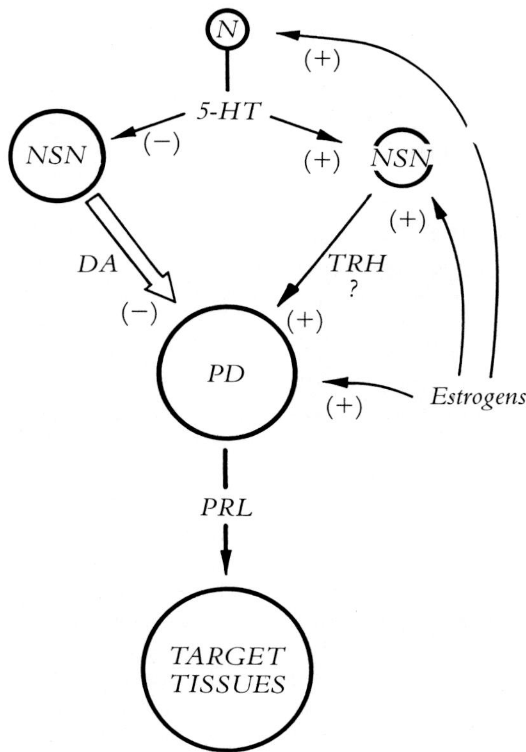

FIG. 4-12. Regulation of prolactin release. Dopamine *(DA)* is the prolactin release-inhibiting hormone. In addition, estrogens can stimulate prolactin *(PRL)* release directly or indirectly, possibly through thyrotropin-releasing hormone *(TRH).* No feedback loop is required since the inhibitory mechanism must be overridden to get release. For key to other abbreviations see Figs. 4-6 and 4-8.

TABLE 4-11. *Neurohypophysial Octapeptide Hormones in Vertebrates*[a]

OCTAPEPTIDE HORMONE	WHERE FOUND
Arginine vasotocin	Agnatha, Chondrichthyes, Osteichthyes, Amphibia, Reptilia, Aves
Glumitocin	Chondrichthyes: skates
Aspargtocin	Chondrichthyes: sharks
Valitocin	Chondrichthyes: sharks
Isotocin (ichthyotocin)	Osteichthyes: Actinopterygii
Mesotocin	Osteichthyes: Dipnoi; Amphibia, Reptilia, Aves, marsupials
Arginine vasopressin	Most mammals
Lysine vasopressin	Suiform mammals, marsupials
Phenypressin	Marsupials
Oxytocin	Mammalia (not marsupials)

[a]See Chapter 7 for details of amino acid sequences.

process. Ejection of milk from the mammary gland is caused by OXY released from the pars nervosa in response to suckling at the breast by the young.

A more detailed discussion of the roles of the octapeptide neurohormones can be found in Chapter 7.

Clinical Aspects of the Hypothalamo-Hypophysial System

The Hypothalamus

The most common clinical disorder of the hypothalamus is *diabetes insipidus*. The patient produces an abnormally large volume (3 to 8 liters/day) of dilute urine. This diuresis is due to the absence of AVP which normally controls water reabsorption in the kidney (see Chapter 7 for more details on the action of AVP). Forty to 50% of such patients are *idiopathic* (denoting a disease of unknown cause) and exhibit no other evidence of neuroendocrine dysfunction. Some individuals have been identified at autopsy as having degeneration of the supraoptic and paraventricular nuclei. About 15% of the cases are related to the presence of tumors within the brain which indirectly affect production of AVP. Physical damage (such as a lesion) or infections (e.g., encephalitis) account for the remainder. Nephrogenic diabetes insipidus is the result of a failure of the kidney tubules to respond to normal levels of AVP.

The syndrome of inappropriate antidiuresis (SIAD) is caused by excessive AVP release. High levels of AVP result in reduced urine production. Drugs such as demeclocycline block the action of AVP on the kidney and are used to treat this condition. Such drugs induce nephrogenic diabetes insipidus. Medications that control AVP release from the pars nervosa often are not uniformly effective.

Tumors within the central nervous system are responsible for a number of other disorders. One of the more dramatic consequences is precocity (accelerated sexual maturation; see Chapter 11 for a technical description of precocity). Precocity is much more common in males. About one-fourth of precocity cases are correlated with the presence of a pineal tumor, and 95% of these occur in males. A number of other cases are associated with hypothalamic tumors, most of which also are found in males. One type of tumor, associated with precocity, the *harmatoma*, occurs in the posterior hypothalamus. It consists of masses of partially disoriented glial and ganglion cells or of normal cells located in abnormal sites. Harmatomas may secrete GnRH which could explain their effects. Other causes for precocity are found in Chapter 11.

Several other pathologies have been identified including the following:

1. Hyponatremia: Low blood sodium may be correlated with a number of factors including brain carcinoma, basal skull fractures, meningitis and encephalitis.

2. Hypernatremia: Excessive levels of sodium may occur as a result of aneurysms in the brain, pineal tumors and so forth. This condition is not accompanied by fluid imbalance.

The Adenohypophysis

Acromegaly is a spectacular disorder of GH regulation leading to gigantism. This is a rare disorder affecting from 3 to 40 individuals per million people in the United States each year. Acromegaly was the first disorder of the pituitary gland to be recognized. It is caused by overproduction of GH due either to the absence of adequate somatostatin to suppress GH release or by the absence of negative feedback to suppress release. Growth hormone-secreting tumors release GH autonomously, but such tumors are uncommon. Approximately half of acromegalic patients are deficient in one or more additional pituitary hormones, usually the gonadotropins. Not only do such patients exhibit excessive growth, but body proportions become distorted. Cartilage tends to proliferate in joints resulting in abnormally proportioned hands and elongate jaws. There are also marked effects on other systems. For example, the skin exhibits excessive sweating and secretion of sebum, the heart is enlarged and hypertension may develop.

Pituitary *chromophobe adenomas* are the most common source of pituitary-related problems. (Any benign or noncarcinogenic glandular tumor can be termed an adenoma.) They rarely secrete any hormones (occasionally GH and seldom TSH or ACTH) and their effects are usually due to pressure on the brain or optic chiasm caused by growth of the adenoma. Most patients experience severe headaches and visual disturbances. Sometimes the production of one or more pituitary hormones may be reduced.

Partial or total *hypopituitarism* refers to selective or total absence of pituitary hormones. These defects may reside in the adenohypophysis itself (primary disorder) or be due to hypothalamic dysfunction (secondary disorder).

There has been considerable interest in the role(s) of endogenous opiates on mental disturbances such as depression and schizophrenia. Clinical studies have yielded mixed results and it is not clear whether mental illness is associated with endogenous opiates.

Comparative Aspects of the Hypothalamo-Hypophysial System in Nonmammalian Vertebrates

The Fishes

The piscine hypothalamo-hypophysial system is separable into the same major divisions as that of mammals: hypothalamus, neurohypophysis and adenohypophysis. Some marked differences occur as well. There is no pars tuberalis in fishes, although there is possibly a homologous structure in the elasmobranchs (Chondrichthyes). The pars distalis of the adenohypophysis, with the possible exception of the hagfishes (Agnatha), shares a common blood supply with the median eminence, the hypothalamo-hypophysial portal system. The pars distalis is differentiated into two subregions or zones. The pars intermedia is posterior to the par distalis and is intimately interdigitated with the pars nervosa of the neurohypophysis to form a *neurointermediate lobe*. This structure is characteristic of all but two groups of fishes, the hagfishes and the lungfishes (Dipnoi). Finally, posterior to the neurointermediate lobe in cartilaginous fishes and most bony fishes is a unique structure formed from the floor of the diencephalon. This structure is known as the *saccus vasculosus*. It is especially well developed in some groups, but its function is unknown.

Two different terminologies have been proposed for the subregions that are recognized in the piscine adenohypophysis. The nomenclature proposed by Green will be used in favor of the alternative system proposed by Pickford and Atz because the Green system is more similar to mammalian terminologies (Fig. 4-13).[48,112] There are three distinct zones recognized by both schemes. The most anterior and rostral (dorsal) portion of the piscine adenohypophysis typically consists of follicles and is termed the *rostral pars distalis* (proadenohypophysis). The remainder of the pars distalis comprises the *proximal pars distalis* (mesoadenohypophysis). The *pars intermedia*

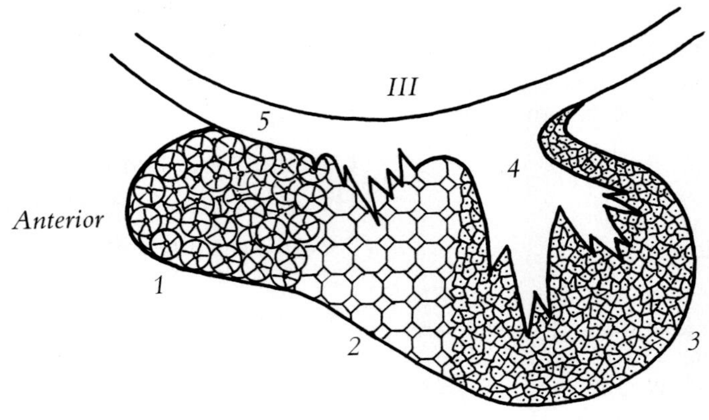

	Zone	Green (1951)	Pickford and Atz (1957)
Adeno hypophysis	1	*Rostral pars distalis*	*Proadenohypophysis*
	2	*Proximal pars distalis*	*Mesoadenohypophysis*
	3	*Pars intermedia*	*Metaadenohypophysis*
Neuro hypophysis	4	*Pars nervosa*	*Pars nervosa*
	5	*Median eminence*	*Median eminence*

Fig. 4-13. Terminology for designating regions of the piscine adenohypophysis. Comparison of Green's nomenclature with that of Pickford and Atz. Zones 3 and 4 are sometimes referred to as the neurointermediate lobe. The Green terminology is used throughout this textbook.

is termed the metaadenohypophysis according to the Pickford and Atz nomenclature. Each of these regions of the adenohypophysis is readily distinguished cytologically because each contains different types that produce different tropic hormones. The cellular types found in each region and the hormones they are thought to produce are discussed for each taxonomic grouping in the following sections.

Class Agnatha

Family Myxinoidea (Hagfishes). The Atlantic and Pacific hagfishes possess the most primitive hypothalamo-hypophysial system among the vertebrates (Fig. 4-14). Consequently it is lacking many of the features characteristic of other piscine groups. Futhermore, they are much more primitive than their living agnathan relatives, the lampreys (Petromyzontidae). There is a single NS center in the hagfish hypothalamus, the *preoptic nucleus*, located dorsal to the optic chiasm at the anterior end of the hypothalamus. This nucleus appears to produce NS product that is stored in the neurohypophysis.[94] There is no anterior neurohemal region in the Atlantic hagfish comparable to the median eminence, although a neurohemal area has been described for the Pacific hagfish and has been termed a median eminence.[30] There is no evidence, however, to support homology to the mammalian median eminence. The origin of the adenohypophysis of hagfishes appears to be from endoderm rather than from ectoderm.[47] If this observation proves to be correct, it represents an additional puzzle with respect to the origin of the pituitary. Furthermore, it raises the question of possible homology of the hagfish adenohypophysis to that of other vertebrates and supports the viewpoint that hagfishes are abberant vertebrates and are not on the mainline evolutionary pathway.

The hagfish adenohypophysis is not differentiated into subregions. It is composed primarily of chromophobic cells and rare PAS(+) basophils or an occasional acidophil. Electron micrographs of the hagfish adenohypophysis show rare granular cells with cytoplasmic granules of 100–200 nm diameter. These granular cells are believed to represent the two rare stainable cellular types identifiable with the light microscope. When hagfish adenohypophysial tissue is cultured in vitro, no observable changes take place in either granular or agranular cells.

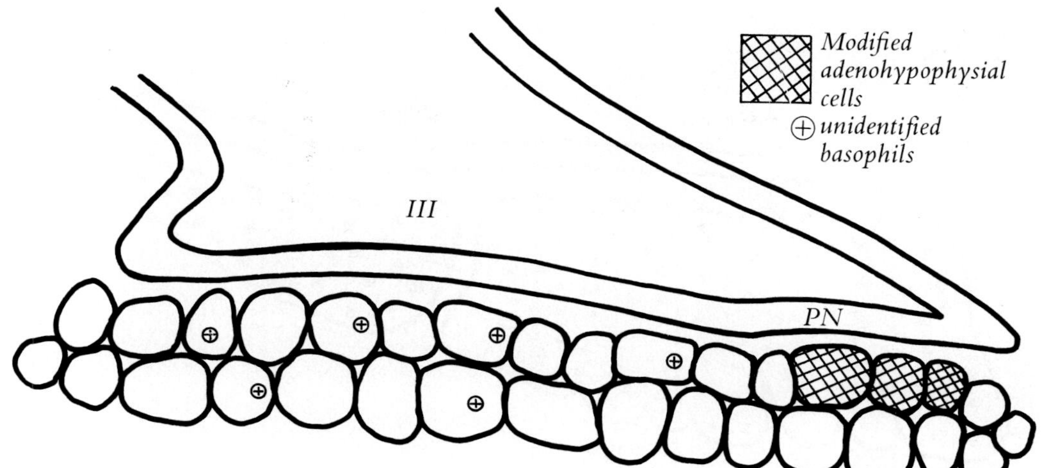

Fig. 4-14. The hagfish hypophysis (Agnatha: Cyclostomata: Myxinoidea). Midsagittal section of the pituitary of *Myxine* showing the distribution of a rare, unidentified basophilic cellular type and the occurrence of modified adenohypophysial cells posteriorly where the adenohypophysis makes contact with the brain. *III,* third ventricle; *PN,* pars nervosa. Anterior is to the left; dorsal, above.

Bioassays of hagfish pituitaries for PRL activity have proven negative,[92] and antiovine PRL antibody does not bind to hagfish adenohypophysial cells.[1] Furthermore, hypophysectomy of Pacific hagfish produces no convincing alterations in either thyroid or gonadal tissue.[84] Gonadotropin activity has been demonstrated in the pituitary of *Eptatretus burgeri,* a shallow water, seasonally breeding hagfish.[106]

Certain cells of the myxinoid adenohypophysis exhibit cytological modifications where they make contact with the neurohypophysis. These altered cells are termed *modified adenohypophysial tissue,* and it has been proposed that this apparent induction by neurohypophysial tissue may represent phylogenetically the origin of the pars intermedia.[30]

Family Petromyzontidae (Lampreys). In the lampreys three regions are distinguished in the adenohypophysis as they are in jawed fishes (Fig. 4-15). The more anterior rostral pars distalis is composed of basophils and chromophobes. These same cellular types as well as azocarmine(+) cells, carminophils, are found in the proximal pars distalis, which is located between the rostral pars distalis and the pars intermedia. Only one PbH(+) cell occurs in the pars intermedia. The tropic hormones associated with the adenohypophysis are discussed in Chapter 5.

The distinct pars nervosa and the pars intermedia form a well-developed neurointermediate lobe. Peptidergic neurons terminate in the pars nervosa where the single octapeptide neurohormone AVT is stored. The lamprey may possess a second neurohemal region associated with the pars distalis. Although this structure has been referred to as a median eminence,[64] this interpretation has not been accepted universally.[36]

Class Chondrichthyes

Selachii (Sharks, Rays, Skates). The selachian (elasmobranch) hypothalamo-hypophysial system possesses two features not found in agnathan fishes. The *pars ventralis* represents a fourth subdivision of the adenohypophysis that is unique to selachians (Fig. 4-16). This unique region is located ventral to the proximal pars distalis to which it is connected by a stalk. Some investigators have suggested that the pars ventralis is homologous to the pars tuberalis of the tetrapod adenohypophysis. Localization of GTH and TSH activity in the pars ventralis supports such a homology.[63,126] The proximal pars distalis also has been found to have GTH activity.[33] Prolactin activity and ACTH activity have been local-

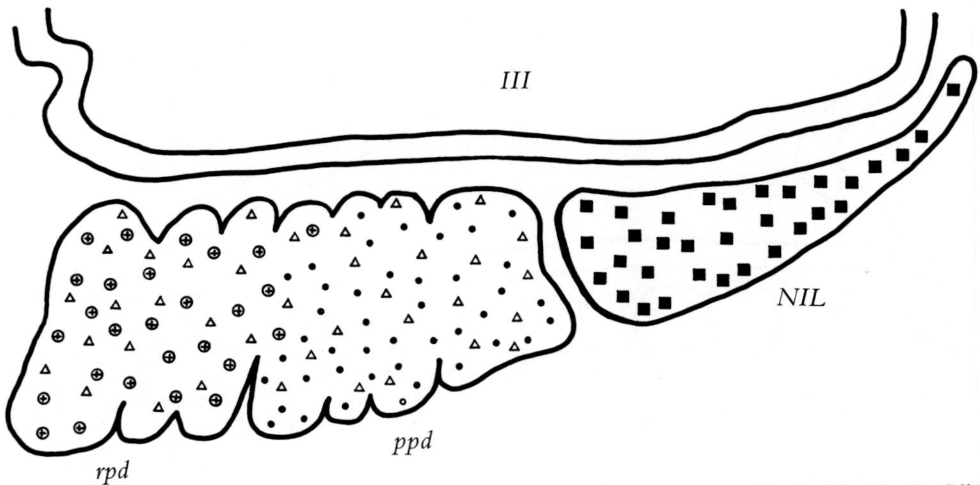

Fig. 4-15. The lamprey hypophysis (Agnatha: Cyclostomata: Petromyzontidae). Midsagittal section showing the differentiation of the adenohypophysis into rostral *(rpd)* and proximal *(ppd)* pars distalis as well as a distinct pars intermedia. The pars nervosa and pars intermedia form a neurointermediate lobe *(NIL)*. *III,* third ventricle. Cellular types on the figure are identified by the following symbols:

● = Gonadotropic basophils (GTH)
■ = MSH-secreting cells
△ = Unidentified acidophils
⊕ = Unidentified basophils

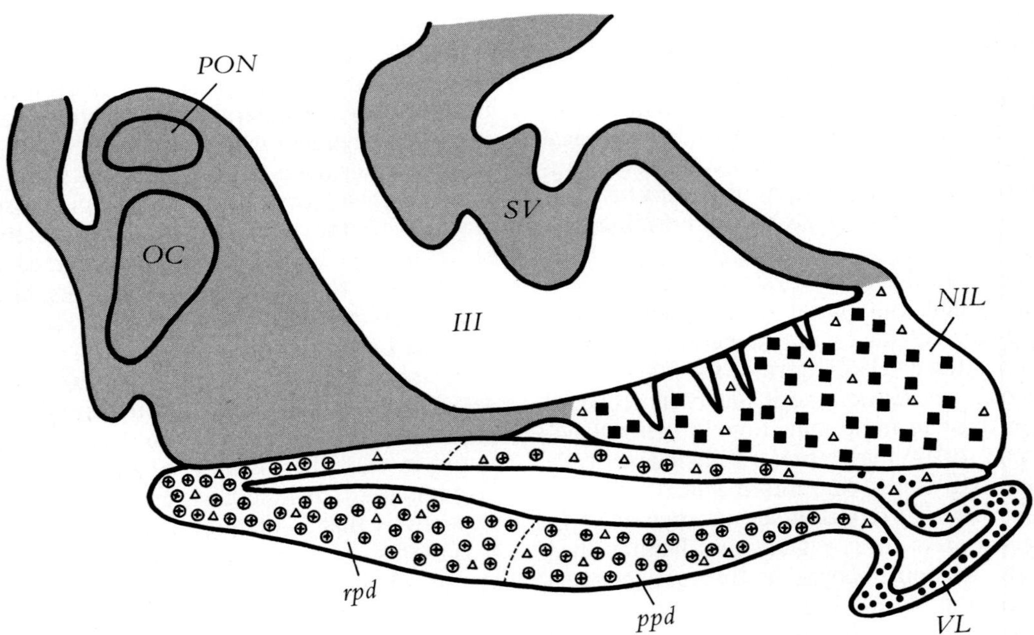

Fig. 4-16. The elasmobranch hypophysis (Chondrichthyes: Selachii). Note the prominent ventral lobe *(VL)* and the appearance of the saccus vasculosus *(SV)* in this midsagittal drawing. *PON,* preoptic nucleus; *OC,* optic chiasm; *III,* third ventricle; *NIL,* neurointermediate lobe; *rpd,* rostral pars distalis; *ppd,* proximal pars distalis.

Cellular types on the figure are identified by the following symbols:

● = Thyrotropic basophils (TSH)
• = Gonadotropic basophils (LH, FSH)
■ = MSH-secreting cells
△ = Unidentified acidophils
⊕ = Unidentified basophils

ized in the rostral pars distalis.[85,122] Growth hormone activity has been demonstrated in the proximal pars distalis.

Seven cellular types have been identified in the pars distalis of the shark *Scyliorhinus caniculus,* on the basis of ultrastructural criteria.[69] The rostral pars distalis possesses two cellular types believed to produce PRL and ACTH. Thyrotropes do not appear to be confined to any particular region of the pars distalis although most of the TSH activity demonstrated by bioassay resides in the ventral lobe. Possibly two types of gonadotrope have been identified in the proximal and ventral lobes respectively, but they may only be variants of a single cellular type. Somatotropic activity has been assigned to a single cellular type localized in the proximal pars distalis. A stellate chromophobe similar to the mammalian stellate cell is found throughout the pars distalis, and it may play a similar role to its mammalian counterpart.

The terms rostral and proximal may be somewhat misleading when applied to the selachian pars distalis because of the presence of the ventral lobe homologous to part of the proximal pars distalis of other fishes or possibly to the pars tuberalis of tetrapods. Consequently these regions are sometimes designated as the rostral, median and ventral lobes of the pars distalis.

The second feature appearing for the first time in selachians is the *saccus vasculosus* derived from the hypothalamus and located immediately posterior to the neurointermediate lobe. It is not as well developed as its homologue in bony fishes, but it does possess the unique *coronet* cellular type characteristic of the saccus vasculosus of bony fishes (Fig. 4-17).

The neurointermediate lobe is well developed. The pars nervosa portion contains unique octapeptide hormones in addition to AVT (see Chap. 7). These hormones are presumably produced in the preoptic nucleus. The pars intermedia contains only one cellular type associated with MSH activity.

In selachians there is a well-developed median eminence with a hypothalamo-hypophysial portal system connecting it to the pars distalis. The median eminence consists of anterior and posterior neurohemal areas.[69] The posterior region receives both peptidergic and aminergic NS axons and appears to be linked by portal vessels to the proximal pars distalis and probably the ventral lobe. There is considerably less NS material in the anterior neurohemal area, which appears to be connected by capillaries to the rostral pars distalis. It is tempting to suggest that the median eminence has differentiated to increase the efficiency of delivering hypothalamic neurohormones to specific adenohypophysial cells.

The occurrence of a highly developed hypothalamo-hypophysial connection suggests that the median eminence and its regulatory relationship to the adenohypophysis probably evolved in the ancestral placoderm fishes. The presence of a similar system in bony fishes would support this view.

Holocephali (Ratfishes). The hypothalamo-hypophysial system of ratfishes has been well studied structurally;[59,124] its general features are depicted in Figure 4-18. The holocephalan adenohypophysis is readily subdivided cytologically into rostral pars distalis, proximal pars distalis and pars intermedia. Although several cellular types have been demonstrated with selective staining procedures, no experimental studies have determined which cells produce tropic hormones.

Holocephalans possess a unique region associated with the adenohypophysis called the *pharyngeal lobe.* This structure is located in the roof of the mouth outside the cranium as though a portion of Rathke's pouch had stayed behind and had not become incorporated into the adenohypophysis proper. The pharyngeal lobe consists of follicles, and may be homologous to the follicular rostral pars distalis of bony fishes.[124] Their extreme dissimilarities ontogenetically, however, make this an unlikely homology.[60] It may be homologous to the ventral lobe of the elasmobranch and the buccal lobe of the coelacanth pituitary.[6]

The ratfish neurohypophysis includes a prominent median eminence connected to the rostral pars distalis and the proximal pars distalis by the hypothalamo-hypophysial portal system. Somatostatin, TRH and GnRH immunoreactivity is present in the hypothalamus.[6] The pars nervosa is mingled with the pars intermedia of the adenohypophysis to form a typical neurointermediate lobe. A well-devel-

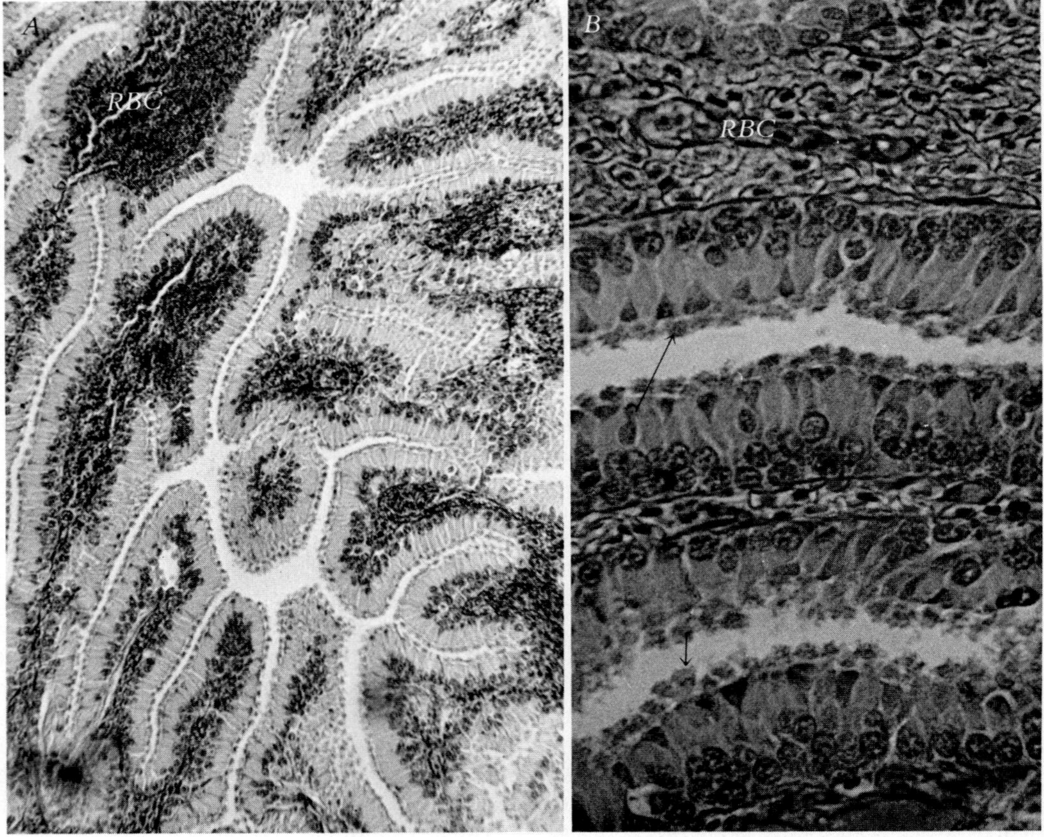

Fig. 4-17. Coronet cells in the saccus vasculosus of a teleost, *Salmo gairdneri. A.* Sagittal section of saccus vasculosus of sexually mature male. *B.* Higher magnification showing cellular details. Note mucoid secretion *(arrows)* of unknown importance on luminal borders of "secretory" cells. *RBC,* red blood cells.

oped saccus vasculosus is present.

Class Osteichthyes: The Primitive Actinopterygii

Polypteri (Polypterus and Erpetoichthyes). The polypterid fishes have been examined structurally and possess all the typical piscine features.[72] These primitive African fishes retain as adults a connection between the hypophysis and the mouth cavity, the *buccohypophysial canal* (*bucco* mouth), which is believed to be a remnant originally connecting Rathke's pouch to the oral cavity (Fig. 4-19). The suggestion that Rathke's pouch may have originated from neural ectoderm rather than oral ectoderm should be carefully considered in these fishes. The buccohypophysial canal or duct is lined with chromophobic cells that have a small quantity of PAS(+) and AB(+) cytoplasm. This cellular type does not appear to be associated with production of any tropic hormones, however.

The pars distalis consists of separate rostral and proximal portions. A number of cellular types have been identified in these two areas, including various basophils acidophils and chromophobes. Experimental studies are needed, however, to identify these cells as sources for particular tropic hormones. Acidophilic cells in the rostral and proximal pars distalis react positively to antibodies against sheep PRL, suggesting that they are a source of PRL or a PRL-like molecule.[1] Growth hormone activity has been demonstrated in the adenohypophysis of *Polypterus,* but no specific cellular type is implicated.[56]

The pars intermedia is closely associated

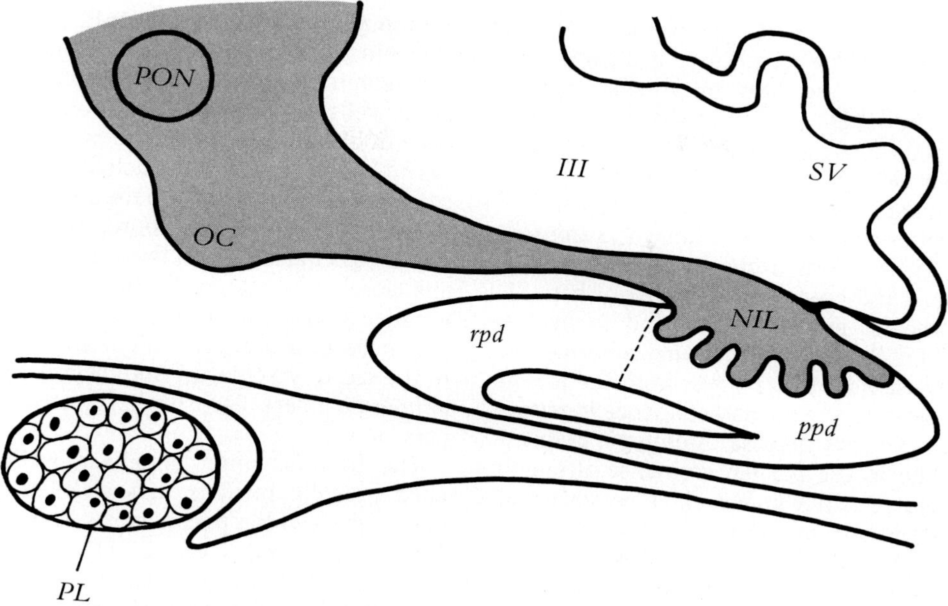

FIG. 4-18. The ratfish hypophysis (Chondrichthyes: Holocephali). Note the unique pharyngeal lobe *(PL)*. For key to symbols and explanation of other abbreviations see Figs. 4-15 and 4-16.

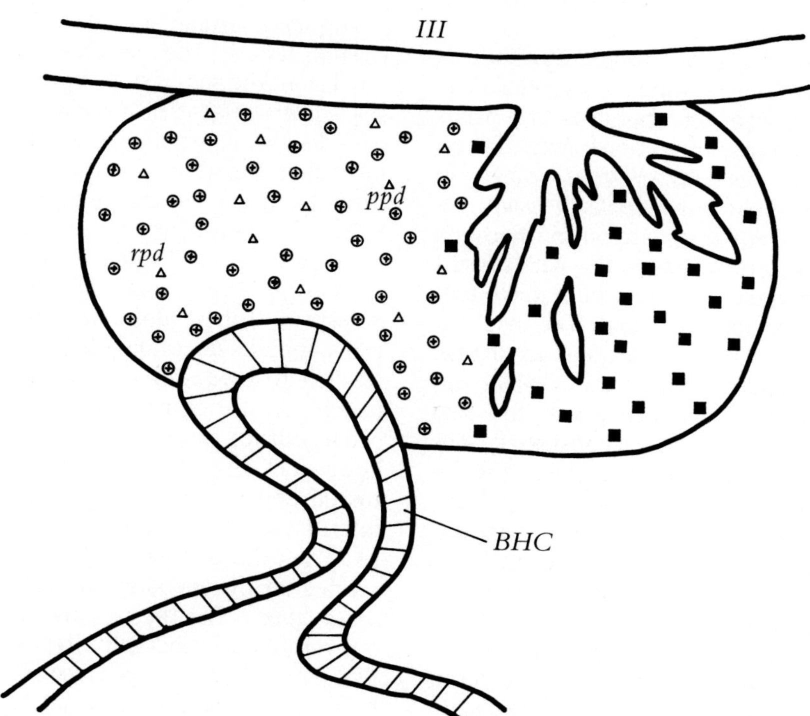

FIG. 4-19. The hypophysis of *Polypterus* (Osteichthyes: Actinopterygii: Polypteri). Note the retention of a connection to the oral cavity, the buccohypophysial canal *(BHC)*. *rpd,* rostral pars distalis; *ppd,* proximal pars distalis. Cellular types on the figure are identified by the following symbols:
■ = MSH-secreting cells
▲ = Unidentified acidophils
⊕ = Unidentified basophils

with the pars nervosa, producing a typical neurointermediate lobe. There is a single cellular type in the pars intermedia that is PAS(+) but PbH(−). This observation is curious since cells responsible for secreting MSH in other vertebrates are all PbH(+).

The pars nervosa contains AVT and another octapeptide neurohormone known as *isotocin* (IST). These two neurohormones are characteristic of the ray-finned fishes (see Chap. 7). The preoptic nucleus is believed to be the source for these octapeptide neurohormones. Peptidgeric fiber tracts travel from the preoptic nucleus via the median eminence to terminate in the pars nervosa. Aminergic neurons terminate in the median eminence although their source is not known. It is possible that peptidergic and aminergic fibers both originate in the preoptic nucleus. The hypothalamo-hypophysial portal system is well developed, and there are no neural fibers penetrating into the pars distalis. As will be seen, direct innervation of adenohypophysial cells becomes common in the more advanced bony fishes.

Chondrostei (Sturgeon, Spoonbill). There is less information concerning the hypothalamo-hypophysial system of chondrostean fishes than for any other ray-finned bony fishes. There is no buccohypophysial canal in chondrosteans, but a hypophysial cavity remains to represent the space within Rathke's pouch. This cavity separates the pars distalis and pars intermedia and may be homologous to the buccohypophysial canal. The pars distalis consists of a rostral zone and a proximal zone (rostral and proximal pars distalis). Numerous follicles occur throughout the pars distalis, and their lumina are considered to be remnants of the hypophysial cavity. The lumina of these follicles are filled with a basophilic colloidal material. The entire pars distalis may be homologous to the proximal pars distalis of teleostean fishes, although the follicles themselves may be homologous to the follicles of the teleostean rostral pars distalis.[59] If this interpretation proves correct the terms rostral pars distalis and proximal pars distalis may no longer be applicable to the two zones of the chondrostean pars distalis.

The cytology of the pars distalis is poorly understood. Acidophils in the rostral portion are thought to be the source for PRL.[121] Gonadotropin activity has also been demonstrated and tentatively assigned to one of the basophilic cells distributed throughout the pars distalis, although the evidence is circumstantial.[8,9] Growth hormone activity has been demonstrated by bioassay in the sturgeon pituitary,[58] but the cellular source is unknown.

The pars intermedia of the sturgeon is large and closely associated with the pars nervosa to produce a typical neurointermediate lobe. The pars nervosa is basically hollow and is similar to the saccus vasculosus. Both peptidergic and aminergic fibers have been reported in the pars nervosa.

The hypothalamus contains a well-developed preoptic nucleus that provides peptidergic fibers to the pars nervosa. The *nucleus lateralis tuberis* consists of peptidgeric, aminergic, and NS neurons, and it may have separated from the preoptic nucleus of the more primitive bony fishes, as suggested by the situation described for *Polypterus*. There is a well-developed median eminence consisting of aminergic axonal endings from the nucleus lateralis tuberis. The median eminence is separated from the pars distalis by a connective tissue sheath so that no neurons penetrate the pars distalis. A hypothalamo-hypophysial portal system possibly conducts neurohormones from the median eminence to the pars distalis, although experimental verification of this hypothesis is not available.

Holostei (Gars and the Bowfin). Adult holostean fishes do not exhibit a buccohypophysial duct nor is there any hypophysial cleft to suggest a relationship to Rathke's pouch. A transient hypophysial cleft does occur during development of the pituitary, however.[59] The adenohypophysis consists of a rostral and proximal pars distalis and a pars intermedia. The rostral pars distalis is follicular. The cellular types have been carefully described for the adenohypophysis of the bowfin *Amia calva*.[7] The rostral pars distalis consists of erythrosinophilic cells (type 1 acidophils) that are believed to produce PRL. Bioassays have confirmed the presence of PRL in the adenohypophysis,[121] but the specific cellular type responsible for its production has not been identified. The follicular lumina contain a colloidal solution that is PAS(+), AB(+) and

AF(+). A second PbH(+) acidophil in the rostral pars distalis is thought to be the source for corticotropin, although there is no experimental evidence that ACTH is present.

At the interface of the rostral and proximal pars distalis occurs an amphophilic cell reputed to produce GTH. Another acidophilic type of cell located in the proximal pars distalis stains positively with orange G (OG[+]) and may be the source of GH that has been demonstrated by bioassay.[56] Two basophilic cells have been differentiated in the proximal pars distalis. One is believed to be the source of TSH, but the role of the other is unknown.

The pars intermedia interdigitates with the pars nervosa to form a neurointermediate lobe. There are two distinguishable cellular types in the pars intermedia of *Amia*. The predominant cell is PbH(+) and presumably secretes MSH. The second cell is a rare PAS(+) cell of unknown significance.[59]

The preoptic nucleus has separated into two distinct portions, the dorsal *pars magnocellularis* and the ventral *pars parvocellularis*. This differentiation of the preoptic nucleus had begun to some degree in *Polypterus*, but complete separation has occurred in the holosteans. The significance of this separation is not clear. Peptidergic fibers from the preoptic nucleus pass to the pars nervosa where octapeptide hormones (AVT and IST) are stored. Aminergic fibers also appear in the pars nervosa and are believed to come from the nucleus lateralis tuberis.[59]

The median eminence is connected to the pars distalis by a well-developed portal system. In addition, there are a limited number of peptidergic and aminergic axons that penetrate the pars distalis.[73] However, only aminergic fibers are associated with the median eminence of *Amia*. Here, in these near-relatives of the teleostean fishes, is the modest beginning of a direct neural innervation of pars distalis cells so well developed in teleosts.[35] In the holostean fishes is the beginning of a shift from neurovascular control to neuroglandular control of the adenohypophysis directly by the hypothalamus.

Class Osteichthyes: Teleostei. The hypothalamo-hypophysial systems of several teleostean species have been studied in detail. In view of the vast adaptive radiation that teleosts have undergone, it is not surprising to find considerable variation in this system. Two major patterns are indicated for "lower" and "higher" teleosts (Figs. 4-14, 4-20, 4-21). However, the major features of the systems in teleosts are rather similar, including cytological features of cells related to the different tropic hormones (Table 4-5). Although only a few species have been examined, they have been examined in greater detail than other piscine groups, and experimental efforts have been made to determine the function of the various cellular types. The tendency to localize cellular types in particular regions of the adenohypophysis is very strong in teleosts and has aided their identification.

In general, the teleostean rostral pars distalis consists of follicles filled with PAS(+) colloidal material. Two cellular types have been identified in the rostral pars distalis, and they have been linked experimentally to secretion of two tropic hormones. The *eta cell* (a carminophil or erythrosinophil; type 1 acidophil) produces PRL.[5,82] These cells are best developed in freshwater fishes. The activity of these cells increases when euryhaline fishes are held in fresh water, a correlation with the osmoregulatory role for PRL in freshwater fishes (see Chap. 16). Treatment of fishes with the drug metyrapone interferes with the synthesis of corticosteroids in the teleostean homologue of the adrenal cortex, the interrenal gland. A reduction in circulating corticosteroids results in stimulation of corticotropic cells and hence identifies the epsilon cells (type 3 basophils) of the rostral pars distalis as the source of ACTH.[82,96,143]

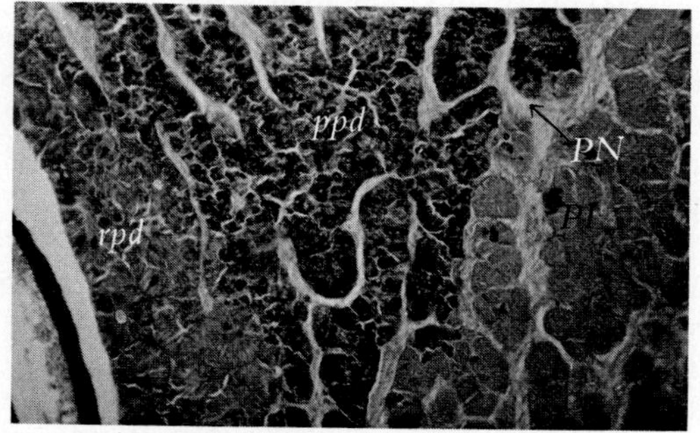

Fig. 4-20. Regions of adenohypophysis of rainbow trout *Salmo gairdneri: rpd,* rostral pars distalis; *ppd,* proximal pars distalis; *PN,* pars nervosa; *PI,* pars intermedia.

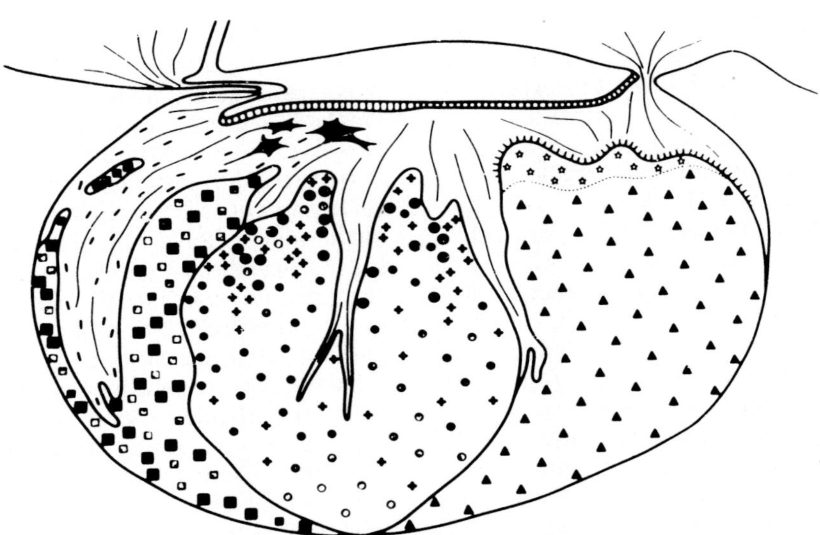

Fig. 4-21. The hypophysis of a "higher" teleost (Osteichthyes: Actinopterygii; Teleostei: Poecilidae). Cellular types on the figure are identified by the following symbols:
● = Thyrotropic basophils (TSH) ▲ = Lactotropes (PRL)
✚ = Somatotropes (GH) ☆ = Corticotropes (ACTH)
○ = Gonadotropes □ = PAS-positive cells, unknown function
■ = MSH-secreting cells
(Reprinted with permission from J. Doerr-Schott (1976). Immunohistochemical detection by light and electron microscopy of pituitary hormones in cold-blooded vertebrates. I. Fishes and amphibians. Gen. Comp. Endocrinol. 28:487–512.)

Thyrotropin-secreting cells (delta cells) have been identified in the proximal pars distalis of several species by using thyroid inhibitors and thyroidectomy.[83,96,98,101] Two kinds of GTH-secreting cells have been demonstrated with selective staining in the proximal pars distalis of chinook salmon and the European eel,[77,95,96,100,133] and it has been suggested they are the cells responsible for secretion of LH and FSH respectively. However, experimental studies support the existence of only one GTH that is LH-like in activity.[37,80] A nonglycoprotein factor is present in teleostean pituitaries that stimulates uptake of yolk precursors by the ovary.[110] Growth hormone activity is associated with the OG(+) alpha cell of the proximal pars distalis.[68,97]

There is a strong tendency to regionalize the various cellular types as unitype clusters within the proximal pars distalis. For example, in *Xiphophorus* the cellular types of the proximal pars distalis are segregated. Thyrotropes and somatotropes are restricted to the dorsal portion of the proximal pars distalis, and the gonadotropes occupy the ventral portion.

The pars intermedia is intimately associated with the pars nervosa of the neurohypophysis to form a neurointermediate lobe. Only one cellular type is found in the pars intermedia of some species, for example, salmonids,[143] but two cellular types are found in other species.[83,99] Type 1 cells are PbH(+), and they are found in all species examined. This cellular type contains granules of 250–400 nm diameter and is believed to secrete MSH. Type 2 pars intermedia cells contain PAS(+) granules (120–200 nm), but their function is unknown.[36]

Neurosecretory centers for regulating secretion of TSH, ACTH, GTH and PRL appear to be localized in the nucleus lateralis tuberis.[111] Release of both TSH and PRL is under inhibitory hypothalamic control, whereas release of ACTH and GTH is under stimulatory control. In contrast, stimulatory control of GH release would seem to reside in the nucleus anterior tuberis located near the preoptic nucleus. The nucleus lateralis tuberis is composed of peptidergic and aminergic neurons. Some of these neurons terminate in the median eminence,

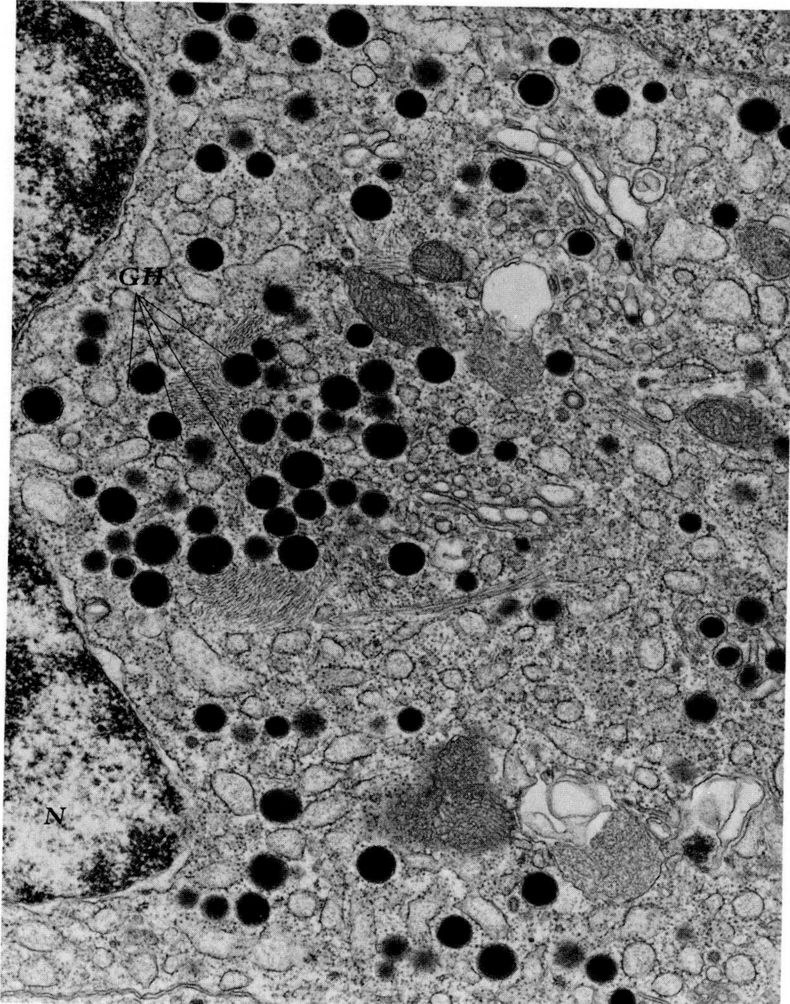

Fig. 4-22. Cellular types from the teleostean pars distalis. Electron micrograph of a somatotrope from a seawater-adapted coho salmon, *Oncorhynchus kisutch*. Courtesy of Howard A. Bern and Richard Nishioka. Nucleus, N; secretion granules containing growth hormone, GH.

but others terminate (synapse) directly on pars distalis cells (Fig. 4-23), providing cytological evidence for direct neural control over adenohypophysial function.[59] The preoptic nucleus in the teleostean hypothalamus consists of peptidergic cells and is responsible for the synthesis of AVT and IST that are stored in the pars nervosa.

Class Osteichthyes: Subclass Sarcopterygii. The hypothalamo-hypophysial system of the lungfishes (Dipnoi) is basically like that of tetrapods, especially the amphibians, although a pars tuberalis is absent in lungfishes (Fig. 4-24). It is not like actinopterygian fishes in that it lacks many of the features that characterize the piscine system. There is less regionalization of cellular types in the lungfish adenohypophysis than in other bony fishes. Furthermore, both the neurointermediate lobe and the saccus vasculosus are absent in lungfishes.

The coelacanth, *Latimeria chalumnae,* which is considered to be closer to the ancestral line of the tetrapods than are the lungfishes, is much more piscinelike than it is tetrapodlike.[75,140] The anatomy of the adeno-

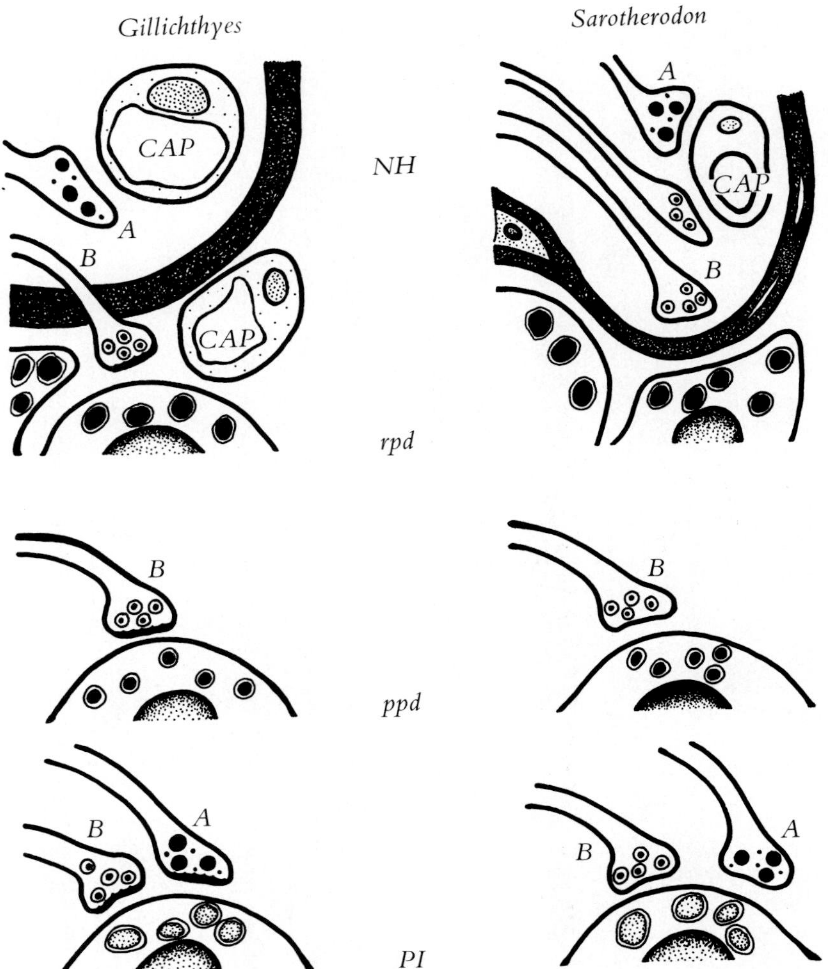

Fig. 4-23. Patterns of direct innervation of adenohypophysial cells in teleostean fishes. *A,* type A neurosecretory fibers; *B,* type B neurosecretory fibers; *CAP,* capillary; *NH,* neurohypophysis; *rpd,* rostral pars distalis; *ppd,* proximal pars distalis; *PI,* pars intermedia. In *Gillichthyes mirabilis,* there is close contact between type B neurons and adenohypophysial cells in all regions, but this does not occur in the rostral portion for tilapia *(Sarotherodon mossambicus).* (After Holmes and Ball.[59])

hypophysis is much like that of the elasmobranch fishes. There is a buccal lobe in the pars distalis which may be homologous to the ventral lobe of elasmobranchs.[6] The pars distalis may be subdivided into rostral and proximal portions with stainable cellular types appearing that are similar to those of teleosts. No experimental studies have been performed, however, to link stainable cellular types with specific tropic functions. Growth hormone is present in the coelacanth adenohypophysis according to bioassay and immunological tests, but this activity has not been assigned to either region of the pars distalis.[57] Only one stainable cellular type has been demonstrated in the pars intermedia, which is probably the source of MSH. The pars intermedia forms a typical neurointermediate lobe characteristic of fishes. The median eminence of the neurohypophysis is connected by a well-developed hypothalamo-hypophysial portal system to the adenohypophysis, particularly the proximal region. Neurosecretory axons appear to penetrate the proximal pars distalis similar to the situation described for the holostean fish *Amia calva.*[74]

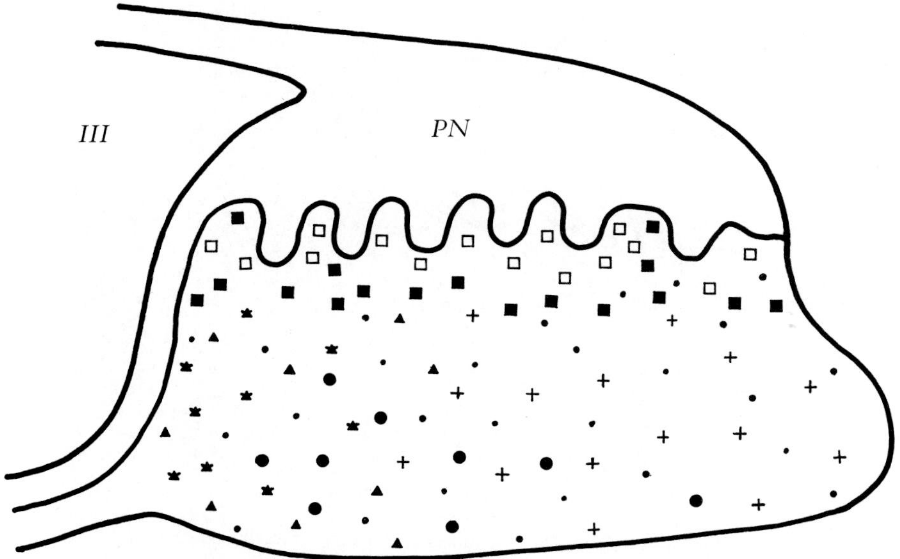

FIG. 4-24. The lungfish pituitary (Osteichthyes: Sarcopterygii: Dipnoi). This pituitary is more like that of the tetrapods than like other fishes. Both the piscine saccus vasculosus and the tetrapod pars tuberalis are absent. *III*, third ventricle; *PN*, pars nervosa. Cellular types on the figure are identified by the following symbols:

□ = PAS-positive cells, unknown function
■ = MSH-secreting cells
+ = Somatotropes (GH)
✱ = Corticotropes (ACTH)
● = Thyrotropic basophils (TSH)
• = Gonadotropic basophils (LH, FSH)
▲ = Lactotropes (PRL)

Although the sarcopterygian fishes represent the closest living relatives to the tetrapods, extant members of this group provide no transitional stages with respect to changes in the hypothalamo-hypophysial system. The living coelacanth appears to be completely fish-like, whereas the lungfishes are like the tetrapods, with the exception of the missing pars tuberalis. Perhaps some embryological studies of pituitary development in lungfishes might reveal a transient homologue to the pars tuberalis.

The Tetrapod Vertebrates

CLASS AMPHIBIA. The amphibian hypothalamo-hypophysial axis has most of the features characteristic of the tetrapod system,[59] including the presence of a pars tuberalis (Figs. 4-25, 4-26). The prominent preoptic nucleus is a major bipartite NS center although other NS nuclei are important as well. At least two kinds of peptidergic fibers originate in the preoptic nucleus, but the significance of this finding is not clear. The *infundibular nucleus* located in the basal hypothalamus supplies aminergic and peptidergic fibers to the median eminence. This nucleus is homologous to at least part of the major hypophysiotropic region of the mammalian hypothalamus, although its relationship to the nucleus lateralis tuberis of fishes is uncertain. A *gonadotropic center* has been identified that contributes aminergic and peptidergic axons to the median eminence. The pars nervosa of the neurohypophysis receives peptidergic fibers originating in the preoptic nucleus. At least two octapeptide hormones are stored in this well-developed neurohemal organ (see Chap. 7). There is no tendency for development of a neurointermediate lobe, nor is a saccus vasculosus or any comparable structure found in amphibians.

The adenohypophysis consists of pars tuberalis, pars intermedia and pars distalis. There is no known function for the pars tuberalis. Based upon ultrastructural comparison of cytoplasmic granules and other features, what appear to be two separate cellular types have been observed in the anuran pars tuberalis[34]

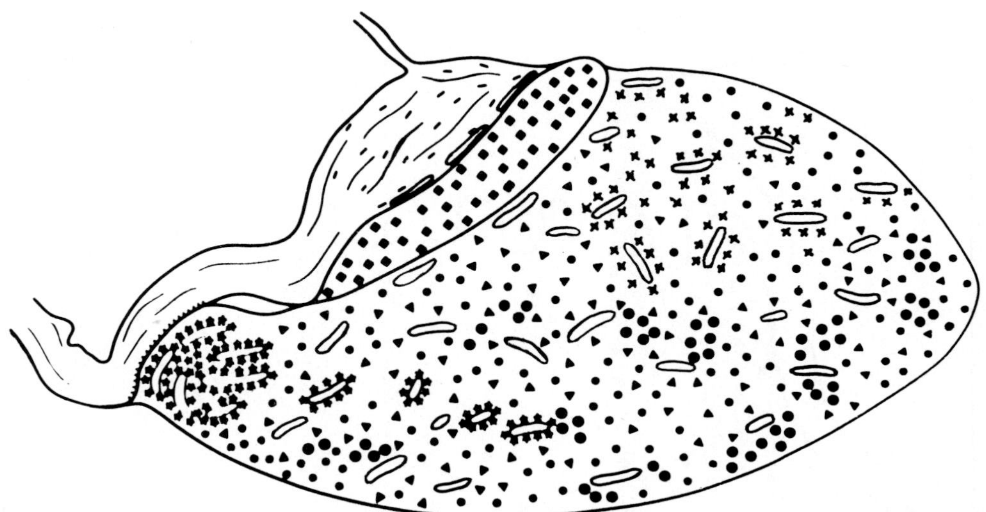

Fig. 4-25. The anuran hypophysis (Amphibia). The pars tuberalis is not shown. Cellular types on the figure are identified by the following symbols:

■ = MSH-secreting cells
▲ = Lactotropes (PRL)
● = Thyrotropic basophils (TSH)
• = Gonadotropic basophils (LH, FSH)
✱ = Corticotropes (ACTH)
+ = Somatotropes (GH)

(Reprinted with permission from J. Doerr-Schott (1976). Immunohistochemical detection by light and electron microscopy of pituitary hormones in cold-blooded vertebrates. I. Fishes and amphibians. Gen. Comp. Endocrinol. 28: 487–512.)

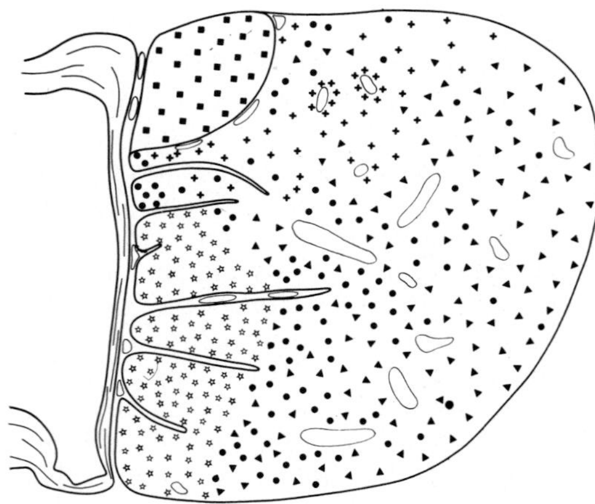

Fig. 4-26. The hypophysis of a caudate amphibian. Cellular types on the figure are identified by the following symbols:

■ = MSH-secreting cells
● = Gonadotropic basophils (LH, FSH)
▲ = Lactotropes (PRL)
+ = Somatotropes (GH)
☆ = Corticotropes (ACTH)

(Reprinted with permission from J. Doerr-Schott (1976). Immunohistochemical detection by light and electron microscopy of pituitary hormones in cold-blooded vertebrates. I. Fishes and amphibians. Gen. Comp. Endocrinol. 28: 487–512.)

(Fig. 4-27). There appears to be a neural pathway extending from the ependymal lining of the third ventricle to the pars tuberalis, but no functional correlations have been reported.

The pars intermedia has a poor vascular supply, but it is directly innervated by aminergic neurons thought to originate in the *caudal aminergic nuclei* of the hypothalamus. Release of MSH appears to be under direct neural control (see Chap. 6).

The pars distalis is not separable into discrete regions although there is a tendency for some regionalization of cellular types. Urodele amphibians exhibit greater regionalization than do anuran species. Careful cytological studies have been performed on many amphibian species, often coupled with experimental manipulations, bioassays or correlations with specific life history events.[26,59,141] Unfortunately there has been considerable disagreement among researchers in this area with respect to establishment of specific sources for the various tropic hormones. The following account of the cytology of *Rana temporaria*[141] will serve as the basic amphibian type for purposes of this text.

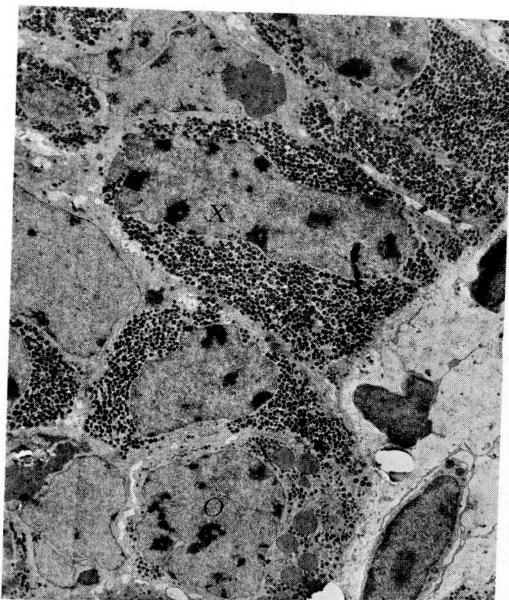

FIG. 4-27. Granular cells in the pars tuberalis of the frog, *Rana pipiens*. One apparent cellular type *(X)* contains both very large and smaller cytoplasmic droplets, whereas another *(O)* contains only the smaller granules which are similar to those seen in tropic hormone-secreting cells of the pars distalis. (Courtesy of Kevin T. Fitzgerald.)

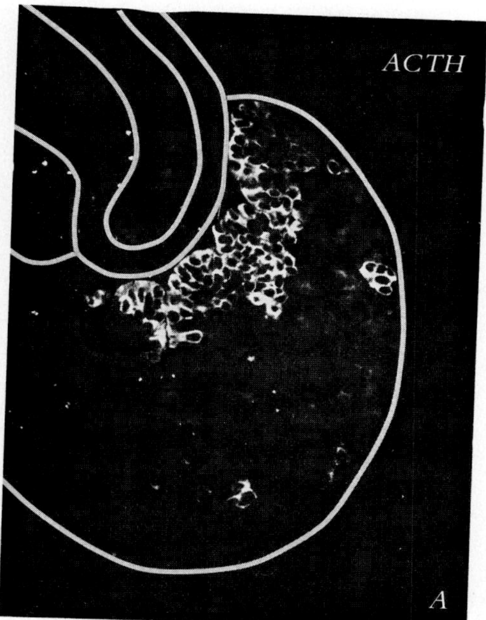

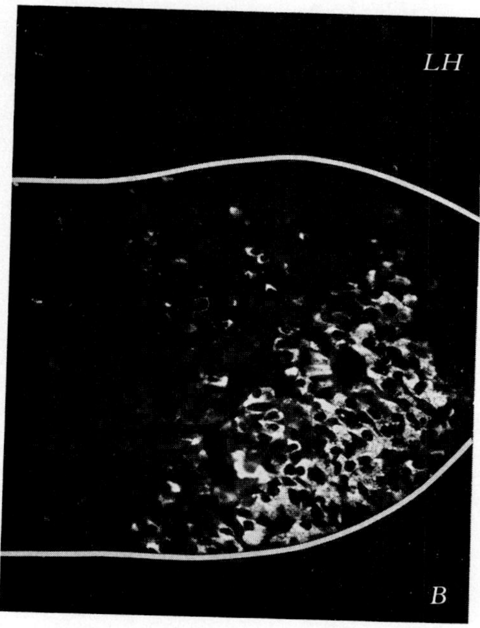

FIG. 4-28. Immunofluorescent localization of corticotropic cells *(ACTH)* and gonadotropes *(LH)* in the pars distalis of the newt *Triturus marmoratus*. The corticotropes in the rostral zone are positively immunofluorescent when antibody specific for mammalian ACTH is conjugated with a fluorescing compound and applied to a section of the pars distalis *(A)*. Similarly, LH-producing cells are demonstrated in the posterior part of the gland *(B)*. (Courtesy of Dr. J. Doerr-Schott.)

Five stainable cellular types can be distinguished in the pars distalis of *R. temporaria* (Table 4-5). There are three basophilic cells and two acidophils plus a number of chromophobic cells.

Type 1 basophils possess granules that stain positively with PAS, AF and AB procedures and are considered to be thyrotropes. Type 2 basophils stain rather weakly with the same procedures but contain cytoplasmic granules that are stainable with OG. This cell is believed to be the source of GTHs (Fig. 4-28). Type 3 basophils are similar to type 1, except they do not stain with AB. This cell is thought to be the source of ACTH (Figs. 4-28, 4-29).

Acidophils of type 1 are large erythrosinophilic and orangeophilic cells. These cells bind antibody to sheep PRL and presumably are the source for PRL in amphibians (Fig. 4-30). Type 2 acidophils are OG(+) and have been suggested to be the source of a GH. There is no evidence, however, to support this contention. Furthermore, there is considerable

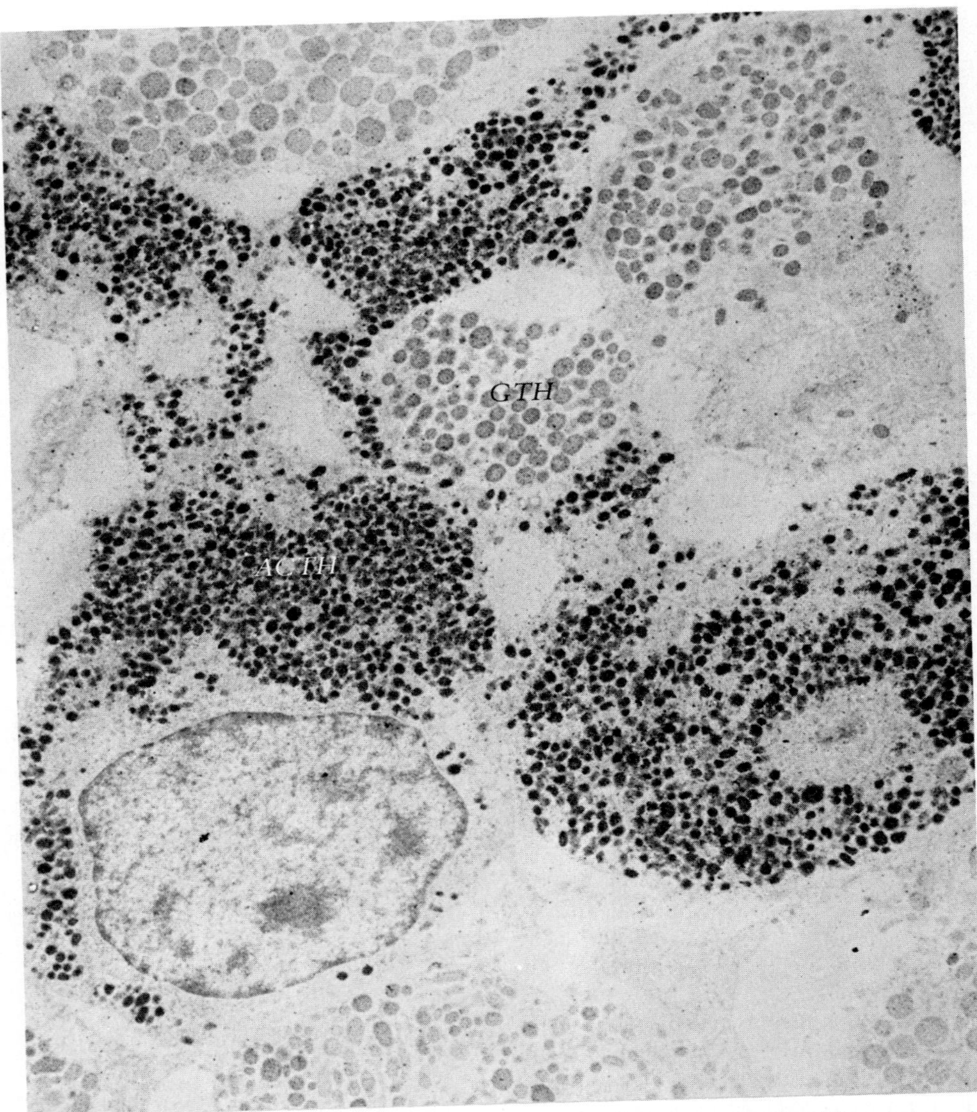

FIG. 4-29. Immunocytochemical demonstration of ACTH-secreting cells in the pars distalis of *Rana temporaria* (Amphibia: Anura). The secretory granules of the corticotrope *(ACTH)* are stained by this highly selective procedure, but the secretory granules of an adjacent gonadotrope *(GTH)* are not stained. (Courtesy of Dr. J. Doerr-Schott.)

evidence to support a role for PRL as a larval GH.[40] The relationship of PRL and GH to amphibians is discussed more fully in Chapter 5.

CLASS REPTILIA. The reptilian hypothalamo-hypophysial system is outlined in Figure 4-31. In reptiles the preoptic nucleus has become two separate nuclei: the *supraoptic nucleus* and the *paraventricular nucleus* (Fig. 4-32). These nuclei consist of peptidergic NS neurons that terminate in the pars nervosa. They produce the octapeptide neurohormones that are stored in the pars nervosa. A separate hypophysiotropic region, the *infundibular nucleus,* is considered to be homologous to the nucleus of the same name in amphibians and birds as well as to the hypophysiotropic area of the mammalian hypothalamus. Aminergic and peptidergic NS fibers originate

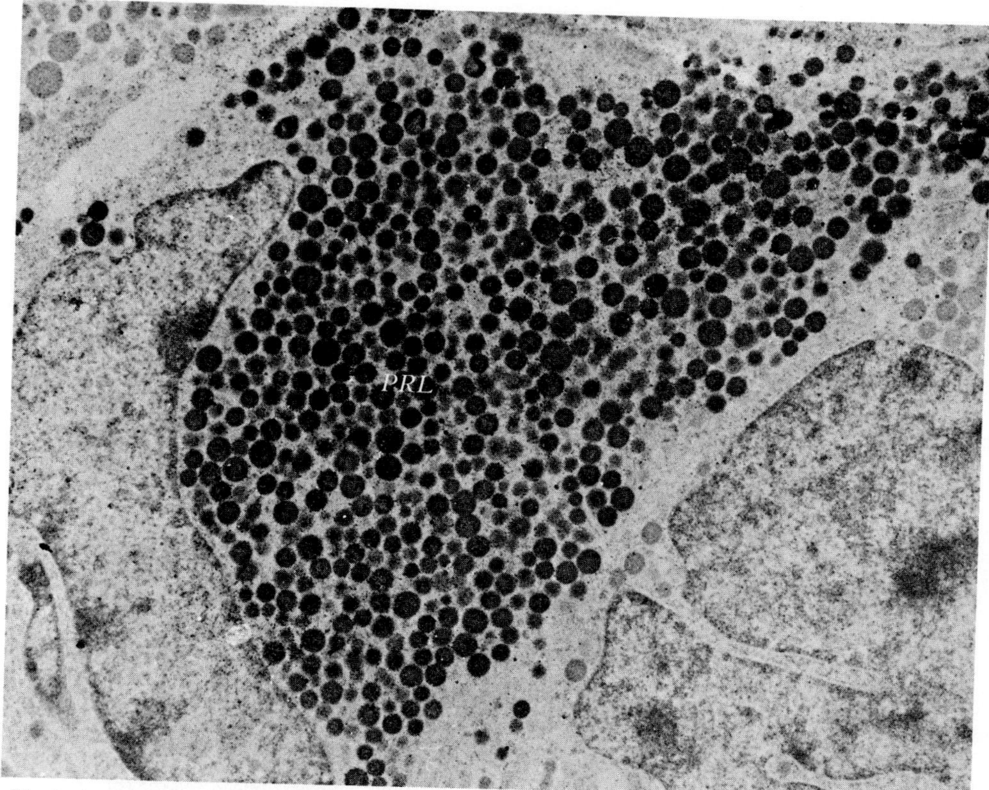

FIG. 4-30. Immunocytochemical demonstration of a PRL-secreting cell in the pars distalis of the frog, *Rana temporaria*. (Courtesy of Dr. J. Doerr-Schott.)

in this nucleus and terminate in the median eminence.

The adenohypophysis is well developed in most reptiles, and it consists of a pars distalis, a pars tuberalis and a pars intermedia. The primitive reptilian condition probably is best represented by the Rhynchocephalia *(Sphenodon)*, Chelonia (turtles) and Crocodilia. The pars distalis appears as two distinct regions reminiscent of the condition in bony fishes. There is a rostral or *cephalic lobe* and a *caudal lobe*. The distribution of cellular types in these lobes of the pars distalis is similar to that described for fishes. The pars tuberalis is well developed in the Rhynchocephalia, Chelonia and Crocodilia, but it is greatly reduced and sometimes absent in lizards. In adult snakes, the pars tuberalis is completely absent. Reptiles have the best developed pars intermedia of any vertebrate group. It is especially elaborate in chelonians, crocodilians, snakes and many lizards.

There are five stainable cellular types in the reptilian pars distalis similar to those described for the amphibians.[59,123] More than one scheme has been proposed for their nomenclature, but a system similar to that adopted for the Amphibia is used here (Table 4-5).

Type 1 acidophils are carminophilic cells located in the cephalic lobe that presumably secrete PRL. Bioassays of the two portions of the pars distalis indicate that PRL activity resides in the cephalic lobe.[121] Type 2 acidophils are located in the caudal lobe. These cells are OG(+) in most reptiles and are believed to secrete GH. Bioassays of the caudal lobe indicate GH activity is present.

Type 1 basophils are somewhat scattered throughout the pars distalis but are more concentrated in the caudal lobe. These cells stain similarly to the thyroptropic type 1 basophils of amphibians and probably secrete TSH. Cytologically these cells are sensitive to thyroidec-

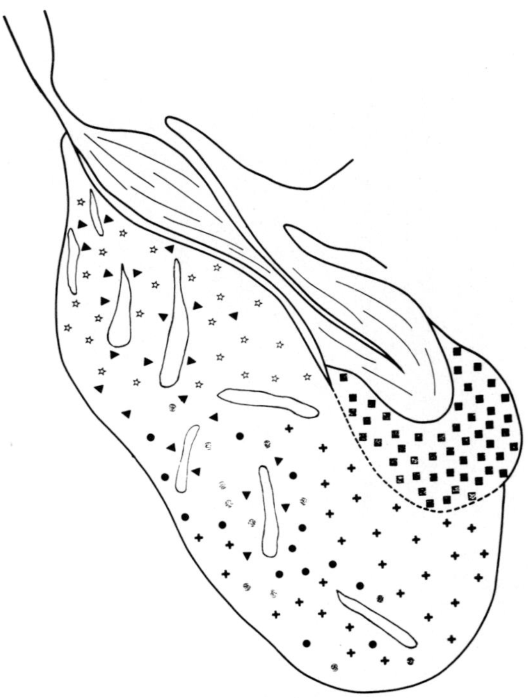

Fig. 4-31. General organization of the reptilian hypophysis. Cellular types on the figure are identified by the following symbols:
■ = MSH-secreting cells
● = Gonadotropic basophils (LH, FSH)
☆ = Corticotropes (ACTH)
▲ = Lactotropes (PRL)
✚ = Somatotropes (GH)
(Courtesy of Dr. J. Doerr-Schott.)

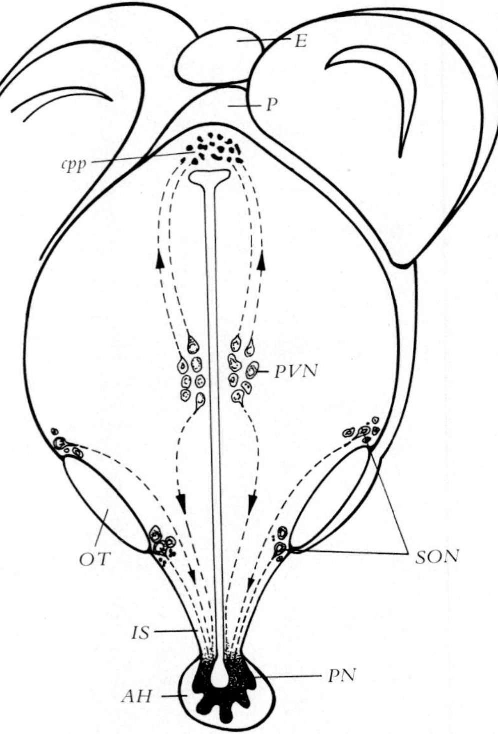

Fig. 4-32. Neurosecretory connections between reptilian (snake) hypothalamic nuclei and the epithalamus and hypophysis. *E,* epiphysis; *P,* paraphysis; *cpp,* commissura palii post; *PVN,* paraventricular nucleus; *SON,* supraoptic nucleus; *OT,* optic tract; *IS,* infundibular stalk; *AH,* adenohypophysis; *NH,* neurohypophysis. Modified from Scharrer.[128]

tomy. Bioassay of the separate lobes of the pars distalis of a lizard, *Anolis carolinensis,* reveals that TSH activity is in the caudal lobe where the majority of type 1 basophils are found in this species.[81]

Type 2 basophils tend to be scattered throughout the pars distalis. These cells are localized ventrally toward the midline in most snakes and some lizards but are limited to the cephalic lobe of other lizards. Gonadotropes as well as some thyrotropes occur in the pars tuberalis of turtles.[108] Type 2 basophils vary greatly in size among different species, but all stain like the gonadotropes of amphibians. Furthermore, these cells respond to castration or treatment with gonadal steroids, making it likely that they secrete GTHs (Fig. 4-33).[59]

The last basophilic type consists of amphophilic cells located in the cephalic lobe. They exhibit similar staining properties to the corticotropes described for amphibians. Bioassays have localized ACTH activity in the cephalic lobe,[79] and the type 3 basophils respond to experimental manipulations such as administration of metyrapone, which blocks corticosteroid synthesis in the adrenal (Fig. 4-34).[24]

The reptilian pars distalis contains chromophobic cells in addition to the stainable cellular types. Reptilian chromophobes appear as agranular, stellate cells and may function as a transport system carrying nutrients from the blood to the hormone-producing cells.[38]

The pars intermedia contains only one stainable cellular type, which is the presumed source for MSH. The skin of many rep-

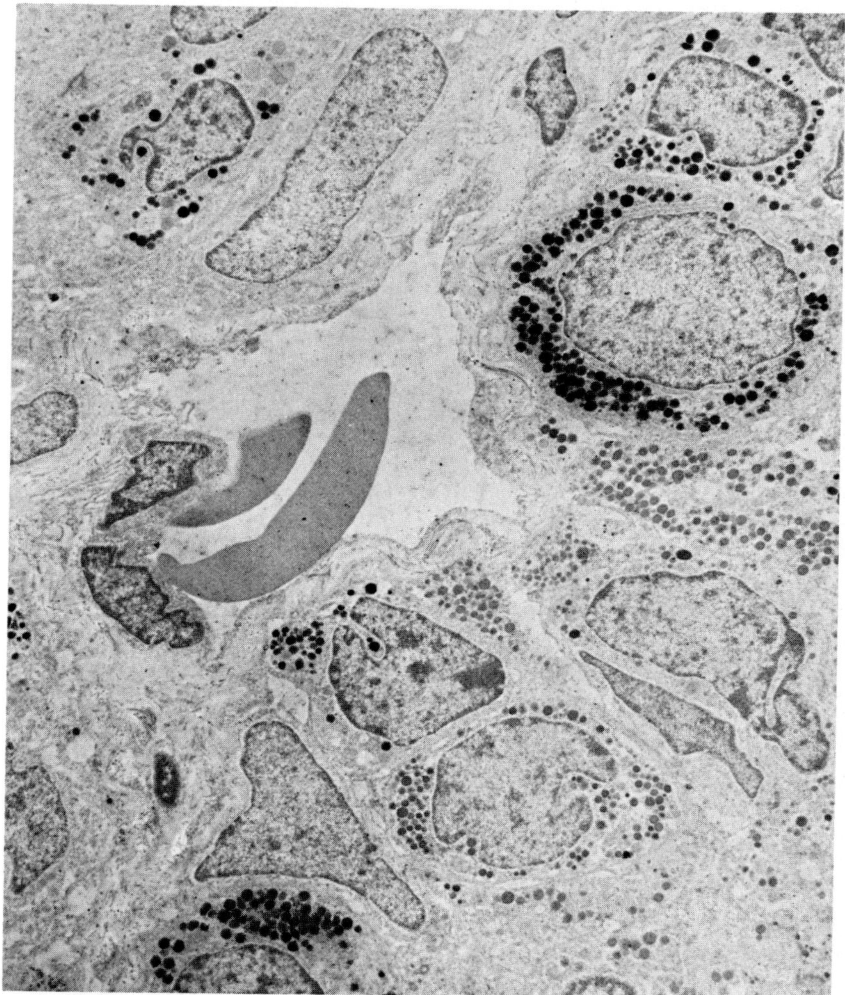

Fig. 4-33. Luteinizing hormone-secreting cell in the pars distalis of a turtle, *Emys leprosa*. Only cells with LH-containing granules are stained histochemically. (Courtesy of Dr. J. Doerr-Schott.)

tiles is sensitive to MSH, and the American chameleon *Anolis carolinensis* is used for a sensitive MSH bioassay (see Chap. 6). This lizard can change from green to brown under the influence of MSH, which allows it to color adapt to different backgrounds in its environment. Color changes in the true chameleon, *Chamaeleo* spp., are under direct neural control, however, and MSH is not involved.

Class Aves. The avian hypothalamo-hypophysial system differs from that of other tetrapods (and fishes) in that the pars intermedia is absent in all species. A well-developed pars tuberalis is present, and the pars distalis consists of cephalic and caudal lobes homologous to those described for reptiles (Fig. 4-3).

The median eminence differs from mammals in that the primary capillaries of the portal system lie superficially or in grooves on the surface rather than penetrating to form the complex vascular bed seen in mammals. This anatomical difference allows an investigator to sever the portal connection with the pars distalis without interrupting fiber tracts. The hypophysiotropic region of the hypothalamus supplies aminergic and peptidergic fibers to the median eminence. The supraoptic nucleus and the paraventricular nucleus are responsi-

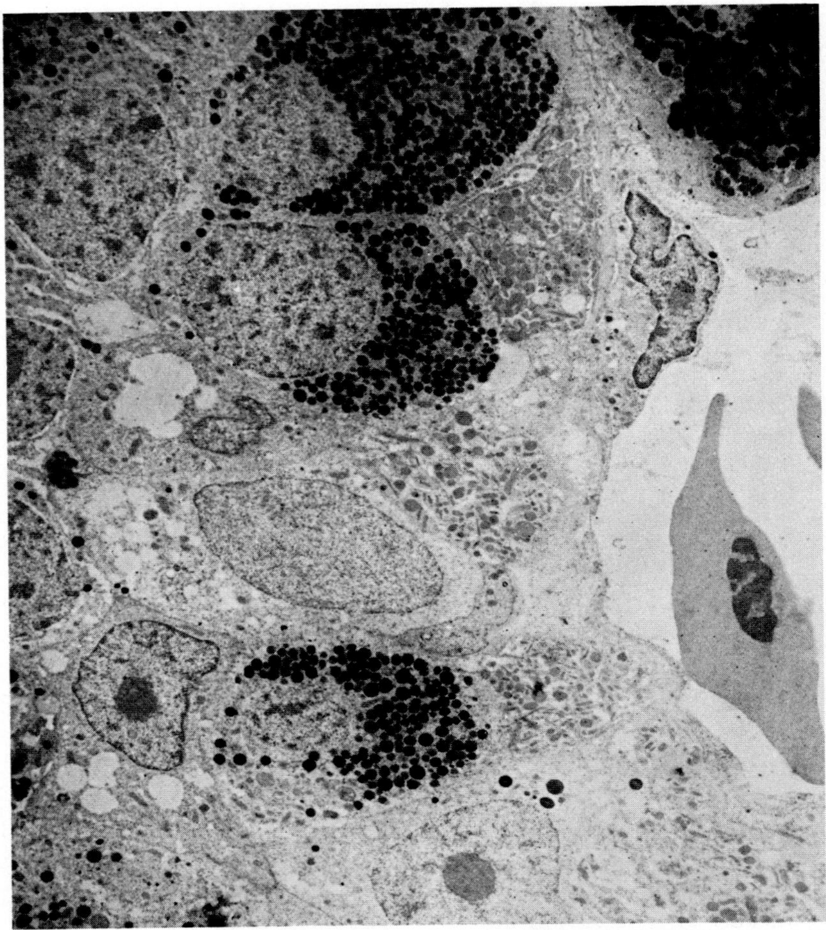

FIG. 4-34. Corticotropes in the pars distalis of a lizard, *Lacerta muralis.* The secretory granules are stained immunohistochemically only in cells producing ACTH. (Courtesy of Dr. J. Doerr-Schott.)

ble for secretion of the octapeptide neurohormones (see Chap. 7).

In some birds, i.e., the pigeon, the Japanese quail and the white-crowned sparrow, the median eminence is separable into an anterior neurohemal area and a more posterior neurohemal area similar to that described for elasmobranchs[129,131,144](Figs. 4-3, 4-35). Each of these areas has is own portal connection to the pars distalis, which consists of a cephalic and a caudal lobe. It is not certain how widespread this phenomenon of two median eminences is among other avian species;[136] however, such potential regionalization of both the median eminence and the pars distalis could represent a mechanism to increase the efficiency of delivery of hypothalamic neurohormones to cellular types regionalized in various parts of the pars distalis. This neurovascular specialization is analogous to the system of direct innervation of pars distalis cells that was observed in teleosts.

The nomenclature for the cytological features of the avian adenohypophysis is somewhat different from the schemes used for other vertebrates. The avian pars distalis contains seven stainable cellular types as well as chromophobic cells. The stainable cells have been grouped into three categories: *serous cells, glycoprotein-containing cells* and *PbH(+) cells*. Some features of these cells are summarized in Table 4-5.

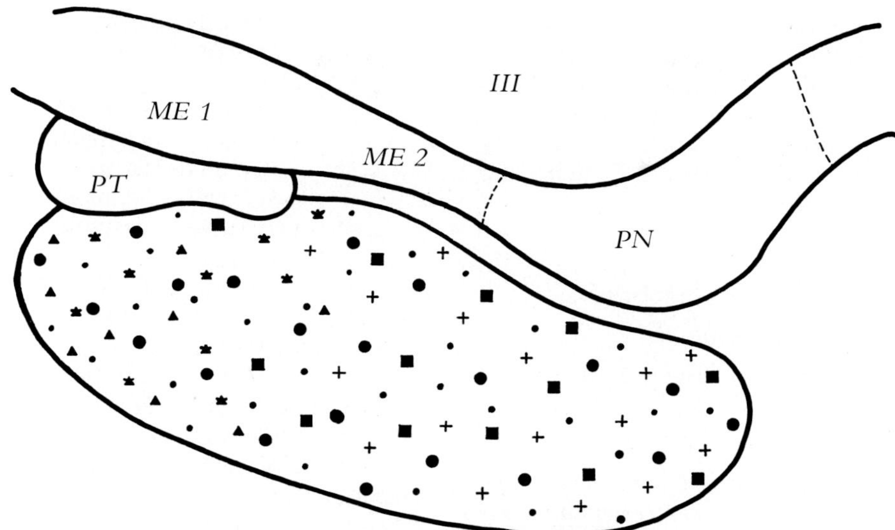

FIG. 4-35. The avian hypophysis. Note the presence of two separate neurohemal areas associated with the pars distalis *(ME 1, ME 2)* and the absence of a pars intermedia. *III,* third ventricle; *PT,* pars tuberalis; *PN,* pars nervosa. Cellular types on the figure are identified by the following symbols:

■ = MSH-secreting cells
● = Thyrotropic basophils (TSH)
• = Gonadotropic basophils (LH, FSH)
+ = Somatotropes (GH)
★ = Corticotropes (ACTH)

The serous cells include the OG(+) alpha cell (type 2 acidophil) located in the caudal lobe and possibly responsible for GH secretion. The second serous cellular type is the erythrosinophilic eta cell (type 1 acidophil) located in the periphery of the cephalic lobe. The eta cell is synonymous with the so-called *broody cell* of egg-incubating birds and is the source of PRL.

Three types of glycoprotein-containing cells can be distinguished in the avian pars distalis. The beta cell of the cephalic lobe is strongly PAS(+) and supposedly produces FSH. The gamma cell is found in the caudal lobe. It is acidophilic and PAS(+) and has been claimed to be the probable source of LH. Both of these cellular types respond in the same manner to experimental manipulations such as castration and administration of synthetic GnRH.[87,145] If separate gonadotropic cells for LH and FSH do exist in birds, this would be the only vertebrate group in which one cellular type did not appear to produce both GHs. Future studies may reveal that these beta and gamma cells of birds are only variants of a single type of cell comparable to the type 2 basophil of other vertebrates.

The delta cell appears to be a type 1 basophil on the basis of its stainability features and is thought to be the source of TSH. This cellular type has been reported to occur throughout the pars distalis;[136] however, only those delta cells of the cephalic lobe of the Japanese quail show cytological changes following thyroidectomy.[87,115] Bioassay data obtained for this same species indicate that TSH activity is restricted to the cephalic lobe. These data suggest that the actual distribution of thyrotropes may be highly dependent upon the species.

There are two PbH(+) cells in the avian pars distalis: the kappa cell and the epsilon cell. The kappa cell presumably secretes MSH.[136] Cytologically the kappa cell is similar to the MSH-secreting PbH(+) cells of other vertebrates, including the PbH(+) cell in the human pars distalis that is also believed to produce MSH. Bioassays for MSH activity support the proposal that MSH-secreting cells are present in the avian pars distalis, but since ACTH also has MSH activity in these bioassays (see Chap. 5) this is not conclusive proof. The epsilon cell located in the cephalic lobe has stainability characteristics like the type 3 basophils of other vertebrates. This cell responds to experimental manipulations such as adrenalectomy and metyrapone treatment,[87,136] indicating that it secretes ACTH.

Some Comparative Aspects of Hypothalamic Control of Adenohypophysial Function in Nonmammals

Since some hypothalamic hypophysiotropic substances of nonmammalian vertebrates have not been identified many researchers refer to them only as factors. For consistency, however, they will be referred to as hormones throughout this text.

The Fishes

Immunoreactive GnRH has been demonstrated in the hagfish, lamprey and shark. Somatostatin is present in the brains of hagfish and sharks and TRH has been found in lampreys and sharks. There is no evidence of any functional roles for these peptides, however.[6]

Numerous studies of releasing hormones have been conducted on teleosts.[6] Teleostean GnRH differs structurally from mammalian GnRH, but is effective in sheep bioassays for mammalian GnRH. Similarly, mammalian GnRH induces ovulation in teleosts.[76] Thyroid function appears to be under inhibitory hypothalamic control, and administration of mammalian TRH depresses thyroid activity. Dopamine blocks PRL release, and TRH stimulates release. Somatostatin is present and can block GH release. Dopamine also blocks GH release. There is some evidence to suggest presence of CRH.

The Tetrapod Vertebrates

Class Amphibia. Hypothalamic control over TSH release in amphibians may be of a stimulatory nature as in mammals,[28,45,119] or it may have no influence as demonstrated for some adult amphibians.[119] Molecules identical to mammalian TRH are present in relatively large amounts in the amphibian hypothalamus,[61] and even greater amounts are found in the skin.[62] However, synthetic mammalian TRH has proven ineffective as a stimulator of thyroid function in a number of species.[43,134,139] Intravenous injection of TRH did elevate plasma levels of the thyroid hormones in one species, *Rana ridibunda,*[22] but a similar approach failed for the Mexican axolotl.[23]

Release of PRL and MSH is considered to be under inhibitory control in amphibians.[65,92] Release of MSH appears to be under direct aminergic neural control in anurans,[90,102] but the situation for PRL release is less clear. The similarity in regulatory mechanisms for MSH and PRL release is reflected also by the actions of certain pharmacological agents on their release. Drugs that affect PRL or MSH release in mammals have similar actions in amphibians. For example, ergot derivatives such as ergocornine or ergocryptine inhibit release of both PRL and MSH.[89,113,114] These agents are alpha-adrenergic blocking agents and support the hypothesis that aminergic substances are involved in the release of both PRL and MSH.

There is also evidence for a PRL-releasing hormone (PRH). Extracts prepared from the hypothalamus of *Xenopus laevis,* the clawed frog, stimulate PRL release from chicken, rat and anuran pituitaries in vitro.[52,53] Hypothalamic content of both PRH and PRIH activities shows a seasonal variation in *Rana temporaria,*[71] and such variations if common to other species could explain conflicting results obtained by various researchers. It is not clear whether any of the reported effects of hypothalamic activities influencing PRL release are due to their TRH content or to substances such as aminergic neurotransmitters present in these extracts.

In mammals TRH causes release of PRL, which is a known antagonist of thyroid hormones in amphibians.[25] No effect of synthetic TRH on PRL release could be demonstrated in the red-spotted newt *Notophthalmus viridescens,*[44] but PRL release was stimulated following injection into bullfrogs[21] and by addition of synthetic TRH to pituitaries of *Xenopus laevis* cultured in vitro.[52] Synthetic TRH also causes release of MSH in frogs.[137]

Gonadotropin release is under positive hypothalamic control. Amphibian GnRH appears to be similar to mammalian GnRH which is effective in both anurans and urodeles.[6] Seasonal changes in hypothalamic GnRH reflect changes in gonadal function.[66,149]

Growth hormone release is autonomous in urodeles but is under stimulatory hypothalamic control in anurans. Immunoreactive somatostatin is present in amphibian brains, but its role in regulating GH release is not clear.

There is evidence for a CRH in the anuran preoptic nucleus,[27] but release of ACTH in urodeles seems to be autonomous.[6]

Class Reptilia. No generalization can be formulated about hypothalamic control in reptiles because very little research has been conducted in this area. Corticotropin release is probably under a mammalian pattern of control. The regulatory pattern for PRL is not clear as some conflicting data have been reported. Release of MSH is under inhibitory control. Thyrotropin release has not been examined but is presumed to be under stimulatory control. Synthetic mammalian TRH does not stimulate the thyroid of the turtle.[125]

Gonadotropin release is under stimulatory hypothalamic control.[6] Immunoreactive GnRH is present in the preoptic area but is not identical to mammalian GnRH. Synthetic mammalian GnRH induces ovulation in some species. Immunoreactive somatostatin is present in turtles and lizards, but its role is not clear.[6] Release of GH is primarily under stimulatory control.

Lesions in the infundibular nucleus of the lizard *Sceloporus cyanogenys* result in reduced adrenal weight, probably due to reduction in ACTH levels.[15] Corticosteroid administration produces similar reductions in adrenal weight, presumably due to negative feedback on ACTH release via the hypothalamus.[16]

It is not clear whether PRL release in turtles is under stimulatory hypothalamic control as in birds or under inhibitory control as in most vertebrates. Cultured pituitaries of *Malaclemys terrapin* release PRL,[11] but extracts prepared from the median eminence of female *Pseudemys scripta* or male rats stimulate PRL release from cultured *Pseudemys* pituitaries.[93] Hypothalamic extracts from another turtle, *Chrysemys picta,* similarly evoke PRL release from either avian or mammalian pituitaries.[51,52] Cultured pituitaries of a lizard, *Dipsosaurus dorsalis,* also release PRL following addition of an extract of rat median eminence.[32] These extracts may have been rich in a legitimate PRH or some other substance such as a neurotransmitter or even the TRH tripeptide. Synthetic mammalian TRH does stimulate PRL release from *C. picta* pituitaries,[55] supporting the interpretation that these effects are due to presence of TRH in the extracts. Whether or not endogenous TRH tripeptide is a physiological regulator of PRL release remains to be seen.

Class Aves. Some of the first studies of hypothalamic control in birds involved lesions in the hypothalmus paralleling mammalian work. Placement of lesions in the hypothalmus produces testicular atrophy in the duck.[70] Similar experiments have resulted in localization of hypothalamic centers regulating release of GTHs, TSH and ACTH.

Release of adenohypophysial hormones appears to be influenced by a mammalian pattern of hypothalamic control except for PRL. The pattern of PRL release in birds is under direct stimulatory control by the hypothalmus, which is unlike the condition in other vertebrates. The avian PRH might be similar if not identical to mammalian TRH since TRH causes PRL release from the bird pituitary in vivo and in vitro.[54]

Thyroid glands of the lesser snow goose, *Anser caerulescens caerulescens,* and the duck, *Anas platyrhynchos* are activated within 20 minutes following injection of synthetic mammalian TRH. Injections of GnRH were without effect on thyroid hormone secretion.[10]

Ovulation can be induced in the Japanese quail with synthetic mammalian GnRH,[17] and mammalian GnRH activates gonadotropes in the avian pars distalis.[87,145] Although some correlations have been noted between amine levels in the avian hypothalamus and tropic hormone release, the role of aminergic substances in hormone release is poorly understood.[7]

Possible Role for the Epiphysial Complex in Hypothalamic Function

The epiphysial complex (see Chap. 15) includes the pineal gland, which is believed to secrete its products into the blood and possibly into the cerebrospinal fluid.[118] The pineal gland may secrete the amine melatonin or small peptides, including AVT, or both. Numerous studies have documented antigonadal actions of pineal extracts, melatonin, or both in fishes, amphibians, reptiles, birds and mammals (see Chap. 11). In addition, effects on thyroid function have been noted in some of these groups (see Chap. 8). It is possible that these pineal actions are mediated via effects on the hypothalamus, or the specific sites of action may be at the target endocrine glands themselves.

Summary

The Adenohypophysis

The adenohypophysis consists of a pars distalis, a pars intermedia and a pars tuberalis.

The origin of the adenohypophysis from Rathke's pouch is reflected in various cavities that are considered to be homologous to the original lumen of the ancestral pouch, such as the buccopharyngeal canal and the lumina of the follicles of the pars distalis of many fishes. The hypophysial cleft appearing in other adult vertebrates may also be a remnant of Rathke's pouch. The embryonic origin of Rathke's pouch is generally assumed to be from oral ectoderm, but recent studies suggest a neural origin similar to the neurohypophysis and hypothalmus.

The major portion of the adenohypophysis consists of a pars distalis which produces GH, PRL, GTHs, (FSH, LH), ACTH, TSH, and, at least in mammals, LPH. The piscine pars distalis consists of distinct rostral and proximal zones that may be homologous to the cephalic and caudal lobes of reptiles and birds. The pars distalis of lungfishes, amphibians and mammals exhibits little or no regionalization.

Cytologically there is considerable unity among the vertebrates with respect to the pars distalis. In spite of the variability in affinities for specific dyes and the multitude of staining techniques employed to identify cellular types, a general classification of vertebrate tropic hormone-secreting cells can be formulated (Table 4-3). The PRL-secreting cell (type 1 acidophil) tends to be rostrally located and has an affinity for azocarmine or erythrosin. The cell believed to be responsible for secretion of GH (type 2 acidophil) is universally OG(+). Type 1 basophils are PAS(+), AB(+) and AF(+) and are the thyrotropes. Type 2 basophils are PAS(+), AB(+) and AF(−) with some acidophilic granules (usually OG[+]) and are gonadotropic cells. Type 3 basophils are weak basophils (may even be chromophobic) and in some cases somewhat PbH(+). This cellular type believed to be responsible for ACTH secretion is generally located rostrally near the PRL cells.

The posterior portion of the adenohypophysis is the pars intermedia, which is responsible for synthesis of MSH. In the fishes, with the exception of the agnathan hagfishes and the lungfishes, the pars intermedia becomes interdigitated with the pars nervosa of the neurohypophysis to form the neurointermediate lobe. The pars intermedia appears to have its beginning via an inductive effect of the infundibulum on the embryonic adenohypophysial cells. The cellular type responsible for secretion of MSH appears to have an affinity for PbH, even in those species that lack a distinct pars intermedia and in which MSH-secreting cells are found in the pars distalis. The class Aves lacks a pars intermedia as do a few mammals.

In addition to the pars distalis and pars intermedia, the tetrapods possess a pars tuberalis that may contain GTH and possibly TSH-producing cells. Fishes lack a pars tuberalis.

The Neurohypophysis

The neurohypophysis consists of an anterior neurohemal area, the median eminence, and a more posterior neurohemal structure, the pars nervosa. The median eminence stores the neurohormones produced in the hypothalamus that regulate tropic hormone release from the adenohypophysis. The hypothalamo-hypophysial portal system connects the median eminence to the adenohypophysis. The median

TABLE 4-12. *Summary of Anatomical Features of Vertebrate Hypothalamo-hypophysial Systems*

GROUP	HYPOTHALAMUS					ADENOHYPOPHYSIS					NH			SPECIAL FEATURES
	PON	NLT	SON	PVN	IFN	PT	RPD	PPD	PI	NIL	ME	PN	SV	
Agnatha: Hagfish	+										?			MAH
Lamprey	+						+	+	+	+	+	+		
Chondrichthyes	+	+					+	+	+	+	+	+	+	Ventral lobe
Osteichthyes														
Polypteri	+	+					+	+	+	+	+	+	+	Buccopharyngeal canal
Teleostei	+	+					+	+	+	+	+	+	+	Neuroglandular control
Latimeria	+						+	+	+	+	+	+	+	Basically fish-like
Dipnoi	+								+		+	+		Basically tetrapod-like, neuroglandular?
Amphibia	+				+	+			+		+	+		PI innervated
Reptilia			+	+	+	+	×	×	+		+	+		Best PI when present
Aves			+	+	+	+	×	×			+	+		Two ME; PI absent
Mammalia			+	+	**	+			+		+	+		

+=present; ×=similar regions but homology not clear; **homologous structures present
PON, preoptic nucleus
SON, supraoptic nucleus
IFN, infundibular nucleus
NLT, nucleus lateralis tuberis
PVN, paraventricular nucleus

PRH	?	?	TRH (+/−)	TRH (+)	TRH (+)
MSHRIH	?	Dopamine	Dopamine?	?	
CRH	?	(+) control	(+) control	(+) control	(+) control

eminence is not a universal component of the neurohypopysis of all vertebrates; its presence is disputed in agnathan fishes. The pars nervosa has no common blood supply with the adenohypophysis. It is responsible for storage of octapeptide neurohormones produced in the hypothalamus until they are released into the general circulation.

The saccus vasculosus is a unique piscine structure posterior to the pars nervosa that might prove to be a component of the neurohypophysis. Its function is unknown, however.

The Hypothalamus

The preoptic nucleus of anamniotes is responsible for production of the octapeptide neurohormones that are stored in the pars nervosa. It consists primarily of peptidergic NS neurons. In bony fishes there is progressive separation of the preoptic nucleus resulting in two distinct nuclei in holosteans and teleosts: pars magnocellularis and pars parvocellularis. A similar tendency is observed in amphibians. In reptiles separation of the preoptic nucleus into the supraoptic nucleus and paraventricular nucleus is complete. Birds and mammals exhibit these separate nuclei, and in mammals, at least, they each specialize in the production of a different octapeptide neurohormone (see Chap. 7).

The NS nuclei controlling adenohypophysial hormone release are generally located in the ventral region of the hypothalmus (*nucleus lateralis tuberis* of fishes; infundibular nucleus of amphibians, reptiles and birds; and the hypophysiotropic region of mammals). Aminergic and peptidergic neurons terminate in the median eminence and are believed to elaborate hypothalamo-hypophysiotropic regulating hormones. These regulating hormones are transferred to the adenohypophysis via the hypothalamo-hypophysial portal system.

Hypothalamic control of adenohypophysial function is a general rule in vertebrates although there is considerable variation as to how that control may be manifest. The control of tropic hormone release via release of hypothalamic regulatory neurohormones that travel through the portal vessels to the adenohypophysis is known as the neurovascular hypothesis. This appears to be the nature of regulation except in teleostean fishes in which direct innervation of pars distalis cells has been observed (neuroglandular hypothesis for regulation of tropic hormone release).

Certain birds and sharks exhibit two separate neurohemal regions in the median eminence that appear to be connected by portal vessels to separate regions of the pars distalis. This condition may represent a neurovascular specialization toward increasing the efficiency of delivering a given hypothalamic hypophysiotropic regulating hormone to the appropriate tropic hormone cell.

Control of the release of GH, GTHs and ACTH is stimulatory in all vertebrates, although there is also strong inhibitory control of GH in mammals by somatostatin. Regulation of TSH release is stimulatory in amniotes, but it may be inhibitory in teleosts and some amphibians. Prolactin release is under inhibitory control by the hypothalamus except in birds and possibly in certain reptiles. Mammals may produce a PRH and PRIH. The

TABLE 4–13. *Summary of Some Information Concerning Hypothalamic Control over Adenohypophysial Function in Nonmammals*

HORMONE	AGNATHA	TELEOSTEI	AMPHIBIA	REPTILIA	AVES
TRH	Present No effect	Present (−) TSH	Present No effect	? ?	Present (+) TSH
GnRH	Present No effect	Present (+) GTH	Present (+) GTH	? (+) GTH	Present (+) GTH
PRIH	?	Dopamine	Dopamine?	(+/−)?	None
PRH	?	?	TRH (+/−)	TRH (+)	TRH (+)
MSHRIH	?	Dopamine	Dopamine?	?	
CRH	?	(+) control	(+) control	(+) control	(+) control

former activity may be due to the tripeptide known as TRH, however. Similar effects of mammalian TRH on PRL release have been reported for birds, reptiles and amphibians. Melanotropin is under inhibitory control in all vertebrates. Although peptides have been reported that will inhibit MSH release in mammals, endogenous control may be neuroglandular. It is not clear whether the MSH activity assayed in avian pituitaries is due to MSH and not ACTH, however.

References

1. Aler, G.M., G. Bage and B. Fernholm (1971). On the existence of prolactin in cyclostomes. Gen. Comp. Endocrinol. 16:498–503.
2. Baker, B.L. (1974). Functional cytology of the hypophysial pars distalis and pars intermedia. Handbook of Physiology, Sec. 7, Endocrinology. Williams & Wilkins, Baltimore, Vol. 4, Part 1, pp. 45–80.
3. Baker, B.L., F.J. Karsch, D.L. Hoffman and W.C. Beckman, Jr. (1977). The presence of gonadotropic and thyrotropic cells in the pituitary pars tuberalis of the monkey *(Macaca mulatta)* Biol. Reprod. 17:232–240.
4. Baker, B.L. and Y.–Y. Yu (1975). Immunocytochemical analysis of cells in the pars tuberalis of the rat hypophysis with antisera to hormones of the pars distalis. Cell Tissue Res. 156:443–449.
5. Ball, J.N. (1969). Prolactin (fish prolactin or paralactin) and growth hormone. In W.S. Hoar and D.J. Randall, eds. Fish Physiology. Academic Press, New York, Vol. 2, pp. 207–240.
6. Ball, J.N. (1981). Hypothalamic control of the pars distalis in fishes, amphibians and reptiles. Gen. Comp. Endocrinol. 44:135–170.
7. Ball, J.N. and B.I. Baker (1969). The pituitary gland: anatomy and histophysiology. In W.S. Hoar and D.J. Randall, eds., Fish Physiology. Academic Press, New York, Vol. 2., pp. 1–111.
8. Barannikova, I.A. (1949). Localization of gonadotropic function in the hypophysis of the sturgeon (*Acipenser stellatus*). Dokl. Akad. Nauk. SSSR 69:117–120.
9. Barannikova, I.A. (1954). Completion of sexual maturation in autumn-running female sturgeons after exclusion of the period of the river spawning migration. Dokl. Akad. Nauk. SSSR 99:641–644.
10. Barrington, E.J.W. (1975). An Introduction to General and Comparative Endocrinology. Clarendon Press, Oxford.
11. Bern, H.A. and C.S. Nicoll (1968). The comparative endocrinology of prolactin. Recent Prog. Horm. Res. 24:681–720.
12. Birk, J., G. Rothenbuchner, U. Loos, S. Raptis, S. Fletcher and E.F. Pfeiffer (1973). The preparation of ^{125}I–TRH: Its distribution, half–life and excretion in mice. In C. Gual and E. Rosenberg, eds., Hypothalamic Hypophysiotropic Hormones. Excerpta Medica, Amsterdam, pp. 141–145.
13. Breton, B., B. Jalabert and C. Weil (1975). Caracterisation partielle d'un facteur hypothalamique de liberation des hormones gonadotropes chez la carpe (Cyprinus carpio L.). Etude *in vitro*. Gen. Comp. Endocrinol. 25:405–415.
14. Burgus, R., M. Amoss, P. Brazeau, M. Brown, N. Ling, C. Rivier, J. Rivier, W. Vale and J. Villarreal (1976). Isolation and characterization of hypothalamic peptide hormones. In F. Labrie, J. Meites and G. Pelletier, eds., Hypothalamus and Endocrine Functions. Plenum Press, New York, pp. 335–372.
15. Callard, I.P., S.W.C. Chan and G.V. Callard (1973). Hypothalamic-pituitary-adrenal relationships in reptiles. In A. Brodish and E.S. Redgate, eds., Brain-Pituitary-Adrenal Interrelationships, Karger, Basel, pp. 270–292.
16. Callard, I.P. and I. Chester Jones (1970). The effect of hypothalamic lesions and hypophysectomy on adrenal weight in *Sceloporus cyanogenys*. Gen. Comp. Endocrinol. 17:194–202.
17. Campbell, G.T. and A. Wolfson (1974). Hypothalamic norepinephrine, luteinizing hormone releasing factor activity and reproduction in the Japanese quail, *Coturnix coturnix japonica*. Gen. Comp. Endocrinol. 23:302–310.
18. Campbell, R.R. and J.F. Leatherland (1979). Effect of TRH, TSH, and LHRH on plasma thyroxine and triiodothyronine in the lesser snow goose *(Anser caerulescens caerulescens)* and plasma thyroxine in the Rouen duck *(Anas platyrhynchos)*. Can. J. Zool. 57:271–274.
19. Carrer, H.F. and S. Taleisnik (1970). Effect of mesencephalic stimulation on the release of gonadotrophins. J. Endocrinol. 48:527–539.
20. Chauvet, M.T., D. Hurpet, J. Chauvet and R. Acher (1980). Phenypressin (Phe^2-Arg^8-vasopressin), a new neurohypophysial peptide found in marsupials. Nature 287:640–642.
21. Clemons, G.K., S.M. Russell and C.S. Nicoll (1979). Effect of mammalian thyrotropin releasing hormone on prolactin secretion by bullfrog adenohypophyses *in vitro*. Gen. Comp. Endocrinol. 38:52–67.

22. Darras, V.M. and E.R. Kuhn (1982). Increased plasma levels of thyroid hormones in a frog *Rana ridibunda* following intravenous injections of TRH. Gen. Comp. Endocrinol. 48:469–475.

23. Darras, V.M. and E.R. Kuhn (1983). Effects of TRH, bovine TSH, and pituitary extracts on thyroidal T_4 release in *Ambystoma mexicanum*. Gen. Comp. Endocrinol. 51:286–291.

24. Del Conte, E. (1969). The corticotroph cells of the anterior pituitary gland of a reptile: *Cnemidophorus 1. lemniscatus* (Sauria, Teiidae). Experientia 25:1330–1332.

25. Dodd, M.H.I. and J.N. Dodd (1976). The biology of metamorphosis. In B. Lofts, ed. Physiology of the Amphibia. Academic Press, New York, Vol. 3, pp. 467–599.

26. Doerr-Schott, J. (1976). Immunohistochemical detection by light and electron microscopy of pituitary hormones in cold-blooded vertebrates. I. Fishes and amphibians. Gen. Comp. Endocrinol. 28:487–512.

27. Dupont, W. (1971). Évolution de la formation corticotrope chez la grenouille verte, *Rana esculenta* L. après transplantation ectopique du lobe distale de l'hypophyse. Ann. Endocrinol. 32:639–652.

28. Etkin, W. and W. Sussman (1961). Hypothalamo-pituitary relation in metamorphosis of *Ambystoma.* Gen. Comp. Endocrinol. 1:70–79.

29. Fawcett, D.W., J.A. Long and A.L. Jones (1969). The ultrastructure of endocrine glands. Recent Prog. Horm. Res. 25:315–380.

30. Fernholm, B. (1972). Neurohypophysial-adenohypophysial relations in hagfish (Myxinoidea, Cyclostomata). Gen. Comp. Endocrinol. Suppl. 3:1–10.

31. Ferrand, R. and S. Hraoui (1973). Origine exclusivement ectodermique de l'adenophypophyse de la Caille: demonstration par la méthode des associations tissulaires interspécifiques. C.R. Soc. Biol. 167:740–743.

32. Fiorindo, R.P. and C.S. Nicoll (1968).[93]

33. Firth, J.A. and L. Vollrath (1973). Determination of the distribution of luteinizing hormone-like gonadotrophic activity within the dogfish pituitary gland by means of the *Xenopus* oocyte meiosis assay. J. Endocrinol. 58:347–348.

34. Fitzgerald, K. (1978). Examination of the pars tuberalis in *Rana pipiens* with light and electron microscopy. M.A. thesis, University of Colorado, pp. 62.

35. Follenius, E. (1965). Bases structurales et ultrastructurales des corrélations diencéphalo-hypophysaires chez les sélaciens et les téléostéens. Arch. Anat. Microsc. Morphol. Exp. 54:195–216.

36. Fontaine, M. and M. Olivereau (1975). Aspects of the organization and evolution of the vertebrate pituitary. Am. Zool. 15, Suppl. 1:61–80.

37. Fontaine, Y–A., and E. Burzawa–Gerard (1977). Esquisse de l'evolution des hormones gonadotropes et thyreotropes des vertebres. Gen. Comp. Endocrinol. 32:341–347.

38. Forbes, M.S. (1972). Observations on the fine structure of the pars intermedia in the lizard *Anolis carolinensis.* Gen. Comp. Endocrinol. 18:146–161.

39. Frohman, L.A., L.E. Bernardis, K.J. Kant (1968). Hypothalamic stimulation of growth hormone secretion. Science 162:580–582.

40. Frye, B.E., P.S. Brown and B.W. Snyder (1972). Effects of prolactin and somatotropin on growth and metamorphosis of amphibians. Gen. Comp. Endocrinol. Suppl. 3:209–220.

41. Fuxe, K., T. Hofelt, P. Eneroth, J–A. Gustafson, and P. Skett (1977). Prolactin-like immunoreactivity: Localization in nerve terminals of rat hypothalamus. Science 196:899–900.

42. Goldstein, A. (1976). Opioid peptides (endorphins) in pituitary and brain. Science 193:1081–1086.

43. Gona, A.G. and O. Gona (1974). Failure of synthetic TRF to elicit metamophosis in frog tadpoles or red-spotted newts. Gen. Comp. Endocrinol. 24:223–225.

44. Gona, A. and O. Gona (1974). Prolactin-releasing effects of centrally acting drugs in the red-spotted newt, *Notophthalmus viridescens.* Neuroendocrinology 14:365–368.

45. Goos, H.J.T. (1969). Hypothalamic neurosecretion and metamorphosis in *Xenopus laevis*. IV. The effect of extirpation of the presumed TRF cells and of a subsequent PTU treatment. Z. Zellforsch. 97:449–458.

46. Gorbman, A. (1980). Endocrine regulatory patterns in agnatha: Primitive or degenerate? In S. Ishii, T. Hirano and M. Wada, eds., Hormones, Adaptation and Evolution, Japan Sci. Soc. Press, Tokyo/Springer Verlag, Berlin, pp. 81–92.

47. Gorbman, A. (1983). Early development of the hagfish pituitary gland: evidence for the endodermal origin of the adenohypophysis. Am. Zool. 23:639–654.

48. Green, J.D. (1951). The comparative anatomy of the hypophysis with special reference to its blood supply and innervation. Am. J. Anat. 88:225–311.

49. Guillemin, R. (1977). The expanding significance of hypothalamic peptides, or, is endocrinology a branch of neuroendocrinology. Recent Prog. Horn. Res. 33:1–28.

50. Guillemin, R. and J.E. Gerich (1976). Somatostatin: Physiological and clinical significance. Annu. Rev. Med. 27:379–388.

51. Hadley, M.E. and V.J. Hruby (1977). Neurohypophysial peptides and the regulation of melanophore stimulating hormone. Am. Zool. 17:809–821.

52. Hall, T.R. and A. Chadwick (1976). Control of prolactin release in the toad, *Xenopus laevis*, Gen. Comp. Endocrinol. 29:246.

53. Hall, T.R., A. Chadwick and N.J. Bolton (1976). Assay of prolactin releasing and inhibiting activities in the hypothalami of vertebrates. Gen. Comp. Endocrinol. 29:242–243.

54. Hall, T.R., A. Chadwick, N.J. Bolton and C.G. Scanes (1975). Prolactin release *in vitro* and *in vivo* in the pigeon and the domestic fowl following administration of synthetic thyrotrophin-releasing factor (TRF). Gen. Comp. Endocrinol. 25:298–306.

55. Hall, T.R., A. Chadwick and I. Callard (1975). Control of prolactin secretion in the terrapin *(Chrysemys picta)*. J. Endocrinol. 67:52p–54p.

56. Hayashida, T. (1971). Biological and immunochemical studies with growth hormone in pituitary extracts of holostean and chondrostean fishes. Gen. Comp. Endocrinol. 17:275–280.

57. Hayashida, T. (1977). Immunoassay and biological studies with growth hormone in a pituitary extract of the coelacanth, *Latimeria chalumnae* Smith. Gen. Comp. Endocrinol. 32:221–229.

58. Hayashida, T. and M.D. Lagios (1969). Fish growth hormone: A biological, immunochemical and ultrastructural study of sturgeon and paddlefish pituitaries. Gen. Comp. Endocrinol. 13:403–411.

59. Holmes, R.L. and J.N. Ball (1974). The Pituitary Gland, A Comparative Account. Cambridge University Press, London.

60. Honma, Y. (1969). Some evolutionary aspects of the morphology and role of the adenohypophysis in fishes. Gunma Symp. Endocrinol. 6:19–36.

61. Jackson, I.M.D. and S. Reichlin (1974). Thyroid-releasing hormone (TRH): Distribution in hypothalamic and extra-hypothalamic brain tissue of mammalian and submammalian chordates. Endocrinology 95:854–862.

62. Jackson, I.M.D. and S. Reichlin (1977). Thyrotropin-releasing hormone: Abundance in the skin of the frog, *Rana pipiens*. Science 198:414–415.

63. Jackson, R.G. and M. Sage (1973). Regional distribution of the thyroid stimulating hormone activity in the pituitary gland of the Atlantic stingray, *Dasyatis sabina*. Fishery Bull. 71:93–97.

64. Jasinski, A. (1969). Vascularization of the hypophyseal region in lower vertebrates (cyclostomes and fishes). Gen. Comp. Endocrinol. Suppl. 2:510–521.

65. Kastin, A.J., S. Viosca and A.V. Schally (1974). Regulation of melanocyte-stimulating hormone release. Handbook of Physiology, Sec. 7, Endocrinology. Williams & Wilkins, Baltimore, Vol. 4, Part 2, pp. 551–562.

66. King, J.A. and R.P. Millar (1979). Hypothalamic luteinizing hormone-releasing hormone content in relation to the seasonal reproductive cycle of *Xenopus laevis*. Gen. Comp. Endocrinol. 39:309–312.

67. Knowles, F. and T.C.A. Kumar (1969). Structural changes related to reproduction in the hypothalamus and in the pars tuberalis of the rhesus monkey. Part 2. The pars tuberalis. Philos. Trans. R. Soc. Lond. 256:357–375.

68. Knowles, F. and L. Vollrath (1966). Neurosecretory innervation of the pituitary of the eels *Anguilla* and *Conger*. II. The structure and innervation of the pars distalis at different stages of the life-cycle. Philos. Trans. R. Soc. Lond. 250:311–342.

69. Knowles, F., L. Vollrath and P. Meurling (1975). Cytology and neuroendocrine relations of the pituitary of the dogfish, *Scyliorhinus canicula*. Proc. R. Soc. Lond. 191:507–525.

70. Kobayashi, H. and M. Wada (1973). Neuroendocrinolgy in birds. In D.S. Farner and J.R. King, eds., Avian Biology. Academic Press, New York, Vol. 3, pp. 287–347.

71. Kuhn, E.R. and H. Engelen (1976). Seasonal variation in prolactin and TSH releasing activity in the hypothalamus of *Rana temporaria*. Gen. Comp. Endocrinol. 28:277–282.

72. Lagios, M.D. (1968). Tetrapod-like organization of the pituitary gland of the polypterformid fishes, *Calamoichthyes calabaricus* and *Polypterus palmas*. Gen. Comp. Endocrinol. 11:300–315.

73. Lagios, M.D. (1970). The median eminence of the bowfin, *Amia calva* L. Gen. Comp. Endocrinol. 15:453–463.

74. Lagios, M.D. (1972). Evidence for a hypothalamo-hypophysial portal vascular system in the coelacanth, *Latimeria chalumnae* Smith. Gen. Comp. Endocrinol. 18:73–82.

75. Lagios, M.D. (1975). The pituitary gland of the coelacanth *Latimeria chalumnae* Smith. Gen. Comp. Endocrinol. 25:126–146.

76. Lam, T.J., S. Pandey and W.S. Hoar (1975). Induction of ovulation in goldfish by synthetic luteinizing hormone-releasing hormone (LH–RH). Can. J. Zool. 53:1189–1192.

77. Leray, C. and N. Carlon (1963). Sur la présence d'une dualité parmi les cellules cyanophiles de l'adenohypophyse de *Mugil cephalus* L. (Téléostéen, Mugilidae). C.R. Soc. Biol. 157:572–575.

78. Licht, P. (1974). Luteinizing hormone (LH) in the reptilian pituitary gland. Gen. Comp. Endocrinol. 22:463–469.

79. Licht, P. and S.D. Bradshaw (1969). A demonstration of corticotropic activity and its distribution in the pars distalis of the reptiles. Gen. Comp. Endocrinol. 13:226–239.

80. Licht, P., H. Papkoff, S.W. Farmer, C.H. Muller, H.W. Tsai and D. Crews (1977). Evolution of gonadotropin structure and function. Recent Prog. Horm. Res. 33:169–248.

81. Licht, P. and L.L. Rosenberg (1969). Presence and distribution of gonadotropin and thyrotropin in the pars distalis of the lizard *Anolis carolinensis*. Gen. Comp. Endocrinol. 13:439–454.

82. McKeown, B.A. and A.P. Van Overbeeke (1969). Immuno-histochemical localization of ACTH and prolactin in the pituitary gland of adult migratory sockeye salmon *(Oncorhynchus nerka)*. J. Fish. Res. Bd. Can. 26:1837–1846.

83. Mattheij, J.A.M., F.J. Kingma and H.W.J. Stroband (1971). The identification of the thyrotropic cells in the adenohypophysis of the cichlid fish *Cichlasoma biocellatum* and the role of these cells and of the thyroid in osmoregulation. Z. Zellforsch. 121:82–92.

84. Matty. A.J., K. Tsuneki, W.W. Dickhoff and A. Gorbman (1976). Thyroid and gonadal function in hypophysectomized hagfish, *Eptatretus stouti*. Gen. Comp. Endocrinol. 30:500–516.

85. Mellinger, J. and M.P. Dubois (1973). Confirmation, par l'immunofluorescence de la fonction corticotrope du lobe rostral et de la fonction gonadotrope du lobe ventral de l'hypophyse d'un poisson cartilagineux, la torpille marbrée (Torpedo marmorata). C.R. Acad. Sci. 276:1879–1881.

86. Mezey, E. and M. Palkovits (1982). Two-way transport in the hypothalamo-hypophysial system. In W.F. Ganong and L. Martini, eds., Frontiers in Endocrinology, Vol 7, pp. 1–29.

87. Mikami, S., T. Kurosu and D.S. Farner (1975). Light- and electron-microscopic studies on the secretory cytology of the adenohypophysis of the Japanese quail, *Coturnix coturnix japonica*. Cell Tissue Res. 159:147–165.

88. Mizunuma, H., W.K. Samson, M.D. Lumpkin, J.H. Moltz, C.P. Fawcett and S.M. McCann (1983). Purification of a bioactive FSH-releasing factor (FSHRF). Brain Res. Bull. 10:623–629.

89. Morgan, C.M. and M.E. Hadley (1976). Ergot alkaloid inhibition of melanophore stimulating hormone (MSH) secretion. Neuroendocrinology 21:10–19.

90. Nakai, Y. and A. Gorbman (1969). Evidence for a doubly innervated secretory unit in the anuran pars intermedia. II. Electron microscopic studies. Gen. Comp. Endocrinol. 13:108–116.

91. Nalbandov, A.V. (1963). Advances in Neuroendocrinology. University of Illinois Press, Urbana.

92. Nicoll, C.S. (1974). Physiological actions of prolactin. Handbook of Physiology, Sec. 7, Endocrinology. Williams & Wilkins, Baltimore. Vol. 4, Part 2, pp. 253–292.

93. Nicoll, C.S. and R.P. Fiorindo (1969). Hypothalamic control of prolactin secretion. Gen. Comp. Endocrinol. Suppl. 3:26–31.

94. Nishioka, R.S. and H.A. Bern (1966). Fine structure of the neurohemal area associated with the hypophysis in the hagfish *Polistotrema stoutii*. Gen. Comp. Endocrinol. 7:457–462.

95. Olivereau, M. (1961). Maturation sexuelle de l'anguille male en eau douce. C.R. Acad. Sci. 252:3660–3662.

96. Olivereau, M. (1963). Action de la reserpine sur l'hypophyse, interrenal et les cellules chromaffines de l'Anguille *Anguilla anguilla* L. C.R. Soc. Biol. 157:1357–1360.

97. Olivereau, M. (1965). Action de la métopirone chez l'anguille normale et hypophysectomisée en particulier sur le système hypophyso-corticosurrenalien. Gen. Comp. Endocrinol. 5:109–128.

98. Olivereau, M. (1972). Identification des cellules thyreotropes dans l'hypophyse du saumon du Pacifique *(Oncorhynchus tshawytscha* Walbaum) après radiothyroidectomie. Z. Zellforsch. 128:175–187.

99. Olivereau, M. and J.N. Ball (1964). Contribution à l'histophysiologie de l'hypophyse des téléostéens en particulier de celle de *Poecilia* species. Gen. Comp. Endocrinol. 4:523–532.

100. Olivereau, M. and M. Herlant (1960). Etude de l'hypophyse de l'anguille male au cours de la reproduction. C.R. Soc. Biol. 154:706–709.

101. Olivereau, M., G. La Roche and A.N. Woodall (1964). Modifications cytologiques de l'hypophyse de la truite à la suite d'une carence en iode et d'une radiothyroidectomie. Ann. Endocrinol. 25:481–490.

102. Oshima, K. and A. Gorbman (1969). Evidence for a doubly innervated secretory unit in the anuran pars intermedia. I. Electrophysiological studies. Gen. Comp. Endocrinol. 13:98–107.

103. Otzan, N. (1966). The fine structure of the adenohypophysis of *Zoarces viviparus* L. Z. Zellforsch. 69:699–718.

104. Pacold, S.T., L. Kirstens, S. Hojvat, A.M. Lawrence and T.C. Hagen (1978). Biologically active pituitary hormones in the rat brain amygdaloid nucleus. Science 199:804–806.

105. Pasteels, J.L., A. Danguy, M. Frerotte and F. Ectors (1971). Inhibition de la secretion de prolactine par l'ergocornine et la 2-Br-α-ergocryptine: action directe sur l'hypophyse en culture. Ann. Endocrinol. 32:188–192.

106. Patzner, R.A. and T. Ichikawa (1977). Effects of hypophysectomy on the testis of the hagfish, *Eptatretus burgeri* Girard (Cyclostomata). Zool. Anz. 199:371–380.

107. Pearse, A.G.E. and T. Takor Takor (1976). Neuroendocrine embryology and the APUD concept. Clin. Endocrinol. 5, Suppl. 229s–244s.

108. Pearson, A.K. and P. Licht. (1982). Morphology and immunocytochemistry of the turtle pituitary gland with special reference to the pars tuberalis. Cell Tiss. Res. 222:81–100.

109. Perks, A.M. (1977). Developmental and evolutionary aspects of the neurohypophysis. Am. Zool. 17:833–850.

110. Peter, R.E. and L.W. Crim (1979). Reproductive endocrinology of fishes: gonadal cycles and gonadotropin in teleosts. Annu. Rev. Physiol. 41:323–335.

111. Peter, R.E. and J.N. Fryer (1980). Endocrine functions of the hypothalamus of actinopterygians. In R.G. Northcutt and R.E. Davis, eds., Fish Neurobiology and Behavior. University of Michigan Press, Ann Arbor.

112. Pickford, G.E. and J.W. Atz (1957). The Physiology of the Pituitary Gland of Fishes. New York Zoological Society, New York.

113. Platt, J.E. (1976). The effects of ergocornine on tail height, spontaneous and T_4-induced metamorphosis and thyroidal uptake of radioiodide in neotenic *Ambystoma tigrinum*. Gen. Comp. Endocrinol. 28:71–81.

114. Platt, J.E. and D.O. Norris (1974). The effect of ergocornine on melanophores of *Ambystoma tigrinum*: Evidence for suppression of pituitary MSH release. J. Exp. Zool. 189:7–12.

115. Radke, W.J. and R.B. Chaisson (1975). Thyroid stimulating hormone distribution in the pars distalis of the Japanese quail. Gen. Comp. Endocrinol. 26:274–276.

116. Reichlin, S., R. Saperstein, I.M.D. Jackson, A.E. Boyd III and Y. Patel (1976). Hypothalamic hormones. Annu. Rev. Physiol. 38:389–424.

117. Rivier, J., J. Spiess, M. Thorner and W. Vale (1982). Characterization of a growth hormone-releasing factor from a human pancreatic islet tumor. Nature 300:276–278.

118. Rollag, M.D., R.J. Morgan and G.D. Niswender (1978). Route of melatonin secretion in sheep. Endocrinology. 102:1–8.

119. Rosenkilde, P. (1972). Hypothalamic control of thyroid function in Amphibia. Gen. Comp. Endocrinol. 3:32–40.

120. Saffaran, M. (1974). Chemistry of hypothalamic hypophysiotropic factors. Handbook of Physiology, Sec. 7, Endocrinology. Williams & Wilkins, Baltimore, Vol. 4, Part 2, pp. 563–588.

121. Sage, M. and H.A. Bern (1972). Assay of prolactin in vertebrate pituitaries by its dispersion of xanthophore pigment in the teleost *Gillichthyes mirabilis*. J. Exp. Zool. 180:169–174.

122. Sage, M. and R.J. Parrott (1969). The control of teleost ACTH cells. Z. Vergl. Physiol. 63:85–90.

123. Saint Girons, H. (1970). The pituitary gland. In C. Gans and T.S. Parsons, eds., Biology of the Reptilia, Morphology C., Academic Press, New York, Vol. 3, pp. 135–200.

124. Sathyanesan, A.G. (1965). The hypophysis and hypothalamo-hypophysial system in the chimaeroid fish *Hydrolagus colliei* (Lay and Bennett) with a note on their vascularization. J. Morphol. 166:413–449.

125. Sawin, C.T., P. Bacharach and V. Lance. (1981). Thyrotropin-releasing hormone and thyrotropin in the control of thyroid function in the turtle, *Chrysemys picta*. Gen. Comp. Endocrinol. 45:7–11.

126. Scanes, C.G., S. Dobson, B.K. Follett and J.M. Dodd (1972). Gonadotrophic activity in the pituitary gland of the dogfish *(Scyliorhinus canicula)*. J. Endocrinol. 54:343–344.

127. Schally, A.V., A. Arimura and A.J. Kastin (1973). Hypothalamic regulatory hormones. Science 179:341–350.

128. Scharrer, E. (1951). Neurosecretion. X. A relationship between the paraphysis and the paraventricular nucleus in the garter snake (*Thamnopis* spp.). Biol. Bull. 101:106–113.

129. Sharp, P.J. and B.K. Follett (1968). The blood supply to the pituitary and basal hypothalamus in the Japanese quail. J. Anat. 104:227–232.

130. Shin, S.H. and J. Kracier (1974). LH-RH radioimmunoassay and its applications: Evidence of antigenically distinct FSH-RH and a diurnal study of LH-RH and gonadotropins. Life Sci. 14:281–288.

131. Singh, R.M. and C.J. Dominic (1970). Disposition of the portal vessels of the avian pituitary in relation to the median eminence and the pars distalis. Experientia. 26:962–964.

132. Siperstein, E.R. and K.J. Miller (1970). Further cytophysiologic evidence for the identity of the cells that produce adrenocorticotropic hormone. Endocrinology 86:451–486.

133. Stahl, A. (1963). Cytophysiologie de l'adenohypophyse des poissons (spécialement en relation avec la fonction gonadotrope). In J. Benoit and C. Da Lage, eds., Cytologie de l'adenohypophyse. C.N.R.S., Paris, pp. 331–344.

134. Taurog, A., C. Oliver, R.L. Eskat, J.C. Porter, and J.M. McKenzie (1974). The role of TRH in the neoteny of the Mexican axolotl, *Ambystoma mexicanum*. Gen. Comp. Endocrinol. 24:267–279.

135. Thornton, V.F. and I.I. Geschwind (1974). Hypothalamic control of gonadotropin release in Amphibia: Evidence from studies of gonadotropin release *in vitro* and *in vivo*. Gen. Comp. Endocrinol. 23:294–301.

136. Tixier-Vidal, A. and B.K. Follet (1973). The adenohypophysis. In D.S. Farner and J.R. King, eds., Avian Biology, Academic Press, New York, Vol. 3, pp. 109–182.

137. Tonon, M.C., P. Leroux, M.E. Stoeckel, P. Saulot, S. Jegou, G. Pelletier and H. Vaudry. (1983). Catechoaminergic control of α-melanocyte-stimulating hormone (α-MSH) release by frog neurointermediate lobe *in vitro*. Evidence for a direct stimulation of α-MSH release by thyrotropin-releasing hormone (TRH). Endocrinology 112:133–141.

138. Vale, W., J. Spiess, C. Rivier and J. Rivier (1981). Characterization of a 41-residue ovine hypothalamic peptide that stimulates secretion of corticotropin and β-endorphin. Science 213:1394–1397.

139. Vandescande, F. and M.-R. Aspeslagh (1974). Failure of thyrotropin releasing hormone to increase ^{125}I uptake by the thyroid in *Rana temporaria*. Gen. Comp. Endocrinol. 23:355–356.

140. Van Kemenade, J.A.M. and J.W. Kremers (1975). The pituitary gland of the coelacanth fish *Latimeria chalumnae* Smith: General structure and adenohypophysial cell types. Cell Tissue Res. 163:291–311.

141. Van Oordt, P.G.W.J. (1974). Cytology of the adenohypophysis. In B. Lofts, ed., Physiology of the Amphibia. Academic Press, New York, Vol. 2, pp. 53–106.

142. Van Oordt, P.G.W.J. and J. Peute (1983). The cellular origin of pituitary gonadotropins in teleosts. In W.S. Hoar, D.J. Randall and E.M. Donaldson, eds., Fish Physiology, Academic Press, NY, Vol. 9A, pp. 137–186.

143. Van Overbeeke, A.P. and J.R. McBride (1967). The pituitary gland of the sockeye *(Oncorhynchus nerka)* during sexual maturation and spawning. J. Fish. Res. Bd. Can. 24:1791–1810.

144. Vitums, A.S., S. Mikami, A. Oksche and D.S. Farner (1964). Vascularization of the hypothalamo-hypophysial complex in the white-crowned sparrow, *Zonotrichia leucophys gambelii,* Z. Zellforsch. 64:541–569.

145. Wada, M. (1975). Cell types in the adenohypophysis of the Japanese quail and effects of injections of luteinizing hormone-releasing hormone. Cell Tissue Res. 159:167–178.

146. White, W.F., M.T. Hedlund, G.F. Weber, R.H. Rippel, E.S. Johnson and J.F. Wilber (1974). The pineal gland: A supplemental source of hypothalamic-releasing hormones. Endocrinology 94:1422–1426.

147. Wilber, J.F., E. Montoya, N.P. Plotnikoff, W.F. White, R. Gendrich, L. Renaud and J.B. Martin (1976). Gonadotropin-releasing hormone: Distribution and effects in the central nervous system. Recent. Prog. Horm. Res. 32:117–159.

148. Yoshimura, F., K. Harumiya, H. Ishikawa and Y. Ohtsuka (1969). Differentiation of isolated chromophobes into acidophils or basophils when transplanted into the hypophysiotropic area of hypothalamus. Endocrinol. Jap. 16:531–540.

149. Zoeller, R.T. (1984). The role of luteinizing hormone-releasing hormone in the neuroendocrine control of seasonal reproduction in the rough-skinned newt, *Taricha granulosa.* Ph.D. Dissertation, Oregon State University.

5·Tropic Hormones of the Adenohypophysis

The adenohypophysial tropic hormones are separable into three distinct categories. The hormones within each category exhibit considerable overlap in chemical structures (that is, amino acid sequences) and in some cases overlap in biological activities as well. Category 1 includes the glycoprotein hormones: thyrotropin (TSH), follicle-stimulating hormone (FSH) and luteinizing hormone (LH). Each of these hormones is comprised of two polypeptide subunits, which each contain specific carbohydrate moieties. Growth hormone (GH) and prolactin (PRL) constitute the category 2 tropic hormones. Both PRL and GH are fairly large, single polypeptide chains, and they exhibit considerable structural and some functional overlap. Category 3 includes the smallest adenohypophysial peptides: corticotropin (ACTH), melanotropin (MSH), lipotropin (LPH) and the endorphins. These molecules are similar chemically, and there is overlap in some of their biological activities.

In addition to the three categories of pituitary tropic hormones, certain tropic hormones of similar chemical structure and biological activity are produced in the placental mammals. As many as five tropic-like hormones are produced by the chorionic (fetal) portion of the placenta, including *chorionic gonadotropin* (CG), which is LH-like in both structure and function, and *chorionic somatomammotropin* (CS), which has some GH but mostly PRL-like activity. Both a *chorionic thyrotropin* (CT) and a *chorionic corticotropin* (CC) have been isolated from human placentas and may occur in other mammals as well. Pregnant mares produce large quantities of a placental gonadotropin that has both FSH-like and LH-like properties. This glycoprotein hormone is termed *pregnant mare serum gonadotropin.* The importance of these placental hormones is discussed in Chapter 11.

An additional type of gonadotropin has been obtained from postmenopausal women, *menopausal gonadotropin* (MG). Human MG is basically FSH-like and is produced by the postmenopausal adenohypophysis in large amounts because of the failure of the ovaries to produce adequate levels of estrogens; that is, the normal negative feedback loop is absent. Menopausal gonadotropin has been employed in both clinical and experimental studies, but the advent of synthetic gonadotropins and synthetic gonadotropin-releasing hormone (GnRH) may soon make its use obsolete.

Initially the activities of the various tropic hormones were determined by bioassays. The most commonly employed bioassays are described below. These biological approaches are still used in the biochemical isolation and characterization of tropic hormones, especially in nonmammals. Once highly purified hormones became available, radioimmunoassays (RIA) were developed for several of the mammalian tropic hormones and are routinely employed to measure circulating levels. There are, however, a number of drawbacks to widely employing RIA for measurement of circulating hormone levels. Production of antibodies against hormones purified from pituitary glands may result in an antibody against a prohormone or some portion of the prohormone rather than against the circulating biologically active form. Use of such an antibody might yield results that do not correlate with biological bioassay data. The close similarities in structure among the various tropic hormones of a given category (for example, PRL, GH and CS all have gross structural similarities) may result in cross-reactivities to the antibody produced against only one hormone. The specificity of the antibody for the structure of the purified hormone antigen makes it difficult to use one antibody prepared against sheep FSH to estimate circulating levels of FSH in another species. For example, the endogenous gonadotropins of the sheep and the alligator may be sufficiently different in structure that it is impossible to know whether one is measuring FSH or LH activity or both when assessing the presence of some immunologically active substance in the blood. These problems of structural similarities make it absolutely essential that any RIA be validated against bioassay, especially if the species used for the antibody preparation is not phylogenetically close to the species in which it is being used.

Greater specificity in immunoassay of hormones may be provided by the newer radioreceptor assays. In these assays, hormone receptors are extracted from target tissues removed from animals of the same species. These receptors theoretically should bind preferentially the endogenous circulating hormone with a much higher affinity than for nonhomologous hormones (that is, hormones of other species). Extracted receptors are used in place of the antihormone antibody of the RIA. A radioreceptor assay can readily distinguish between GH and PRL because the receptors are extracted from tissues that will bind only one of the two hormones.[103] Such procedures may have great potential for studies in species in which it is not yet practical to obtain purified hormones for developing a RIA. Because of technical problems, however, it may be some time before this procedure achieves its full potential.[65]

Much of our initial knowledge concerning structures and functions of tropic hormones has come about as a result of the availability of pituitary glands and placentas from slaughtered domestic livestock. Since many differences may occur in the structure of polypeptides with similar but not identical biological activity, it has become increasingly important to designate the source of the hormone used in experimental studies. This is especially true when using mammalian hormones in nonmammals where two different molecules may function similarly in mammals but might provide different results in a nonmammal. Investigators who study mammalian tropic hormones usually designate the source of the hormone such as bovine (cow), ovine (sheep), porcine (pig), equine (horse). An additional lower case letter preceding the abbreviation of a tropic hormone designates the species source. For example, bovine growth hormone would be designated bGH, whereas growth hormone prepared from humans would be hGH. This system is useful only so long as there remain relatively few purified hormones.

Category 1 Tropic Hormones

All of the mammalian glycoprotein tropic hormones examined to date are composed of two peptide subunits with an assortment of carbohydrate moieties attached (see Figs. 5-1, 5-2; Tables 5-1, 5-2). Molecular weights for these glycoproteins are about 32,000 daltons.

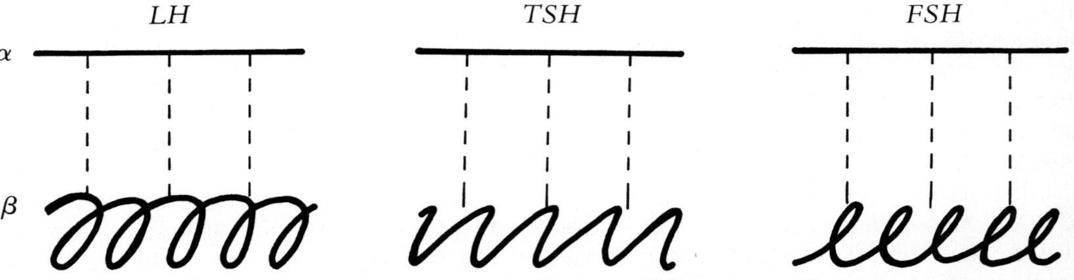

Fig. 5-1. Schematic representation of the structures for the three pituitary glycoprotein hormones. Each hormone consists of a dimer of an alpha peptide that is similar in all three hormones and a beta peptide that is specific for each.

TSH-β: NH_2- Phe- Cys - Ile - Pro - Thr - Glu - Tyr - Met- Met- His - Val - Glu - Arg- Lys -

CHO (attached to Asn)

LH-β: Acyl-Ser - Arg- Gly -Pro- Leu- Arg- Pro - Leu- Cys - Glu - Pro - Ile - Asn - Ala - Thr- Leu - Ala - Ala - Gln - Lys - Glu-

30 CHO (attached to Asn); 40

TSH-β: Glu- Cys- Ala -Tyr- Cys - Leu- Thr - Ile - Asn - Thr- Thr- Val - Cys - Ala - Gly - Tyr - Cys - Met- Thr- Arg-

LH-β: Ala - Cys- Pro -Val - Cys - Ile - Thr - Phe- Thr- Thr- Ser - Ile (Cys, Ala, Gly, Tyr) Cys - Pro - Ser - Met-

50; 60

TSH-β: Asx- Val - Asx -Gly- Lys - Leu- Phe - Leu- Pro - Lys - Tyr- Ala - Leu - Ser - Gln - Asp - Val - Cys - Thr- Tyr - Arg-

LH-β: Lys- Arg- Val -Leu- Pro - Val (Ile, Leu, Pro, Pro) Pro - Met- Pro - Gln - Arg - Val - Cys - Thr- Tyr - His -

70; 80

TSH-β: Asp- Phe- Met-Tyr- Lys - Thr- Ala - Glu- Ile - Pro - Gly - Cys - Pro - Arg- His - Val - Thr- Pro - Tyr - Phe - Ser -

LH-β: Glu- Leu- Arg-Phe- Ala - Ser - Val - Arg- Leu - Pro - Gly (Cys, Pro, Pro, Gly, Val, Asp, Pro) Met- Val - Ser -

90; 100

TSH-β: Tyr- Pro- Val -Ala - Ile - Ser - Cys - Lys - Cys - Gly - Lys - Cys - Asx - Thr- Asx - Tyr - Ser - Asx - Cys - Ile - His -

LH-β: Phe- Pro- Val -Ala - Leu - Ser (Cys, His, Cys, Gly, Pro, Cys) Arg - Leu - Ser - Ser - Thr- Asp - Cys - Gly - Pro-

110; 120

TSH-β: Glu- Ala - Ile -Lys- Thr- Asn- Tyr - Cys- Thr- Lys - Pro - Gln - Lys - Ser - Tyr - Met- COOH

LH-β: Gly- Arg- Thr-Glu- Pro - Leu- Ala - Cys- Asp - His - Pro - Pro - Leu - Pro - Asp - Ile - Leu - COOH

Fig. 5-2. Comparison of amino acid sequences for beta subunits of mammalian TSH and LH. (Modified from Pierce, J.G.[92]).

TABLE 5-1. *Amino Acid Composition (Number of Residues per Molecule) of Subunits Isolated from Human Thyrotropin and Gonadotropins*

AMINO ACID	TSH-α	LH-α	FSH-α	TSH-β	LH-β	FSH-β
Lys	5.5	6.4	5.4	7.7	7.8	3.6
Hist	3.0	3.0	3.0	3.0	—	1.6
Arg	3.1	4.7	3.3	5.5	10.0	2.6
Asp	5.6	6.4	9.3	11.8	8.0	10.3
Thr	7.7	8.7	7.6	11.3	7.3	9.4
Ser	7.1	8.2	7.0	5.7	6.8	6.4
Glu	8.8	10.7	11.1	8.2	8.7	12.0
Pro	6.7	9.7	9.1	8.4	16.3	16.7
Gly	4.5	5.7	6.4	4.8	8.4	4.6
Ala	4.2	4.8	7.7	6.8	5.6	8.2
Cys ($^1/_2$)	10.2	10.4	6.0	12.5	11.9	15.9
Val	7.1	8.4	7.1	5.0	11.8	7.9
Met	3.1	2.7	6.1	2.0	1.8	1.4
Ile	1.8	1.7	3.9	9.8	4.6	4.9
Leu	4.7	5.3	5.3	6.6	8.9	6.1
Tyr	4.8	3.8	3.6	10.5	2.4	3.8
Phe	4.9	4.7	3.8	4.8	2.3	3.8
Trp	—	—	—	—	—	—

Modified from Pierce, J.G.[92]

NOTE: Alpha subunits are arbitrarily expressed relative to histine at 3.0 residues. Beta subunits are expressed to LH-β with 120 residues.

Each hormone consists of an *alpha subunit* that is identical in all three adenohypophysial glycoproteins as well as chorionic gonadotropin. The *beta subunit* is specific to each hormone and is responsible for its unique biological activity. Each subunit is synthesized as a separate pre-subunit, modified and eventually coupled. There is considerable overlap between beta subunits of LH and CG, which have very similar biological activity.

The carbohydrate components of the glycoprotein hormones also slow considerable specificity. Follicle-stimulating hormones contain larger quantities of sialic acid than do the others, and the sialic acid is largely associated with the beta subunit. Sialic acid protects FSH from rapid degradation by the liver. Treatment of FSH with the enzyme *neuraminidase* selectively removes sialic acid and allows it to be degraded rapidly.

It is relatively easy to dissociate these glycoproteins into their respective subunits. These subunits have little if any biological activity by themselves when administered to mammals. It is possible to recombine the dissociated subunits and restore full biological activity. Any

TABLE 5-2. *Percent Carbohydrate Composition of Subunits Isolated from Pituitary Gonadotropins and Thyrotropins*

	ALPHA SUBUNITS			BETA SUBUNITS		
CARBOHYDRATE	TSH-α	LH-α	FSH-α	TSH-β	LH-β	FSH-β
Hexose	7.3	8.3	2.8	3.0	4.3	13.8
Hexosamine	13.3	8.6	2.3	6.9	5.8	7.1
Sialic acid	—	—	0.8	—	—	3.7

Modified from Papkoff, H.[88]

Table 5-3. *Relative Potencies of FSH and LH Purified from Different Vertebrates and Tested in the* Anolis *and* Xenopus *Gonadotropin Bioassays*[65]

HORMONE	RELATIVE POTENCY *ANOLIS* BIOASSAY	*XENOPUS* BIOASSAY
Ovine FSH	100.0[a]	<0.005
Ovine LH	0.04	2.0[b]
Snapping turtle FSH	3.0[a]	0.002
Snapping turtle LH	0.13	1.8[b]
Chicken FSH	4.3[a]	<0.0015
Chicken LH	0.85	0.08[b]
Bullfrog FSH	7.0[a]	0.004
Bullfrog LH	1.2	0.33[b]

[a] *Anolis* Bioassay for FSH: maintenance of testis weight in hypophysectomized lizard.
[b] *Xenopus* bioassay for LH: in-vitro ovulation.

alpha subunit combined with any beta subunit results in a fully active hormone characteristic of the source of the beta subunit. Thus, an alpha subunit isolated from TSH when combined with a beta subunit from FSH yields a glycoprotein with FSH activity and not TSH activity.

Bioassays for FSH

In male mammals FSH typically stimulates spermatogenesis in the testis. In females FSH stimulates follicular growth in the ovary. Follicle-stimulating hormone may also stimulate steroidogenesis in the testis although there is little if any contribution to circulating levels (see Chap. 11).

The major bioassay for FSH prior to development of RIAs was the increase in testis or ovarian weight in hypophysectomized rats.[114] Another specific bioassay for FSH is the maintenance of testis weight in male lizards *Anolis carolinensis* following hypophysectomy. The lizard testis is very unresponsive to LH, and this bioassay is very specific for small quantities of highly purified FSH (Tables 5-3, 5-4).

Bioassays for LH

In contrast to FSH, LH stimulates circulating androgens and estrogens in males and females and causes ovulation and subsequent formation of the corpus luteum in females (see Chap. 11). Luteinizing hormone may also be

Table 5-4. *Relative Effectiveness of Purified Ovine Gonadotropin (FSH and LH) in Some Gonadotropin Bioassays*[65]

BIOASSAY	MINIMAL EFFECTIVE DOSE (μg/ML OR μg/INJECTIONS[a]) FSH	LH	RELATIVE POTENCY
A. Testis weight maintenance in hypox lizard (*Anolis carolinensis*)	0.01	20.0	FSH>>LH
B. In-vitro ovulation of frog ovary (*Xenopus laevis*)	>200.0	0.5	LH>>>FSH
C. Spermiation response by frog (*Hyla regilla*)	0.5	1.0	FSH ≅ LH

[a] Injection for bioassays A and C.

responsible for progesterone synthesis and release by the corpus luteum. In males, LH causes release of mature spermatozoa from the testes (spermiation). Major actions for LH are the stimulation of steroid secretion and gamete release, whereas FSH is primarily involved with gamete preparation (follicle development in females and spermatogenesis in males). Since three pituitary tropic hormones are named for their actions in females (PRL, FSH and LH), it seems reasonable that at least one of these, LH, might be renamed for its action on the androgen-producing cells that occur between the seminiferous tubules of the testis rather than for inducing corpus luteum formation (luteinization) in the female. Hence it was suggested that LH be named the *interstitial cell-stimulating hormone* for its action on the steroidogenic *interstitial cell* (Leydig cell) of the testis. Equality of the sexes has not been realized, however, and the feminist name of LH has remained.

Numerous bioassays have been developed for quantitatively measuring LH activity. One of the first bioassays was the spermiation response observed following injection of pituitary extracts or purified LH into frogs or toads.[46] At one time this bioassay was widely employed to detect the presence of CG in urine of women. The structural and functional similarity of the hCG and hLH to amphibian gonadotropins is the basis for this bioassay. A spermiation test, however, responds to highly purified FSH and cannot be considered a specific bioassay for LH-like hormones.[65] Pregnancy is now determined from urine samples with a simple immunoassay involving an antibody produced against hCG.

A popular bioassay for LH is the *ovarian ascorbic acid depletion test* (OAAD), which is based upon a quantitative reduction of ascorbic acid in ovarian tissue following administration of LH.[90] The degree of depletion is proportional to the dose of LH, and this bioassay is not affected by FSH. The relationship of ascorbic acid to hormone secretion is not understood, however. The pigment response to LH by feathers of the African weaver finch *Euplectes franciscanus* is also specific for LH or CG,[93] but it is not employed routinely.

The specific response of amphibian ovaries in vitro to LH or CG (ovulation) has resulted in development of several similar bioassays.[65,100,105,113] Administration of pituitary LH or progesterone is the most potent stimulator of ovulation in isolated fragments of anuran or urodele ovaries. Luteinizing hormone causes progesterone synthesis in follicular cells surrounding the oocyte, and it is progesterone that induces the ovulatory event.[110] The system is responsive to some other steroids but is unresponsive to other tropic hormones.

Bioassays for TSH

Stimulation of thyroid gland function can be quantified cytologically by means of the TSH dose-dependent increase in epithelial height of the thyroid follicles in hypophysectomized animals. A more rapid technique involves measurement of the rate at which an injected dose of radioactive iodide (radioiodide) is accumulated by thyroid follicles.[114] This bioassay can also be performed in vitro so that other variables can be eliminated. These parameters indicate only the degree of TSH-stimulation proportional to circulating TSH levels but provide no consistent information concerning rates of thyroid hormone synthesis and release from the stimulated thyroid gland (see Chap. 8).

The human has been shown to produce variant TSHs, one of which is associated with a pathological condition known as Graves' disease. Normal TSH has a biological half-life of about 0.25 hours, and maximum radioiodide uptake in thyroids of hypophysectomized rats is observed 4 hours after TSH administration. The abnormal TSH has a biological half-life of 7.5 hours and causes maximum radioiodide uptake 12 hours after administration. This so-called *long-acting thyroid-stimulator* is frequently employed in mammalian studies of thyroid function.

Category 2 Tropic Hormones

Two pituitary tropic hormones, GH and PRL, plus one placental tropic hormone, CS, comprise category 2. Prolactin and GH are large single polypeptide hormones of similar structure (Fig. 5-3) and molecular weight (about 23,000). Human CS is extremely similar to both hGH and PRL (Fig. 5-3). There is an 85% homology between hGH and hCS as well as a 48% overlap with ovine PRL. Both GH and PRL produce a number of common effects on osmoregulation (renal function, intestinal fluid absorption), selective tissue growth (prostate gland, sebaceous gland), lactation and other processes.[81] Ovine PRL and hCS have only weak effects on body growth, however.[17] The human placenta also produces PRL which accumulates in amniotic fluid. This placental PRL is indistinguishable from pituitary PRL.[32]

Growth Hormone

Growth hormone is often termed a protein anabolic hormone because it stimulates incorporation of amino acids into proteins. It is assayed biologically by means of the somewhat cumbersome measurement of the thickness of the epiphysial cartilage in the tibia of the hypophysectomized rat or mouse.[114] Currently RIA techniques are employed routinely to measure blood and pituitary content of GH in mammals.

Growth hormone represents about one half of the total hormone content of the human adenohypophysis. It has been characterized as a protein composed of 191 amino acids (MW = 21,500)[56] having a biological half life in blood of 20 to 40 minutes. Human GH has been synthesized in the laboratory. Crude GH preparations consist of a collection of protein isohormones. Each form is thought to have its own actions, and collectively they produce all the effects normally attributed to pituitary GH activity. The gene responsible for synthesis of the 21,500 dalton form of GH has been constructed and inserted successfully into the genome of mice.[87] Growth rates of mice with the inserted genes and growth rates of their offspring are about twice that of normal mice.

Growth hormone secretion can be increased by rising levels of certain amino acids (for example, arginine), and GH in turn lowers blood levels of amino acids through stimulation of protein synthesis. Secretion of GH is also stimulated by low blood glucose levels and is inhibited by high ones. Growth hormone cooperates with insulin to channel utilization of these nutrients following a meal (see Chaps. 13 and 19). Furthermore, GH becomes an important regulator of blood glucose and amino acid utilization during short-term and long-term starvation.

Circulating levels of hGH are highest during the period of maximum growth (ages 2 to 17 years). A daily secretory rhythm becomes established at about 4 years of age and continues throughout adult life. This pattern of GH secretion is both irregular and spontaneous, depending upon the physiological state of the individual, but episodes of GH release are frequently correlated with the onset of deep sleep.[17]

Optimum growth-promoting actions of GH are obtained in hypophysectomized animals only when thyroid hormones are administered together with GH. This relationship between thyroid hormones and GHs has been described as a synergism (Chap. 1), that is, the growth response elicited by combined therapy with thyroid hormones and GH is greater than predicted by adding together the responses obtained with each hormone administered alone. Either thyroid hormones or GH will reinitiate some growth in hypophysectomized animals, but complete resumption of normal growth requires combined therapy. Furthermore, animals that exhibit thyroid deficiencies grow slowly and abnormally (see Chap. 8).

Thyroid hormones may influence growth in two ways. They stimulate synthesis of GH in intact rats, but their action pertinent to the effect in hypophysectomized animals is a peripheral one.[95] Thyroid hormones maintain a "responsive state" in the target cells so that they are more sensitive to GH (see Chap. 8 for more details of this "permissive" effect). Androgens and estrogens to a lesser extent can increase the responsiveness of human tissues to hGH, but the mechanism is not understood. The influence of steroids on amino acid and carbohydrate metabolism is discussed in Chapter 19.

Another growth-related action of GH is the liberation of small peptides (mol wt = 6000–9000) from circulating plasma proteins. These peptides were first called sulfation factors because of effects on incorporation of sulfate into cartilage. They are now known as *somatomedins.*[17,108] Several peptides have been isolated

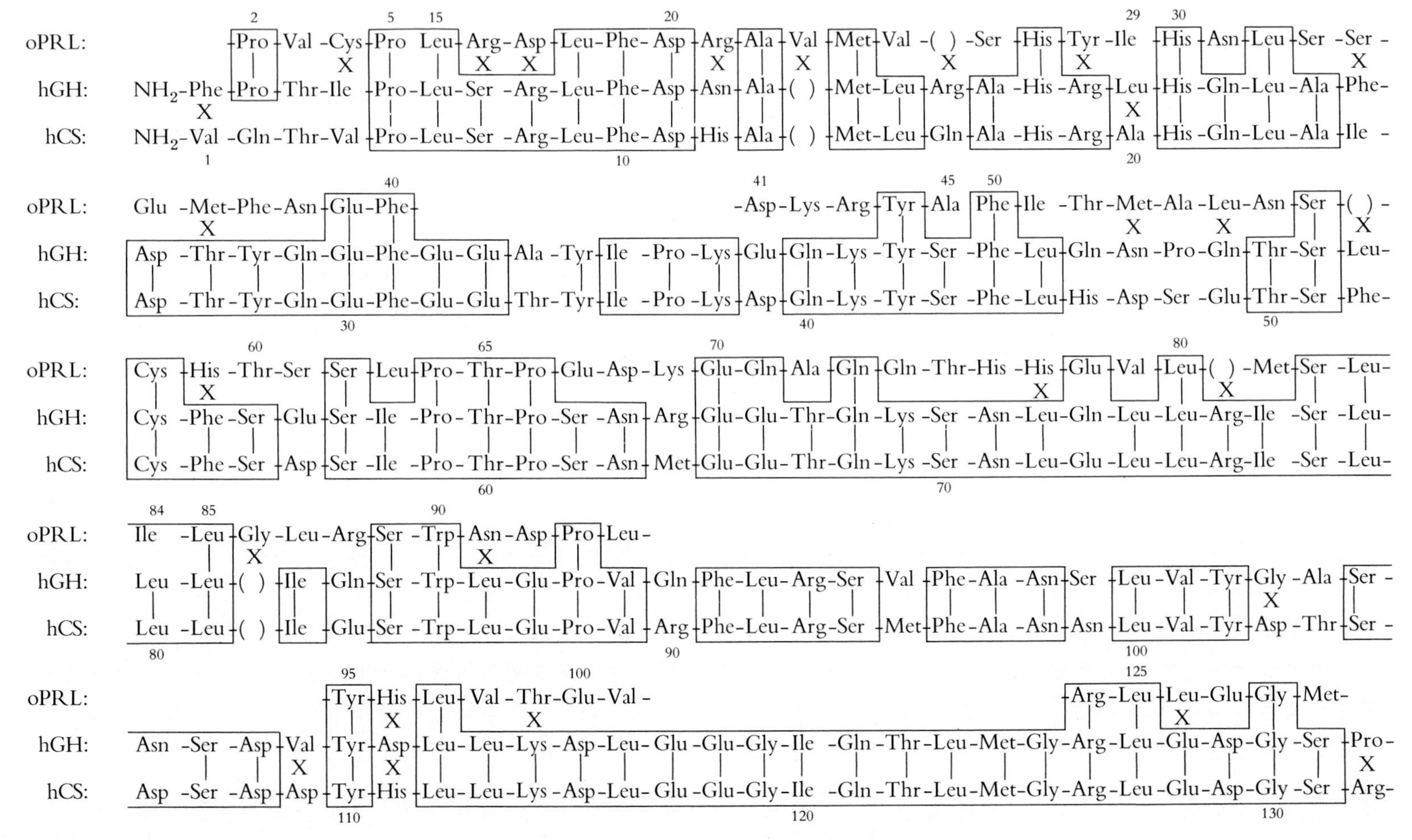

oPRL: Pro Val Cys Pro Leu Arg Asp Leu Phe Asp Arg Ala Val Met Val ( ) Ser His Tyr Ile His Asn Leu Ser Ser
hGH: NH2-Phe Pro Thr Ile Pro Leu Ser Arg Leu Phe Asp Asn Ala ( ) Met Leu Arg Ala His Arg Leu His Gln Leu Ala Phe
hCS: NH2-Val Gln Thr Val Pro Leu Ser Arg Leu Phe Asp His Ala ( ) Met Leu Gln Ala His Arg Ala His Gln Leu Ala Ile
oPRL: Glu Met Phe Asn Glu Phe Asp Lys Arg Tyr Ala Phe Ile Thr Met Ala Leu Asn Ser ( )
hGH: Asp Thr Tyr Gln Glu Phe Glu Glu Ala Tyr Ile Pro Lys Glu Gln Lys Tyr Ser Phe Leu Gln Asn Pro Gln Thr Ser Leu
hCS: Asp Thr Tyr Gln Glu Phe Glu Glu Thr Tyr Ile Pro Lys Asp Gln Lys Tyr Ser Phe Leu His Asp Ser Glu Thr Ser Phe
oPRL: Cys His Thr Ser Ser Leu Pro Thr Pro Glu Asp Lys Glu Gln Ala Gln Gln Thr His His Glu Val Leu ( ) Met Ser Leu
hGH: Cys Phe Ser Glu Ser Ile Pro Thr Pro Ser Asn Arg Glu Glu Thr Gln Lys Ser Asn Leu Gln Leu Leu Arg Ile Ser Leu
hCS: Cys Phe Ser Asp Ser Ile Pro Thr Pro Ser Asn Met Glu Glu Thr Gln Lys Ser Asn Leu Glu Leu Leu Arg Ile Ser Leu
oPRL: Ile Leu Gly Leu Arg Ser Trp Asn Asp Pro Leu
hGH: Leu Leu ( ) Ile Gln Ser Trp Leu Glu Pro Val Gln Phe Leu Arg Ser Val Phe Ala Asn Ser Leu Val Tyr Gly Ala Ser
hCS: Leu Leu ( ) Ile Glu Ser Trp Leu Glu Pro Val Arg Phe Leu Arg Ser Met Phe Ala Asn Asn Leu Val Tyr Asp Thr Ser
oPRL: Tyr His Leu Val Thr Glu Val Arg Leu Leu Glu Gly Met
hGH: Asn Ser Asp Val Tyr Asp Leu Leu Lys Asp Leu Glu Glu Gly Ile Gln Thr Leu Met Gly Arg Leu Glu Asp Gly Ser Pro
hCS: Asp Ser Asp Asp Tyr His Leu Leu Lys Asp Leu Glu Glu Gly Ile Gln Thr Leu Met Gly Arg Leu Glu Asp Gly Ser Arg

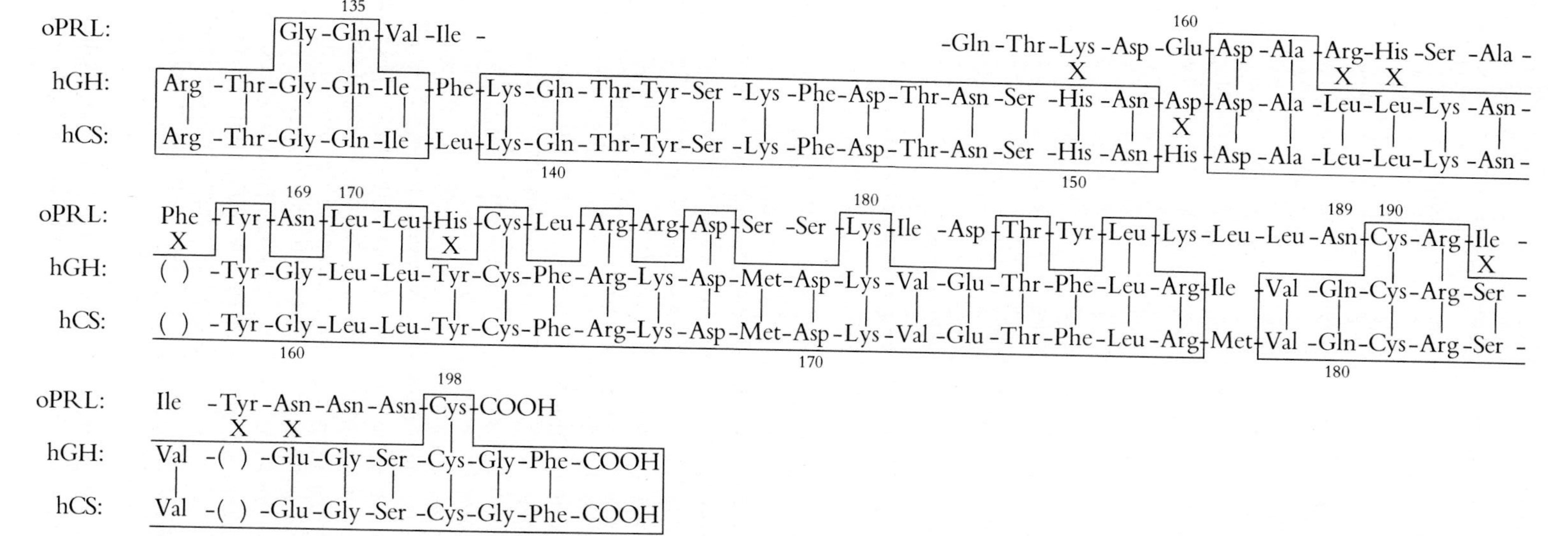

Fig. 5-3. Comparison of the amino acid sequences of some Category 2 pituitary hormones: ovine prolactin *(oPRL)*, human growth hormone *(hGH)* and human somatomammotropin *(hCS)*. Unrelated amino acid pairs, X. (Modified from Li, C.H. (1974). Chemistry of ovine prolactin. Handbook of Physiology, Sec. 7, Endocrinology. Williams & Wilkins, Baltimore, Vol. 4, Part 2, pp. 103–110).

TABLE 5-5. *Comparison of Amino Acid Composition of Some Growth Hormones*

AMINO ACID	HUMAN	BOVINE	OVINE	EQUINE	PORCINE	CANINE	RABBIT	RAT
Lys	9	11.5	13	9.5	11	11.5	10	10
His	3	3	3	3	3	3	3	3
Arg	11	13	13	12	12	12	12	9.5
Asp	20	16	16	14	15	17	14	14.5
Thr	10	12	12	7	7	9	7	7
Ser	18	12.5	12	13	14	16	12	11.5
Glu	26	24.5	25	21	24	25	22	22
Pro	8	6	8	7	7	9.5	6	7
Gly	8	10	10	9	8	9	9	8.5
Ala	7	14	14	14.5	16	18.5	13	14
Cys (½)	4	4	4	3	4	4	3	2.5
Val	7	6	7	7	8	7.5	6	6
Met	3	4	4	2.5	3	3	3	4
Ile	8	7	7	5.5	6	6	4	6.5
Leu	26	25.5	22	21	24	25	21	18
Tyr	8	6	6	5.5	7	7	6	5.5
Phe	13	13	13	9	12	12.5	10	9
Trp	1	1	1	2	1	—	1	1

After Wilhelmi.[111]
NOTE: Values calculated in terms of moles of amino acid per 22,000 g protein.

that exhibit somatomedin activities. Two of these (somatomedins A and C) stimulate formation of cartilage, whereas another (somatomedin B) stimulates incorporation of ^{3}H-thymidine by glial cells and fibroblasts (that is, stimulates new DNA synthesis and cellular division). Two of these growth stimulators are structurally related to insulin and have some insulin activity (see Chap. 13) in addition to their growth-promoting actions. They are known as insulinlike growth factors I and II (IGF I, IGF II). Thus, GH controls proliferation of cartilage that serves as the matrix for bone formation via release of plasma-bound somatomedin. A bioassay for somatomedin has been developed using costal cartilage from pigs in vitro.[102] Somatomedin activity has been demonstrated in plasma from three primates, including man, as well as from domestic pigs, cows, sheep, goats, horses, donkeys, dogs, rabbits, guinea pigs and rats.

Prolactin

Prolactin also occurs in multiple isohormones and has been shown to produce a variety of distinctive actions in animals, including effects associated with reproduction, growth, osmoregulation and the integument (Table 5-6). In addition, PRL may produce synergistic actions with ovarian, testicular, thyroid and adrenal hormones. The best-known action for PRL is the lactogenic effect on the mammary gland of female animals for which the hormone was named. Prolactin stimulates the synthesis of milk proteins by the mammary gland. A similar effect is produced by CS from the placenta. In some species PRL may also influence the synthesis of progesterone by the corpus luteum. There is evidence in male mammals for effects of PRL on certain sex accessory structures. These actions of PRL are discussed more extensively in Chapter 11 with respect to the overall regulation of reproduction in mammals.

PROLACTIN BIOASSAYS. Several specific bioassays for PRL have been reported utilizing animals representing four major vertebrate classes (teleosts, amphibians, birds and mammals):

1. The sodium-retaining bioassay in the cichlid teleost, tilapia, *Sarotherodon (Tilapia) mossambicus*[14]

TABLE 5-6. *Actions of Mammalian Prolactins in Vertebrates*

A. Actions related to reproduction

Teleosts

- Skin mucous secretion (e.g., discus "milk")
- Reduction of toxic effects of estrogen
- Growth and secretion of seminal vesicles
- Parental behavior (nest building, fin fanning, buccal incubation of eggs)
- Maintenance of brood pouch in male seahorse
- Gonadotropic

Amphibians

- Water-drive (prior to reproduction)
- Secretion of oviductal jelly
- Spermatogenic and/or antispermatogenic
- Ovulation
- Stimulation of cloacal gland development

Reptiles

- Antigonadotropic

Birds

- Production of crop "milk"
- Formation of brood patch
- Antigonadal
- Premigratory restlessness
- Parental behavior
- Synergism with steroids on female reproductive tract
- Suppression of sexual phase of reproductive cycle

Mammals

- Mammary development and lactation
- Preputial gland size and activity
- Synergism with androgen on male sex accessory glands
- Luteotropic in rodents
- Fertility in dwarf mice
- Increased testis cholesterol
- Increased androgen binding in human prostate
- Stimulation of glucuronidase activity in rodent testis
- Parental behavior
- Decreased copulatory activity in male rabbits
- Advanced puberty in rats
- Vaginal mucification in rats
- Antiovulatory and antiluteinizing actions in rats
- Relaxation of uterine cervix in rats
- Reduced catabolism of progesterone by rat uterus
- Inhibition of myometrial contractions
- Increased estradiol binding by rat uterus
- Decreased GTH release

B. Actions related to growth and development

Teleosts

- Proliferation of melanocytes
- Growth of seminal vesicles
- Renal glomerular growth, tubule stimulation and proliferation

Amphibians

- Tail and gill growth
- Limb regeneration
- Proliferation of melanophores
- Structural changes accompanying water drive
- Brain growth in tadpoles
- Cloacal gland development
- Ultimobranchial stimulation

Reptiles

- Tail regeneration
- Skin sloughing

Birds

- Proliferation of pigeon crop-sac mucosa
- Epidermal hyperplasia in brood patch
- Feather growth
- Development of female reproductive tract

Mammals

- Mammary development
- Sebaceous and preputial gland growth
- Hair growth
- Erythropoietic actions
- Renotropic actions
- Spermatogenic actions
- Male sex accessory development

C. Actions related to water and electrolyte balance

Cyclostomes

- Electrolyte metabolism in hagfish

Teleosts

- Survival of hypophysectomized euryhaline freshwater species
- Restoration of water turnover in hypophysectomized *Fundulus kansae*
- Restoration of plasma Na^{+} and Ca^{++} in hypophysectomized eels when given with cortisol
- Skin, buccal and gill mucous secretion
- Reduced gill Na^{+} efflux (reduced permeability)
- Reduced gill permeability to water
- Inhibition of gill Na^{+}-K^{+} ATPase
- Renotropic action (increased glomerular size)
- Increased urinary water elimination and decreased salt excretion

TABLE 5-6. *Actions of Mammalian Prolactins in Vertebrates (Continued)*

Stimulation of renal Na^+-K^+ ATPase
Decreased water absorption and increased Na^+ absorption in flounder bladder
Decreased salt and water absorption from eel gut
Amphibians
Skin and electrolyte changes associated with water drive, metamorphosis
Sodium and water transport across toad bladder
Restoration of plasma Na^+ in hypophysectomized newts
Possible hypercalcemia in toads
Reptiles
Restoration of plasma Na^+ levels in hypophysectomized lizard
Birds
Stimulation of nasal (orbital) salt gland secretion
Mammals
Lactation
Increased Na^+ retention at renal level
Corticotropic

D. Actions on integumentary structures
Teleosts
Reduced gill Na^+ efflux
Reduced gill permeability to water
Inhibition of gill Na^+-K^+ ATPase
Restoration of water turnover in hypophysectomized *Fundulus kansae*
Skin, buccal and gill mucous secretion
Melanogenesis and proliferation of melanocytes (synergism with MSH)
Dispersal of yellow pigment in cutaneous xanthophores (?)
Maintenance of brood pouch in male seahorse
Amphibians
Skin changes associated with water drive
Proliferation of melanophores
Effects on toad bladder
Skin yellowing in frogs
Reptiles
Epidermal sloughing
Birds
Production of crop "milk"
Formation of brood patch
Stimulation of feather growth
Stimulation of nasal gland secretion
Mammals
Mammary development and lactation
Sebaceous and preputial gland size and activity
Hair maturation

E. Actions on steroid-dependent targets or synergisms with steroids on targets
Cyclostomes
Electrolyte metabolism in hagfish
Teleosts
Na^+ retention by gills (corticosteroids)
Na^+ retention by kidney (corticosteroids)
Salt and water movement in gut (corticosteroids)
Synergism with androgens on catfish seminal vesicles
Dispersal of yellow pigment in xanthophores (corticosteroids) (?)
Maintenance of brood pouch in male seahorse (corticosteroids)
Amphibians
Stimulation of oviductal jelly secretion (estrogens and progestogens)
Na^+ transport across anuran bladder (aldosterone)
Water-drive structural changes (sex steroids)
Spermatogenesis (androgens)
Cloacal gland development (androgens)
Reptiles
Restoration of plasma Na^+ levels in hypophysectomized lizard (corticosteroids)
Antigonadotropic actions (sex steroids?)
Birds
Formation of brood patch (synergism with ovarian or testicular steroids)
Parental behavior (possible progesterone synergism)
Synergism with estrogens and progestogens on female reproductive tract
Stimulation of nasal (orbital) gland secretion (corticosteroids)
Stimulation of feather growth (sex steroids in some species)
Antigonadotropic actions (sex steroids?)
Mammals
Mammary growth (ovarian steroids)
Milk secretion (corticosteroids)
Sebaceous and preputial gland secretion (gonadal and cortical steroids)
Growth and secretion of male sex accessory glands (androgens)
Luteotropic action (estrogens?)
Renal Na^+ reabsorption (aldosterone?) and renotropic action (androgens)
Spermatogenesis (androgens)
Advanced puberty (gonadal steroids)
Hair growth (androgens, corticosteroids)
Vaginal mucification in rats (estrogen and progesterone)

Modified from Nicoll[79] with additions from other sources.

2. The xanthophore-expanding bioassay in the teleost *Gillichthyes mirabilis*[97]
3. The red-eft water drive performed in the newt *Notophthalmus viridescens*[35]
4. The crop-sac assay performed in the domestic pigeon[78]
5. The in-vitro mouse mammary gland assay[52,68,106]

The extremely similar structures of GHs and PRLs within and among species makes specific RIA for either PRL or GH difficult, and extreme caution should be used when interpreting RIA data, especially the use of mammalian PRL antibodies in nonmammals.[80] This point will be emphasized by the discussions of these hormones in nonmammals that follow.

Sodium-Retaining Bioassay in Teleosts. This bioassay stresses the osmoregulatory actions of PRL in teleostean fishes (see Chap. 16), and particularly its effect on sodium uptake across the gill and resultant alterations in plasma sodium levels. Only some pituitaries from teleostean species, however, will produce a measurable response in this bioassay, and all other piscine and other nonmammalian preparations are inactive. Purified mammalian PRLs, curiously, work very well in this bioassay. A similar bioassay was developed prior to this one that employed hypophysectomized guppies, *Poecilia latipinna.*[23] The intact tilapia bioassay is simpler because of the larger size of the assay animal and because hypophysectomy is unnecessary. Adaptation of these fishes to seawater almost eliminates PRL from the circulation.[14]

Xanthophore-Expanding Bioassay in Gillichthyes. This bioassay is performed in the gobiid fish *Gillichthyes mirabilis,* the long-jawed mud sucker. It is an all-or-none bioassay for determination of the smallest dose of purified hormone or the greatest dilution of pituitary homogenate or extract that will cause local yellowing in 50% of the fish tested following injection of the test material beneath the preopercular skin. The bioassay does have the distinct advantage, however, of being extremely sensitive to piscine (including agnathan) and amphibian pituitary homogenates. For example, teleostean pituitaries are more than 100,000 times more effective in the assay than is ovine PRL that is used as a standard.[98] As little as 1/100th of a tiger salamander pituitary gives a positive response in the xanthophore-expanding bioassay, whereas an entire pituitary of the same size is required to produce a minimal response in the pigeon crop-sac bioassay.[86] The specificity of this bioassay is questioned by the failure of purified tilapia (teleost) PRL to produce a typical response, suggesting that the bioassay may be measuring some contaminant rather than PRL.

Red-Eft Water-Drive Bioassay. Prolactin induces a second metamorphosis or "water drive" in newts (see Chaps. 8, 17) that is characterized by migration of the juvenile terrestrial form, the eft, back to water where breeding will occur. Water-drive behavior is accompanied by a series of physiological and morphological changes as well, but these are not related to the bioassay per se. Following injection of PRL the efts will leave the dry areas of their laboratory containers and submerge themselves in water. No other hormone has been found to induce water-drive behavior. This bioassay has the disadvantage of being an all-or-none response. Pituitary preparations for all classes of vertebrates except the class Agnatha, possess water-drive–inducing activity (Table 5-7).

Pigeon Crop-Sac Bioassay. The pigeon crop-sac bioassay was briefly described in Chapter 1. This bioassay has the advantage over the previously described assays of being a quantitative, dose-related bioassay. Consequently a standard curve may be prepared and relative activities of unknown preparations quantitatively assessed. The disadvantages of the crop-sac bioassay are the time involved in performing it and the fact that most piscine PRLs will produce only an atypical response or no response at all (Table 5-7). Positive results have been obtained with lungfish pituitaries as well as pituitaries from all tetrapod groups[79] (Table 5-7).

Mammary Gland In-vitro Bioassay. Mammary gland explants from pseudopregnant or midpregnant mice (or rabbits) are cultured in a precise medium that includes some other hormones. The addition of PRL or pituitary homogenates to the culture medium causes cytological changes that can be quantified according to a numerical index (Fig. 5-4). These cytological changes are correlated with the ability of PRL to stimulate milk synthesis.

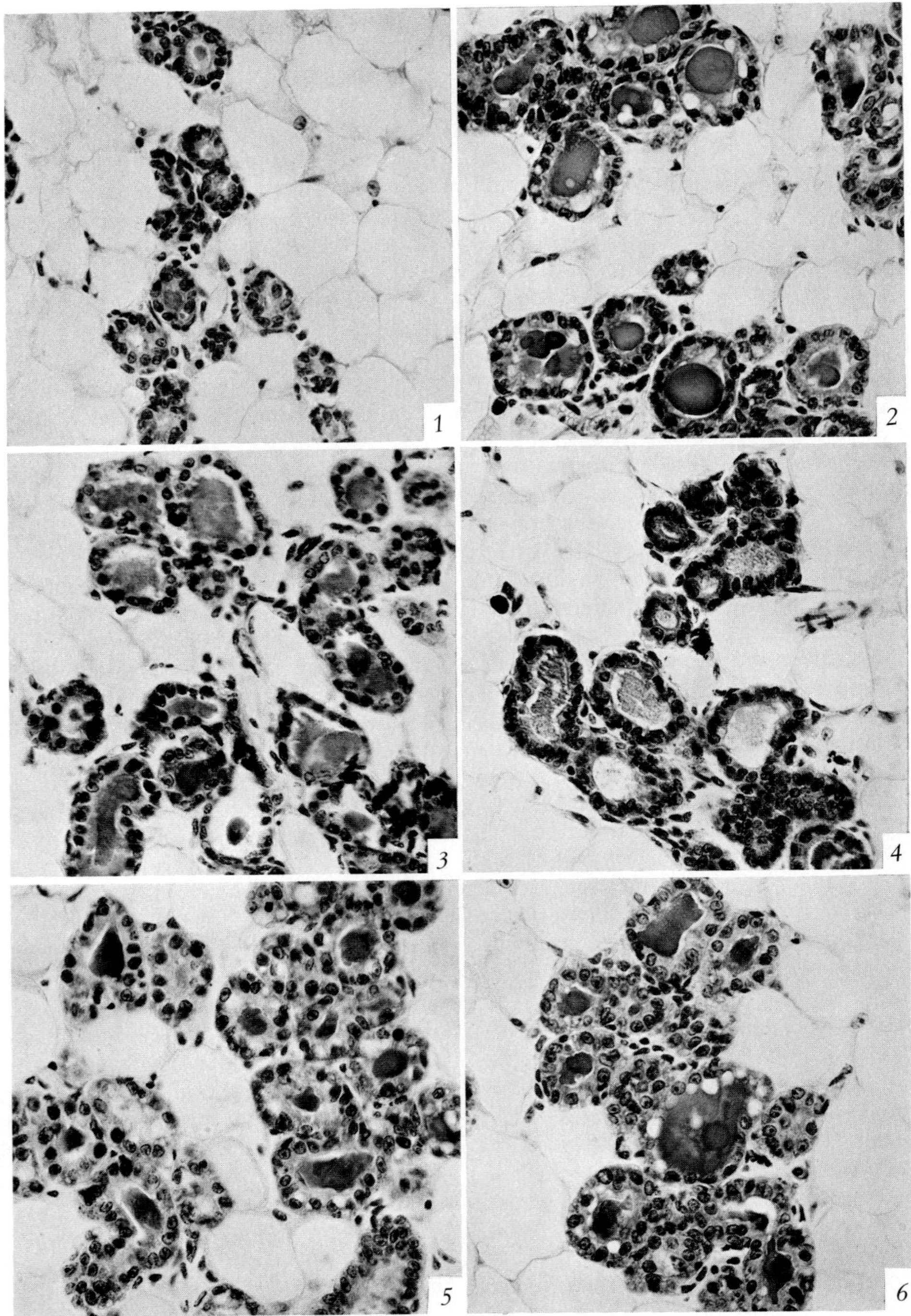
1
2
3
4
5
6

FIG. 5-4. Mouse mammary gland in vitro bioassay for tetrapod prolactins. Secretion rating (SR) is on a scale of 1 to 5. (Reprinted with permission from Nicoll, C.S., H.A. Bern and D. Brown (1966). Occurrence of mammotrophic activity [prolactin] in the vertebrate adenohypophysis. J. Endocrinol. 34:343–354.)

1. Control explant in maintenance culture medium containing insulin and aldosterone. The alveoli of the cultured gland are not distended and contain only a small amount of secretion. SR = 1.
2. Addition of Necturus pituitaries (Amphibia). SR = 5.
3. Addition of turtle pituitaries (Reptilia). SR = 4.
4. Addition of pigeon pituitaries (Aves). SR = 3.
5. Addition of guinea pig pituitaries (Mammalia). SR = 4.
6. Addition of purified mammalian prolactin. SR = 5.

Mammotropic (lactogenic) activity is present in the pituitaries of all tetrapod species, but piscine pituitary preparations yield minimal responses, if any (Table 5-7). Like the other bioassays the mammary gland response is not a rapid assessment.

An Electrophoretic Assay. An assay for PRLs has been developed involving electrophoresis of hormone-containing extracts on polyacrylamide gels (Fig. 5-5) followed by densitometric quantification.[13,83,84] Prolactin molecules migrate as a distinguishable band of protein in the gel, and the position of the PRL band in a gel prepared from an "unknown" source can be compared to purified PRL in another gel. Migration to identical positions is evidence of the presence of PRL in the unknown. The protein bands in the gel may be stained with a general protein stain (for example, amido Schwartz). The intensity of staining, which is proportional to the quantity of PRL in the band, can be determined with the aid of a densitometer. Growth hormone can be readily distinguished from PRL because the latter migrates through the gel well ahead of GH. This technique is utilized to prepare relatively pure preparations of tropic hormones as well. Initially, however, it was essential to locate and quantitate PRL activity and GH activity by bioassaying the banded proteins.

Category 3 Tropic Hormones

Corticotropin and lipotropin are associated with the pars distalis components of the adenohypophysis, whereas MSH is found primarily in the pars intermedia. All of these hormones are similar in structure (Fig. 5-6) and overlap considerably with respect to biological activities.

TABLE 5-7. *Bioassayable Prolactin in Vertebrate Pituitaries*

VERTEBRATE GROUP	*GILLICHTHYES*[a] XANTHOPHORE–YELLOWING RESPONSE	TILAPIA NA^{+}–RETAINING RESPONSE	RED–EFT WATER DRIVE	PIGEON CROP–SAC ASSAY	MOUSE MAMMARY IN VITRO
Agnatha	+	–	–	–	–
Chondrichthyes	+	–	+	–	–
Chondrostei	+	–	?	–	–
Holostei	+	–	?	–	–
Teleostei	+	+, –	+	–	–[b]
Dipnoi	+	–	+	+	+
Amphibia	+	–	+	+	+
Reptilia	+	?	+	+	+
Aves	+	?	+	+	+
Mammalia	+	+, –	+	+	+

[a] This assay system may not be specific for prolactin (see text).
[b] Purified tilapia PRL stimulates casein synthesis in the rabbit mammary gland.[45]

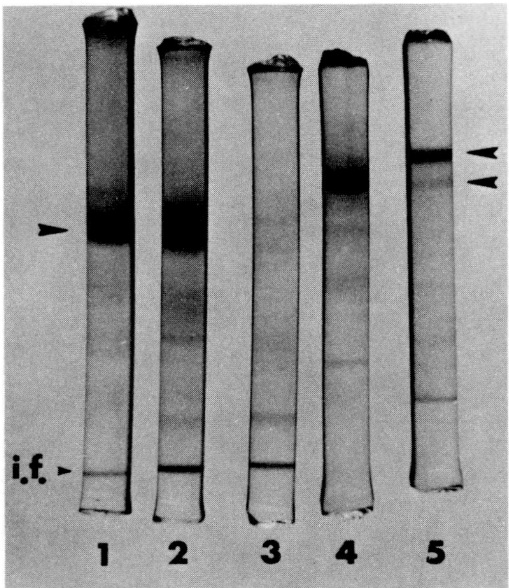

Fig. 5-5. Identification of pituitary prolactin in teleosts using polyacrylamide gel electrophoresis. Prolactin is indicated for homogenates of rostral *(1)* and proximal *(2)* pars distalis and from pars intermedia *(3)* from tilapia *(Sarotherodon mossambicus)* and from rostral *(4)* and proximal *(5)* pars distalis of *Cichlasoma labiatum. i.f.*, solvent front. A single prominent band of stained prolactin appears in both pars distalis preparations from tilapia, but two different bands appear in the rostral *(4)* and proximal *(5)* pars distalis homogenates from *Cichlasoma.* These stained bands can be quantified densitometrically. Reproduced by permission of the National Research Council of Canada from the Canadian Journal of Zoology, Volume 51, pp. 687–695, 1973. A copy of the original photograph was provided by Dr. W. Craig Clarke.)

Corticotropin

Mammalian ACTH has been purified from several mammalian sources (bovine, porcine, ovine, human). It has 39 amino acids in a single peptide chain with a molecular weight of about 4500. Amino acids 1–23 of ACTH have full biological activity, 1–19 have 80% of full activity, but fragment 1–16 has very little biological activity. Amino acids 24–39 are obviously outside of that region of the molecule responsible for its biological activity. A synthetic peptide identical to amino acids 1–24 has been prepared; it is known as *beta corticotropin.* The structures of the active fragments of several mammalian ACTHs are provided in Figure 5-7, and comparisons to other category 3 hormones are made in Figure 5-6.

The classical bioassay for ACTH has been the *adrenal ascorbic acid depletion* test (AAAD), which is similar to the OAAD bioassay for LH.[114] The lowest effective dose of purified ACTH in this bioassay is 0.2 mU or about 1.2×10^{-9}g (about 1 ng). The adrenal cortex secretes certain corticosteroids in response to ACTH stimulation (see Chap. 10), but the relationship of ascorbic acid to steroid secretion is not understood. The AAAD test is rather cumbersome, however, and it has generally been replaced by measurement of either circulating ACTH or corticosteroids with RIA.

Melanotropin

The name of this tropic hormone stems actually from its actions in amphibians and reptiles where it causes dispersion of melanin pigment granules contained within a specialized cell, the melanophore, located in the skin. Dispersal of these melanin granules causes the animal to appear darker. Consequently the standard bioassays for MSH have been developed in amphibians and reptiles utilizing their ability to adapt to dark or light backgrounds. One bioassay involves measurement of the quantity of light reflected (using a reflectometer) from an isolated piece of skin removed from a light-adapted frog. A similar bioassay employs isolated pieces of skin from the light-background-adapted *Anolis carolinensis,* the American chameleon. A rapid all-or-none response (darkening) occurs in vitro.[20]

The adenohypophyses of all vertebrates tested possess MSH activity, including birds that lack a pars intermedia. However, physiological roles for MSH have not been shown in birds or in most mammals. A physiological role has not been established for MSH in fishes, but their pigmentary changes apparently are under dual sympathetic-parasympathetic innervation, allowing for rapid responses. The physiological roles for MSH are discussed in Chapter 6.

Three mammalian MSH molecules have been identified, and a given mammal typically possesses two of these. *Alpha MSH* consists of only 13 amino acids, and *beta MSH* has about 22. Beta-Ser-MSH has been isolated from sheep. The structure of human beta MSH is compared to alpha MSH and other category 3 hormones in Figures 5-6.

Hormone	Source	Common amino acid sequences																	
		1	2	3	4	5	6	7	8	9	10	11	12	13	14	15	16	17	18
β-MSH	porcine	Asp	Glu	Gly	Pro	Tyr	Lys	Met	Glu	His	Phe	Arg	Tyr	Gly	Ser	Pro	Pro	Lys	Asp
ACTH	porcine, ovine				1	2	3	4	5	6	7	8	9	10	11	12	13	14	15
					Ser	Tyr	Ser	Met	Glu	His	Phe	Arg	Tyr	Gly	Lys	Pro	Val	Gly	Lys. . .
α-MSH	porcine, equine				1	2	3	4	5	6	7	8	9	10	11	12	13		
				CH_3CO—	Ser	Tyr	Ser	Met	Glu	His	Phe	Arg	Tyr	Gly	Lys	Pro	Val—NH_2		
β-LPH & γ-LPH	sheep	41	42	43	44	45	46	47	48	49	50	51	52	53	54	55	56	57	58
		. . .Asp	Ser	Gly	Pro	Tyr	Lys	Met	Glu	His	Phe	Arg	Tyr	Gly	Ser	Pro	Pro	Lys	Asp. . .

Common heptapeptide core (positions boxed: 7–13 of β-MSH; 4–10 of ACTH and α-MSH; 47–53 of β-LPH & γ-LPH)

FIG. 5-6. Partial amino acid sequences of some Category 3 pituitary hormones: corticotropin, *ACTH;* melanotropin, *α-MSH* and *β-MSH;* lipotropin, *β-LPH* and *γ-LPH.*

Source of ACTH	Amino acid sequence								
	1 25	26	27	28	29	30	31	32	33 39
Porcine	Ser. . . . Asn	Gly	Ala	Glu	Asp	Glu	[Leu-]	Ala	Glu. . . . Phe
Ovine	Ser. . . [Asp]	Gly	Ala	Glu	Asp	Glu	Ser	Ala	[Gln]. . . Phe
Bovine	Ser. . . . Asn	Gly	Ala	Glu	Asp	Glu	Ser	Ala	[Gln]. . . Phe
Human	Ser. . . . Asn	Gly	Ala	Glu	Asp	Glu	Ser	Ala	Glu. . . . Phe

FIG. 5-7. Comparison of the partial amino acid sequences for some mammalian corticotropins. (Modified from Hofmann, K.[44]).

Lipotropin

Lipotropin is believed to be an adenohypophysial hormone that stimulates lipolysis (that is, hydrolysis of fats to free fatty acids and glycerol) in adipose tissue. The standard bioassay for LPH is to culture mouse or rabbit epididymal (testis) fat pads and measure the release of glycerol or free fatty acids or both into the culture medium. Another technique employs measurement of the inhibition of incorporation of ^{14}C-labeled acetate into lipid following addition of LPH to the culture medium. This is, in effect, a measurement of lipogenesis, which is inversely related to lipolysis.

Two different LPHs have been characterized. The first peptide consists of 58 amino acids and has been termed gamma LPH. The larger peptide is known as beta LPH and consists of the 58 amino acids as gamma LPH plus 33 additional ones (Fig. 5-6). Lipotropin, presumably of pituitary origin, has been identified in the systemic circulation, and its release can be stimulated by arginine vasopressin. Aldosterone release may be stimulated by LPH,[69] but circulating LPH has not been linked to changes in lipid metabolism, leaving open the question of the physiological role for LPH.

The Endorphins and Enkephalins

A search for endogenous compounds that produce analgesic opiate-like (morphine) effects on the central nervous system has resulted in identification and chemical characterization of two groups of biologically active peptides.[37,94] The four larger peptides (16–31 amino acid residues) are known as the *endorphins,* so named because they are endogenous and produce morphine-like effects.[36,57] Two smaller peptides with opioid activity were identified by other workers as pentapeptides. These latter opioids were named *enkephalins,* meaning "in the head." It was soon observed that the endorphins have a chemical structure identical to a large fragment of ovine beta LPH (beginning with residue 61; Fig. 5-8) and that one of the enkephalins is identical to residues 61–65 of LPH. The other enkephalin is identical except for the substitution of leucine for methionine at position 65 (Fig. 5-8). Hence these enkephalins are known as Met-enkephalin and Leu-enkephalin respectively. This same sequence of five amino acids in Met-enkephalin is found in the amine terminus of all four endorphin molecules, suggesting that its presence in brain extracts may be an artifact of partial hydrolysis of an endorphin molecule. The distribution of endorphins in the central nervous system parallels that observed for ACTH and LPH.[6,37,94] The enkephalins, however, are localized in different neurons, suggesting that their structural relationship to LPH and the endorphins is coincidence and not an artifact of preparation. Another potent endorphin, called *dynorphin,* has been isolated. Dynorphin contains a peptide sequence identical to Leu-enkephalin in its amino terminal end (Fig. 5-8).

The endorphins have also been localized in cells of the pars intermedia and the pars distalis that react positively to antibodies prepared against both ACTH and LPH.[6,37,94] The distribution of these same compounds as well as of the enkephalins within the central nervous system is not affected by hypophysectomy, and it is assumed that the pituitary is not the source for these neural peptides. Endorphins

Hormone	Amino acid sequence																													
	61	62	63	64	65	66	67	68	69	70	71	72	73	74	75	76	77	78	79	80	81	82	83	84	85	86	87	88	89	90	91
Ovine β-LPH	Tyr	Gly	Gly	Phe	Met	Thr	Ser	Gly	Lys	Ser	Gln	Thr	Pro	Leu	Val	Thr	Leu	Phe	Lys	Asn	Ala	Ile	Ile	Lys	Asn	Ala	His	Lys	Lys	Gly	Gln
α-Endorphin	Tyr	Gly	Gly	Phe	Met	Thr	Ser	Gly	Lys	Ser	Gln	Thr	Pro	Leu	Val	Thr															
β-Endorphin	Tyr	Gly	Gly	Phe	Met	Thr	Ser	Gly	Lys	Ser	Gln	Thr	Pro	Leu	Val	Thr	Leu	Phe	Lys	Asn	Ala	Ile	Ile	Lys	Asn	Ala	His	Lys	Lys	Gly	Gln
γ-Endorphin	Tyr	Gly	Gly	Phe	Met	Thr	Ser	Gly	Lys	Ser	Gln	Thr	Pro	Leu	Val	Thr	Leu														
δ-Endorphin	Tyr	Gly	Gly	Phe	Met	Thr	Ser	Gly	Lys	Ser	Gln	Thr	Pro	Leu	Val	Thr	Leu	Phe	Lys	Asn	Ala	Ile	Ile	Lys	Asn	Ala	His				
Met-enkephalin	Tyr	Gly	Gly	Phe	Met																										
Leu-enkephalin	Tyr	Gly	Gly	Phe	Leu																										

Fig. 5-8. Amino acid sequences of a portion of ovine β-LPH (fragment 61–91) compared to the opioid peptides (endorphins and enkephalins). The ovine β-LPH sequence is from Li and Chung,[57] and the opiate peptide structures are based on Guillemin.[36,37]

as well as ACTH and LPH have been identified in both cerebrospinal fluid and in the blood. Factors such as arginine vasopressin that increase ACTH and beta-LPH blood levels do not enhance endorphin release, however.

Painful stimuli elevate levels of endorphins and enkephalins in the cerebrospinal fluid, and they appear to exhibit the features required for endogenous opiate-like agents. There is little doubt that these compounds probably function as neurotransmitters within the central nervous system related to their morphine-like actions. The action of morphine, a non-peptide, is blocked by closely related molecules such as *naloxone*. The effects of endorphins also are blocked by naloxone implying closeness in mechanisms of action for morphine and the endorphins. These endogenous opioids can influence release of GH and PRL,[37] an effect also induced by morphine (see Table 4-8). Endogenous opioids may be involved in stress responses by mediating stress-induced eating. The possible roles for endorphins and enkephalins as regulators of behavior, especially as related to painful stimuli, and their possible endocrine implications represent one of the most exciting areas of neuroendocrinology to appear since the discovery of the first hypothalamo-hypophysiotropic hormone.

Most of the category 3 peptides are produced by post-translational processing of a large prohormone known as *pro-opiomelanocortin*, POMC (Fig. 5-9).[53] Dynorphin and the enkephalins apparently have separate prohormones. The pattern of the subsequent cleavage of POMC depends on the type of cell. For example, in corticotropes the cleavage fragments include a 16K fragment, ACTH and LPH. The 16K fragment includes the sequence of γ-MSH which probably is released only as a consequence of extraction procedures used to isolate the peptides. In melanotropes, ACTH is cleaved further to produce α-MSH and the fragment of ACTH known as CLIP (corticotropin-like peptide).

Functional Overlap of Category 3 Hormones

There is a common heptapeptide core (seven amino acids) in α-MSH, ACTH and LPH (see Fig. 5-6). This similarity in structure is re-

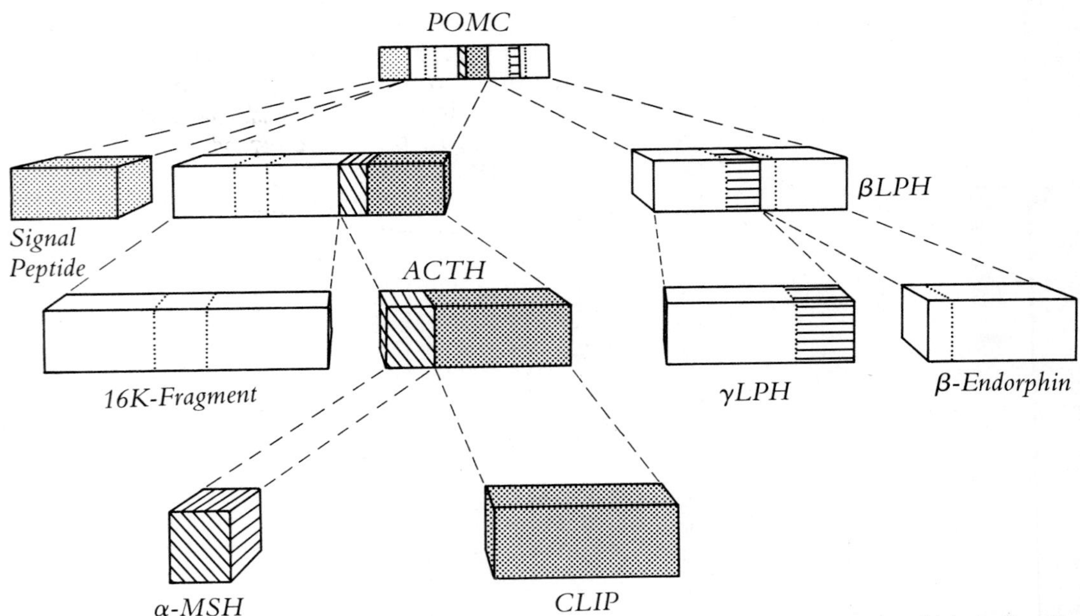

FIG. 5-9. Pro-opiomelanocortin (POMC) is a preprohormone from which various cells can produce biologically active peptides by enzymatically cleaving the parent molecule at predetermined sites. A corticotrope in the pars distalis would cleave POMC at β-LPH, ACTH and a 16K-fragment. A melanotrope in the pars intermedia would release β-LPH, 16K-fragment, MSH and CLIP. The 16-K fragment and β-LPH contains the α-MSH and β-MSH peptides, respectively. The met-enkephalin peptide (ENK) is present in β-endorphin.

flected clearly by overlapping biological activity. Corticotropin has considerable MSH activity and some lipolytic activity. Lipotropin has rather low ACTH activity but strong MSH action. Melanotropin has both weak ACTH and LPH activity. These overlaps in function affect interpretation of bioassayable data on MSH activity. Which peptide is the bioassay measuring, MSH or ACTH?

Comparative Aspects of Tropic Hormones in Nonmammalian Vertebrates

Gonadotropins

Some purified GTHs have been isolated from nonmammalian species, and they have been partially characterized (Table 5-8). Although more GTHs are being isolated each year, no clear phylogenetic pattern has yet emerged.[58]

Mammalian GTHs have been examined extensively for activity in lower vertebrates, and many recent reviews of this work are available for fishes, amphibians, reptiles and birds.[19,58,65-67] Generally the hormonal control of reproduction involves two GTHs with LH-like and FSH-like activities. The apparent failure to find two GTHs in some vertebrate groups (squamate reptiles, teleostean fishes and some birds) may be due to derived secondary reliance on only one GTH with repression of synthesis of the other. Specific activity for both mammalian FSH and LH may be related to biological half-life differences between the two hormones when they are examined in vivo[96] and emphasizes the need for good in-vitro bioassays in a variety of vertebrates. The question concerning the number of GTHs in all groups must be left incompletely answered at this time, however.

It has been proposed that the primitive glycoprotein hormone was an LH-like molecule that became modified into a TSH-like hormone[28] (Fig. 5-10). Follicle-stimulating hormone presumably diverged later from TSH. This scheme was suggested from studies of purified subunit structure. Part of this proposal resides on the presence of only an LH-like hormone in teleosts. Certain contradictory data must be resolved, however, such as the belief that both FSH and LH are produced by the same cell but TSH is produced by another cellular type.

Fishes

Class Chondrichthyes. Gonadotropin activity is present in both the proximal pars distalis and the ventral lobe of selachians. Antibody to mammalian GTHs binds to cells of the ventral lobe.[73] Bioassay of the proximal pars distalis reveals the presence of an LH-like GTH that will stimulate oocyte maturation in the clawed frog *Xenopus laevis*.[25]

Class Osteichthyes. The first observation suggesting a single LH-like GTH in teleosts was that mammalian FSH appeared to be inactive in teleosts and that mammalian LH could support the entire reproductive process. Gonadotropins purified from salmon, carp and rainbow trout have high LH-like activity when tested with the frog spermiation bioassay,[7,11,21,29] as do pituitary extracts prepared from

Table 5-8. *Percent Carbohydrate Composition of Purified Vertebrate Luteinizing Hormones and Follicle-Stimulating Hormones*[65]

HORMONE	SPECIES	HEXOSE	HEXOSAMINE	SIALIC ACID	TOTAL CARBOHYDRATE
LH	Sheep	7.2	9.1	0.4	16.7
	Chicken	5.2	7.1	1.4	13.7
	Sea turtle	6.4	8.9	1.9	17.2
	Bullfrog	3.6	5.5	0.2	9.3
FSH	Sheep	5.7	4.5	2.8	13.0
	Chicken	3.1	3.2	0.8	7.1
	Sea turtle	4.9	6.6	0.6	12.1
	Bullfrog	7.2	9.8	3.0	20.0

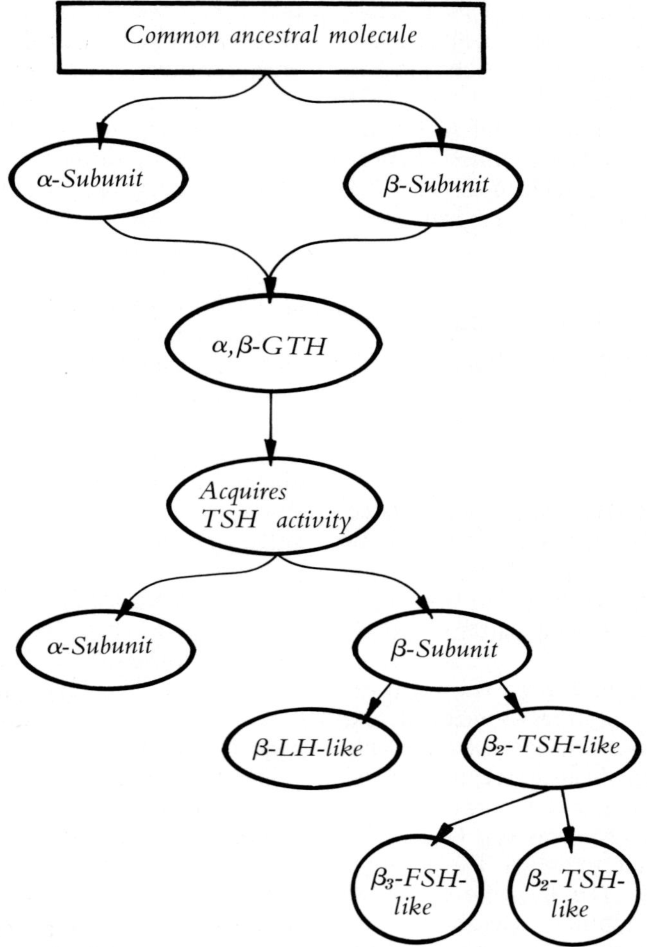

Fig. 5-10. Proposed scheme for glycoprotein hormone evolution based upon analysis of subunit peptide sequences for teleostean and mammalian gonadotropins. (After Fontaine and Burzawa-Gerard.[28])

lungfishes.[11] The spermiation reaction, however, is not as specific for LH as was previously supposed and will respond to highly purified FSH.[65] Sialic acid is not reported to be essential for the biological activity of teleostean GTH, but salmon GTH lost much of its activity following removal of sialic acid prior to its assay in the lizard testicular bioassay.[63] Crude extracts of salmon pituitaries, however, had no effect on chicken Sertoli cells, which are highly sensitive to FSH.[49] The observation that antibody prepared against mammalian LH was bound by salmon gonadotropic basophils but not antibody against mammalian FSH lends further support to the contention that the gonadotropin of teleosts and possibly of lungfishes is LH-like.

Further extraction of certain teleostean GTH preparations yields a nonglycoprotein fraction that stimulates uptake from the blood of protein precursors utilized in yolk synthesis by growing oocytes.[91] The official status of this "nonglycoprotein-gonadotropin" awaits further study.

Highly purified LH has been reported to have intrinsic TSH activity in teleosts,[69,76] supporting the suggestion that an LH-like hormone was the primitive hormone that later gave rise to TSH.[28]

Class Amphibia. Two distinct GTHs have

been isolated and purified from the bullfrog, the tiger salamander *Ambystoma tigrinum*, and the leopard frog *Rana pipiens*.[24,61,64] Purified bullfrog LH and FSH both stimulate spermatogenesis and spermiation in bullfrogs, but only bullfrog LH elevated plasma levels. *Ambystoma* LH was not as effective as bullfrog LH in raising plasma androgen levels in bullfrogs. Conversely, *Ambystoma* LH was more effective than bullfrog LH in *Ambystoma*, although the latter was considerably more effective than *Ambystoma* FSH. Bullfrog LH is more effective than ovine LH in stimulating progesterone synthesis in amphibians.[59] These data strongly support the existence of two structurally and functionally separate GTHs in amphibians. Bullfrog LH also stimulates reptilian and avian thyroids emphasizing the closeness of LH and TSH.

Class Reptilia. Studies employing injections of mammalian hormones into squamate reptiles have emphasized a role for FSH-like GTHs but suggest no role for LH-like hormones. Earlier data might be interpreted as a consequence of a very short biological half-life for injected mammalian LH or that mammalian FSH might be similar enough to both a squamate FSH and LH to possess both activities. Purification of gonadotropic activity from squamate reptiles, however, has shown only one FSH-like molecule, although both FSH-like and LH-like GTHs have been isolated from chelonians and crocodilians.[65] Presence of only one molecular species of GTH in squamates does not rule out the possibility that this molecule has intrinsic FSH-like and LH-like activities. Recent studies suggest snake GTH may not be homologous to either FSH or LH.[60] Since both GTHs are found in other reptiles the squamate condition is probably secondarily derived and does not represent a primitive condition.

There is great variability in the responses of reptilian tissues to GTHs purified from different vertebrate groups. Testicular weight maintenance in hypophysectomized *Anolis carolinensis* is readily maintained by FSH-like hormones purified from mammals, birds, reptiles or amphibians, but this testicular parameter is very insensitive to LH-like gonadotropins. Nevertheless, plasma androgen levels in hypophysectomized *A. carolinensis* may be elevated by either FSH-like or LH-like GTHs from almost any source.[54,65] Similar effects on plasma levels of androgens or on androgen synthesis by minced testes in vitro have been observed for crocodilians.[65] The situation in chelonians is not clear as testes of some species do not respond to LH-like hormones in vitro,[65] whereas at least one species (*Chrysemys picta*) does respond to in-vivo injections of mammalian LH but not as well as to FSH.[54] This observation may be related to contamination of the LH preparation with FSH, or it could be due to species differences. Purified salmon GTH, which is LH-like in most bioassays, had no effect on circulating androgen levels in *C. picta*,[54] however, supporting the possibility of contamination of the mammalian LH used.

The reptilian ovary, like the testis, exhibits broad sensitivity to FSH and LH. Follicle-stimulating hormones are generally the most effective, although there are some conflicting reports. In *C. picta* both partially purified ovine LH and chicken LH stimulated synthesis of estrogens and progesterone by preovulatory and postovulatory follicles respectively.[12] Only minimal response to ovine or chicken LH was observed. In contrast, other studies have found that turtle ovaries respond best to FSH-like GTHs but that highly purified oLH is ineffective.[65]

Obviously the story of the reptilian GTHs is incomplete. Although the squamates appear to possess only one FSH-like GTH, crocodilians and chelonians clearly possess two. The apparent lack of specificity by reptilian tissues for nonhomologous GTHs emphasizes the importance of working with purified GTHs from the species being studied or from very closely related species.

Class Aves. Birds are believed to conform to the typical mammalian pattern of two GTHs, LH and FSH, although avian species are rather insensitive to mammalian FSH and LH.[67,75] Two separate GTHs have been extracted and partially purified from domestic galliform birds.[27,99] Preliminary studies of the duck support existence of only one GTH.[65] More species need to be examined.

Chicken LH stimulates interstitial cells in the testis of chickens or Japanese quail, and the seminiferous tubules are stimulated by chicken FSH.[48] Mammalian LH and avian LH are reported to be more effective than FSHs in stimulating androgen production by chicken interstitial cells in vitro.[71] Some conflicting reports suggest that avian FSH and LH are more nearly equal in their actions on minced pigeon or chicken testes, however.[65] Reptilian LH is more effective than reptilian FSH in stimulating the avian testis. Purified amphibian GTHs (both LH-like and FSH-like) are equally effective, although their overall activity in birds is low. Purification of additional avian GTHs and development of specific RIAs for avian GTHs will provide more precise answers about the involvement of GTHs in avian reproduction.

Thyrotropins

Mammalian TSHs have been shown to stimulate thyroid function in all vertebrates examined with the usual exception of the hagfishes. Similarly pituitaries from most nonmammals exhibit TSH-like activity when tested in mammals. The specific actions of TSH on thyroid glands and the functions of thyroid hormones in nonmammals are discussed in Chapter 8.

Although little is known about the structures of nonmammalian TSHs, it is apparent that there is great similarity to those of mammals. Purified bullfrog TSH is thyrotropic in both anurans and urodeles but is ineffective on thyroids of reptiles and birds. Curiously, bullfrog LH exhibits thyrotropic activity in reptiles and birds (see Licht[58]). Purified LHs of tetrapods have also been shown to exert a TSH-like action in teleosts.[69,76] This overlap in function has been used as support for the origin of TSH from an LH-like primitive glycoprotein hormone.[28]

Growth Hormones and Prolactins

Prolactin. Prolactin has so many different actions in vertebrates that it is almost impossible to describe them all. Indeed, people have suggested a variety of names for this hormone that might be more descriptive, such as versitilin, ubiquitin, panaceanin and miscellanin. Many of the reported actions of PRL, however, may be grouped into a few general types: 52% of the reported actions are related to growth phenomena; 38% are related to reproduction; 25% involve water and electrolyte balance; 26% are concerned with integumentary structures; and 35% concern actions synergistic with other hormones.[82] The most primitive role for PRL may be related to osmotic-ionic balance,[4] with the other actions being acquired during vertebrate evolution. Certainly the major role for PRL in teleostean fishes is related to osmotic regulation in fresh water (see Chap. 16), and even in man PRL release can be induced following alterations in blood osmotic pressure.[10] Regardless of the multiplicity of roles or even the establishment that it may be an osmoregulatory hormone, the term prolactin is here to stay.

Prolactin provides an excellent example for the evolution of endocrine systems from a variety of viewpoints. There have been evolutionary changes in the structure of the PRL molecule as evidenced by the failure of fish PRLs to work in mammalian bioassays, although mammalian PRLs retain piscine activity. The antigenic portion of the piscine PRLs is similar to mammals as evidenced by the binding of mammalian PRL antibodies to the lactotropes of the piscine rostral pars distalis. Furthermore, new target tissues have evolved (for example, the crop sac of birds and the mammary glands of mammals) that possess receptors specific for the "newer" portions of the molecules. This is evidenced by the failure of the piscine PRLs to activate responses in avian and mammalian tissues. It is unfortunate that there are no bioassays employing reptilian tissues and that purified reptilian PRLs are not available to fill in this part of the evolutionary changes that appear to be supported by studies with the bioassays of the other major groups.

Class Agnatha. Immunochemical studies suggest that the pituitaries of hagfish contain a molecule that binds antibody prepared against mammalian PRL,[1] but only negative bioassays have been reported.[79] Some cyclostome pituitaries, however, do contain bioassayable PRL, based on responses observed for lamprey pituitaries in the xanthophore-expanding *Gillichthyes* bioassay.[98]

Class Chondrichthyes. The xanthophores of *Gillichthyes* expand following application of pituitary extracts from selachians,[98] indicating the possible presence of PRL activity in the rostral pars distalis. No bioassays of holocephalan pituitaries have been reported.

Class Osteichthyes. As mentioned previously, PRL plays an important role in osmotic regulation in freshwater teleosts (see also Chap. 16). Teleostean PRLs have little biological activity in amniote bioassays, but they work well in amphibians and teleosts (Table 5-6). Purified PRLs have been prepared from five species of teleosts, and all chemically resemble mammalian GH more closely than mammalian PRL.[5] However, both highly purified tilapia GH and PRL can stimulate synthesis of milk proteins in cultured rabbit mammary gland cells.[45] Some investigators have proposed that since the structures of teleostean and other piscine PRLs are different from those of amphibians and the amniotes, they should be given a separate name. Thus, *paralactin* is sometimes used to refer to the piscine PRL-like substance in the rostral portion of the pars distalis.

Class Amphibia. Prolactins from most amphibians cross-react with antibody to rat growth hormone,[38] and PRL is thought by some to be the larval GH of amphibians.[31] Tiger salamanders were the only animals tested whose PRL did not cross-react with rat GH antibody.[38] In addition to possible influences on larval growth, PRL is antimetamorphic in both anurans and urodeles, that is, it blocks metamorphosis from the aquatic larva to the semiterrestrial or terrestrial juvenile form (see Chap. 17). Prolactin induces water-drive behavior in newts and possibly in salamanders and influences secondary sexual characters associated with breeding.[18,22,35,109] Integumentary effects of PRL have been observed on the skin of newts and salamanders.[18,93,112] Prolactin also affects water balance in anurans and urodeles as it does in fishes.[9,33,34]

Class Reptilia. The reptiles are the only major vertebrate groups in which a good bioassay has not been developed, and little work has been done with PRL in reptiles. Prolactin stimulates growth in juvenile snapping turtles *Chelydra serpentina* and lizards *Lacerta s. sicula.*[62,77] Appetite is also stimulated in *Lacerta* by PRL. A possible effect on water balance has been reported in turtles in which PRL influenced glomerular filtration.[8] Reptilian PRLs give positive responses in other vertebrates (Table 5-6), and this PRL activity appears to be confined to the cephalic (rostral) lobe of the pars distalis.[98] Considerable research remains to be done with respect to PRL in reptiles.

Class Aves. Prolactin plays several essential roles in avian reproduction. In some cases PRL synergizes with other hormones, as in formation of the broodpatch for incubating eggs, fat deposition and induction of migratory restlessness.[50,72] This last behavior appears just prior to the actual migration of birds. The involvement of PRL in reproduction and migration is discussed in Chapters 11 and 18 respectively.

Prolactin has been purified from chickens.[99] Chicken PRL is similar in amino acid composition and electrophoretic properties to mammalian PRLs and appears to be distinct from chicken GH.

Growth Hormone. Compared to PRL, there are few comparative data on structure and function of vertebrate growth hormones (Table 5-9). Mammalian GHs are effective in most nonmammals, and most nonmammalian preparations exhibit GH activity in mammals. Immunological studies of GHs prepared from different vertebrates have not clarified any relationships. Comparative studies are hampered by the similarities of GH and PRL, especially in the amphibians in which prolactin seems to be the larval growth factor.

Class Chondrichthyes. Growth hormone activity can be demonstrated in the selachian pars distalis with the rodent tibia bioassay.[2] Somatomedin activity has also been demonstrated for two sharks, *Squalus acanthias* and *Mustelus canis,* although no definite link to GH has been established.[102] No data on holocephalans are available.

Class Osteichthyes. Polypterid, chondrostean, holostean and teleostean pituitaries exhibit GH activity in the tibia bioassay.[2] Furthermore, by means of immunochemical techniques employing anti-rat GH antibody, GH activity has been demonstrated in the pituitaries of chondrostean, holostean and teleostean fishes.[38,39] Mammalian GHs are very active in promoting growth of fishes.[42] Growth hormone isolated from tilapia is structurally unlike other GHs, but GH from sturgeon is mammalianlike.[5]

There is a marked influence of thyroid hormones on growth in teleosts. Thyroid hor-

TABLE 5-9. *Amino Acid Composition (Number of Residues) of Vertebrate Growth Hormones as Compared to Ovine GH*

AMINO ACID	BULLFROG[a]	LEOPARD FROG[b]	SEA TURTLE[c]	SNAPPING TURTLE[d]	DUCK[e]	SHEEP
Lys	11.0	12.5	11.7	12.0	12.3	11
His	6.2	6.7	4.8	4.2	4.9	3
Arg	16.7	17.2	11.6	12.9	9.9	13
Asp	29.5	28.4	20.2	20.3	21.2	16
Thr	11.9	11.7	7.9	9.2	9.8	12
Ser	11.8	11.8	15.0	13.9	11.7	13
Glu	18.2	17.5	24.7	24.0	25.0	24
Pro	6.3	5.3	8.9	7.3	9.6	6
Gly	7.0	9.3	8.2	9.0	9.8	10
Ala	5.8	8.0	12.9	10.7	11.2	15
Cys (½)	4.1	3.6	4.0	4.1	3.6	4
Val	10.8	10.8	7.6	7.7	8.4	6
Met	4.1	3.8	4.2	4.2	4.3	4
Ile	7.9	7.9	7.3	7.0	6.0	7
Leu	18.0	17.8	25.6	26.3	25.6	27
Tyr	10.2	7.6	5.4	6.6	6.3	6
Phe	10.8	9.9	10.5	11.7	10.2	13
Trp	0.9	ND	1.3	0.9	1.0	1

Modified from Farmer et al.[25]
[a] *Rana catesbeiana.*
[b] *R. pipiens.*
[c] *Chelonia mydas.*
[d] *Chelydra serpentina.*
[e] *Anas platyrhynchos.*

mones accelerate growth in fishes,[3] and thyroid hormone treatment restores growth rates to normal in radiothyroidectomized rainbow trout.[85] Although it has not been conclusively demonstrated it is reasonable to assume a synergistic relationship of thyroid hormones and GHs similar to that reported for mammals. Androgens also produce a positive effect on growth of salmonid fishes,[42] suggesting a protein anabolic action for these steroids that is probably independent of the action of GH.

The presence of somatomedin activity is reported in two teleosts examined by means of the porcine costal cartilage bioassay.[102] No relationship between somatomedin and GH has been indicated, however.

Class Amphibia. The amphibians are complicated by the observation that PRL may be a larval growth hormone, whereas GH per se may operate only in transformed or metamorphosed individuals.[31] Both GH and PRL have been isolated from frogs, *Rana catesbeiana,* and *Rana pipiens.*[15,16,25] Purified frog GHs are not as effective as bovine GH in the rat tibia bioassay, however (Table 5-10). The large number of similarities in the physical properties between amphibian and mammalian GHs and the similarities in amino acid composition suggest that there has been considerable conservatism expressed in the evolution of tetrapod GHs.[25]

Cross-reaction occurs between antibody prepared against rat GH and PRLs prepared from most amphibian species,[40] and only the tiger salamander of those species examined appears to produce GH distinctly different from mammalian PRL. Nevertheless, antibody prepared against bullfrog PRL does not cross-react immunologically with bullfrog GH.[16] This observation supports the interpretation that inability to distinguish a distinct tropic hormone, such as PRL, in a nonmammal with antibody prepared against some mammalian tropic hormone, such as GH, does not mean the endogenous hormones (PRL and GH) are not separate and distinct hormones.

TABLE 5-10. *Effects of Bovine (bGH) and Purified Bullfrog (fGH) Growth Hormones on Thickness of the Epiphysial Cartilage in the Rat Tibia Bioassay*

HORMONE	DOSE	NO. RATS TESTED	MEAN WIDTH OF EPIPHYSIAL PLATE[a]
None	—	5	142.3 ± 2.7
bGH	5 μg	5	185.1 ± 4.1
bGH	25 μg	5	252.3 ± 3.1
fGH	5 μg	4	155.6 ± 2.1
fGH	25 μg	4	220.4 ± 17.6
fGH + fGH-antibody	25 μg	4	156.4 ± 2.1

Data from Clemons.[15]
[a] μm ± SEM

Somatomedin activity has been demonstrated in *Xenopus laevis,* but no link to either PRL or GH has been proposed.[102]

Class Reptilia. Mammalian GH, like PRL, stimulated growth in juvenile snapping turtles and in the lizard *Lacerta,*[62,77] although the sites of action for GH and PRL in the lizard appear to be different. Growth hormone stimulated appetite in *Lacerta,* as reported for PRL, and also produced marked increase in growth of the digestive tract (splanchnomegaly), an action reported for PRL in other vertebrate groups (Table 5-5).

Purified GH has been prepared from the caudal lobe of adult snapping turtle pituitaries and sea turtles.[25,89] Many characteristics of these GHs are similar to those of other tetrapods. Turtle GHs are very effective in the rat tibia bioassay.[25]

Class Aves. Growth hormone activity has been demonstrated in pituitaries of chickens and turkeys by means of the mouse tibia bioassay.[41,43,104] Antibovine GH antibody apparently does not cross-react with chicken pituitary extracts.[74] Purified GH from duck pituitaries does cross-react with rat GH antibody, however,[89] and the apparent failure to observe cross-reactivity between chicken and bovine GH should be reexamined.

Corticotropins, Lipotropin and Melanotropin

Little comparative literature about the structures of ACTH and MSH exist for nonmammalian hormones. Peptides appear to be present in the pituitaries of all vertebrates (except hagfishes) that possess ACTH-like and MSH-like activities. Purified MSH has been prepared from the pituitary of the dogfish shark (Table 5-8), but this is the only case of verified structure for nonmammalian category 3 tropic hormones.

The functional roles for mammalian ACTH and homologous pituitary extracts or homogenates in various vertebrate groups are discussed in Chapter 10. Adrenal production of corticosteroids appears to be under control of a corticotropic factor in nonmammals. Corticotropins prepared from mammals are sometimes used to investigate melanophore responses in nonmammals, especially amphibians, since it has strong MSH activity. This action of ACTH as well as the actions of endogenous MSH-like factors are discussed in Chapter 6.

Opiate activity (endorphins?) has been demonstrated in both the neurointermediate lobe and pars distalis of rainbow trout in amounts comparable to the pars intermedia of guinea pigs.[47] Presumably data for other nonmammals will be available soon.

Summary

There are three categories of tropic hormones based on chemical structure. Category 1 includes the glycoproteins, LH, FSH and TSH. Category 2 includes the large peptides, GH and PRL. Category 3 includes the very similar smaller peptides, ACTH, MSH and LPH. Structural similarities suggest that LPH may be related to the endorphins, which are linked to opiate actions on the mammalian central nervous system. Placentas of mammals produce up to four tropic-like hormones, including CG (LH-like), CS (PRL-like and GH-like to some degree), CT (TSH-like) and CC (ACTH-like). Pregnant mare serum gonadotropin is a chorionic-type GTH with both FSH- and LH-like properties.

The established occurrence of at least one hormone from each category in all gnathostomes (jawed vertebrates) suggests that early in vertebrate evolution three cellular types (basophil, acidophil and possibly PbH(+) cells respectively) differentiated, and each began elaboration of one of three types of molecules (glycoproteins, large peptides and small peptides respectively). These three primitive molecules attained functional significance as tropic hormones and gave rise via amino acid substitution, cleavage of fragments from larger molecules or both to the additional hormones that characterize each category.

Careful studies of agnathan fishes and of the so-called protochordates (urochordates and cephalochordates) may provide clues to the origins of tropic hormones. Isolation of tropic hormones from additional species of nonmammals should provide greater understanding of the molecular aspects of tropic hormone evolution as well as evolution of receptors for these hormones.

References

1. Aler, G.M., G. Bage and B. Fernholm (1971). On the existence of prolactin in cyclostomes. Gen. Comp. Endocrinol. 16:498–503.
2. Barrington, E.J.W. (1975). An Introduction to General and Comparative Endocrinology, Clarendon Press, Oxford.
3. Barrington, E.J.W., N. Barron and D.J. Piggens (1961). The influence of thyroid powder and thyroxine upon the growth of rainbow trout (*Salmo gairdnerii*). Gen. Comp. Endocrinol. 1:170–178.
4. Bern, H. (1975). On two possible primary activities of prolactins: Osmoregulatory and developmental. Verh. Dtsch. Zool. Ges. 1975:40–46.
5. Bern, H.A. (1983). Functional evolution of prolactin and growth hormone in lower vertebrates. Amer. Zool. 23:663–671.
6. Bloom, F.E., E. Battenberg, J. Rossier, N. Ling, J. Leppaluoto, T.M. Vargo and R. Guilleman (1977). To spritz or not to spritz: The doubtful value of aimless ionotophoresis. Life Sci. 14:1819–1834.
7. Breton, B., B. Jalabert and P. Reinaud (1976). Purification of gonadotropin from rainbow trout (*Salmo gairdnerii* Richardson) pituitary glands. Ann. Biol. Anim. Biochem. Biophys. 16:25–36.
8. Brewer, K.J. and D.M. Ensor (1976). Prolactin and osmoregulation of the terrapin, *Chrysemys picta.* Gen. Comp. Endocrinol. 29:285.
9. Brown, P.S. and S.C. Brown (1982). Effects of hypophysectomy and prolactin on the water-balance response of the newt, *Taricha torosa.* Gen. Comp. Endocrinol. 46:7–12.
10. Buckman, M.T. and G.T. Peake (1973). Osmolar control of prolactin secretion in man. Science 181:755–757.
11. Burzawa-Gerard, E. (1969). Quelques propriétés des hormones gonadotropes des poissons comparée a celles des mammifères. Colloq. Int. Centre Nat. Rech. 177:351–356. Cited by E.M. Donaldson (1973), Reproductive endocrinology of fishes. Am. Zool. 13:909–927.
12. Callard, I.P., I. McChesney, C. Scanes, and G.V. Callard (1976). The influence of mammalian and avian gonadotropins on *in vitro* ovarian steroid synthesis in the turtle (*Chrysemys picta*). Gen. Comp. Endocrinol. 28:2–9.
13. Clarke, W.C. (1973). Disc-electrophoretic identification of prolactin in the cichlid teleosts *Tilapia* and *Cichlasoma* and densitometric measurement of its concentration in Tilapia pituitaries during salinity transfer experiments. Can. J. Zool. 51:687–695.
14. Clarke, W.C. (1973). Sodium-retaining bioassay of prolactin in the intact teleost *Tilapia mossambica* acclimated to sea water. Gen. Comp. Endocrinol. 21:498–512.
15. Clemons, G.K. (1976). Development and preliminary application of a homologous radioimmunoassay for bullfrog growth hormone. Gen. Comp. Endocrinol. 30:357–363.
16. Clemons, G.K. and C.S. Nicoll (1977). Effects of antisera to bullfrog prolactin and growth hormone on metamorphosis of *Rana catesbeiana* tadpoles. Gen. Comp. Endocrinol. 31:495–497.

17. Daughaday, W.H., A.C. Herington and L.S. Phillips (1975). The regulation of growth by endocrines. Annu. Rev. Physiol. 37:211–244.

18. Dent, J.N. (1975). Integumentary effects of prolactin in lower vertebrates. Am. Zool. 15:923–935.

19. deVlaming, V.L. (1974). Environmental and endocrine control of teleost reproduction. In C.B. Schreck, ed., Control of Sex in Fishes. VPI, Blacksburg, Va., pp. 13–83.

20. Dickhoff, W.W. (1977). A rapid, high-efficiency bioassay of melanocyte-stimulating hormone. Gen. Comp. Endocrinol. 33:304–306.

21. Donaldson, E.M. and Y. Yamazaki (1968). Preparation of gonadotropic hormone from salmon pituitary glands. 51st Annual Conference Chemical Institute of Canada. Cited by E.M. Donaldson (1973), Reproductive endocrinology of fishes. Am. Zool. 13:909–927.

22. Duvall, D. and D.O. Norris (1977). Prolactin and substrate stimulation of locomotor activity in adult tiger salamanders. (Ambystoma tigrinum). J. Exp. Zool. 200:103–106.

23. Ensor, D.M. and J.N. Ball (1968). A bioassay for fish prolactin (paralactin). Gen. Comp. Endocrinol. 11:104–110.

24. Farmer, S.W., P. Licht, H. Papkoff and E.L. Daniels (1977). Purification of gonadotropins in the leopard frog (*Rana pipiens*). Gen. Comp. Endocrinol. 32:158–162.

25. Farmer, S.W., H. Papkoff and T. Hayashida (1976). Purification and properties of reptilian and amphibian growth hormones. Endocrinology 99:692–700.

26. Firth, J.A. and L. Vollrath (1973). Determination of the distribution of luteinizing hormone-like gonadotropic activity within the dogfish pituitary gland by means of the *Xenopus* oocyte meiosis assay. J. Endocrinol. 58:347–348.

27. Follett, B.K., C.G. Scanes and T.J. Nicholls (1972). The chemistry and physiology of the avian gonadotropins. In Hormones Glycoproteiques Hypophysaires. INSERM, Paris, pp. 193–211.

28. Fontaine, Y.A. and E. Burzawa-Gerard (1977). Esquisse de l'évolution des hormones gonadotropes et thyreotropes des vertebres. Gen. Comp. Endocrinol. 32:341–347.

29. Fontaine, Y.A. and E. Gerard (1963). Purification d'un facteur gonadotrope de l'hypophyse d'un Teléostéen, la carpe (*Cyprinus carpio*). C.R. Acad. Sci. 256:5634–5637.

30. Freiden, E. and H. Lipner (1963). Biochemical Endocrinology of the Vertebrates. Prentice-Hall, Englewood Cliffs, N.J.

31. Frye, B.E., P.S. Brown and B.N. Snyder (1972). Effects of prolactin and somatotropin on growth and metamorphosis of amphibians. Gen. Comp. Endocrinol. Suppl. 3:209–220.

32. Golander, A., T. Hurley, J. Barrett, A. Hizi and S. Handwerger (1978). Prolactin synthesis by human chorion-decidual tissue: a possible source of prolactin in the amniotic fluid. Science 202:311–313.

33. Goldenberg, S. and M.R. Warburg (1976). Changes in the response to oxytocin followed throughout ontogenesis in two anuran species. Comp. Biochem. Physiol. 53C:105–113.

34. Goldenberg, S. and M.R. Warburg (1977). Changes in the effect of vasotocin on water balance of *Rana ridibunda* during ontogenesis. Comp. Biochem. Physiol. 57A:451–456.

35. Grant, W.C. Jr. and J.A. Grant (1958). Water drive studies on hypophysectomized efts of *Diemictylus viridescens*. I. The role of the lactogenic hormone. Biol. Bull. 174:1–9.

36. Guillemin, R. (1977). The expanding significance of hypothalamic peptides, or, is endocrinology a branch of neuroendocrinology. Recent Prog. Hormone Res. 33:1–28.

37. Guillemin, R. (1978). Peptides in the brain: The new endocrinology of the neuron. Science 202:390–402.

38. Hayashida, T. (1970). Immunological studies with rat pituitary growth hormone (RGH). II. Comparative immunochemical investigation of GH from representatives of various vertebrate classes with monkey antiserum to RGH. Gen. Comp. Endocrinol. 15:432–452.

39. Hayashida, T. and M.D. Lagios (1969). Fish growth hormone: A biological, immunochemical and ultrastructural study of sturgeon and paddlefish pituitaries. Gen. Comp. Endocrinol. 13:403–411.

40. Hayashida, T., P. Licht and C.S. Nicoll (1973). Amphibian pituitary growth hormone and prolactin: Immunochemical relatedness to rat growth hormone. Science 182:169–171.

41. Hazelwood, R.L. and B.S. Hazelwood (1961). Effects of avian and rat pituitary extracts on tibial growth and blood composition. Proc. Soc. Exp. Biol. Med. 108:10–12.

42. Higgs, D.A., U.H.M. Fagerlund, J.R. McBride, H.M. Dye and E.M. Donaldson (1977). Influence of combinations of bovine growth hormone, 17 α-methyl testosterone and L-thyroxine on growth of yearling coho salmon (*Oncorhynchus kisutch*). Can. J. Zool. 55:1048–1056.

43. Hirsch, L.J. (1961). A study of the growth promoting principle in the domestic fowl. Ph.D. thesis, University of Illinois, Urbana.

44. Hofmann, K. (1974). Relations between chemical structure of adrenocorticotropin and melanocyte-stimulating hormones. Handbook of Physiology, Sec. 7, Endocrinology, Williams & Wilkins, Baltimore, Vol. 4, Part 2, pp. 29–58.

45. Houdebine, L.-M., S.W. Farmer and P. Prunet (1981). Induction of rabbit casein synthesis in organ

culture by tilapia prolactin and growth hormone. Gen. Comp. Endocrinol. 45:61–65.

46. Houssay, B.A. (1949). Hypophyseal functions in the toad *Bufo arenarum* Hensel. Qt. Rev. Biol. 24:1–27.

47. Hunter, C. and B.I. Baker (1979). The distribution of opiate activity in the trout pituitary gland. Gen. Comp. Endocrinol. 37:111–114.

48. Ishii, S. and T. Furuya (1975). Effects of purified chicken gonadotropins on the chick testis. Gen. Comp. Endocrinol. 25:1–8.

49. Ishii, S. and K. Yamamoto (1976). Demonstration of follicle-stimulating hormone (FSH) activity in hypophyseal extracts of various vertebrates by the response of the Sertoli cells of the chick. Gen. Comp. Endocrinol. 29:506–510.

50. Jones, R.E. (1971). The incubation patch of birds. Biol. Rev. 46:315–339.

51. Kastin, A.J., S. Viosca and A.V. Schally (1974). Regulation of melanocyte-stimulating hormone release. Handbook of Physiology, Sec. 7, Endocrinology. Williams & Wilkins, Baltimore, Vol. 4, Part 2, pp. 551–562.

52. Kleinberg, D.L. and A.G. Frantz (1971). Human prolactin: Measurement in plasma by *in vitro* bioassay. J. Clin. Invest. 50:1557–1568.

53. Krieger, D.T. (1983). Brain peptides: what, where and why? Science 222:975–985.

54. Lance, V., C. Scanes and I.P. Callard (1977). Plasma testosterone levels in male turtles, *Chrysemys picta,* following single injections of mammalian, avian and teleostean gonadotropins. Gen. Comp. Endocrinol. 31:435–441.

55. Lewis, U.J., R.N.P. Singh, G.F. Tutwiler, M.B. Sigel, E.F. VanderLaan and W.P. VanderLaan (1980). Human growth hormone: a complex of proteins. Rec. Prog. Horm. Res. 36:477–504.

56. Li, C.H. (1974). Chemistry of ovine prolactin. Handbook of Physiology, Sec. 7, Endocrinology, Vol. 4, Part 2, pp. 103–110.

57. Li, C.H. and D. Chung (1976). Isolation and structure of an untriakontapeptide with opiate activity from camel pituitary glands. Proc. Natl. Acad. Sci. 73:1145–1148.

58. Licht, P. (1983). Evolutionary divergence in the structure and function of pituitary gonadotropins of tetrapod vertebrates. Am. Zool. 23:673–683.

59. Licht, P. and D. Crews (1976). Gonadotropin stimulation of *in vitro* progesterone production in reptilian and amphibian ovaries. Gen. Comp. Endocrinol. 29:141–151.

60. Licht, P., S.W. Farmer, A. Bona Gallo and H. Papkoff (1979). Pituitary gonadotropins in snakes. Gen. Comp. Endocrinol. 39:34–52.

61. Licht, P., S.W. Farmer, and H. Papkoff (1975). The nature of the pituitary gonadotropins and their role in ovulation in a urodele amphibian (*Ambystoma tigrinum*). Life Sci. 17:1049–1054.

62. Licht, P. and H. Hoyer (1968). Somato-tropic effects of exogenous prolactin and growth hormone in juvenile lizards (*Lacerta s. sicula*). Gen. Comp. Endocrinol. 11:338–346.

63. Licht, P. and H. Papkoff (1972). Relationship of sialic acid to biological activity of vertebrate gonadotropins. Gen. Comp. Endocrinol. 19:102–113.

64. Licht, P. and H. Papkoff (1974). Separation of two distinct gonadotropins from the pituitary gland of the bullfrog, *Rana catesbeiana.* Endocrinology 94:1587–1594.

65. Licht, P., H. Papkoff, S.W. Farmer, C.H. Muller, H.W. Tsui and D. Crews (1977). Evolution of gonadotropin structure and function. Recent Progr. Horm. Res. 33:169–248.

66. Lofts, B. (1974). Reproduction. In B. Lofts, ed., Physiology of the Amphibia, Academic Press, New York, Vol. 2, pp. 107–218.

67. Lofts, B. and R.K. Murton (1973). Reproduction in birds. In D.S. Farner and J.R. King eds., Avian Biology. Academic Press, New York, Vol. 3, pp. 1–107.

68. Loewenstein, J.E., I.K. Mariz, G.T. Peake and W.H. Daughaday (1971). Prolactin bioassay by induction of N-acetyl-lactosamine synthetase in mouse mammary gland explants. J. Clin. Endocrinol. Metab. 33:217–224.

69. MacKenzie, D.S. (1982). Stimulation of the thyroid gland of a teleost fish, *Gillichthyes mirabilis,* by tetrapod pituitary glycoprotein hormones. Comp. Biochem. Physiol. 72A:477–482.

70. Matsuoka, H., P.J. Mulrow, and C.H. Li (1980). β-Lipotropin: a new aldosterone-stimulating factor. Science 209:307–308.

71. Maung, Z.W. (1976). Effect of LH and cAMP on steroidogenesis in interstitial cells isolated from the testis of the Japanese quail. Gen. Comp. Endocrinol. 29:254.

72. Meier, A.H., J.T. Burns and J.W. Dusseau (1969). Seasonal variations in the diurnal rhythm of pituitary prolactin content in the white-throated sparrow, *Zonotrichia albicollis.* Gen. Comp. Endocrinol. 12:282–289.

73. Mellinger, J. and M.P. Dubois (1973). Confirmation, par l'immunofluorescence de la fonction corticotrope du lobe rostral et de la fonction gonadotrope du lobe ventral de l'hypophyse d'un poisson cartilagineux, la torpille marbrée (*Torpedo marmorata*). C.R. Acad. Sci. 276:1879–1881.

74. Moudgal, N.R. and C.H. Li (1961). Immunochemical studies of bovine and ovine pituitary growth hormone. Arch Biochem. Biophys. 93:122–127.

75. Nalbandov, A.V. (1976). Reproductive Physiology. Comparative Reproductive Physiology of Domestic Animals, Laboratory Animals and Man, 3rd ed. Freeman, San Francisco.

76. Ng, T.B., D.R. Idler and J.G. Eales (1982). Pituitary hormones that stimulate the thyroidal system in teleost fishes. Gen. Comp. Endocrinol. 48:372–389.

77. Nichols, C.W. Jr. (1973). Somatotropic effects of prolactin and growth hormone in juvenile snapping turtles (*Chelydra serpentina*). Gen. Comp. Endocrinol. 21:219–224.

78. Nicoll, C.S. (1967). Bioassay of prolactin. Analysis of the pigeon crop-sac response to local prolactin injection by an objective and quantitative method. Endocrinology 80:641–655.

79. Nicoll, C.S. (1974). Physiological actions of prolactin. Handbook of Physiology, Sec. 7, Endocrinology. Williams & Wilkins, Baltimore, Vol. 4, Part 2, pp. 253–292.

80. Nicoll, C.S. (1975). Radioimmunoassay and the radio-receptor assays for prolactin and growth hormone: A critical appraisal. Am. Zool. 15:881–904.

81. Nicoll, C.S. (1982). Prolactin and growth hormone: specialists on the one hand and mutual mimics on the other. Pers. Biol. Med. 25:369–381.

82. Nicoll, C.S. and H.A. Bern (1971). On the actions of prolactin among the vertebrates: Is there a common denominator? In G.E.W. Wolstenholme and J. Knight, eds., Ciba Foundation Symposium on Lactogenic Hormones. Livingston, London, pp. 299–324.

83. Nicoll, C.S. and C.W. Nichols, Jr. (1971). Evolutionary biology of prolactins and somatotropins. I. Electrophoretic comparison of tetrapod prolactins. Gen. Comp. Endocrinol. 17:300–310.

84. Nicoll, C.S., J.A. Parsons, R.P. Fiorindo and C.W. Nichols, Jr. (1969). Estimation of prolactin and growth hormone levels by polyacrylamide disc electrophoresis. J. Endocrinol. 45:183–196.

85. Norris, D.O. (1969). Depression of growth following radiothyroidectomy of larval chinook salmon and steelhead trout. Trans. Am. Fish. Soc. 98:104–106.

86. Norris, D.O., R.E. Jones and B.B. Criley (1973). Pituitary prolactin levels in larval, neotenic and metamorphosed salamanders (*Ambystoma tigrinum*). Gen. Comp. Endocrinol. 20:437–442.

87. Palmiter, R.D., G. Norstedt, R.E. Gelinas, R.E. Hammer and R.L. Brinster (1983). Metallothionein-human GH fusion genes stimulate growth in mice. Science 222:809–814.

88. Papkoff, H. (1972). Subunit relationships among the pituitary glycoprotein hormones. Gen. Comp. Endocrinol. Suppl. 3:609–616.

89. Papkoff, H. and T. Hayashida (1972). Pituitary growth hormone from the turtle and duck: Purification and immunochemical studies. Proc. Soc. Exp. Biol. Med. 140:251–255.

90. Parlow, A.F. (1961). Bioassay of pituitary luteinizing hormone by depletion of ovarian ascorbic acid. In A. Albert, ed., Human Pituitary Gonadotropins. Charles C Thomas, Springfield, Ill., pp. 300–310.

91. Peter, R.E. and L.W. Crim (1979). Reproductive endocrinology of fishes: Gonadal cycles and gonadotropin in teleosts. Annu. Rev. Physiol. 41:323–335.

92. Pierce, J.G. (1974). Chemistry of thyroid-stimulating hormone. Handbook of Physiology, Sec. 7, Endocrinology. Williams & Wilkins, Baltimore, Vol. 4, Part 2, pp. 79–102.

93. Platt, J.E. and M.A. Christopher (1977). Effects of prolactin on the water and sodium content of larval tissues from neotenic and metamorphosing *Ambystoma tigrinum*. Gen. Comp. Endocrinol. 31:243–248.

94. Rees, L.H. (1977). Human adrenocorticotropin and lipotropin (MSH) in health and disease. In L. Martini and G.M. Besser, eds., Clinical Neuroendocrinology. Academic Press, New York, pp. 401–441.

95. Reichlin, S. (1974). Regulation of somatotrophic hormone secretion. Handbook of Physiology, Sec. 7, Endocrinology. Williams & Wilkins, Baltimore, Vol. 4, Part 2, pp. 405–448.

96. Roos, J. and C.B. Jorgensen (1974). Rates of disappearance from blood and biological potencies of mammalian gonadotropins (HCG and ovine LH) in the toad *Bufo bufo bufo* (L.). Gen. Comp. Endocrinol. 23:432–437.

97. Sage, M. (1970). Control of prolactin release and its role in color change in the teleost *Gillichthyes mirabilis*. J. Exp. Zool. 173:121–128.

98. Sage, M. and H.A. Bern (1972). Assay of prolactin in vertebrate pituitaries by its dispersion of xanthophore pigment in the teleost *Gillichthyes mirabilis*. J. Exp. Zool. 180:169–174.

99. Scanes, C.G. and S. Harvey (1981). Growth hormone and prolactin in avian species. Life Sci. 28:2895–2902.

100. Schuetz, A. W. (1971). In vitro induction of ovulation and oocyte maturation in *Rana pipiens* ovarian follicles: Effects of steroidal and nonsteroidal hormones. J. Exp. Zool. 178:377–386.

101. Segal, S.J. (1957). Response of weaver finch to chorionic gonadotropin and hypophyseal luteinizing hormone. Science 126:1242–1243.

102. Shapiro, B. and B.L. Pimstone (1977). A phylogenetic study of sulfation factor activity in 26 species. J. Endocrinol. 74:129–135.

103. Shin, B.P.C., P.A. Kelly and H.G. Friesen (1973). Radioreceptor assay for prolactin and other lactogenic hormones. Science 180:968–971.

104. Solomon, J. and R.O. Greep (1959). The growth hormone content of several vertebrate pituitaries. Endocrinology 65:334–335.

105. Thornton, V.F. (1971). A bioassay for progesterone and gonadotropins based on the meiotic division of *Xenopus* oocytes *in vitro*. Gen. Comp. Endocrinol. 16:599–605.

106. Turkington, R.W. (1971). Measurement of prolactin activity in human serum by induction of specific

milk proteins in mammary gland *in vitro*. J. Clin. Endocrinol. Metab. 33:210–216.

107. Turner, C.D. and J.T. Bagnara (1976). General Endocrinology, 6th ed. W.B. Saunders Co., Philadelphia.

108. VanWyk, J.J. (1980). Growth hormone, somatomedins and growth failure. In D.T. Krieger and J.C. Hughes, eds., Neuroendocrinology, Sinauer Assoc. Inc., Sunderland, Mass., pp. 299–309.

109. Vellano, C. (1972). Un neuvo metado per il dosaggio biologico della prolattina. Boll. Soc. Ital. Biol. Sper. 48:360–362.

110. Wasserman, W.J. and L.D. Smith (1978). Oocyte maturation: Non mammalian vertebrates. In R.E. Jones, ed., The Vertebrate Ovary. Plenum Press, New York.

111. Wilhelmi, A.E. (1974). Chemistry of growth hormone. Handbook of Physiology, Sec. 7, Endocrinology, Williams & Wilkins, Baltimore, Vol. 4, Part 2, pp. 59–78.

112. Wittouck, P.J. (1975). Influence de la composition saline du milieu sur la concentration ionique du serum chez l'axolotl, intact et hypophysectomise. Effet de la prolactine. Gen. Comp. Endocrinol. 27:169–178.

113. Wright, P. (1945). Factors affecting *in vitro* ovulation in the frog. J. Exp. Zool. 100:565–575.

114. Zarrow, M.X., J.M. Yochim and J.L. McCarthy (1964). Experimental Endocrinology: A Sourcebook of Basic Techniques. Academic Press, New York.

6·Regulation of Pigmentation: The Pars Intermedia

Many vertebrates show changes in pigmentation or pigmentary patterns that are correlated with environmental factors or particular events in their life histories. Rapid responses are under direct neural control, and the slower responses are generally the result of endocrine control or a combination of neural and endocrine control. Pigmentation patterns mediated through melanotropin (MSH) from the pars intermedia are emphasized in this chapter with some minor reference to other endocrine factors and neural innervation.

Vertebrates possess a variety of specialized, pigmented cells referred to as *chromatophores* (Table 6-1). These cellular types singly or in special combinations are the bases for color patterns associated with the integument. *Physiological color changes* involving displacement of pigments within a pigment cell are characteristic only of fishes, amphibians and reptiles. All vertebrates exhibit increases in the number of chromatophores or increases in the amount of pigment contained within the chromatophores or both. This type of color change is termed *morphological color change.*

The terminologies employed here are from Bagnara and Hadley.[3] These authors do not recognize the term melanocyte as adopted by the Nomenclature Committee of the Sixth International Pigment Cell Conference in 1966 (Fig. 6-1). Mammalian researchers refer to the melanin-containing cells of the skin and other organs as melanocytes. The epidermal melanophore can be considered equivalent to the mammalian melanocyte.

Chromatophores

The types of chromatophores found among the vertebrates include the *melanophores,* usually containing black or brown pigments; *iridophores* (guanophores), appearing silvery or golden when viewed with reflected light; *xanthophores,* containing yellow or orange pigments; and *erythrophores* with red or orange pigments. In many cases a combination of these different chromatophore types occurs in the integument to provide a particular color or to allow for changes in coloration according to environmental conditions.

Structural coloration is due to interference, diffraction or *Tyndall scattering* of light waves. The Tyndall effect results from scattering of light by the reflecting platelets in iridophores. This scattering often imparts a blue coloration to amphibians and reptiles. If these iridophores are overlayed by xanthophores containing yellow pigments, the integument will appear green. Combinations of iridophores and other chromatophores may result in shades of blue, green, yellow, orange, red, bronze or gold.

Epidermal Melanophores

Epidermal melanophores (Fig. 6-2) are common in reptiles and occur at some stage in the life history of amphibians (embryo, larva or adult). They are also present in the hair of mammals and the feathers of birds. Fishes do not prominently exhibit epidermal melano-

TABLE 6-1. *Vertebrate Chromatophores*

CHROMATOPHORE	ORGANELLE	PIGMENT	COLOR
Melanophore	Melanosomes	Melanins	Brown, black (yellow, red)
Iridophore (guanophore, leucophore)	Reflecting platelets	Guanine, adenine, hypoxanthine, uric acid	–
Xanthophore	Pterinosomes	Pteridines	Yellow, orange
	Carotenoid vesicles	Carotenoids	Yellow, orange, red
Erythrophore	Pterinosomes	Pteridines	Red, orange
	Carotenoid vesicles	Carotenoids	Yellow, orange, red

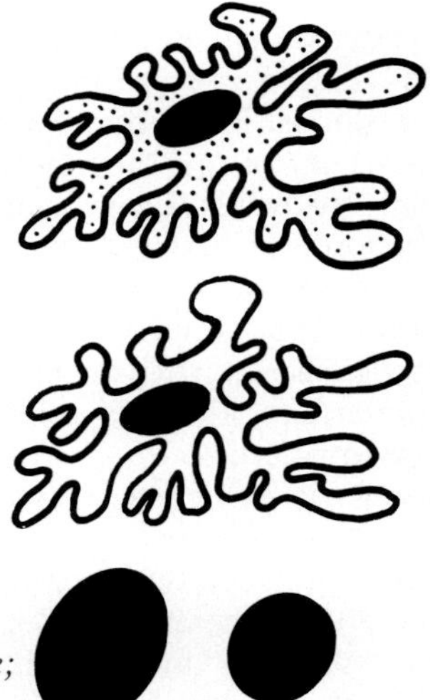

MELANOCYTE
A cell that synthesizes the pigment melanin

MELANOBLAST
Precursor of melanocyte; contains premelanosomes but does not synthesize melanin

MELANOSOME
Melanin-containing organelle in which melanization is complete; no tyrosinase activity present

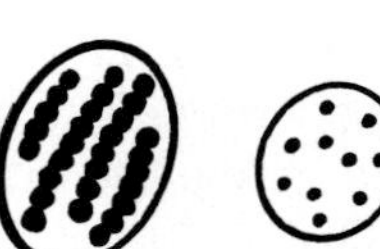

PREMELANOSOME
Active in melanin synthesis; tyrosinase activity present

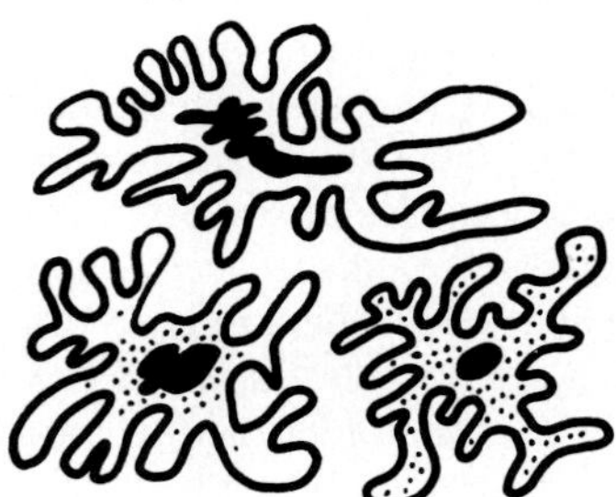

MELANOPHORE
A dermal or epidermal cell that participates with other cells in rapid color changes by intracellular displacement (migration) of melanosomes

FIG. 6-1. Terminology of vertebrate melanin-containing cells based on the Sixth International Pigment Cell Conference, 1966. Note that a melanocyte differs functionally from a melanophore in this terminology.

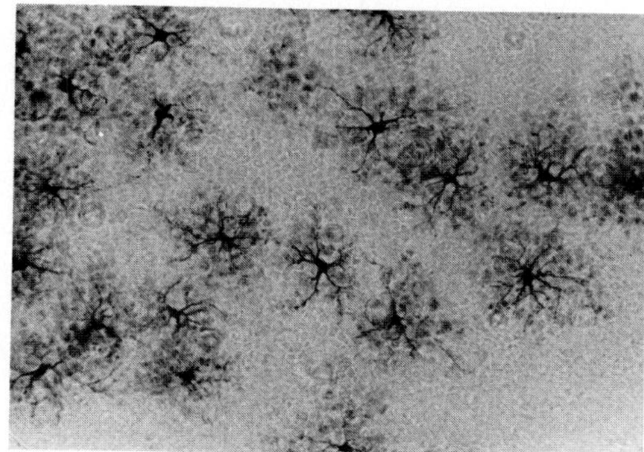

FIG. 6-2. Epidermal melanophores (melanocytes) in skin of *Rana pipiens.* Extracellular melanization is evident and is due to the secretory activities of the melanophores. (Reprinted with permission from J.T. Bagnara and M.E. Hadley (1973). Chromatophores and Color Change, the Comparative Physiology of Animal Pigmentation. Prentice-Hall, Englewood Cliffs, N.J.)

phores. This type of chromatophore typically is fusiform with long, slender processes that have few branches. Epidermal melanophores synthesize the pigment *melanin* and often deposit it extracellularly. These cells are involved in morphological color changes only and do not play a role in physiological color changes.

Dermal Melanophores

Dermal melanophores are found in the dermis, in various organs and on the surfaces of certain blood vessels and nerves. These cells are stellate and are principally involved in physiological color changes in lower vertebrates. Dermal melanophores contain the pigment *melanin* localized in organelles called *premelanosomes* or *melanosomes.* Premelanosomes are organelles that are still synthesizing melanin from its basic precursor, the amino acid tyrosine. These organelles exhibit high tyrosinase activity, the enzyme responsible for melanin synthesis. Melanosomes have ceased melanin synthesis and exhibit no tyrosinase activity. The intracellular origin of melanosomes is depicted in Figure 6-3. When examined with the aid of the electron microscope, melanosomes appear as uniformly electron-dense bodies in the cytoplasm, whereas the premelanosomes may show varying degrees of density even within a given organelle.

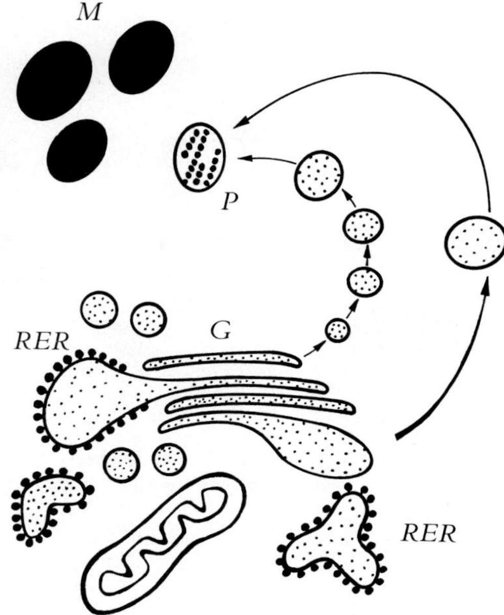

FIG. 6-3. Formation of premelanosomes and melanosomes in a melanophore (melanocyte). *RER,* rough endoplasmic reticulum; *G,* Golgi apparatus; *P,* premelanosomes; *M,* melanosomes.

Dispersion of melanosomes into the stellate processes of the melanophore causes a darkening of the integument. Aggregation of melanosomes near the nucleus of the melanophores will cause the integument to lighten. Migration of melanosomes is the principal mechanism employed whereby fishes, amphibians and reptiles adapt to light or dark backgrounds. These melanosome migrations may be under neural or endocrine control or both.

The ability to adapt to dark or light backgrounds is used as an index for endocrine state with respect to MSH. The degree of dispersion of melanosomes within a given melanophore may be quantified on an arbitrary scale from 1 to 5 where 1 indicates complete aggregation and 5 indicates maximum dispersion. This index of melanophore expansion is referred to as the *Hogben* or *melanophore index* (Figs 6-4, 6-5). This index is useful in examining intact animals when it is not feasible to utilize the MSH bioassays (see Chap. 5).

Iridophores

Iridophores are found in the dermis (Fig. 6-6), and they are highly variable in general

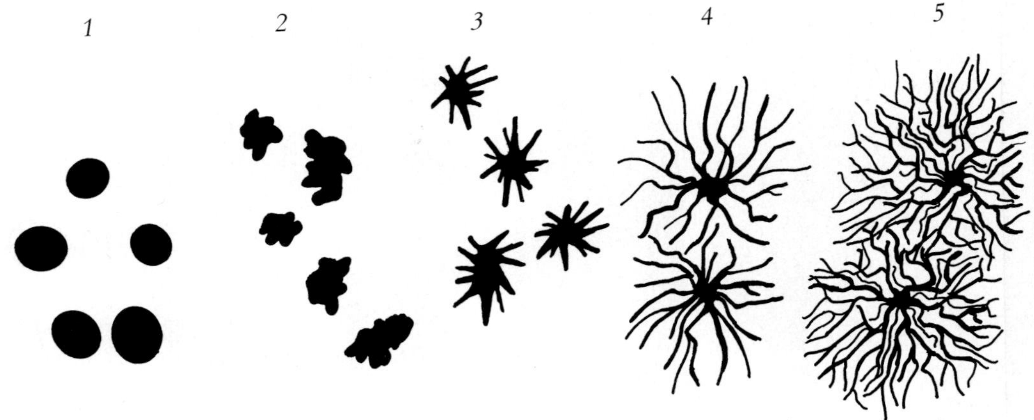

FIG. 6-4. The melanophore index for determining the degree of dispersion of the melanosomes within the stellate dermal melanophores of amphibian larvae. Maximum dispersion = 5. (After Hogben and Slome.[18])

appearance in different vertebrate groups. They reflect light because of the presence of *reflecting platelets* in their cytoplasm. These flat, reflecting platelets contain *purines,* especially guanine, although hypoxanthine, adenine or uric acid may be employed. Reflecting platelets are arranged in oriented stacks (Fig. 6-6). Iridophores are sometimes involved with morphological and physiological color changes as well as with structural color patterns, but their regulation is not fully understood.

Xanthophores and Erythrophores

Xanthophores typically contain yellow pigments, and erythrophores contain red pigments, although either of them may possess orange pigments. These chromatophores are dermal, although they are occasionally located in the epidermis, as in the red spots of the red-spotted newt *Notophthalmus viridescens.*

The pigments contained within these chromatophores are usually *carotenoids* but may be *pteridines.* Pteridines are found in distinct

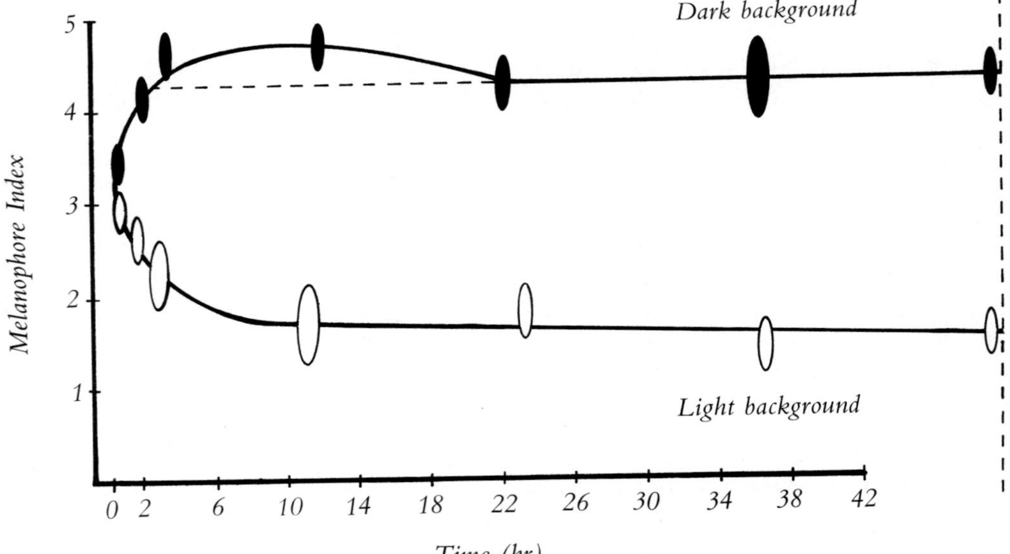

FIG. 6-5. Melanophore index for animals transferred from darkness into light and placed on a black or white background. *1* = complete aggregation; *5* = maximum dispersion. (Redrawn from Novales.[40])

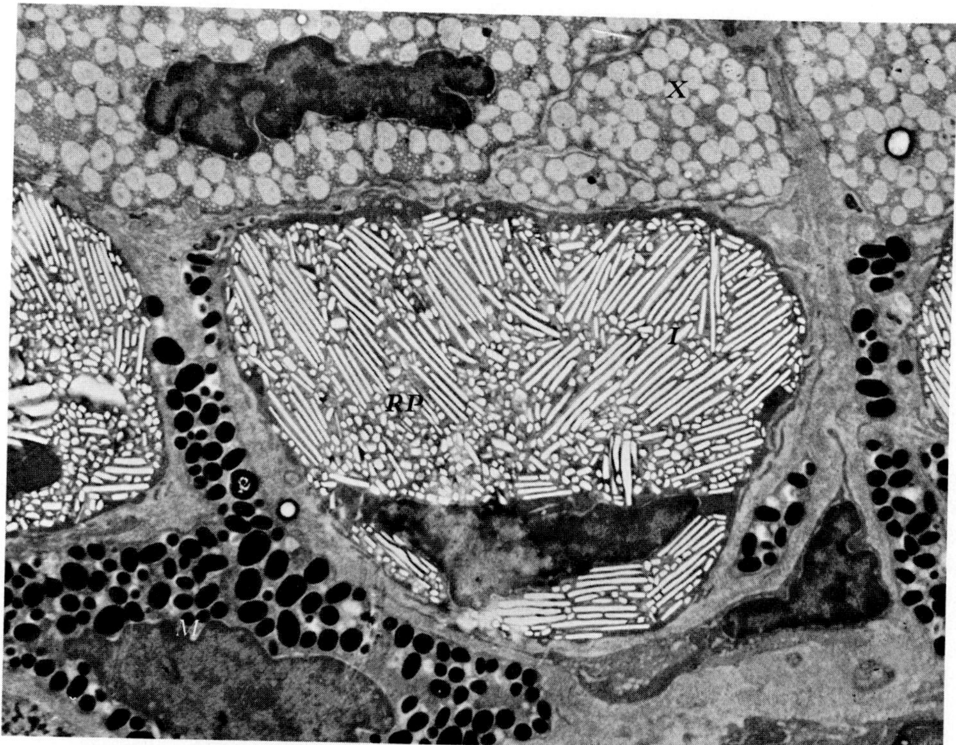

FIG. 6-6. Iridophore. This section from the skin of *Hyla cineria* (Amphibia: Anura) shows an iridophore *(I)* with reflecting platelets *(RP)* overlain by a xanthophore *(X)*. Portions of a melanophore *(M)* containing melanosomes are also shown. (Reprinted with permission from J.T. Bagnara, M.E. Hadley, and J.D. Taylor (1969). Regulation of bright colored pigmentation of amphibians. Gen. Comp. Endocrinol. Suppl. 2:425–438.)

cytoplasmic organelles called *pterinosomes* that are derived presumably from smooth endoplasmic reticulum. These organelles are spherical or ellipsoidal (about 0.5 mm diameter) and are composed of a series of concentric lamellae (Fig. 6-7). Pterinosomes are evenly distributed throughout the cytoplasm of certain xanthophores and erythrophores of fishes, amphibians and reptiles. The *carotenoid vesicles* are organelles containing carotenoid pigments. These organelles are much smaller than pterinosomes and are not lamellar in structure (Fig. 6-7).

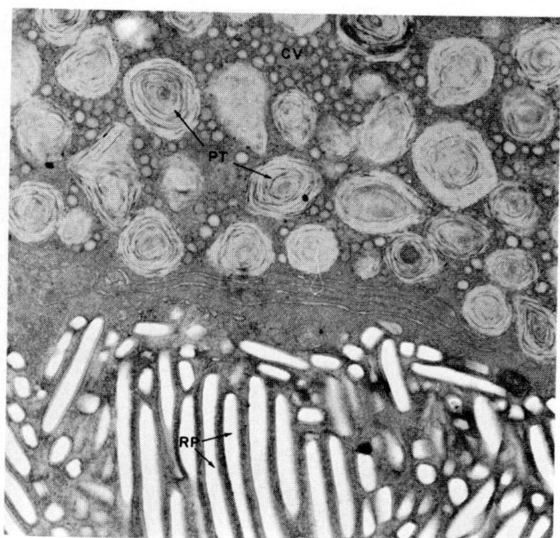

FIG. 6-7. Pterinosomes *(PT)* and carotenoid vesicles *(CV)* in a xanthophore. An iridophore with reflecting platelets *(RP)* appears below the xanthophore. From the skin of *Hyla cineria* (Amphibia: Anura). (Reprinted with permission from J.T. Bagnara, M.E. Hadley, and J.D. Taylor (1969). Regulation of bright colored pigmentation of amphibians. Gen. Comp. Endocrinol. Suppl. 2:425–438).

Overlapping of Characteristics in Chromatophores

Melanophores are sometimes observed that contain reflecting platelets (characteristic of iridophores) or pterinosomes (containing pteridine pigments as found in xanthophores and erythrophores). Either xanthophores or iridophores may contain melanosomes in addition to their characteristic organelles. Some chromatophores have been described that contain both pterinosomes and reflecting platelets. Obviously the descriptive categories outlined above are not mutually exclusive. These categories, however, are useful in characterizing the majority of chromatophores and in discussing their neural and endocrine regulation.

The Dermal Melanophore Unit

Dermal melanophores appear in some amphibians in a precise arrangement with xanthophores and iridophores to form a functional entity that has been termed the *dermal melanophore unit*[3] (Fig. 6-8). Similar associations of chromatophores may occur in lizards as well. This unit consists of an iridophore surrounded by extensions of a more basal dermal melanophore. Both of these cells are overlain by a xanthophore. The interactions of xanthophore pigments and Tyndall scattering caused by reflecting platelets of the iridophore can be altered by the movement of melanosomes in the dermal melanophore. The distribution of melanosomes in the skin of light-adapted and dark-adapted frogs is illustrated in Figures 6-9 and 6-10. Such alterations in position of the melanosomes can result in gradations of color.

Pigmentation Patterns

Coloration patterns in some vertebrates may be determined by the distribution of types of chromatophores and by the relationship of dermal chromatophore units to other chromatophores. For example, the dark spots on the skin of the frog *Rana pipiens* are due to concentrations of epidermal melanophores and extracellular deposition of melanin, whereas adjacent regions of the skin that may vary from light green to black are occupied exclusively by dermal chromatophore units (Fig. 6-11).

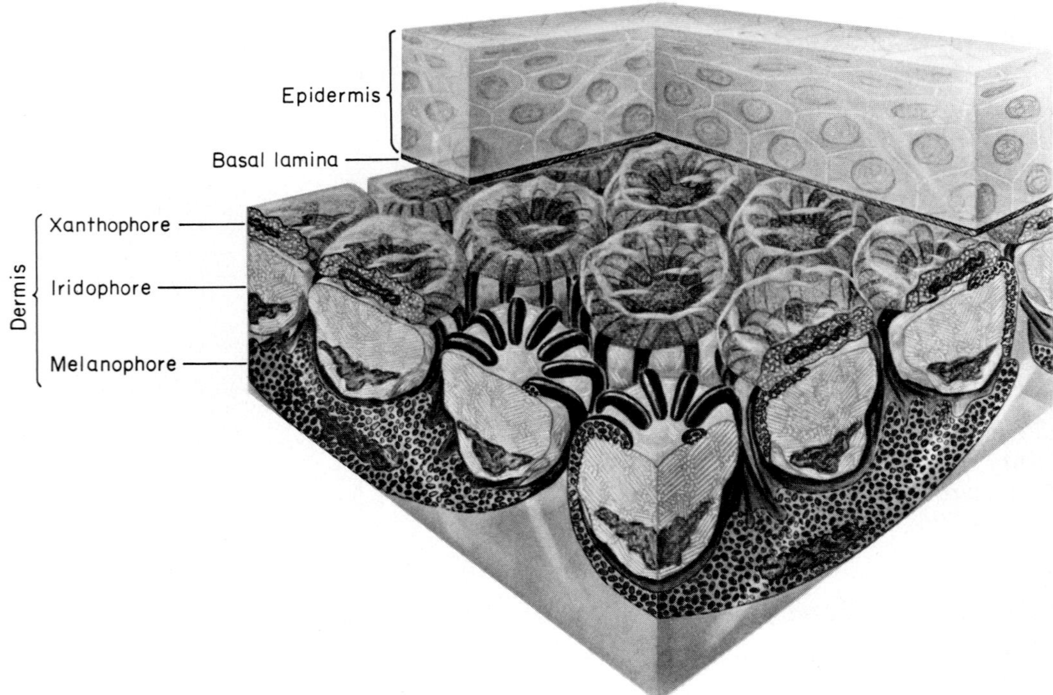

Fig. 6-8. The dermal chromatophore unit. This is a composite scheme based upon several anuran species. (Reprinted with permission from J.T. Bagnara, M.E. Hadley, and J.D. Taylor (1969). Regulation of bright colored pigmentation of amphibians. Gen. Comp. Endocrinol. Suppl. 2:425–438).

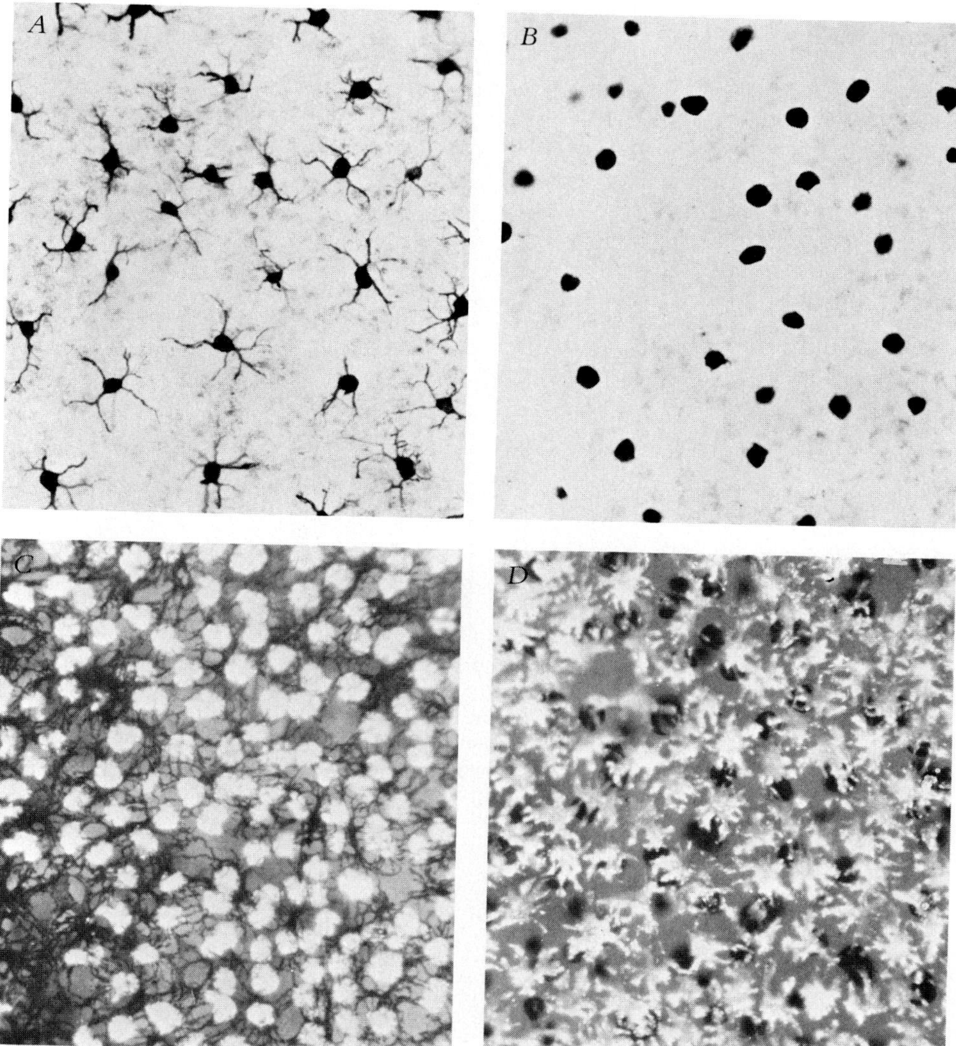

FIG. 6-9. Adaptation to a dark background or MSH treatment causes melanosome dispersion in both epidermal *(A)* and dermal *(C)* melanophores, but melanophores are aggregated in the light or in the absence of MSH *(B, D)*. Note that the white-colored iridophores in the dermis are punctate (reflecting platelets are aggregated) in dark-adapted or MSH-treated skin *(C)* but are dispersed in the opposite condition *(D)*. (Reprinted with permission from J.T. Bagnara and M.E. Hadley (1973). Chromatophores and Color Change, The Comparative Physiology of Animal Pigmentation. Prentice-Hall, Englewood Cliffs, N.J.)

Regulation of Chromatophores by Melanotropin

The pars intermedia is the primary endocrine regulator of pigmentary responses in vertebrates through elaboration of MSH. Development of the pars intermedia and factors controlling the secretion of MSH are outlined in Chapter 4. Recall that MSH release is under inhibitory hypothalamic control and that MSH belongs to the family of adenohypophysial polypeptides that includes lipotropin, corticotropin (ACTH) and the endorphins.

The major target for MSH is the dermal melanophore, and in a few cases, other chromatophores may be affected.

Adenyl cyclase activity is enhanced by MSH

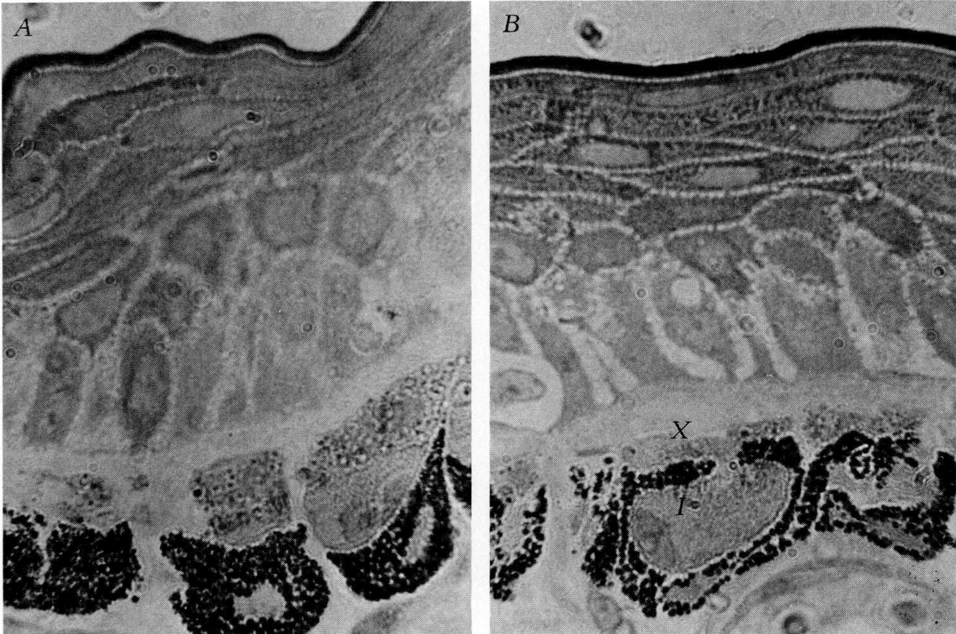

Fig. 6-10. Cytological comparison of dermal melanophore units in the dermis of light- and dark-adapted frogs, *Agalychnis dacnicolor* (Amphibia: Anura). In the light-adapted frog *(left)* the melanosomes are concentrated in the perinuclear region of the melanophore. In the dark-adapted frog *(right),* the melanosomes are dispersed into the processes of the melanophore that separates the xanthophore *(X)* from the iridophore *(I)*. (Reprinted with permission from J.T. Bagnara, M.E. Hadley, and J.D. Taylor (1969). Regulation of bright colored pigmentation of amphibians. Gen. Comp. Endocrinol. Suppl. 2:425–438.)

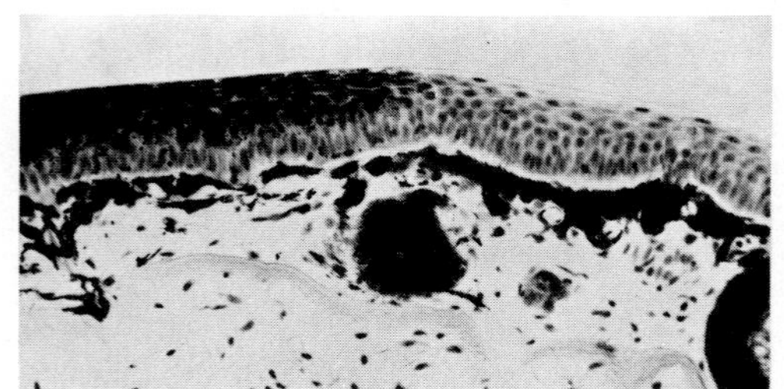

Fig. 6-11. Comparative pattern effects in skin produced by epidermal and dermal chromatophore distribution. To the *left* of this transverse section of adult *Rana pipiens* skin is a pigment spot deposited by the activities of epidermal melanophores. Note the absence of epidermal melanophores and extracellular melanin in the epidermis overlying dermal chromatophore units *(right).* (Reprinted with permission from J.T. Bagnara and M.E. Hadley (1973). Chromatophores and Color Change, The Comparative Physiology of Animal Pigmentation. Prentice-Hall, Englewood Cliffs, N.J.)

in melanin-synthesizing cells of fish, amphibians and mammals.[40] Melanotropin activates adenyl cyclase in the melanophore plasmalemma, which in turn produces cyclic adenosine 3′, 5′-monophosphate (cAMP). Melanosome dispersion is effected by cAMP and is enhanced by caffeine through its inhibition of the cAMP-degrading enzyme phosphodiesterase (see Chap. 1 for a review of the cAMP mechanism of hormone action). Corticotropin also causes melanosome dispersion by activating adenyl cyclase. Cyclic guanosine 3′, 5′-monophosphate (cGMP) however, is without effect.[39] Melanophore regulation by nervous elements may operate by inhibiting the action of MSH on cAMP formation. For example, norepinephrine, the neurotransmitter of postganglionic sympathetic neurons, inhibits the MSH-induced increase in cAMP.[2] A scheme for the mechanisms of MSH action on the melanophore is provided in Figure 6-12.

The actual mechanism of how melanosomes migrate in and out of the stellate processes of

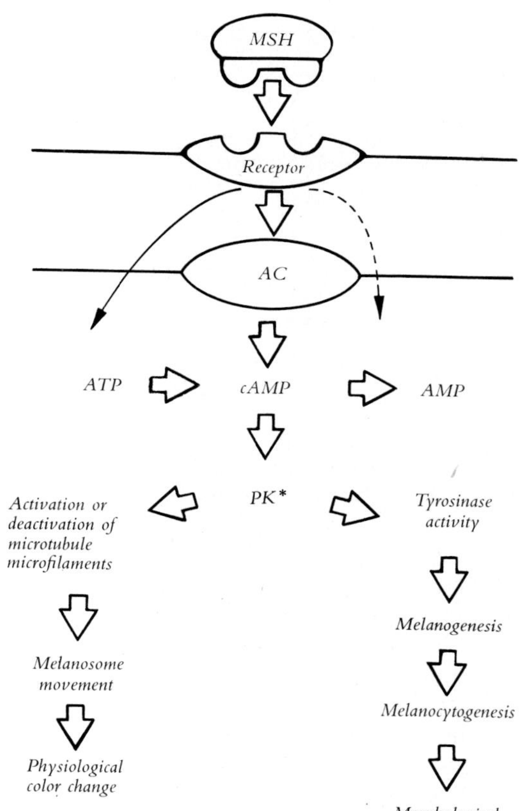

FIG. 6-12. Mechanism of action by MSH on the melanophore. This scheme incorporates physiological and morphological color changes. *AC*, adenyl cyclase; *PK**, activated or phosphorylated protein kinase. (Modified from Hadley and Bagnara.[13])

the melanophore is unknown. It appears that microtubules are essential for aggregation of the melanosomes, and these may be activated by cAMP. Any experimental treatment known to interfere with microtubule formation, such as application of the drug colchicine, blocks melanosome aggregation. Ultrastructural observations, however, in some amphibian melanophores do not support the presence of microtubules oriented properly to cause melanosomes to disperse, and the role of microtubules needs further clarification.[40]

Class Agnatha

Hagfishes (*Myxine glutinosa*) show no ability to adapt to different backgrounds,[1] suggesting no role for MSH with respect to background adaptation. However, hypophysectomy of lampreys (Petromyzontidae) produces permanent paling, presumably due to loss of MSH.[6] Exogenous MSH causes melanosome dispersion in lampreys.[56] Nothing is known about factors controlling MSH release in cyclostomes.[22]

Class Chondrichthyes

Sharks do adapt to background but very slowly, requiring up to 100 hours to achieve maximum adaptation.[53] Hypophysectomy abolishes this ability to "background adapt," whereas ectopic transplants of the neurointermediate lobe cause permanent darkening regardless of the background upon which the shark is placed.

The dogfish shark pituitary contains α-MSH,[32] and sharks darken following injection of either α- or β-MSH.[33] Melanophore responses to MSH are paralleled by similar responses in xanthophores.[16]

Both aminergic and peptidergic fibers penetrate into the dogfish pars intermedia. Possibly peptidergic fibers control synthesis of MSH by the pars intermedia cells, and aminergic fibers are responsible for controlling MSH release.[27] The pars intermedia of the holocephalan *Hydrolagus colliei* also exhibits NS innervation, although the type of innervation has not been determined.[19] The vascular arrangement between the hypothalamus and the pars intermedia of the dogfish shark implies neurovascular control rather than direct neural innervation or neurohumoral control.[35] It is not clear what mechanism predominates in controlling release of MSH in these fishes.

Class Osteichthyes: Teleostei

The pigmentary responses of fishes are under control of direct aminergic innervation of melanophores and other chromatophores (Tables 6-2, 6-3) and MSH does not play a major role in physiological color changes.[1,3,40] The melanophores of most species do not respond to either hypophysectomy or exogenous MSH, whereas others show only a limited response to MSH following denervation of the melanophores. Dispersion of pigments in mel-

TABLE 6-2. *Drugs Causing Melanosome Aggregation When Injected Subcutaneously in the Opercular Area of the Fish* Scopthalmus aquosus

DRUG	MED[a] (μg)	AFTER PYROGALLOL[b] TREATMENT (μg)
Epinephrine	0.04	0.00010
Isoproterenol	0.08	0.00002
Dopamine	0.02	0.02
Dopa	Inactive	Inactive
Phenylephrine	0.0002	0.0004
Melatonin	0.06	0.06
5-HT	0.1	2.0

Modified from Scott, G.T. (1972).[51]
[a] Minimum effective dose (3 or 4 fish responding of 5 tested).
[b] Pyrogallol is an inhibitor of the enzyme catechol-o-methyl transferase, which inactivates epinephrine and norepinephrine.

anophores of goldfish *Carassius auratus* and erythrophores of the European minnow *Phoxinus phoxinus* occurs following treatment with MSH. Melanophore dispersion can be induced only in denervated melanophores of the killfish *Fundulus heteroclitus* because of the presence of overriding neural stimuli in intact fish.

MSH may play some role in morphological color changes in teleosts. Treatment of xanthic goldfish (goldfish normally lacking any melanophores) with MSH stimulates melanophore differentiation and melanogenesis. Hypophysectomy of *Fundulus heteroclitus* causes a reduction in the number of melanophores,[43] and treatment with MSH results in an increase in

TABLE 6-3. *Drugs Causing Melanosome Dispersion When Injected Subcutaneously in the Opercular Area of the Fish* Scopthalmus aquosus

DRUG	MED[a] (μg)
Serotonin blockers	
LSD-25	0.8
Dibenamine	0.2
Adrenergic blockers	
Dihydroxyergotamine	0.6
Propranolol	6.0
Depressants	
Pentobarbital sodium	80.0
Phenothiazine ataractics	
Chlorpromazine	0.8
Cholinergic substances	
Acetylcholine	No effect up to 500 μg

Modified from Scott, G.T. (1972).[51]
[a] Minimum effective dose (3 or 4 fish responding out of 5 fish tested)

the number of melanophores.[28] A conflicting report suggests melanophore differentiation in xanthic goldfish is caused by ACTH and not by MSH,[5] but this difference has not been resolved.

Class Amphibia

Melanophores. Direct control of amphibian melanophores is under endocrine regulation, and there is no evidence for innervation of amphibian melanophores with the possible exception of limited neural control in *Rana pipiens.*[3] There is, however, evidence for neural control of MSH release (see also Chap. 4).

It was once claimed that there were two hormones controlling pigmentation in *Xenopus laevis,* a B or darkening substance and a W or lightening substance.[18] The B substance is MSH, and the existence of the W substance believed to be produced by the pars tuberalis has been disproved.[21]

There have been reports of dual "innervation" of the pars intermedia in amphibians of a different type than in the cartilaginous fishes. Adrenergic fibers have been shown to penetrate the pars intermedia of *Rana temporaria* and *Bufo arenarum,*[7,8] and two types of adrenergic fibers synapse with pars intermedia cells of *Rana pipiens.*[36,41] No innervation of the pars intermedia is observed in the African clawed frog *Xenopus laevis,* however.[11] Dual control of MSH release as suggested for some anurans may operate through the presence of alpha and beta adrenergic receptors in the plasmalemma of the pars intermedia cells.[13] The catecholamines, dopamine, norepinephrine, and epinephrine, as well as alpha receptor agonists such as phenylephrine all inhibit MSH release from the pars intermedia. Isoproterenol stimulates MSH release by activating beta adrenergic receptors. Known antagonists of alpha receptors (for example, dibenamine and dihydroergotamine) block the inhibitory actions of the catecholamines. Finally, antagonists of beta receptors, such as propranolol, block the action of isoproterenol.

Certain cautions must be employed when one is attempting to interpret the actions of various drugs on MSH release from the pars intermedia. Epinephrine, for example, inhibits MSH release when applied at higher doses (10^{-5} M) but stimulates MSH release when applied at lower doses (10^{-6} or 10^{-7} M). Apparently at higher doses epinephrine saturates both alpha and beta receptors, but the alpha effect predominates. At lower doses, epinephrine is more readily bound to the beta receptors so that the beta effect predominates, and MSH is released. The observation that a certain compound stimulates release of MSH does not necessarily imply a normal in-vivo role for that substance or for the type of innervation it might suggest.

Dopamine is the most potent inhibitor of MSH release, and several investigators have proposed that it is the hypothalamic MSH release-inhibiting hormone (MSHRIH) in amphibians as in mammals.[15] The actions of the other catecholamines under experimental conditions may only reflect an influence on the normal mechanism whereby dopamine controls MSH release.

Other Amphibian Chromatophores. Pigment organelles of xanthophores are normally in an expanded state in most amphibians. In the tree frog *Hyla arenicolor,* however, the xanthophores are normally in an aggregated condition, and they may be dispersed by the application of MSH.[3] An endogenous role for MSH on xanthophore pigment organelles has not been confirmed.

The aggregation of reflecting platelets in the iridophores of *Rana pipiens* skin is stimulated by cAMP or MSH.[14,40] These iridophores possess alpha and beta adrenergic receptors, and stimulation of the alpha receptors produces dispersion of the reflecting platelets. These data suggest a possible role for catecholamines in iridophore regulation.

Class Reptilia

Reptiles exhibit a variety of mechanisms for regulating dermal pigment cells, including neural and endocrine mechanisms. Unlike the well-established pattern of adrenergic innervation in most amphibians, no innervation of the pars intermedia has been observed at either the light or electron microscopic level in several lizard species.[9,37,48] Even the primitive tuatara of New Zealand, *Sphenodon punctatus,* exhibits no innervation of the pars intermedia.[55] Innervation of pigment cells does occur in some reptiles, and pigmentary control of dermal melanophores may be neural, endocrine or both.

Color changes in the true chameleon *Chameleo pumilis* are under direct neural control, and MSH has no effect on the skin chromatophores.[17] Melanophores of *Chameleo jacksoni,* however, respond to both MSH and ACTH.[4] The opposite extreme is found in the American chameleon *Anolis carolinensis,* in which there is no neural control over melanophore responses,[23-25] and melanosome dispersion can be readily induced in vitro by application of MSH or cAMP to isolated pieces of *Anolis* skin.[34] Pretreatment with alpha adrenergic-blocking agents obliterates the response of *Anolis* melanophores to MSH. Horned lizards, *Phrysonoma* spp., exhibit both neural and hormonal regulation of melanophores.[42]

Neither xanthophores nor iridophores of *A. carolinensis* show any response to MSH.[52] It is not known whether any non-melanin-containing chromatophores of other reptiles show any regulatory control.

Class Aves

Feather pigments (including melanin) are under the control of gonadal, thyroidal and gonadotropic hormones.[46] The only reported action for MSH in birds is related to a developmental action. Embryonic implants of chicken pituitaries cause formation of black feathers where normally only white feathers would develop.[12] This effect can be mimicked by treatment with either α-MSH or ACTH.

Class Mammalia

The first report for an action of MSH in mammals was the observation that injection of a highly purified MSH preparation into humans caused a darkening of skin and nevi (a nevus is a congenital mole).[30] This action was due both to dispersion of melanosomes in melanophores and an increase in free melanin contained within surrounding keratinocytes.

Hypophysectomy of the short-tailed weasel results in regrowth of white hair characteristic of the winter coat even in animals possessing summer pelage (brown) at the time of hypophysectomy.[49] Treatment of hypophysectomized weasels with MSH or ACTH causes regrowth of brown pelage. Ectopically transplanted pituitaries also result in production of brown pelage in hypophysectomized weasels. Similar actions of MSH on pelage of mice have been reported.[10]

Alpha MSH cooperates with testosterone to stimulate lipogenesis and the synthesis of wax esters in the sebaceous glands of rats.[53] This observation suggests that other roles for MSH should be sought in mammals in addition to actions on melanophores.

Influence of the Epiphysial Complex on Regulation of Chromatophores

The epiphysial complex consists of one or more dorsal evaginations from the epithalamic portion of the brain (see Chap. 15). These epithalamic structures include the pineal gland or pineal organ, the *epiphysis cerebri.* In fishes and amphibians the epiphysial complex includes a photoreceptor as well as a glandular component. In amniotes there is a progressive tendency to reduce the photoreceptive function and emphasize the endocrine function of the pineal. Avian and mammalian pineal organs completely lack any photoreceptive structures.

Many studies have demonstrated an influence of the epiphysial complex on pigmentary responses. The blanching that had been observed in amphibian larvae maintained in the dark is due to melatonin produced in the pineal gland. Melatonin may inhibit MSH release or directly influence the distribution of melanosomes in the melanophores, causing the animals to lighten, or it may do both (Fig. 6-13).

Fishes

There is little evidence to support a role for the pineal of fishes in pigmentary responses.[3] Pinealectomy does abolish the diurnal rhythm of color change in lampreys,[6] but the effects of melatonin and pineal implants are inconsistent in different species. No role for the pineal has been reported for members of the class Chondrichthyes. Some teleosts exhibit differential day and night coloration patterns, and

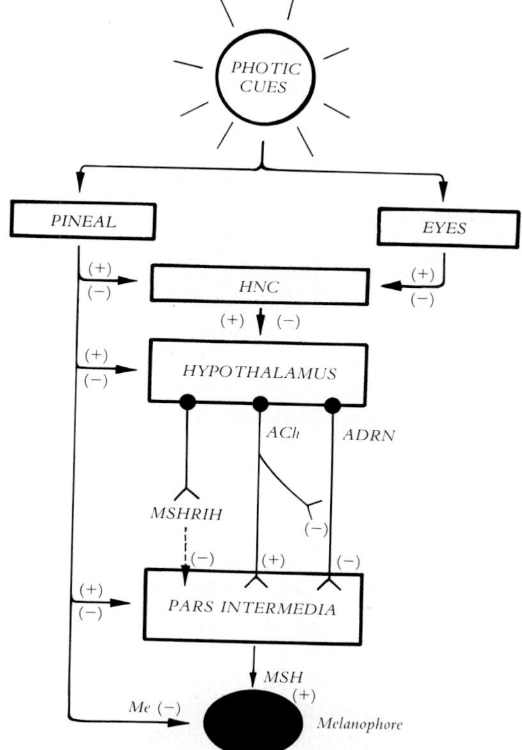

FIG. 6-13. Influence of photoreceptors *(pineal, eyes)* on release of MSH from the pars distalis. *Photic cues* influence higher neural centers *(HNC)* via the pineal or the lateral eyes or both. These neural centers control the activity of hypothalamic centers that innervate the pars intermedia or influence a neurosecretory center that produces MSHRIH. Pineal melatonin *(Me)* may antagonize the activity of MSH on the melanophore. *ACh,* acetylcholine; *ADRN,* adrenergic transmitters. (Modified from Hadley and Bagnara.[13])

melatonin can influence dispersion in some melanophores and aggregation in others to produce the typical "night pattern."[1] In general, no physiological role for the pineal in color changes has been established in teleosts.[3]

Class Amphibia

Melatonin does cause blanching of dark-adapted frogs and is equally effective in hypophysectomized frogs treated with MSH.[3,13] Pinealectomized larvae do not blanch when placed in the dark as do intact larvae, and it is concluded that the influences of light on pigment dispersion and aggregation in amphibian melanophores is mediated through the pineal gland.

Amniotes

There is no evidence to support a role for epithalamic structures as regulators of pigmentary responses in either reptiles or birds. In mammals, however, several examples of color change have been investigated and a role for pineal influence established. The production of the white winter coat in the weasel *Mustela erminea bangsi* can be induced in the spring molt with melatonin treatment.[50] This action of melatonin is believed to occur at the hypothalamus where it influences the output of hypothalamic MSHRIH. Normally the production of brown pigment in the hair of this mammal is dependent upon pituitary MSH.

Influence of Other Hormones on Pigmentation

Prolactin (PRL) preparations cause marked expansion of the xanthophores of the teleost *Gillichthyes mirabilis* and are the basis for the *Gillichthyes* xanthophore-expanding bioassay described in Chapter 5. In addition, prolonged treatment with mammalian PRL has been shown to cause darkening of the integument of fishes and amphibians.[28,45] Expansion of the xanthophores of *Gillichthyes* can also be induced with MSH and ACTH, and some reports of pigmentary changes with crude preparations of PRL on melanophores may be attributable to contamination with either or both of these peptides. Purified tilapia PRL is ineffective in the *Gillichthyes* xanthophore-expanding bioassay, but the assay responds to PRL obtained from eels.[26]

Gonadotropins and gonadal steroids have been reported to influence pigmentation in fishes, amphibians, birds and mammals. The direct action of luteinizing hormone on melanization of bird feathers was mentioned in Chapter 5 (weaver finch bioassay). Follicle-stimulating hormone preparations induce integumentary darkening in tiger salamander larvae and in the American chameleon. A summary of the actions of gonadal steroids and gonadotropins on pigmentation is provided in Table 6-4.

Thyroid hormones stimulate the deposition of guanine in the scales of teleosts and induce silvering in radiothyroidectomized and intact juvenile trout.[38,44] The increased darkening observed in radiothyroidectomized trout and salmon may be due in part to stimulation of melanophores following their concentration of radioactive iodide used to destroy the thyroid tissue.[29,38]

Summary

There are four basic types of chromatophores involved in pigmentary changes: melanophores (both dermal and epidermal), iridophores, xanthophores and erythrophores. The different pigments associated with these chromatophores are contained in specific organelles. Melanin is found in the melanosomes of the melanophore. The reflecting platelets of iridophores contain guanine and other purines. Pteridines are found in pterinosomes and carotenoid pigments are found in carotenoid vesicles of both xanthophores and erythrophores. Pigmentary responses are a result of migration of these organelles within the chromatophore (that is, dispersion or aggregation), the result of proliferation of chromatophores or new pigment synthesis. The first type of response is referred to as physiological color change and the latter two as morphological color change.

Pigmentary responses are largely under the control of MSH from the pars intermedia except in teleosts in which a considerable amount of direct neural control is manifest. Even in teleosts, however, MSH may affect morphological color changes. Release of MSH is primarily under the inhibitory control of the hypothalamus. Adrenergic fibers may influence release of MSH in some vertebrates. An MSHRIH has been chemically characterized as a small peptide, but it is possible that dopamine is MSHRIH.

The action of MSH on melanophores has been shown to be operating through the second messenger, cAMP. Microtubules appear to be involved in the migration of pigment organelles within the chromatophore, and cAMP may influence microtubule formation.

The pineal complex affects pigmentary patterns in two ways. Numerous studies have shown that the pineal complex acts as a transducer of light stimuli and influences the release of MSH from the pars intermedia. Melatonin, the presumed hormone secreted by the pineal organ, antagonizes the action of MSH on the melanophore by inhibiting cAMP formation normally stimulated by MSH.

Pigmentary responses have been influenced by manipulations involving PRL, gonadal steroids, gonadotropins and thyroid hormones. MSH has not been shown to influence pigments in adult birds.

TABLE 6-4. *Effects of Gonadal Steroids and Gonadotropins on Vertebrate Pigment Cells*

VERTEBRATE	HORMONE	EFFECT	REF.
Teleost	Androgens	Induction of nuptial pigment	3
Frog skin	Progesterone	Dispersion of melanosomes; aggregation of iridophores	3
Tiger salamander larvae	FSH	Prolonged darkening	45
American chameleon	FSH	Prolonged darkening	20
Weaver finches (Aves)	Estrogens, Androgens, LH	Stimulation of melanin production in epidermal melanophores, feathers and beak	3
Mammals	Estrogens	Increase melanin content in epidermal melanophores	3
	Androgens	Molting of castrate showing less melanin in hair	3

References

1. Abbott, F.S. (1973). Endocrine regulation of pigmentation in fish. Am. Zool. 13:885–894.

2. Abe, K., R.W. Butcher, W.E. Nicholson, C.E. Baird, R.A. Liddle and G.W. Liddle (1969). Adenosine 3′, 5′-monophosphate (cyclic AMP) as the mediator of the actions of melanocyte stimulating hormone (MSH) and norepinephrine on the frog skin. Endocrinology 84:362–368.

3. Bagnara, J.T. and M.E. Hadley (1973). Chromatophores and Color Change: The Comparative Physiology of Animal Pigmentation. Prentice-Hall, Englewood Cliffs, N.J.

4. Canella, M.F. (1963). Note di fisiologia dei cromatofori dei vertebrati pecilotermi, particolarmente dei lacertili. Monitore Zool. Ital. 71:430–480.

5. Chavin, W. (1956). Pituitary-adrenal control of melanization in xanthic goldfish, *Carassius auratus* L. J. Exp. Zool. 133:1–45.

6. Eddy, J.M.P. and R. Strahan (1968). The role of the pineal complex in the pigmentary effector system of the lampreys, *Mordacia mordax* (Richardson) and *Geotria australis* Gray. Gen. Comp. Endocrinol. 11:528–534.

7. Enemar, A. and B. Falck (1965). On the presence of adrenergic nerves in the pars intermedia of the frog, *Rana temporaria.* Gen. Comp. Endocrinol. 5:577–583.

8. Enemar, A., B. Falck and F.C. Iturriza (1967). Adrenergic nerves in the pars intermedia of the pituitary in the toad, *Bufo arenarum.* Z. Zellforsch. 77:325–330.

9. Forbes, M.S. (1972). Observations on the fine structure of the pars intermedia in the lizard *Anolis carolinensis.* Gen. Comp. Endocrinol. 18:146–161.

10. Geschwind, I.I. (1966). Change in hair color in mice induced by injection of α-MSH. Endocrinology 79:1165–1167.

11. Goos, H.J. Th. (1969). Hypothalamic control of the pars intermedia in *Xenopus laevis* tadpoles. Z. Zellforsch. 97:118–124.

12. Groenendijk-Huijbers, M.M. (1968). Development of black down feathering in hybrid chick embryos after pituitary implantation. Experientia 24:501–503.

13. Hadley, M.E. and J.T. Bagnara (1975). Regulation of release and mechanism of action of MSH. Am. Zool. 15, Suppl. 1:81–104.

14. Hadley, M.E. and J.M. Goldman (1969). Physiological color changes in reptiles. Am. Zool. 9:489–504.

15. Hadley, M.E. and V.J. Hruby (1977). Neurohypophysial peptides and the regulation of melanophore stimulating hormone (MSH) secretion. Am. Zool. 17:809–821.

16. Hogben, L.T. (1936). The pigmentary effector system. VII. The chromatic function in elasmobranch fishes. Proc. R. Soc. Lond. 120:142–158.

17. Hogben, L.T. and L. Mirvish (1928). The pigmentary effector system. V. The nervous control of excitement pallor in reptiles. J. Exp. Biol. 5:295–308.

18. Hogben, L.T. and D. Slome (1931). The pigmentary effector system. VI. The dual character of endocrine coordination in amphibian colour change. Proc. R. Soc. Lond. 108:10–53.

19. Jasinski, A. and A. Gorbman (1966). Hypothalamo-hypophysial vascular and neurosecretory links in the ratfish, *Hydrolagus colliei* (Lay and Bennett). Gen. Comp. Endocrinol. 6:476–490.

20. Jones, R.E. Unpublished observations.

21. Jorgenson, C.B. and L.O. Larsen (1960). Control of colour change in amphibians. Nature 186:641–642.

22. Kastin, A.J., S. Viosca and A.V. Schally (1974). Regulation of melanocyte-stimulating hormone release. Handbook of Physiology, Sec. 7, Endocrinology. Williams & Wilkins, Baltimore, Vol. 4, Part 2, pp. 551–562.

23. Kleinholz, L.H. (1936). Studies in reptilian color changes. I. A preliminary report. Proc. Natl. Acad. Sci. 22:454–456.

24. Kleinholz, L.H. (1938). Studies in reptilian colour changes. II. The pituitary and adrenal glands in the regulation of melanophores of *Anolis carolinensis.* J. Exp. Biol. 15:474–491.

25. Kleinholz, L.H. (1938). Studies in reptilian colour changes. III. Control of the light phase and behaviour of isolated skin. J. Exp. Biol. 15:492–499.

26. Knight, P.J., A. Chadwick and J.N. Ball (1978). Biological tests of eel "prolactin" separated by gel electrophoresis. Gen. Comp. Endocrinol. 36:30–32.

27. Knowles, F. (1965). Evidence for a dual control, by neurosecretion, of hormone synthesis and hormone release in the pituitary of the dogfish, *Scylliorhinus stellaris.* Philos. Trans. R. Soc. Lond. 249:435–456.

28. Kosto, B., G.E. Pickford and M.R. Foster (1959). Further studies of the hormonal induction of melanogenesis in the killifish, *Fundulus heteroclitus.* Endocrinology 65:869–881.

29. LaRoche, G., A.N. Woodall, C.L. Johnson and J.E. Halver (1966). Thyroid function in rainbow trout (*Salmo gairdnerii* Rich). II. Effects of thyroidectomy on the development of young fish. Gen. Comp. Endocrinol. 6:249–266.

30. Lerner, A.B., K. Shizume and I. Bunding (1954). The mechanism of endocrine control of melanin pigmentation. J. Clin. Endocrinol. Metab. 14:1463–1490.

31. Lowry, P.J. and A. Chadwick (1970). Interrelations of some pituitary hormones. Nature 226:219–222.

32. Lowry, P.J. and A. Chadwick (1970). Purification and amino acid sequence of melanocyte-stimulating hormone from the dogfish *Squalus acanthias.* Biochem. J. 118:713–718.

33. Lundstrom. H.M. and P. Bard (1932). Hypophysial control of cutaneous pigmentation in an elasmobranch fish. Biol. Bull. 62:1–9.

34. Mayer, T.C. (1967). Pigment cell migration in piebald mice. Dev. Biol. 15:521–535.

35. Meurling, P. (1963). Nerves of the intermediate lobe of *Etmopterus spinax* (Elasmobranchii). Z. Zellforsch. 61:183–201.

36. Nakai, Y. and A. Gorbman (1969). Evidence for a doubly innervated secretory unit in the anuran pars intermedia. II. Electron microscopic studies. Gen. Comp. Endocrinol. 13:108–116.

37. Nayar, S. and K.R. Pandalai (1963). Pars intermedia of the pituitary gland and integumentary colour changes in the garden lizard, *Calotes versicolor.* Z. Zellforsch. 58:837–845.

38. Norris, D.O. (1966). Radiothyroidectomy in the salmonid fishes *Salmo gairdnerii* Richardson and *Oncorhynchus tshawytscha* Walbaum. Ph.D. thesis, University of Washington.

39. Novales, R.R. (1971). On the role of cAMP in the function of skin melanophores. Ann. N.Y. Acad. Sci. 185:494–506.

40. Novales, R.R. (1974). Actions of melanocyte-stimulating hormones. Handbook of Physiology, Sec. 7, Endocrinology. Williams & Wilkins, Baltimore, Vol. 4, Part 2, pp. 347–366.

41. Oshima, K. and A. Gorbman (1969). Evidence for a doubly innervated secretory unit in the anuran pars intermedia. I. Electrophysiological studies. Gen. Comp. Endocrinol. 13:98–107.

42. Parker. G.H. (1938). The colour changes in lizards, particularly in *Phrynosoma.* J. Exp. Biol. 15:48–73.

43. Pickford, G.E. and B. Kosto (1957). Hormonal induction of melanogenesis in hypophysectomized killifish (*Fundulus heteroclitus*). Endocrinology 61:177–196.

44. Piggens, D.J. (1962). Thyroid feeding of salmon parr. Nature 195:1017–1018.

45. Platt, J.E. and D.O. Norris (1974). The effect of ergocornine on melanophores of *Ambystoma tigrinum:* Evidence for suppression of pituitary MSH release. J. Exp. Zool. 189:7–12.

46. Ralph, C.L. (1969). The control of color in birds. Am. Zool. 9:521–530.

47. Ralph, C.L. (1975). The pineal complex: A retrospective view. Am. Zool. 15, Suppl. 1:105–116.

48. Rodriguez, E.M. and J. LaPointe (1970). Light and electron microscopy of the pars intermedia of the lizard, *Klauberina riversiana.* Z. Zellforsch. 104:1–13.

49. Rust, C.C. (1965). Hormonal control of pelage cycles in the short-tailed weasel (*Mustela erminea bangsi*). Gen. Comp. Endocrinol. 5:222–231.

50. Rust, C.C. and R.K. Meyer (1969). Hair color, molt and testis size in male, short-tailed weasels treated with melatonin. Science 165:921–922.

51. Scott, G.T. (1972). The action of psychoactive drugs on pigment cells of lower vertebrates. In V. Riley, ed., Pigmentation: Its Genesis and Biologic Control. Appleton-Century-Crofts, New York, pp. 327–342.

52. Taylor, J.D. and M.E. Hadley (1970). Chromatophores and color change in the lizard, *Anolis carolinensis.* Z. Zellforsch, 104:282–294.

53. Thody, A.J., M.F. Cooper, D. Meddis, P.E. Bowden and S. Shuster (1975). The sebaceous gland response to melanocyte-stimulating hormone and testosterone. J. Endocrinol. 67:18–19.

54. Waring, H. (1963). Color Change Mechanisms of Cold-Blooded Vertebrates. Academic Press, New York.

55. Weatherhead, B. (1971). Cytology of the neurointermediate lobe of the tuatara, *Sphenodon punctatus* Gray. Z. Zellforsch. 119:21–42.

56. Young, J.Z. (1935). The photoreceptors of lampreys. II. The function of the pineal complex. J. Exp. Biol. 12:254–270.

7·The Neurohypophysial Octapeptide Neurohormones

The anatomy of the vertebrate neurohypophysis and its relationship to hypothalamic neurosecretory centers were discussed in Chapter 4. In this chapter the specific octapeptide neurohormones stored in the pars nervosa of the major vertebrate groups will be considered.

Biological Activities Associated with the Mammalian Pars Nervosa

Five different biological activities have been associated traditionally with the pars nervosa of the neurohypophysis including a *pressor* effect (increased blood pressure), an *antidiuretic* action (reduced urine volume), *uterotonic* effect (induction of uterine contractions), a *milk-ejection* effect (ejection of milk from mammary glands) and a *depressor* effect (reduction in blood pressure). Diuresis or diuretic effect (increased urine production) has been reported but is believed to be simply a consequence of the pressor effect on renal vessels.

The pressor effect may be more primitive than the antidiuretic action,[31] occurring primarily on the peripheral vasculature. Later the emphasis of octapeptide action shifted to the preglomerular renal vasculature allowing for reduced filtration and thus antidiuresis. Finally, the mechanisms for tubular reabsorption of water evolved and became the predominant antidiuretic mechanism of mammals. The uterotonic effect first appears among the chondrichthyian fishes and has been demonstrated in all gnathostomes. Milk-ejecting activity is possibly a modification of the uterotonic action acquired after the evolution of the mammary gland.

The name *pituitrin* was applied to the first crude preparation from the mammalian pars nervosa that contained these activities. Soon this preparation was separated into *pitocin,* which possessed uterotonic, milk-ejecting, and depressor activity, and *pitressin,* which contained the pressor and antidiuretic activities. *Oxytocin* (OXY) was eventually found to be the active principle of pitocin, whereas *vasopressin* was present in pitressin. Later it was discovered that there are three different vasopressins in mammals: 8-arginine vasopressin (AVP), 8-lysine vasopressin (LVP) and 2-phenylalanine vasopressin or phenypressin (Fig. 7-1). Most mammals possess AVP. In the Suiformes (family Tayassuidae, peccaries; family Hippopotamidae, hippopotami) both AVP and LVP are present in the pars nervosa. The domestic pigs (family Suidae) appear to have only LVP. One strain of mice has been shown to produce only LVP. Marsupials produce the unique variant of vasopressin, *phenypressin* (PVP), as well as LVP and mesotocin (MST).[10]

The Pressor Effect

The first demonstration of biological activity in pars nervosa extracts was made by G. Oliver and E.A. Shafer in 1895.[20] A rapid rise in blood pressure was observed following administration of extracts prepared from whole pituitary

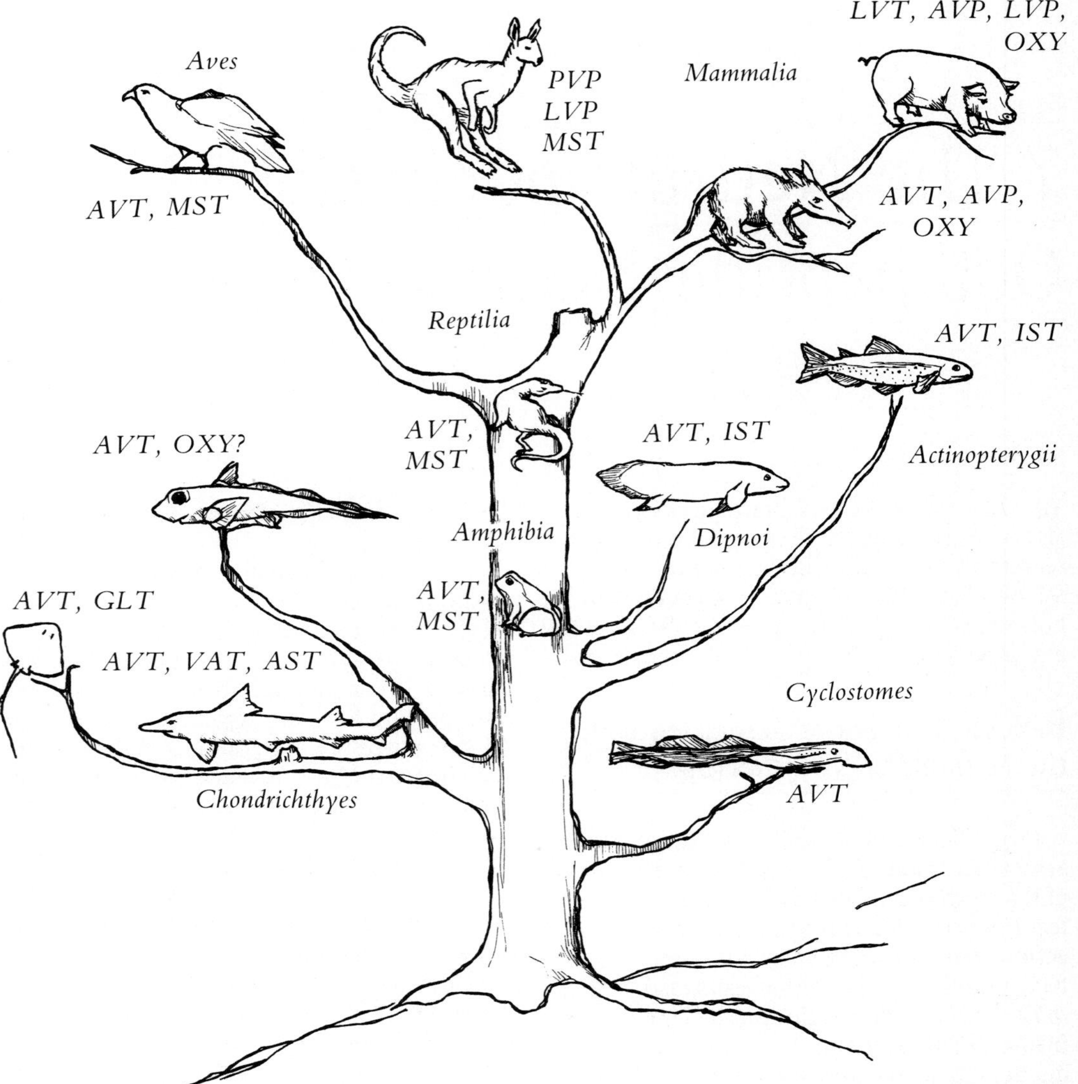

FIG. 7-1. Distribution of neurohypophysial octapeptide neurohormones among vertebrates. *AST,* aspargtocin; *AVP,* arginine vasopressin; *AVT,* arginine vasotocin; *GLT,* glumitocin; *IST,* isotocin; *LVP,* lysine vasopressin; *LVT,* lysine vasotocin; *MST,* mesotocin; *OXY,* oxytocin; *VAT,* valitocin; *PVT,* phenypressin.

glands to anesthetized mammals. Later this activity was localized by W.H. Howell in the pars nervosa.[20] Diuresis (excessive urine production and elimination) was observed by several investigators following administration of pars nervosa extracts. This diuresis was due primarily to increased blood pressure causing an increase in glomerular filtration rate (GFR) in the kidney. Eventually, this principle became known as *vasopressin.* The pressor activity of vasopressins is usually assayed by monitoring blood pressure changes in rats.

The Antidiuretic Effect

The antidiuretic properties of pars nervosa preparations in man were independently reported by F. Farini and R. van den Velden in 1913.[20] A correlation was observed between lesions in the pituitary gland and the occurrence of the clinical syndrome of abnormally high production of dilute urine, *diabetes insipidus*. Administration of pars nervosa extracts decreases urine output (antidiuretic) and increases the specific gravity of urine produced by sufferers of diabetes insipidus. (Increased specific gravity of the urine indicates a less dilute or more concentrated urine.) This antidiuretic effect can be demonstrated in the isolated kidney and is due to increased water reabsorption and not to changes in GFR.[52] The pars nervosa principle responsible for this activity is also vasopressin. The permeability of the cells in the collecting duct of each nephron in the kidney is increased in the presence of vasopressin. This increased permeability to water results in a new diffusion of water from the lumen of the collecting duct into the interstitial spaces and eventually back into the blood vascular system. Artificially increasing the blood osmotic pressure causes release of vasopressin from the neurohypophysis, and urine output is decreased. An increase in blood volume or the presence of ethyl alcohol in the bloodstream reduces vasopressin release, and excess water is added to the urine with a resultant increase in urine volume and considerable dilution of the urine (decrease in specific gravity). The double-barreled action of consuming large quantities of beer on vasopressin release is well known to many individuals.

Antidiuretic activity is often assayed in rats, which are very sensitive to doses that are too low to cause any pressor effect. Obviously any pressor effect would cause diuresis and invalidate the assay. An additional bioassay for the vasopressins is the water-balance effect on urinary bladders of anuran amphibians.[61]

The Uterotonic Effect

Pars nervosa extracts were first observed by Dale in 1906 to stimulate uterine contractions,[20] and this effect became known as the uterotonic effect. This initial observation eventually led to the clinical use of OXY to induce uterine contractions in labor and to reduce postpartum hemorrhage. The uterotonic activity of OXY is measured routinely with an invitro bioassay technique.[61] For example, the contraction of an isolated rat uterus or strips of uterus can be easily quantified following application of purified OXY, and the uterotonic activity of unknown samples or other known substances can be compared quantitatively.

Bioassays for OXY all involve female target tissues, and one may ask what the role, if any, is for OXY in male mammals. Oxytocin has been shown to induce rhythmic contractions in the vas deferens and epididymis of rams.[29] These results are related to earlier observations of increased semen production and semen containing greater numbers of spermatozoa in ejaculates of rams, bulls and rabbits treated with OXY prior to ejaculation. Based upon the actions of OXY on both the female and male genital tracts, some investigators have suggested that OXY release may be responsible for the induction of the rhythmic contractions of these structures associated in humans with the sensation of orgasm.

Milk Ejection

Application of pars nervosa extracts to a cannulated mammary nipple in a goat results in milk ejection.[20] This action was later reported in cows as well although it was also shown that the extract had no effect on the total yield of milk (that is, synthesis of milk). These observations led to development of a sensitive invitro bioassay for OXY, the milk-ejecting principle of mammals. One such bioassay utilizes mammary glands dissected from pregnant mice.[28]

Depressor Activity

Occasionally experimental studies of pars nervosa extracts demonstrated the presence of depressor activity or reduction in blood pressure. This depressor effect is caused by OXY and is usually assayed in the chicken.[61]

Metabolic Actions

Regulation of certain metabolic events may prove to be a physiological action of neurohypophysial octapeptide hormones. The vasopressins depress circulating levels of free fatty acids in most mammals that have been examined, employing inhibitory effects on either lipolysis (hydrolysis of fats) or on release of lipolytic hormones such as growth hormone or epinephrine. They might stimulate the metabolism of free fatty acids by muscle cells although there is no evidence to directly support this suggestion. In contrast, blood glucose is elevated by the vasopressins as well as by OXY. The importance of these metabolic effects of neurohypophysial octapeptides in overall metabolic regulation in vertebrates has not been established, and additional research is needed to verify a physiological role for these hormones in metabolism.[17]

Release of Tropic Hormones

Numerous studies of the effect of exogenous octapeptides on tropic hormone release have been reported, but their physiological significance as potential mediators of tropic hormone release has been debated. The structural similarity of some possible releasing peptides to fragments of the pars nervosa neurohormones was pointed out in Chapter 4. The demonstration of elevated levels of vasopressin and its specific "carrier" protein in hypothalamo-hypophysial portal vessels of rhesus monkeys, however, does support a possible role for vasopressin as a tropic hormone-releasing hormone.[62] Thus the possibility of a physiologically important releasing role for pars nervosa octapeptides remains.

Neural Functions

The distribution of neurohypophysial hormones in the brain suggests that vasopressins and OXY may function as peptide neurotransmitters. Octapeptides have been shown to produce behavioral effects in animals and even to enhance learning in humans.[59]

Characteristics of Mammalian Neurohypophysial Octapeptide Hormones

Chemistry

Each octapeptide molecule consists of a five-membered amino acid ring, including cystine (residues 1–6), and a side chain of three amino acids (residues 7–9). Although a neutral molecule, OXY is very similar in chemical structure to the basic vasopressins (Table 7-1). Oxytocin has little activity in the biological assays for vasopressins, however. Similarly the vasopressins are relatively inactive in OXY-specific bioassays (Table 7-2). Apparently the differences in biological activity reside primarily at position 3 in these molecules. The presence of the amino acid isoleucine (Ile) at position 3 imparts OXY-like activity to the peptide, whereas phenylalanine (Phe) at the same position imparts strong pressor and antidiuretic properties to the molecule (Tables 7-1 and 7-2). Arginine or lysine at position 8 is responsible for the basic properties of the vasopressins.

Source

The production of pars nervosa hormones is accomplished by the supraoptic and paraventricular neurosecretory (NS) nuclei of the hypothalamus,[3] and the pars nervosa acts only as a storage area for these hormones until they are released into the general circulation. Oxytocin is produced primarily by the NS neurons of the paraventricular nucleus, and the vasopressins are synthesized primarily in the supraoptic nucleus. Within the NS cells, neurohypophysial octapeptides are associated with proteins known as *neurophysins,* which have a molecular weight of about 12,000 daltons. In the rat, different neurophysins have been identified in association with OXY and AVP respectively.[7]

The neurophysins are often termed carrier proteins and are transported and stored with the octapeptide hormones in the NS granules. Oxytocin and vasopressin are synthesized as parts of two larger peptides of between 20,000 and 25,000 daltons.[16] As the secretion granules travel through the axons to the pars nervosa, the prohormones are cleaved into the specific hormones and associated neurophysins as well as another large peptide.[58] The respective prohormones for vasopressin and OXY are *propressophysin* and *prooxyphysin*[47] Other studies suggest there are even larger precursors (80,000 daltons) for propressophysin and prooxyphysin which include the sequence identified as proopiomelanocortin.[33]

Blood levels of OXY and AVP vary with the physiological state of the animal. There are no predictable rhythmic patterns of secretion. However, secretion of OXY and AVP into the cerebrospinal fluid shows a definite diurnal

TABLE 7-1. *Structure of Neurohypophysial Octapeptide Hormones in Vertebrates*

HORMONE	AMINO ACID SEQUENCE								
	1	2	3	4	5	6	7	8	9
Oxytocin	Cys -	Tyr -	Ile -	Gln -	Asn -	Cys -	Pro -	Leu -	Gly - NH_2
Mesotocin	Cys -	Tyr -	Ile -	Gln -	Asn -	Cys -	Pro -	Ile -	Gly - NH_2
Isotocin	Cys -	Tyr -	Ile -	Ser -	Asn -	Cys -	Pro -	Ile -	Gly - NH_2
Glumitocin	Cys -	Tyr -	Ile -	Ser -	Asn -	Cys -	Pro -	Gln -	Gly - NH_2
Valitocin	Cys -	Tyr -	Ile -	Gln -	Asn -	Cys -	Pro -	Val -	Gly - NH_2
Aspargtocin	Cys -	Tyr -	Ile -	Asn -	Asn -	Cys -	Pro -	Leu -	Gly - NH_2
Arginine vasopressin	Cys -	Tyr -	Phe -	Gln -	Asn -	Cys -	Pro -	Arg -	Gly - NH_2
Lysine vasopressin	Cys -	Tyr -	Phe -	Gln -	Asn -	Cys -	Pro -	Lys -	Gly - NH_2
Phenypressin	Cys -	Phe -	Phe -	Gln -	Asn -	Cys -	Pro -	Arg -	Gly - NH_2
Arginine vasotocin	Cys -	Tyr -	Ile -	Gln -	Asn -	Cys -	Pro -	Arg -	Gly - NH_2

rhythm in cats and monkeys.[41,43] Daytime levels are elevated implying an important role for octapeptides and demonstrating the use of cerebrospinal fluid as a medium to transport these hormones from one brain region to another.

Mechanism of Action

Arginine vasopressin produces its effects on collecting duct permeability to water in the kidney through stimulation of adenyl cyclase activity[2] and an increase in cyclic adenosine 3′,5′-monophosphate (cAMP) (see Chap. 1 concerning the cAMP mechanism in general). Microtubule and microfilaments may be affected by increased cAMP levels and bring about permeability changes in the responsive cellular membrane.[55]

One might assume OXY operates via a cAMP dependent mechanism as well. However, in uterine muscle OXY depolarizes the plasmalemma whereas agents known to operate via cAMP production (epinephrine, isoproteronol)

TABLE 7-2. *Biological Activity of Neurohypophysial Peptides in Various Bioassays*

	ACTIVITY UNITS[a]				
HORMONE	UTEROTONIC (RAT)	DEPRESSOR (CHICKEN)	MILK EJECTION (RABBIT)	PRESSOR (RAT)	ANTIDIURETIC (RAT)
Oxytocin	450	450	450	5	5
Mesotocin	291	502	330	6	1
Isotocin	145	310	290	0.06	0.18
Glumitocin	10	–	53	0.35	0.41
Valitocin	199	278	308	9	0.8
Aspargtocin	107	201	298	0.13	0.04
Arginine vasotocin	120	300	220	255	260
Arginine vasopressin	17	62	69	412	465
Lysine vasopressin	5	42	63	285	260

SOURCE: Acher, R.[1]
NOTE: For distribution of these hormones among the vertebrates, see Fig. 7-1.
[a] Units are expressed in IU/μ moles pure synthetic substance; 1 mg synthetic oxytocin = 500 USP units.

cause hyperpolarization (decreased contraction). Such observations suggest a different mode of operation for OXY.

Biological Half-Life

The biological half-life for OXY and for AVP in mammals is about 1–5 minutes, although it may be longer in large mammals. Between 4 and 20 minutes are generally required to clear 90% of an injected dose through the activities of the kidneys and the liver. Pregnant mammals produce an enzyme, oxytocinase, that circulates in the blood. The presence of this enzyme in the blood may represent a mechanism to prevent OXY from acting on the uterus should its release be stimulated prior to the normal time of parturition. The dramatic increase in OXY seen in some mammals just prior to birth may be due in part to reduction of oxytocinase.

In the toad (*Bufo marinus*) the biological half-life for AVT and OXY is 32 and 10 minutes respectively.[5] Unexpectedly the biological half-life for these hormones is very similar in the chicken (20 and 10 minutes respectively).[5] Considering the lower body temperature for the toad, it would seem that clearance of these hormones in the toad through the actions of the liver may be actually much more rapid than in birds. This slow inactivation time in birds as compared to toads and mammals deserves closer attention.

Comparative Aspects of Neurohypophysial Octapeptide Hormones

The elucidation of an evolutionary pattern for the origin of the neurohypophysial octapeptides has been exciting for comparative endocrinologists. Comparative studies were initiated as long ago as 1908, when pressor effects were identified in extracts of the avian pars nervosa and the teleostean neurointermediate lobe. Following these initial observations an intricate story unfolded involving the evolution of not only functional aspects, related primarily to water balance and reproduction, but also structural alterations in the hormones themselves. Amino acid substitutions producing changes in molecular structure and function have been traced to single base changes (point mutations) in the sequences of bases in the DNA responsible for directing the synthesis of these neurohormones.[49]

Molecular Evolution

Nine different neurohypophysial octapeptide hormones have been positively identified in vertebrates. The amino acid sequences of these hormones and their abbreviations as used in this chapter are provided in Table 7-1, and the distribution of these peptides among the vertebrate groups is illustrated in Figure 7-1. Scrutiny of these molecules reveals two distinct molecular groupings, the basic *arginine vasotocin* (AVT) and a family of neutral OXY-like octapeptides. The majority of the vertebrates possess the neutral octapeptide known as *mesotocin* (MST) or 8-isoleucine OXY, and some groups exhibit more than one neutral octapeptide. Oxytocin may occur only in eutherian mammals. Arginine vasotocin is present in all nonmammalian vertebrates. This molecule is structurally similar to both the mammalian vasopressins and to OXY. Arginine occurs in position 8 as it does in the vasopressins, but Ile appears in the ring structure at position 3, causing the ring to be the same as for OXY. Consequently AVT has both OXY-like and vasopressin-like activities related to the ring structure and the basic side chain respectively. Although AVT might at first be assumed to be a hybrid molecule, its distribution among the vertebrates would argue that it may be the most primitive neurohypophysial octapeptide and hence "ancestral" to both the vasopressins and OXY as well as to other neutral octapeptides. The appearance of AVT in the pars nervosa of fetal mammals and its later disappearance after birth argues for AVT as an evolutionary precursor. Arginine vasotocin, however, may be present in the pineal glands of some adult mammals, suggesting the assumption of a new role (see Chap. 15).

Distribution and Genetics of Neurohypophysial Octapeptides

As previously mentioned, AVT is present in all nonmammalian neurohypophyses and occurs in the neurohypophysis of fetal mammals as well. Cyclostomes exhibit only AVT and no neutral octapeptide, supporting the hypothesis that AVT represents the most primitive octapeptide. Considerable variation is found with respect to the neutral octapeptides. Elasmobranchs exhibit three different neutral octapeptides: *aspargtocin* (AST), *valitocin* (VAT), *glumitocin* (GLT). The teleostean fishes produce a unique neutral octapeptide, *isotocin* (ichthyotocin, IST), but the lungfishes exhibit MST, as do all of the nonmammalian tetrapods. The vasopressins appear for the first time in the mammals.

A number of investigators have noted the similarities in structures of the various neurohypophysial octapeptides and have proposed evolutionary schemes based upon single base changes in the nuclear DNA (cistron) responsible for directing the synthesis of each octapeptide.[49,57] Some of these schemes are summarized in Figure 7-2 and may be compared to Figure 7-1 (distribution among vertebrates) and Table 7-1 (amino acid sequences of all known octapeptides). The entire phylogeny of these neurohormones, with only a few exceptions, can be accounted for by a single base change in the DNA responsible for determining the amino acid to be placed in position 3 or position 8 of the peptide. The exceptions require two steps, suggesting the existence of an intermediate peptide that either is still unknown or has disappeared with the extinction of some ancestor.

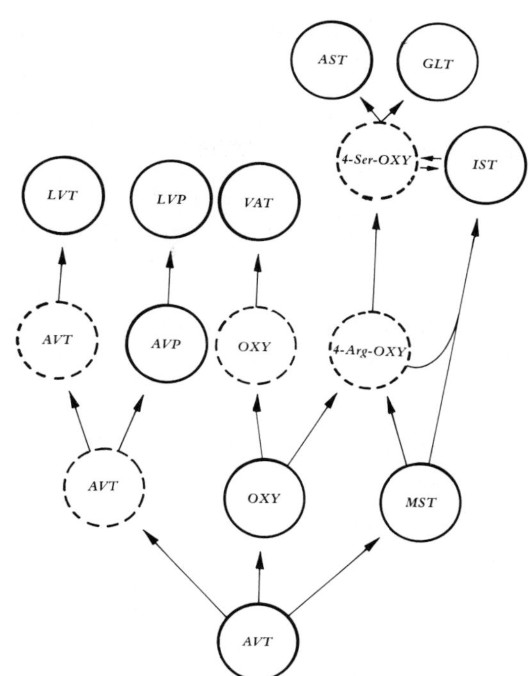

FIG. 7-2. Possible schemes for genetic changes leading to evolution of neurohypophysial octapeptide neurohormones. These pathways are based on gene duplications (*) and single base substitutions. Phenypressin (not shown) appears to be a variant of AVP. Two amino acid substitutions are required to form it from AVT. For key to abbreviations see Fig. 7-1. (From schemes proposed by a number of workers.)

Class Agnatha: Cyclostomata

Larval and adult cyclostomes produce only one neurohypophysial octapeptide, AVT.[46,49] The presence of only AVT in the cyclostomes is considered strong support for believing that AVT is the most primitive octapeptide from which the others have been derived through duplication, mutation and subsequent selection of the gene responsible for directing its synthesis.[1,49,57]

A pressor effect was first reported for neurohypophysial extracts from the hagfish *Myxine glutinosa* in 1913.[25] Since that time extracts prepared from lampreys and hagfishes have been shown to possess milk-ejection activity, antidiuretic effects, uterotonic activity and frog water-balance activity.[49]

Purified AVT has not been shown to produce any effects on water balance or urine production in lampreys,[22] but it does seem to influence renal sodium metabolism (*natriureferic* activity).[6,48] Suggestive effects of AVT on sodium and water balance in hagfishes has been reported.[38]

Class Chondrichthyes

Among these fishes there are several neutral octapeptides present in addition to the basic AVT.[1,49] Sharks have two OXY-like octapeptides, AST and VAT as well as AVT (Table 7-1). These two neutral peptides were formerly known as the elasmobranch OXY-like principles (EOP I and II) until they were finally characterized chemically. A different OXY-like neutral octapeptide, GLT, is characteristic, however, of the closely related skates.

Although AVT has been retained in all of the Chondrichthyes, a gene duplication has probably occurred with subsequent mutations resulting through chance in the establishment of at least four different neutral octapeptides. In the case of sharks they would appear to have been an additional variation, but it is not clear from the literature whether one shark can produce both VAT and AST or whether polymorphism exists in these populations.

Neurohypophysial principles from elasmobranchs have been employed in the normal array of mammalian bioassays ever since the first studies were performed in 1908.[24] Extracts prepared from elasmobranch neurointermediate lobes exhibit milk-ejecting, uterotonic and antidiuretic properties in the ratio of 3:1:0.05.[40] Pressor effects have not been reported.[24,40] Avian depressor activity is present, however.[26]

Neurointermediate lobe extracts devoid of AVT activity cause contraction in vitro of uteri that were isolated from viviparous sharks.[19] The effects of these extracts presumably containing VAT and/or AST suggest a primitive role for neutral octapeptides in the induction of oviductal contractions and oviposition or birth. Crude mammalian preparations of neurohypophysial hormones when administered in large quantities to sharks and skates induce a pressor effect, but the physiological importance of this event is questionable.

Holocephalans *(Hydrolagus colliei)* produce OXY-like and AVT-like hormones associated with their neurointermediate lobe. Pharmacological investigations employing mammalian bioassays indicate that the neutral principle may even be OXY, although chemical confirmation is needed. No information is available concerning the physiological roles for neurohypophysial octapeptides in holocephalans.

Class Osteichthyes: Polypteri, Chondrostei, Holostei

The neurointermediate lobe of *Polypterus senegalis* has uterotonic, milk-ejecting, frog water-balance and natriureferic (sodium) activities.[38] The OXY-like activities are presumably due to the presence of IST, and the iono-osmoregulatory actions are due to AVT.

Chondrostean fishes have AVT stored in their neurointermediate lobes and may also possess an OXY-like molecule, most likely IST.[1]

The holostean fishes probably produce both IST and AVT. Extracts from the neurointermediate lobe exhibit uterotonic, pressor, depressor and milk-ejecting activities. Two fractions have been separated from holostean neurointermediate lobes that qualitatively and quantitatively behave like AVT and IST.[38]

In-vivo studies of neurohypophysial octapeptides in polypterid, chondrostean and holostean fishes have not been reported, and such studies are needed to ascribe physiological roles for these hormones.

Class Osteichthyes: Teleostei

Since the first observation of pressor activity in neurointermediate lobes of teleosts, numerous studies have confirmed it and demonstrated antidiuretic, uterotonic and water-balance activities. All of these activities are believed to be due to AVT, however. What was originally believed to be OXY was later discovered to be 4-serine, 8-isoleucine oxytocin or IST. It may not be possible to ascertain whether the uterotonic activity in extracts is due to IST or AVT since purified molecules both possess this activity. Although IST and AVT are the only neurohypophysial octapeptides reported from the teleostean neurointermediate lobe, it should be kept in mind that only a few of the more than 20,000 species of teleosts have been examined. It is likely that in a few cases, at least, a different neutral octapeptide will be discovered.

Arginine vasotocin generally does not produce a water-conserving action in teleosts. Many investigators have demonstrated a strong diuretic action for AVP, LVP, and AVT.[37] This diuretic action appears to be due to an increase in glomerular filtration rate (pressor effect) rather than a renal action. The attachment of biological significance to the large doses of these hormones required to produce diuresis is questioned by studies with the Atlantic eel, *Anguilla anguilla.*[23] High doses of AVT administered to eels cause a pressor effect, intermediate doses cause diuresis and low doses are antidiuretic. It will not be possible to thoroughly evaluate these interesting data, however, until sufficient information concerning circulating levels becomes available for animals maintained under differing environmental conditions. It is possible that all of these activities of AVT are "physiological," depending upon the type of osmotic stress to which the animal is subjected. These data do emphasize the danger of extrapolating from results obtained following injection of arbitrarily chosen doses of a hormone without regard to dose-response relationships or thorough examination of different physiological states.

Numerous reports have implicated AVT in spawning reflexes. Isolated oviducts of several oviparous and viviparous teleosts contract in the presence of small amounts of AVT, IST or OXY.[19] The ovaries of four species of viviparous teleosts (family Cyprinodontidae) also contract in the presence of neurohypophysial octapeptides, and this may be related to expulsion of the young that develop within the ovarian cavity. There is a progressive increase in the sensitivity of these ovaries to AVT during gestation. These observations certainly support a role for AVT in egg laying as well as in the birth process of at least some viviparous species.

Arginine vasotocin is much more potent than IST at inducing the spawning reflex in oviparous killifish *Fundulus heteroclitus.* This does not rule out a physiological role for IST, however, since the important criterion is which hormone is secreted endogenously (if any) during spawning. If only IST is released, the greater potency for AVT would be meaningless physiologically.

Class Osteichthyes: Sarcopterygii

The pars nervosa of the lungfishes is organized anatomically like that of a tetrapod (Chap. 4), and like the tetrapods it contains AVT and MST. In addition, some pharmacological studies support the presence of small quantities of OXY. No data have been reported for the living crossopterygian, the coelacanth, but its piscine-like hypothalamo-hypophysial organization suggests AVT and IST or a unique neutral octapeptide might be expected.

Only a few studies have been conducted with respect to the physiological roles for these octapeptides in lungfishes. There appear to be no general water-balance effects or antidiuretic actions on the kidney. Sodium levels may be altered following administration of very large doses of various octapeptides, but the physiological importance of this natriureferic action is questionable. Induction of diuresis by arginine vasotocin presumably is due to a pressor effect and resultant increase in GFR,[37] but further investigation is required to establish a true physiological role. It would be of special interest to examine possible roles of AVT as an antidiuretic principle in estivating African lungfishes while in their mud cocoons.

Class Amphibia

Adult amphibians take up water from the aquatic environment following injection of neurohypophysial octapeptides. This water-balance effect is sometimes termed the Brunn effect after Fritz Brunn, who in 1921 demonstrated this phenomenon in frogs.[20] In *Bufo marinus,* AVT is 50 times more potent than OXY and 200 times more potent than MST in producing a water-balance effect. Furthermore, dehydration of *B. marinus* depletes the pars nervosa of NS material, supporting a physiological role for AVT in water conservation.

The Brunn effect is brought about by the action of AVT at three sites: (1) reduction in urinary losses via effects on the kidney, (2) promotion of water reabsorption from the bladder, and (3) promotion of water absorption across the skin.[37] Of these sites the urinary bladder has received the most attention. The urinary bladder is very sensitive to the actions of neurohypophysial octapeptides, and the toad bladder has become a favorite system in which to examine the mechanism of action of neurohypophysial octapeptide hormones, including the vasopressins (Fig. 7-3). The toad bladder is also one of the standard bioassays for vasopressin-like activities.[4]

The action of octapeptides on the amphibian kidney may be more complicated than previously supposed.[37] Although AVT causes constriction of the afferent renal blood vessels (pressor effect) with resultant increase in GFR (diuresis), MST apparently causes vascular dilation (depressor effect) with a decrease in

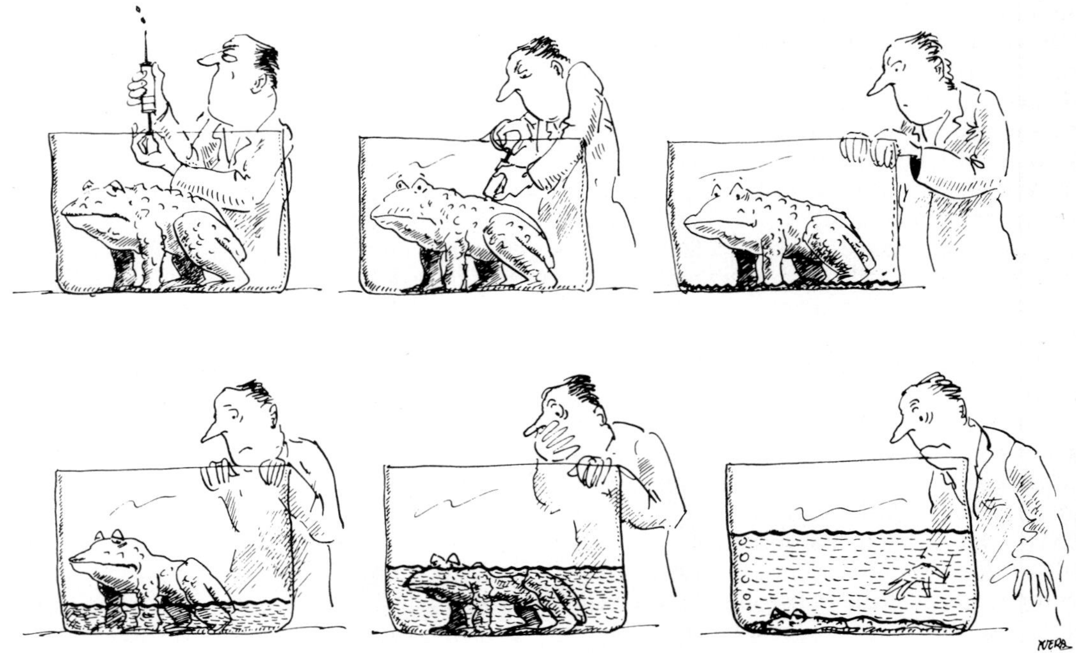

FIG. 7-3. Diuretic action of neurohypophysial peptides in the toad. (Courtesy of Mr. Frans Vera.)

urine formation (antidiuretic). However, MST increases GFR in hypophysectomized salamander larvae.[53] Arginine vasotocin may prove to be diuretic through a pressor effect, whereas MST could be considered antidiuretic because of its depressor activity on the renal vessels. A direct action of AVT on tubular reabsorption has been demonstrated in bullfrogs but does not occur in *Necturus.*[37] Obviously the simple terms antidiuretic and diuretic for neurohypophysial principles should not be loosely applied since the mechanisms of action and target tissues involved may vary greatly.

Totally aquatic amphibians such as tadpoles of *Rana catesbeiana* or *Bufo bufo* and adult *Xenopus laevis* do not exhibit a Brunn effect. Neotenous and larval urodele amphibians also exhibit little or no Brunn effect, and lower quantities of neurohypophysial octapeptides are present in their neurohypophyses than in more terrestrial individuals (Table 7-3).

In addition to employing AVT as a water-conserving hormone, some interesting adaptations have evolved in terrestrial amphibians that are essential for water conservation. Many terrestrial anurans possess a highly vascularized "pelvic patch" that is involved directly in active water absorption.[45] Furthermore, development of this patch in a given species is inversely correlated with the availability of water in their natural habitats.

Arginine vasotocin produces behavioral effects in amphibians. Injections of AVT into male newts causes them to clasp the females (a mating grasp).[34] This action may be mediated by the nervous system. In *Rana pipiens,* AVT stimulates water uptake in females which inhibits the release call.[13] When a female is not ready to spawn, the release call signals the clasping male that he is wasting his time.

Oviductal contractions have been reported in many amphibian species following application of neurohypophysial octapeptides.[22,32] Arginine vasotocin can induce birth of young in viviparous species such as the salamander *Salamandra maculosa,* and AVT induces contractions in the oviducts of a number of oviparous anurans and urodeles. The presence of oviductal receptors for AVT is dependent on prior exposure to progesterone.[36]

TABLE 7-3. *Summary of Physiological Responses to Neurohypophysial Octapeptides Demonstrated in Vertebrates*

VERTEBRATE CLASS	PRESSOR	AVIAN DEPRESSOR	HYDRO-OSMOTIC	NATRIUREFERIC (NA^+)	UTERUS OR OVIDUCT	LIPOLYTIC (AVT)	HYPERGLYCEMIC (AVT)
Agnatha	AVT						
Chondrichthyes	AVT	(OXY)[a] (MST)[a]					
Osteichthyes	AVT	IST, MST	AVT, IST	AVT, IST		AVT	AVT
Amphibia	AVT, MST AVT[b]	MST[b]	AVT	AVT	AVT	AVT	AVT
Reptilia	AVT[c] AVT, MST[d]	AVT, MST[e] MST[f]	AVT		AVT		AVT
Aves	AVT	AVT, MST (OXY)[a]	AVT		AVT		
Mammalia	AVP, AVT[g]		AVP, LVP, AVT[g]	AVP	OXY, AVP	AVP[h], LVP	

Modified from LaPointe J.[32]
NOTE: No physiological functions are indicated for aspargtocin, valitocin or glumitocin.
AVP, arginine vasopressin; AVT, arginine vasotocin; IST, isotocin; LVP, lysine vasopressin; MST mesotocin; OXY oxytocin.
[a] Pharmacologic dose
[b] *Rana*
[c] lizard
[d] turtle
[e] snake
[f] turtle, lizard
[g] fetal
[h] AVP increases lipolysis; LVP decreases lipolysis

Class Reptilia

The physiological roles for neurohypophysial octapeptides in reptiles are very similar to those observed for birds and amphibians that have the same octapeptide hormones, AVT and MST. These neurohormones have been implicated in reproduction, but associations with water balance and vascular effects are not so well established. Oviposition has been induced with neurohypophysial peptides in several species of snakes and lizards.[11,30] Birth of young has been induced with AVT in a viviparous lizard.[18] Arginine vasotocin induces oviductal contractions in isolated oviducts of both lizards and turtles.[31,35] Furthermore, AVT is more effective than either OXY or MST at inducing contractions. No role for endogenous AVT or MST has been reported in relation to oviposition or birth, however.

Some qualitative data have been reported that relate endogenous levels of neurohypophysial octapeptides with dehydration in the ring-necked snake *Diadophis punctatus* and in the garden lizard *Calotes versicolor.*[42,51] In both cases, dehydration was correlated with a decreasing amount of stainable NS material in the hypothalamus and pars nervosa. Plasma AVT levels are greater in salt-loaded and dehydrated lizards than in water-loaded lizards establishing a possible physiological role for regulating water reabsorption.[44]

Both OXY and MST have been shown to bring about a depressor effect in the alligator, lizards and snakes.[12,50,60] A pressor action of OXY, surprisingly, has been reported for turtles as well.[27,60] These data suggest that crocodilians and squamates are more similar to birds in exhibiting a depressor response to OXY than are the turtles.

Class Aves

Water deprivation or administration of saline (NaCl) solutions to domestic or wild bird species results in depletion of stainable NS material from the pars nervosa.[15] Of those birds examined, only the budgerigar *Melopsittacus undulatus,* a desert-dwelling species, shows no change in NS material following several days of water deprivation.[56] Desert-dwelling mammals exhibit similar insensitivity to dehydration with respect to the quantity of NS material in the pars nervosa. This does not necessarily imply that neurohypophysial hormones are not involved as antidiuretic hormones in these birds. Rather, it illustrates that other adaptations to water deprivation have evolved in desert species, and they are not so sensitive to dehydration when measured by the crude parameter of stainability of the pars nervosa.

Both OXY and AVT are antidiuretic in birds, and a possible role for MST in antidiuretic responses may be inferred. However, it appears that AVT is much more potent than OXY,[35] suggesting that AVT is the endogenous antidiuretic principle. In contrast, AVT is only about 60% as effective a depressor agent in birds as is OXY. The physiological importance of the avian depressor effect is questionable since a much larger dose (10 times) is needed to induce a depressor effect than to cause antidiuresis. Nevertheless, the avian depressor effect has proven to be a useful bioassay for characterizing and elucidating the probable structures of unknown octapeptides.

Arginine vasotocin appears to play an important role in oviposition via its stimulatory effect on oviductal contraction.[32] Oviposition can be accelerated by treating birds with neurohypophysial octapeptides during the appropriate stage of the egg-laying cycle.[8,9] Arginine vasotocin has about 50 times the potency of OXY in stimulating the avian oviduct. Definitive support for an endogenous role in oviposition is supplied by the observation that blood levels of AVT are elevated in the domestic hen at the time of ovulation.[54]

Summary

The most primitive neurohypophysial octapeptide hormone appears to be AVT, the only octapeptide hormone identified in larval and adult cyclostomes. Arginine vasotocin has been retained in all nonmammalian vertebrates, and one or more neutral octapeptides has evolved that possess activities similar to OXY. Fetal mammals also produce AVT, which appears to be involved in osmoregulation in the aquatic fetal environment (ontogeny recapitulates phylogeny?). Adult mammals have replaced AVT with AVP, LVP or PVP. The neutral octapeptide hormone of most mammals is OXY. Pineal glands of adult mammals may also produce AVT (except the suiformes who seem to make LVT instead).

Several evolutionary schemes have been proposed for the neurohypophysial octapeptide hormones related to their amino acid content and sequences. All of these schemes involve occurrence of single base substitutions in one of two duplicate DNA cistrons responsible for directing the synthesis of one basic and one neutral octapeptide. In spite of a few gaps in our knowledge and some indecision as to certain steps, these schemes represent the most complete picture of hormonal evolution in the vertebrates.

The major roles for the neurohypophysial octapeptide hormones appear to be related to water balance (the basic peptides) and the induction of muscular contractions in reproductive ducts leading to oviposition or birth (AVT?, MST?, OXY). Milk ejection from the mammary gland in response to suckling by the young is mediated via OXY as well. Neurohypophysial octapeptides may also be involved as tropic hormone-releasing hormones, but more evidence is required to establish this. Some diuretic and antidiuretic effects of these hormones may be produced through pressor and depressor actions respectively. Both the pressor and depressor actions on the vascular system could be considered to be pharmacological actions with respect to everyday physiological regulation. The pressor effects may become important when one considers the homeostatic events related to maintaining normal blood volume and pressure under conditions of dehydration or mild hemorrhage.

References

1. Acher, R. (1974). Chemistry of the neurohypophysial hormones: An example of molecular evolution. Handbook of Physiology, Sec. 7, Endocrinology. Williams & Wilkins, Baltimore, Vol. 4, Part 1, pp. 119–130.
2. Andreoli, T.E. and J.A. Schafer (1977). Some considerations of the role of antidiuretic hormone in water homeostasis. Recent Prog. Horm. Res. 33:387–434.
3. Bargmann, W. and E. Scharrer (1951). The site of origin of the hormones of the posterior pituitary. Am. Sci. 39:255–259.
4. Bentley, P.J. (1958). The effects of neurohypophysial extracts on water transfer across the wall of the isolated urinary bladder of the toad, *Bufo marinus*. J. Endocrinol. 17:201–202.
5. Bentley, P.J. (1974). Actions of neurohypophysial peptides in amphibians, reptiles and birds. Handbook of Physiology, Sec. 7, Endocrinology. Williams & Wilkins, Baltimore, Vol. 4, Part 1, pp. 545–563.
6. Bentley, P.J. and B.K. Follett (1963). Kidney function in a primitive vertebrate, the cyclostome *Lampetra fluviatilis*. J. Physiol. 169:902–918.
7. Burford, G.D., C.W. Jones and B.T. Pickering (1971). Tentative identification of a vasopressin-neurophysin and an oxytocin-neurophysin in the rat. Biochem. J. 124:809–813.
8. Burrows, W.H. and T.C. Byerly (1942). Premature expulsion of eggs by hens following injection of whole posterior pituitary preparations. Poult. Sci. 21:416–421.
9. Burrows, W.H. and R.M. Fraps (1942). Action of vasopressin and oxytocin in causing premature oviposition in domestic fowl. Endocrinology 30:702–705.
10. Chauvet, M.T., D. Hurpet, J. Chauvet and R. Acher (1983). Identification of mesotocin, lysine vasopressin and phenypressin in the eastern gray kangaroo *(Macropus giganteus)*. Gen. Comp. Endocrinol. 49:63–72.
11. Clausen, H.J. (1940). Studies on the effect of ovariectomy and hypophysectomy on gestation in snakes. Endocrinology 27:700–704.
12. Dantzler, W.H. (1967). Glomerular and tubular effects of arginine vasotocin in water snakes *(Natrix sipedon)*. Am. J. Physiol. 212:83–91.
13. Diakow, C. (1978). Hormonal basis for breeding behavior in female frogs: vasotocin inhibits the release call of *Rana pipiens*. Science 199:1456–1457.
14. Follett, B.K. and D.S. Farner (1966). The effects of daily photoperoid on gonad growth, neurohypophysial hormone content, and neurosecretion in the hypothalamo-hypophysial system of the Japanese quail *(Coturnix coturnix japonica)*. Gen. Comp. Endocrinol. 7:111–124.
15. Follett, B.K. and H. Heller (1964). The neurohypophysial hormones of lungfishes and amphibians. J. Physiol. 172:92–106.
16. Gainer, H., Y. Sarne and M.J. Brownstein (1977). Neurophysin biosynthesis: conversion of a putative precursor during axonal transport. Science 195:1354–1356.

17. George, J.C. (1977). Comparative physiology of metabolic responses to neurohypophysial hormones in vertebrates. Am. Zool. 17:787–808.

18. Guillette, L.J. (1979). Stimulation of parturition in a viviparous lizard *(Sceloporus jarrovi)* by arginine vasotocin. Gen. Comp. Endocrinol. 38:457–460.

19. Heller, H. (1972). The effect of neurohypophysial hormones on the female reproductive tract of lower vertebrates. Gen. Comp. Endocrinol Suppl. 3:703–714.

20. Heller, H. (1974). History of neurohypophysial research. Handbook of Physiology, Sec. 7, Endocrinology. Williams & Wilkins, Baltimore, Vol. 4, Part 1, pp. 103–117.

21. Heller, H. (1974). Molecular aspects in comparative endocrinology. Gen. Comp. Endocrinol. 22:315–332.

22. Heller, H. and P.J. Bentley (1965). Phylogenetic distribution of the effects of neurohypophysial hormones on water and sodium metabolism. Gen. Comp. Endocrinol. 5:96–108.

23. Henderson, I.W. and N.A.M. Wales (1974). Renal diuresis and antidiuresis after injections of arginine vasotocin in the fresh-water eel (*Anguilla anguilla* L.) J. Endocrinol. 41:487–500.

24. Herring, P.T. (1908). The physiological action of extracts of the pituitary body and saccus vasculosus of certain fishes. Q. J. Exp. Physiol. 1:187–188.

25. Herring, P.T. (1913). Further observations upon the comparative anatomy and physiology of the pituitary body. Q. J. Exp. Physiol. 6:73–108.

26. Hogben, L.T. and G.R. deBeer (1925). Studies on the pituitary. VI. Localization and phyletic distribution of active materials. Q. J. Exp. Physiol. 15:164–176.

27. Hogben, L.T. and W. Schlapp (1924). Studies on the pituitary. III. The vasomotor activity of pituitary extracts throughout the vertebrate series. Q. J. Exp. Physiol. 14:229–258.

28. Hruby, V.J. and M.E. Hadley (1975). A simple, rapid, and quantitative *in vitro* milk-ejecting assay for neurohypophysial hormones and analogues. In R. Walter and J. Meienhofer, eds., Peptides: Chemistry, Structure and Biology. Ann Arbor Science Publ., Ann Arbor, Mich., pp. 729–736.

29. Knight, T.W. and D.R. Lindsay (1970). Short- and long-term effects of oxytocin on quality and quantity of semen from rams. J. Reprod. Fertil. 21:523–529.

30. La Pointe, J. (1964). Induction of oviposition in lizards with the hormone oxytocin. Copeia 1964:451–452.

31. La Pointe, J. (1969). Effects of ovarian steroids and neurohypophysial hormones on the oviduct of the viviparous lizard, *Klauberina riversiana,* J. Endocrinol. 43:197–205.

32. La Pointe, J. (1977). Comparative physiology of neurohypophysial hormone action on the vertebrate oviduct-uterus. Am. Zool. 17:763–773.

33. Lauber, M., D. Nicolas, H. Boussetta, C. Fahy, P. Beguin, M. Camier, H. Vaudry and P. Cohen (1981). The molecular weight 80,000 common forms of neurophysin and vasopressin from bovine neurohypophysis have ACTH-like and β-endorphin-like sequences and liberate by proteolysis biologically active ACTH. Proc. Natl. Acad. Sci. USA. 78:6086–6090.

34. Moore, F.L., L.J. Miller, S.P. Spielvogel, T. Kubiac and K. Folkers (1982). Luteinizing hormone-releasing hormone involvement in the reproductive behavior of a male amphibian. Neuroendocrinology 35:212–216.

35. Munsick, R.A., W.H. Sawyer and H.B. Van Dyke (1960). Avian neurohypophysial hormones: pharmacological properties and tentative identification. Endocrinology 66:860–871.

36. Norris, D.O., L.J. Guillette and M.F. Norman (1980). Response of urodele oviduct to arginine vasotocin (AVT) in vitro: influence of steroids. Am. Zool. 20:831.

37. Pang, P.K., P.B. Furspan and W.H. Sawyer (1983). Evolution of neurohypophyseal hormone actions in vertebrates. Am. Zool. 23:655–662.

38. Perks, A.M. (1969). The Neurohypophysis. In W.S. Hoar and D.J. Randall, eds., Fish Physiology. Academic Press, New York, Vol. 2, pp. 112–206.

39. Perks, A.M. (1977). Developmental and evolutionary aspects of the neurohypophysis. Am. Zool. 17:833–849.

40. Perks, A.M. and M.H.I. Dodd (1963). Evidence for a neurohypophysial principle in the pituitary gland of certain elasmobranch species. Gen. Comp. Endocrinol. 3:286–299.

41. Perlow, M.J., S.M. Reppert, H.A. Artman, D.A. Fisher, S.M. Seif, and A.G. Robinson (1982). Oxytocin, vasopressin, and estrogen-stimulated neurophysin: daily patterns of concentration in cerebrospinal fluid. Science 216:1416–1418.

42. Philibert, R.L. and F.I. Kamemoto (1965). The hypothalamo-hypophyseal neurosecretory system of the ring-necked snake, *Diadophis punctatus.* Gen. Comp. Endocrinol. 5:326–335.

43. Reppert, S.M., H.G. Artman, S. Swaminathan, and D.A. Fisher (1981). Vasopressin exhibits a rhythmic daily pattern in cerebrospinal fluid but not in blood. Science 213:1256–1257.

44. Rice, G.E. (1982). Plasma arginine vasotocin concentrations in the lizard *Varanus gouldi* (Gray) following water loading, salt loading and dehydration. Gen. Comp. Endocrinol. 47:1–6.

45. Roth, J. (1973). Vascular supply to the ventral pelvic region of anurans as related to water balance. J. Morphol. 140:443–460.

46. Rurak, D.W. and A.M. Perks (1977). The neurohypophysial principles of the western brook lamprey, *Lampetra richardsoni:* Studies in the ammocoete larva. Gen. Comp. Endocrinol. 31:91–100.

47. Russell, J.T., M.J. Brownstein and H. Gainer (1979). Biosynthesis of vasopressin, oxytocin and neurophysins: Isolation and characterization of two common precursors (propressophysin and prooxyphysin). Endocrinology 107:1880–1891.

48. Sawyer, W.H. (1965). Evolution of neurohypophysial principles. Arch. Anat. Microsc. Morphol. Exp. 54:295–312.

49. Sawyer, W.H. (1977). Evolution of active neurohypophysial principles among the vertebrates. Am. Zool. 17:727–738.

50. Sawyer, W.H. and M.K. Sawyer (1952). Adaptive responses to neurohypophysial fractions in vertebrates. Physiol. Zool. 25:84–98.

51. Sheela, R. and K.R. Pandalai (1968). Reaction of the paraventricular nucleus to dehydration in the garden lizard, *Calotes versicolor.* Gen. Comp. Endocrinol. 11:257–261.

52. Starling, E.H. and E.B. Verney (1924). The secretion of urine as studied on the isolated kidney. Proc. R. Soc. Lond. 97:321–363.

53. Stiffler, D. (1981). The effects of mesotocin on renal function in hypophysectomized *Ambystoma tigrinum* larvae. Gen. Comp. Endocrinol. 45:49–55.

54. Sturkie, P.D. and Y. Lin (1966). Release of vasotocin and oviposition in the hen. J. Endocrinol. 35:325–326.

55. Taylor, A., M. Mamelak, E. Reaven and R. Maffly (1973). Vasopressin: Possible role of microtubules and microfilaments in its action. Science 181:347–350.

56. Uemara, H. (1964). Effects of water deprivation on the hypothalamo-hypophysial neurosecretory system in the grass parakeet, *Melopsittacus undulatus.* Gen. Comp. Endocrinol. 4:193–198.

57. Valtin, H., J. Stewart and H.W. Sokol (1974). Genetic control of the production of posterior pituitary principles. Handbook of Physiology, Sec. 7. Endocrinology, Vol. 4, Part 1, pp. 131–172.

58. Watson, S.L., N.G. Seidah and M. Chretien (1982). The carboxy terminus of the precursor to vasopressin and neurophysin: immunocytochemistry in rat brain. Science 217:853–855.

59. Weingartner, H., P. Gold, J.C. Ballenger, S.A. Smallberg, R. Summers, D.R. Rubinow, R.M. Post and F.K. Goodwin (1981). Effects of vasopressin on human memory functions. Science 211:601–603.

60. Wooley, P. (1959). The effect of posterior lobe pituitary extracts on blood pressure in several vertebrate classes. J. Exp. Biol. 36:453–458.

61. Zarrow, M.X., J.M. Yochim and J.L. McCarthy (1964). Experimental Endocrinology: A Sourcebook of Basic Techniques. Academic Press, New York.

62. Zimmerman, E.A., P.W. Carmel, M.K. Husain, M. Ferin, M. Tannenbaum, A.G. Frantz and A.G. Robinson (1973). Vasopressin and neurophysin: High concentrations in monkey hypophysial portal blood. Science 182:925–927.

8·The Thyroid Gland

The thyroid gland is unique among vertebrate endocrine glands in that it stores its secretory products (thyroid hormones) extracellularly. Two separate hormones are synthesized by thyroid cells from the amino acid tyrosine: *triiodothyronine* (T_3) and *tetraiodothyronine* or *thyroxine* (T_4). These hormones contain iodide ions (I^-) bound to the phenolic rings of the tyrosines.

Thyroid hormones influence reproduction, growth, differentiation and metabolism. These actions often occur cooperatively with other hormones, and the thyroid hormones enhance the effectiveness of these other hormones. This cooperative role for thyroid hormones is referred to as a *permissive action* whereby thyroid hormones produce changes in target tissues that "allow" these tissues to be more responsive to another hormone, to neural stimulation or possibly to certain environmental stimuli such as light. The major role for thyroid hormones in adult organisms may be to maintain this state of well-being in many types of tissues so that maximal sensitivity to other regulating agents is retained. Thyroid hormones also are essential for normal development.

Some Historical Aspects

Either deficient or excessive production of thyroid hormones may lead to serious pathological states (Table 8-1). The first description of thyroid disease was of abnormal enlargement of the thyroid in man recognized by Chinese physicians about 3000 B.C.[148] As a remedy they recommended ingestion of seaweed and burned sponge or desiccated deer thyroids. The first two substances contained therapeutic quantities of iodide and the last sufficient thyroid hormones to alleviate the pathological symptoms in most cases. Hypothyroid deficiencies of this sort were recognized in Western culture as clinical disorders many centuries later. In 1526 the *cretinism syndrome* was described clinically in Europe. Cretinism is manifest very early in life as a consequence of severe thyroid deficiency. This syndrome is characterized by dwarfism and a number of other physical abnormalities in addition to severe mental retardation, slow mental and physical activity, bradycardia (slowing of heart beat) and hypothermia. In 1880–1890 another classic clinical disorder in adults, *myxedema*, was linked to hypothyroid function. Myxedematous symptoms in adults are related to abnormal accumulation of water and protein throughout the body as well as to other disturbances in general metabolism. These accumulations of protein and fluid alter facial features, causing the patient to appear expressionless. In later stages of the disorder the sufferer becomes less interested in both self and environment, and if untreated would eventually enter a coma and die. *Juvenile myxedema* is similar to cretinism except that early growth and development are normal but become severely retarded in later childhood. All of these different clinical syndromes have the same basic cause: hypofunction of the thyroid gland.

TABLE 8-1. *Symptoms of Thyroid Deficiency and Hyperactivity in Man*

	HYPOTHYROID	HYPERTHYROID
Appearance	Myxedema; deficient growth	Exophthalmus
Behavioral symptoms	Mental retardation; mentally and physically sluggish; somnolent; sensitive to cold	Often quick mentally; restless, irritable, anxious, hyperkinetic; wakeful; sensitive to heat
Metabolism	Hypophagia; low basal metabolic rate; reduced QO_2 of liver, kidney, and muscle in vitro; decrease in oxidative enzymes; constipation	Hyperphagia; high basal metabolic rate; increased QO_2 of liver, kidney and muscle in vitro; increased oxidative enzymes; diarrhea
Muscle function	Weakness; hypotonia	Weakness; fibrillary twitchings, tremors

Modified from Tepperman.[140]

Bauman discovered in 1896 that an organic iodide-containing compound could be extracted from thyroid glands. Subsequently it was demonstrated that this "thyroidin" substance could reverse the adverse effects of iodide deficiency. In the early 1900s the thyroid gland and its hormones were implicated in elevating basal metabolic rate, primarily through effects on certain tissues, for example, liver, kidney and muscle. This observation has strongly influenced the direction of thyroid research in mammals as well as in many nonmammalian vertebrates. The action of thyroid hormones on metabolism is reflected in clinical thyroid states (Table 8-1).[148]

The iodide-containing hormone, *thyroxine*, was isolated and crystallized by Edward C. Kendall in 1915. This event marked a significant point not only in thyroid research but in endocrinology as a whole for thyroxine was the first hormone to be isolated in pure form. It was not until 1952, however, that the second thyroid hormone, T_3, was identified by J. Gross and R. Pitt-Rivers. The importance of this discovery will become evident as the mechanisms of synthesis and action for thyroid hormones are discussed. It was the discovery of the so-called antithyroid drugs in the early 1940s as well as the ready availability of radioactive isotopes of iodide (radioiodide) following the nuclear fission of uranium that made it possible to elucidate the details of thyroid hormone synthesis, metabolism and mechanisms of action.[148]

Embryonic Development and Organization of the Mammalian Thyroid Gland

The entire mammalian thyroid gland consists of many follicles encapsulated with a connective tissue sheath. The thyroid gland is highly vascularized with a dense capillary network surrounding each follicle. Sympathetic innervation of the thyroid has been described, and it appears that both the vasculature and the follicle cells may be innervated.

Development of the thyroid gland begins by formation of a ventral bud in the floor of the embryonic pharynx (endoderm) between the first and second pharyngeal pouches.[9] The gland initially differentiates as cellular cords that later separate into clusters of cells destined to become thyroid follicles. The cells of a cluster secrete a proteinaceous fluid termed *colloid* that accumulates extracellularly in the center of the cluster. This secretory activity eventually leads to a colloid-filled space, the *lumen* of the follicle, surrounded by a single layer of epithelial cells, the epithelium of the follicle (Figs. 8-1 and 8-2). The portion of the follicular cell that borders on the lumen of the follicle is known as the *apical* part. The nucleus is generally found in the *basal* portion of the cell that is farthest from the lumen and closest to the capillaries.

In addition to capillaries and follicles, *parafollicular* or *C cells* occur in the regions between or adjacent to the follicles. Parafollicular cells may occur within follicles or may even form follicular structures in some species. These cells are derived from another pharyngeal derivative, the *ultimobranchial body*, and secrete a hormone, *calcitonin*, that influences calcium metabolism (see Chap. 12). A comparison of parafollicular cells and follicular cells (Table 8-2) emphasizes their different structural and functional features. In some mammals the parathyroid glands may be embedded within the mass of the thyroid (Fig. 8-2). The parathyroids, like the parafollicular cells, have their origin nearby from the embryonic pharynx and in some species get incorporated into the mass of thyroid follicles during development. The parathyroid glands are also discussed in Chapter 12.

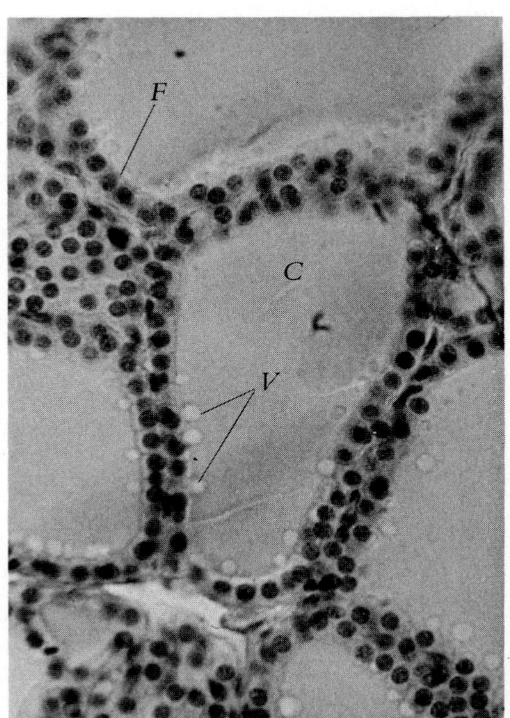

Fig. 8-2. General organization of the mammalian thyroid gland. Section from dog thyroid showing one complete follicle surrounded by portions of other follicles. *C*, colloid; *V*, vacuole in colloid; *F*, follicular epithelium.

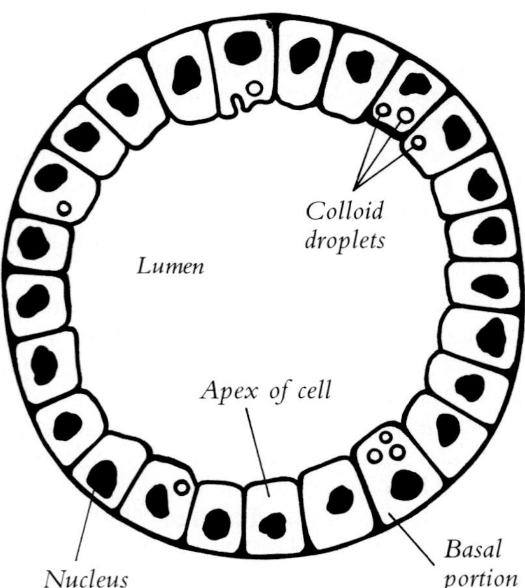

Fig. 8-1. Structure of a thyroid follicle (see text for explanation).

Biochemistry of Thyroid Hormones

The events related to the ability of thyroid follicles to synthesize and release thyroid hormones are discussed separately for simplicity, but it is important to keep in mind that many of these events may be occurring simultaneously. The processes discussed in this section include:

1. Accumulation of inorganic iodide by follicular cells
2. Synthesis of thyroglobulin, a glycoprotein containing tyrosine residues for hormone synthesis
3. Binding of inorganic iodide to tyrosine residues in thyroglobulin
4. Synthesis of T_3 and T_4 from iodinated tyrosines
5. Storage of thyroglobulin containing the

TABLE 8-2. *Comparison of Characteristics of Thyroid Follicular and Parafollicular Cells*

THYROID FOLLICULAR CELL	THYROID PARAFOLLICULAR CELL
Absence of secretion granules	Large number of eosinophilic granules, 0.2 μm diameter; stain with silver nitrate
Endoplasmic reticulum cisternae of larger diameter, containing flocculent precipitate like that found in albumin-secreting cells	Many mitochondria and high level of the mitochondrial enzyme α-glycerophosphate dehydrogenase
Carbohydrate added at Golgi apparatus, which is rather inconspicuous in these cells	No luminal surface present
	Nucleus more irregular in outline than those of follicular cells
Enlargement of Golgi apparatus from TSH treatment	Golgi apparatus prominent
Binds antibody to thyroglobulin but not to calcitonin	Binds antibody to calcitonin
Cytology not altered by high blood calcium level	Degranulation due to high blood calcium level
Readily accumulates iodide	

thyroid hormones in the lumen of the follicle

6. Engulfing of the colloid by follicular cells and hydrolysis of thyroglobulin to release thyroid hormones
7. Diffusion of T_3 and T_4 into the general circulation and their transport to target tissues
8. Mechanisms of action for thyroid hormones
9. Metabolism and excretion of thyroid hormones

Dietary Iodide and Iodide Uptake

The principal source for inorganic iodide is dietary. In certain portions of the world, environmental iodide is in short supply, for example, the Great Lakes and Rocky Mountain regions of the United States and northeastern Europe. Consequently unsupplemented human diets are low in naturally occurring iodide, and hypothyroid states commonly are encountered unless an iodide supplement is used. At one time hypothyroid goiters or enlarged thyroids were common in people who inhabited these low-iodide regions or "goiter belts," but the use of iodized salt has almost eliminated this condition. (The term goiter or goitre originally meant any tumor or abnormal glandular enlargement in the neck but has come to mean an enlarged thyroid.)[52]

Inorganic iodide is readily absorbed from the intestine into the blood, from which it is selectively accumulated by thyroid follicular cells. There is an energy-dependent, active transport mechanism or "iodide pump" in the follicular cell basal membrane that is specific for iodide. This uptake of iodide is enhanced by rapid conversion of inorganic iodide within the follicular cell to organically bound forms (that is, iodinated tyrosines).

The events of iodide uptake, accumulation and binding to tyrosine have been examined with the aid of radioiodide. The radioisotope of iodide employed most frequently for iodide uptake studies is ^{131}I, a strong gamma-emitting isotope with a short radiation half-life (8.3 days). Radioiodide is generally administered in the form of a sodium salt ($Na^{131}I$). This particular isotope of iodide can be detected in blood or tissues with unsophisticated detection equipment because of the high-energy gamma radiation it emits. Another isotope of iodide, ^{125}I, is often employed in thyroid studies that make use of the lower energy radiation produced by this isotope and its longer radiation half-life (57.4 days). This isotope emits beta and gamma radiation and is suitable for high-resolution autoradiography at both the level of the light and electron microscopes. Because of its lower energy emission and longer radiation half-life, ^{125}I is more suited for metabolic studies, for it is much less destructive to cells than ^{131}I. Uptake of radioiodide, like that of the normal isotope (^{127}I), is stimulated by thyrotropin (TSH) from the adenohypophysis, and there is no discrimination among the various isotopes in the formation of organically bound iodide associated with thyroid hormone synthesis.

Calculation of a rate for radioiodide accumulation following administration of a given dose provides a quantitative estimate of the degree of TSH stimulation and a reflection of pituitary TSH release. Hence, measurement of radioiodide uptake and accumulation provides a simple and rapid method for estimating endogenous activities of the hypothalamo-thyroid axis as well as a means to assess responsiveness of thyroid follicular cells to exogenous TSH. Usually radioiodide uptake is expressed as percent uptake of the injected dose at some predetermined time, such as 24 hours following administration of radioiodide (Table 8-3).

The ability to bind iodide is not a feature unique to thyroid follicular cells (Table 8-4), and most cells will accumulate some iodide. Cells such as melanophores (melanocytes), pigmented retinal cells and the epithelial cells of sweat glands, salivary glands, lactating mammary glands and kidney tubules readily accumulate radioiodide following injection of either radioactive isotope. Furthermore, oocytes of many oviparous (egg-laying) vertebrates accumulate large amounts of injected radioiodide. This ovarian accumulation is associated with the normal process of ensuring a source of iodide in the egg that can be used by the young animal for early synthesis of thyroid hormones until an adequate dietary source becomes available. Marsupial and placental mammals and other live-bearing vertebrates probably transfer sufficient iodide to the developing young from the maternal blood or via the milk to suckling newborns.

Thyroid hormones may not be released into the circulation in proportion to the uptake and binding of radioiodide, however. Uptake, binding and release of thyroid hormones are separate events independently influenced by a variety of factors, as evidenced in the following discussions. Nevertheless, measurement of radioiodide uptake is a rapid and convenient method to assay for TSH activity with respect to endogenous levels or exogenous treatments, and it is widely employed in thyroid research.

Biosynthesis of Thyroid Hormones

The actual synthesis of thyroid hormones in the follicular cells involves, first, the synthesis of thyroglobulin containing tyrosine residues and, second, the binding of accumulated inorganic iodide to the tyrosines. The final step in synthesis of thyroid hormones is the linking together (coupling) of two iodinated tyrosines

Table 8-3. *Some Effects of TSH and Thyroid Inhibitors on ^{131}I Uptake by Thyroids of Larval Salamanders,* Ambystoma tigrinum[106]

N	Mean Body Weight (g±SEM)	Daily Injections; Pretreatment for 7 Days	Mean Thyroid Uptake (% Injected Dose ± SEM)
6	11 ± 0.5	None	4.6 ± 1.6
6	8 ± 0.6	0.25 μg TSH[a]	12.4 ± 2.5
6	11 ± 0.6	2.5 μg TSH	29.2 ± 4.7
6	17 ± 1.6	25 μg TSH	38.3 ± 1.0
6	9 ± 0.6	2.5 μg TSH + 10 μg PTU[b]	10.2 ± 2.9
6	7 ± 1.0	2.5 μg TSH + 0.5 mg NaSCN[c]	3.9 ± 0.7

Note: Radioiodide uptake was determined 24 hours after intraperitoneal injection of 5 μCi ^{131}I.
[a] Ovine TSH, NIH-TSH-S6.
[b] Propylthiouracil.
[c] Sodium thiocyanate.

TABLE 8-4. *Accumulation of Radioiodide by Thyroids and Gonads of Sexually Mature Vertebrates*

CLASS	SPECIES	SEX	RADIOIODIDE UPTAKE GONAD/THYROID
Osteichthyes[a]	*Micropterus dolomieu* (smallmouth bass)	M	0.012
		F	3.780
Amphibia[a]	*Ambystoma tigrinum* (tiger salamander, neotene)	M	0.045
		F	0.512
Aves[119]	*Coturnix coturnix japonica* (Japanese quail)	F	4 to 10

[a]Norris, unpublished data.

of thyroglobulin to form the iodinated hormones T_3 and T_4. Most of these events that are described below were elucidated with the aid of ^{125}I.

SYNTHESIS OF THYROGLOBULIN. Thyroglobulin is a large, globular glycoprotein that is not especially rich in tyrosine residues. Actually the term as used here may embrace more than one molecular form of thyroglobulin. Thyroglobulins extractable from follicles occur in several sizes, ranging from 12S to 27S. (*S* stands for Svedberg sedimentation coefficient, which is related to size, shape and, to a lesser degree, electrostatic charge of a molecule. These parameters determine the migration and final position of molecules in a molecular gradient following high-speed centrifugation.) Comparative analysis of thyroglobulins from different vertebrates indicates different proportions in the various size classes of thyroglobulins (Table 8-5). Most mammalian thyroglobulin preparations exhibit a predominant 19S component (88–100% of the total iodinated protein in thyroid preparations) with a small proportion of larger 27S and occasionally a small quantity of 12S thyroglobulin (rabbit, rat and especially the guinea pig). The 19S form consists of two 12S-subunits, and the 27S form is composed of three subunits. Regardless, thyroglobulin will be treated in the following discussions as though it were a single molecular species. An emphasis on the true form of thyroglobulin is irrelevant to its essential role in thyroid hormone synthesis.

Thyroglobulin synthesis occurs at the rough endoplasmic reticulum and is packaged into membrane-bound secretion granules in the Golgi apparatus.[101] It appears that noniodinated tyrosines are incorporated into thyroglobulins first, since no transfer RNAs for iodinated tyrosines have been demonstrated in follicular cells.[15] Iodination of tyrosine residues in the completed thyroglobulin molecule occurs later at the cell-colloid interface.[139]

IODINATION OF TYROSINE RESIDUES IN THYROGLOBULIN. Organic binding of iodide begins with conversion of inorganic iodide to "active iodide," a form of inorganic iodide that readily binds to the phenolic ring of tyrosine. Although the exact chemical nature of active iodide has never been determined with certainty, it is apparently formed in the follicular cell by an enzymatic *peroxidase system* that involves glucose oxidation and reduction of pyridine nucleotides to form hydrogen peroxide, H_2O_2. Inorganic iodide reacts with H_2O_2 to form active iodide, which in turn binds immediately to tyrosine residues in thyroglobulin. Treatment of thyroid hormone-synthesizing systems with the enzyme catalase specifically hydrolyzes H_2O_2 to water and oxygen. This blocks iodination, supporting the role of peroxides in formation of organically bound iodide.

The binding of one active iodide to tyrosine at position 3 on the phenolic ring yields *3-monoiodotyrosine* or MIT. A second active iodide may attach at position 5 of the same tyrosine residue, resulting in conversion of MIT to *3,5-diiodotyrosine* or DIT. The 3 position is always iodinated more readily and 3-monoiodotyrosine but never a 5-monoiodotyrosine is formed. The proportion of MIT to DIT formed will be determined by the amount of active iodide available, which in turn depends upon the size of the inorganic iodide

TABLE 8-5. *Sedimentation Coefficients (S) for Chordate Iodoproteins (Thyroglobulins)*

SPECIES	PERCENT IODOPROTEINS FOUND			
	<12	12s	19s	27s
Urochordata				
Ciona intestinalis (tunicate)	100	–	–	–
Vertebrata				
Agnatha				
Lampetra fluviatilis (river lamprey)	32	68	–	–
Chondrichthyes				
Scyliorhinus stellaris (dogfish shark)	–	16	80	4
Osteichthyes				
Conger conger (Congo eel; teleost)	–	6	73	6
Reptilia				
Thalassochelis caretta (sea turtle)	–	11	84	5
Testudo hermanni (land turtle)	–	12	84	4
Aves				
Anas platyrhynchos (domestic duck)	–	trace	94	6
Gallus gallus (domestic chicken)	–	trace	94	5
Mammalia				
Cavia porcellus (guinea pig)	–	14	83	3
Rattus rattus (rat)	–	trace	93	7
Mus musculus (mouse)	–	–	94	6
Oryctolagus cuniculus (rabbit)	–	trace	98	2
Canis familiaris (dog)	–	–	94	6
Felis catus (cat)	–	–	92	8
Bos taurus (ox)	–	–	91	9
Bubalus bulalis (brahma)	–	–	93	7
Capra hircus (goat)	–	–	90	10
Ovis aries (sheep)	–	–	88	12
Sus scrofa (pig)	–	–	88	12
Equus caballus (horse)	–	–	100	–
Equus asinus (donkey)	–	–	100	–
E. caballus × *E. asinus* (mule)	–	–	100	–
Homo sapiens (man)	–	–	92	8
Macaca mulatta (rhesus monkey)	–	–	92	8

Data from Roche et al.[120] and Ui.[150]

pool. The structures of MIT and DIT are depicted in Figure 8-3 where they may be compared to the structures of T_3 and T_4.

Most of the available evidence supports the interpretation that iodination of tyrosine residues in thyroglobulin occurs at the surface of microvilli present on the apical surface of the follicular cell[139] (Fig. 8-4). The peroxidase enzymatic system believed to be responsible for the formation of active iodide is present in the membranes of the apical surface.[146] Presumably iodination occurs as thyroglobulin is being secreted into the colloid for storage.

THE COUPLING OF IODINATED TYROSINES. The exact way in which thyroid hormones are formed from iodinated tyrosines is not known. Coupling appears to be an enzymatically controlled process that involves two iodinated

Table 8-6. *Comparison of Thyroid Function in a Monotreme (Echidna), Marsupial (Bandicoot) and Placental Mammal (Rabbit)*

	EUTHYROID PARAMETERS			EFFECT OF THYROIDECTOMY	
	IODIDE UPTAKE (% INJECTED DOSE)	PLASMA T_4 (nmol/l)	PLASMA T_3 (nmol/l)	BMR[a]	BODY TEMPERATURE
Echidna, *Tachyglossus aculeatus*	6.4	15.7	0.7	No effect	No effect
Bandicoot, *Perameles nasuta*	13.7	22.0	1.5	Decrease	No effect
Rabbit, *Oryctolagus caniculus*	22.9	57.9	6.9	Decrease	No effect

Data from Hurlbert and Augee (1982), Physiol. Zool. 55:220–228.
[a] BMR = basal metabolic rate.

tyrosines, either two DIT molecules or one DIT plus one MIT. The alanine side chain of one of the iodinated tyrosines is cleaved off, and the remaining iodinated phenolic ring is joined to the other iodinated tyrosine through formation of an ether (—O—) linkage (Fig. 8-3). The resultant structure is known as an iodinated *thyronine*. Appropriate coupling of MIT and DIT yields the resultant 3,5,3′-triiodothyronine or T_3. Similarly, coupling of two DIT molecules results in formation of 3,5,3′,5′-tetraiodothyronine or T_4. The proportion of MIT and DIT available for coupling will influence the proportions of T_4 and T_3 formed. Normally much more T_4 than T_3 is synthesized, but the relative proportion of T_3 may increase markedly if iodide is in short supply.

Coupling of iodinated tyrosines presumably occurs between adjacent residues in the folded, globular thyroglobulin molecule or possibly between iodinated tyrosines in adjacent thyroglobulin molecules. Only a fraction of the iodinated tyrosines are actually coupled, however. Formation of iodinated thyronines occurs for only about 10% of the iodinated tyrosine residues present in thyroglobulin, and about 90% of the extractable organic iodide is still in the form of MIT and DIT.[107]

The specificity of the coupling reaction implies an enzymatic conversion of iodinated tyrosines to thyronines. Only one triiodothyronine is ever formed in the thyroid, although it would be possible to form 3,3′,5′-triiodothyronine, depending upon the relative positions of MIT and DIT and from which molecule the alanine side chain was cleaved. This isomer of T_3 can be formed by deiodination of T_4 in the liver. The other possible combinations are ruled out because formation of 5-MIT does not occur. There is a requirement that DIT be positioned "on the right," whereas either MIT or DIT may occur to the "left" for the coupling reaction to proceed. The stereospecificity for DIT is further supported by the failure of thyroid systems to synthesize, even under conditions of severe iodide deficiency, any diiodothyronines (T_2) utilizing two MIT molecules. Two enzymatic schemes have been proposed to explain observations on the coupling mechanism, and they are outlined in Figure 8-5. One of these schemes employs the same peroxidase system involved in the formation of active iodide, making it the more likely endogenous mechanism.

Hormone Release: Hydrolysis of Thyroglobulin

Release of thyroid hormones following administration of TSH is not linked to thyroid hormone synthesis. Thyrotropin stimulates engulfment of colloid by the follicular cell and its intracellular hydrolysis to amino acids, MIT, DIT, T_3 and T_4 (Fig. 8-6). Autoradiographic studies indicate that the first event observed following TSH administration is the

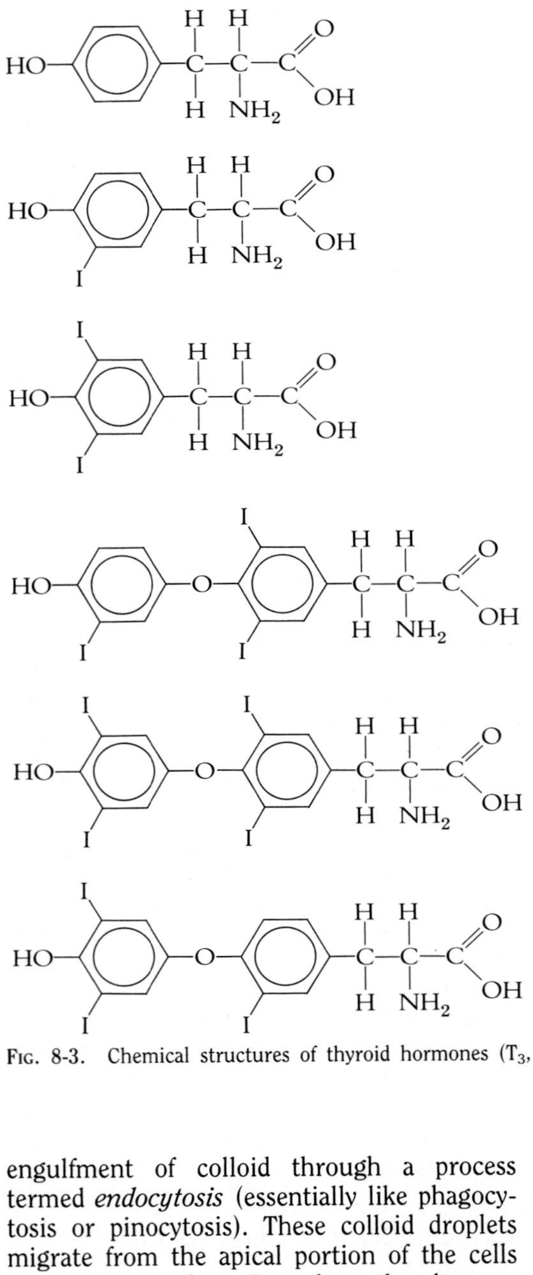

Tyrosine

3-Monoiodotyrosine (MIT)

3,5-Diiodotyrosine (DIT)

3,5,3′-Triiodothyronine (T_3)

3,5,3′,5′-Tetraiodothyronine (T_4, Thyroxine)

3,3′,5′-Triiodothyronine (rT_3, Reverse T_3)

Fig. 8-3. Chemical structures of thyroid hormones (T_3, T_4), precursors (tyrosine, MIT, DIT) and reverse T_3 (rT_3).

engulfment of colloid through a process termed *endocytosis* (essentially like phagocytosis or pinocytosis). These colloid droplets migrate from the apical portion of the cells toward the basal portion where they become associated with electron-dense organelles that appear to be lysosomes. These lysosomes contain a number of hydrolytic enzymes, including acid phosphatase. Fusion of the colloid droplets with lysosomes results in formation of "fusion droplets" or *phagolysosomes*. As the phagolysosomes migrate toward the basal portion of the cell they become progressively degranulated, presumably because of hydrolysis of thyroglobulin and diffusion of the hydrolysis products into the cytosol.

Thyroglobulin hydrolysis within the phagolysosome releases MIT, DIT, T_3, T_4 and amino acids, which diffuse into the cytosol. Essentially it is only T_3 and T_4 that are "allowed" to diffuse from the cell into the vast capillary network surrounding the follicles. A cytoplasmic enzyme, deiodinase, hydrolyzes MIT and DIT to tyrosine and inorganic iodide, which are lacking in any thyroidal hormone activity. Deiodinase may also deiodinate a very

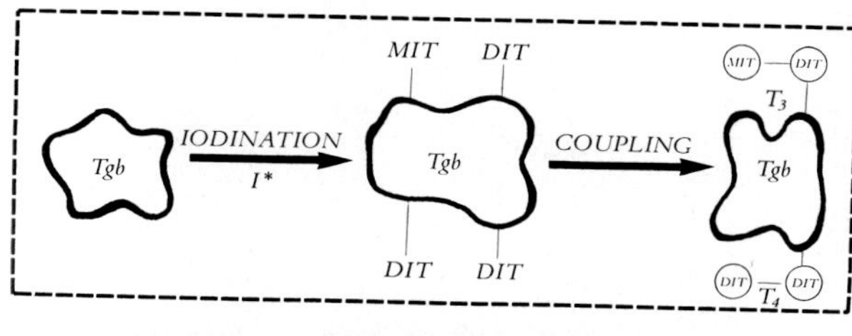

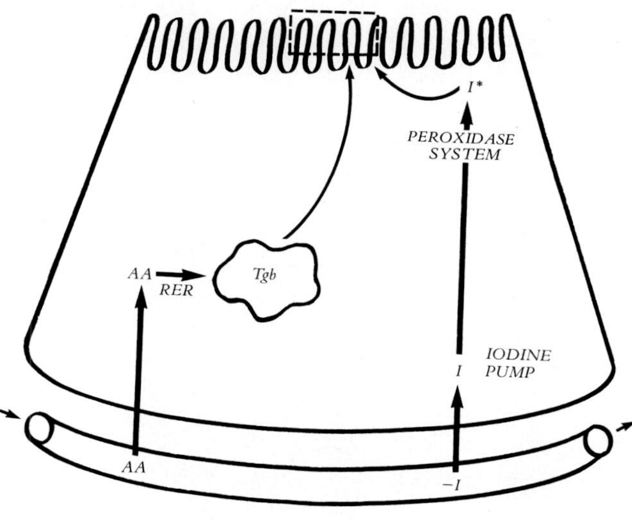

Fig. 8-4. Cytological locations for major events in the biosynthesis of thyroid hormones, MIT and DIT. See text for explanation. *Tgb*, thyroglobulin; I*, active iodide; AA, amino acids including tyrosine; RER, rough endoplasmic reticulum.

small proportion of T_3 and T_4 as well. Deiodination is apparently a conservation mechanism to reuse inorganic iodide for later iodination. The iodinated tyrosines (MIT and DIT) cannot be used in thyroglobulin synthesis, as stated previously, and they must be either deiodinated or allowed to diffuse from the cell. Approximately 85 to 90% of the iodide released through deiodination of MIT and DIT enters a "second iodide pool" within the follicular cell, which is then available for iodination of newly synthesized thyroglobulin. The remainder of this inorganic iodide diffuses out of the cell.

It has been proposed that hydrolysis of thyroglobulin could occur extracellularly in the colloid as well as intracellularly. Hydrolytic enzymes, catheptases, capable of releasing iodinated compounds from thyroglobulin have been localized in the colloid. These catheptases, however, require very low pH (pH 3–4) for optimal activity, and they may not be active in the colloid where the pH conditions are approximately neutral (pH 7.0). Nevertheless, one could argue that localized pH changes sufficient to activate these enzymes might occur in the colloid that would not be detected by standard pH determinations. Although extracellular hydrolysis might contribute to overall thyroglobulin destruction following TSH stimulation, the majority of hydrolysis occurs in the phagolysosomes.

Transport of Thyroid Hormones in the Blood

Most of the circulating thyroid hormones (about 99%) are bound reversibly to serum proteins. Serum binding and transporting of thyroid hormones are essential, because T_3 and T_4, like the steroid hormones, are hydrophobic and are not highly soluble in blood. Being hydrophobic, free thyroid hormones readily cross cell membranes and are rapidly removed from the blood and metabolized, especially by the liver and kidneys. Several different serum proteins are capable of binding and

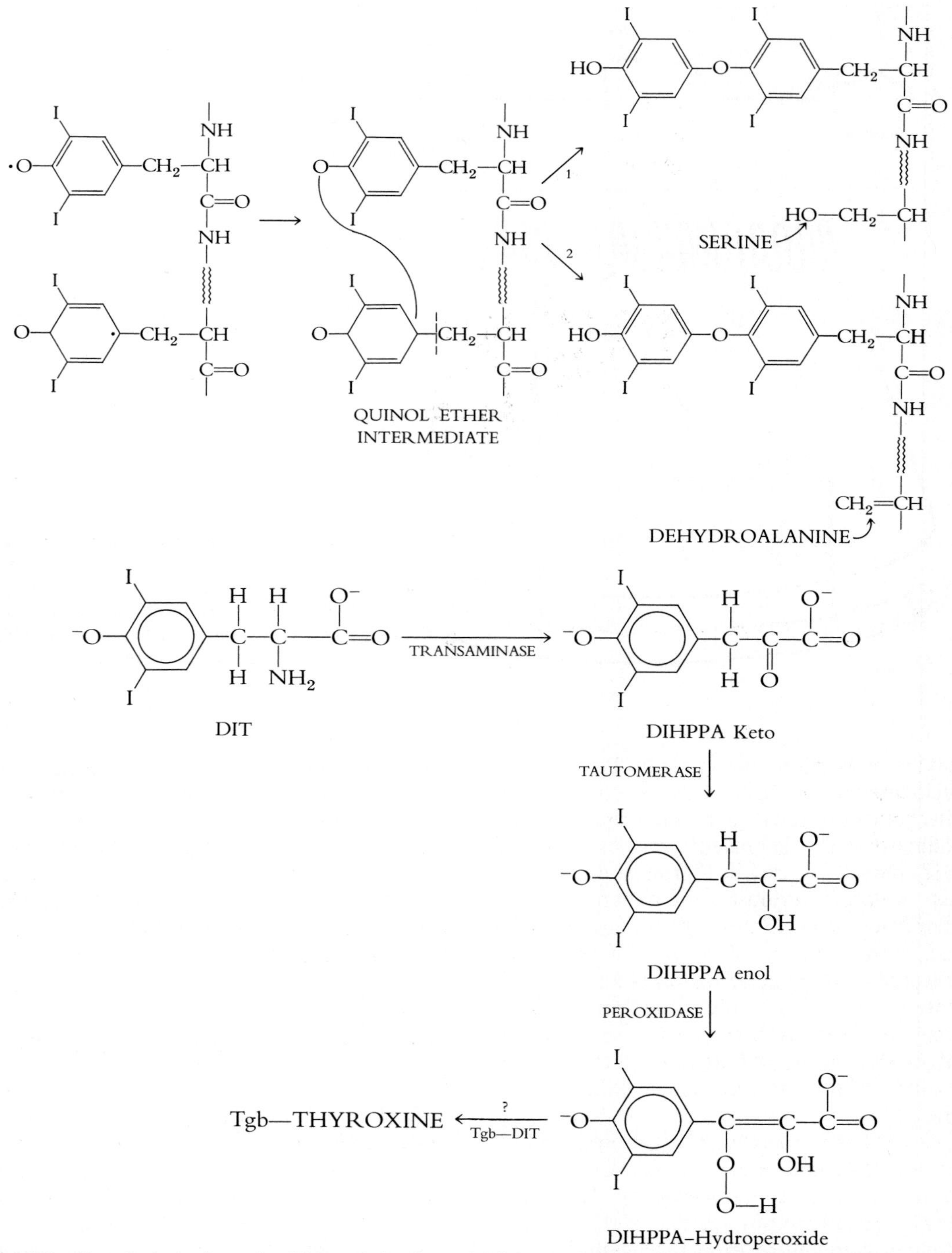

QUINOL ETHER INTERMEDIATE

SERINE

DEHYDROALANINE

DIT

TRANSAMINASE

DIHPPA Keto

TAUTOMERASE

DIHPPA enol

PEROXIDASE

Tgb—THYROXINE

Tgb—DIT

DIHPPA–Hydroperoxide

FIG. 8-5. Hypothetical scheme for *(A)* intramolecular and *(B)* intermolecular coupling of iodinated tyrosines to form thyroxine. *Tgb,* thyroglobulin, DIHPPA, pyruvic acid analog of DIT. DIHPPA has been identified in thyroid cells. Modified from Taurog, A.[139]

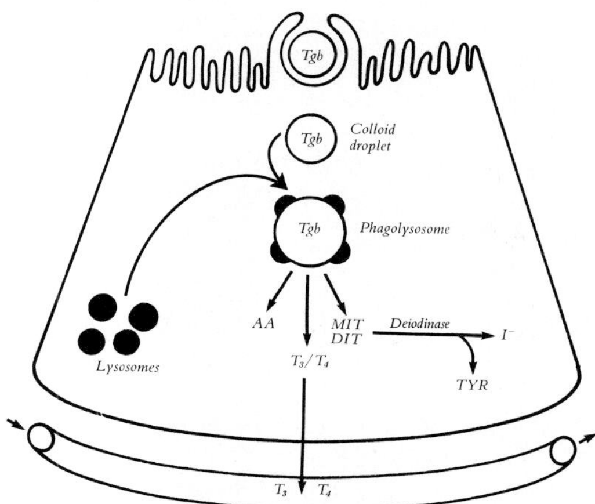

FIG. 8-6. Cytological events in the endocytosis of colloid, hydrolysis of thyroglobulin *(Tgb)* and release of thyroid hormones into the circulation. *AA*, amino acids. TYR, tyrosine. See text for explanation.

transporting thyroid hormones (Table 8-7). In man, for example, about 75% of the bound hormones are linked to the α_2-globulins and 15 and 10% respectively are bound to prealbumin and albumin. Only a very small fraction (<1%) are transported free in the blood.

Prior to development of sensitive radioimmunoassays and competitive protein-binding assays for T_3 and T_4, the standard method for assessing thyroid hormone levels was to determine the total *protein-bound iodide* (PBI) in the plasma. In many species, especially anamniotes, inorganic iodide is also carried by serum proteins. Determination of PBI may provide an overestimate of thyroid hormone levels, which also vary with changes in circulating iodide levels. Extraction of whole serum with butyl alcohol (butanol) removes the iodinated thyronines with the butanol phase and leaves the inorganic iodide behind in the aqueous phase. Thus; the *butanol-extractable iodide* (BEI) is used as a better estimate of circulating thyroid hormone levels, especially in nonmammals. Techniques for radioimmunoassay of T_3 and T_4 in very small volumes of plasma or serum have been developed, and the use of PBI and BEI is becoming of historical interest only.

Under normal conditions, circulating T_4 levels are much greater than T_3 levels (Table 8-8). Only about one-seventh to one-half of the circulating T_3, however, is of thyroid origin, and the remainder is produced through peripheral deiodination of T_4.[109,136] This deiodination is accomplished primarily through the efforts of the liver, kidneys, and skeletal muscle. Free T_3 or T_4 in the serum is in equilibrium with bound hormones so that as free hormones are metabolized there is a proportionate dissociation of bound hormone to replace the free hormone lost through metabolism.

Thyroxine is more tightly bound than T_3 to the serum proteins, and consequently T_3 is more readily eliminated from the blood. The biological half-life for T_3 in humans is about 24 hours, whereas T_4 has a much longer biological half-life (about 7 days), attributable to the greater affinity of T_4 for the serum-binding proteins. The reduced serum protein binding and more rapid clearance of T_3 from the circulation is believed in part to provide the explanation for the observed greater effectiveness of T_3 over T_4 when administered to humans or rats. Thus T_4 may prove to be only a storage reservoir, bound as it is to the serum proteins. Following conversion from T_4 through deiodination, T_3 can readily enter target cells.

TABLE 8-7. *Percentage Distribution of Added ^{125}I-Thyroxine among Serum Proteins of Selected Mammals Demonstrating Binding to Different Fractions*

SPECIES	ALBUMIN	POSTALBUMIN	α_1-GLOBULIN	α_1–α_2 GLOBULIN
Domestic goat	22.0	–	–	78.0
Elephant	26.8	–	–	73.2
Hyena	63.1	36.9	–	–
Jaguar	52.3	47.7	–	–
Polar bear	56.6	–	43.4	–

Modified from Joasoo, A. et al.[69]

TABLE 8-8. *Circulating Levels of Thyroid Hormones for Selected Vertebrate Species*

CLASS/ORDER	SPECIES	T_3	T_4	REF.
Agnatha/Cyclostomata	*Petromyzon marinus*			
	(mature females)	0.5–1.77 nmoles/liter	69.5–139 nmoles/l	64
	(ammocetes)	—	4.9–18.5 μg/dl	171
	(adults)	—	0.46 μg/dl	170
	Eptatretus stouti (Pacific hagfish)	—	2.2–10.5 μg/dl	96
Osteichthyes/Teleostei	*Salvelinus fontinalis* (brook trout)		0.15–3.36 μg/dl	61
	Ictalurus punctatus (channel catfish)		0–0.38 μg/dl	61
	Aplodinotus grunniens (freshwater drum)		0.92–1.80 μg/dl	61
Amphibia/Anura	*Bufo viridis*	—	1.0–19.9 ng/ml	121
	Bufo bufo	—	0.4–5.2 ng/ml	121
Amphibia/Caudata	*Ambystoma tigrinum* (sexually mature larvae)	0.07–0.73 ng/ml	0.25–9.0 ng/ml	[a]
Reptilia/Squamata	*Naja naja* (cobra)	—	1.25–1.55 μg/dl	166
Aves/Galliformes	*Gallus gallus* (domestic chicks, 1 day to 6 weeks old)	—	1.45–3.0 μg/dl	26
Mammalia/Marsupialia	*Macropus eugenii* (tammar wallaby)	—	1.3–2.7 μg/dl	74
/Carnivora	*Phoca vitulina* (harbor seal)	—	0.9–1.7 μg/dl	118
/Primates	*Homo sapiens*	0.9 ng/ml	50 ng/ml	86

[a] Unpublished data of D.O. Norris

Peripheral Metabolism of Thyroid Hormones

Thyroxine has several metabolic fates after being released from the thyroid gland.[136] Approximately 33 to 40% is converted to T_3, and this deiodination may be important in the mechanism of action for thyroid hormones. Peripheral deiodination of T_4 is the major source for circulating T_3. About 15 to 20% of the circulating T_4 is converted to tetraiodothyroacetic acid, which has no significant physiological activity and is excreted in urine or bile. Approximately one half of the circulating T_4 is eventually converted by deiodination to a unique form of T_3 with the structure of 3,3′,5′-triiodothyronine (Fig. 8-3). It has no biological activity. This form of T_3 is known as *reverse* T_3 (rT_3), and it is more rapidly degraded than normal T_3. As a result of this rapid clearance, rT_3 levels in the blood are rather low. Increases or decreases in circulating T_3 levels are always accompanied by reciprocal changes in rT_3 levels.

Mechanism of Action of Thyroid Hormones

The molecular mechanism of action for thyroid hormones appears to be similar to that described for steroids (Chap. 1). Thyroid hormones, because of their hydrophobic nature, readily enter target cells where they bind to receptor proteins. Following binding to receptors they may influence the synthesis of new proteins via an effect on nuclear gene transcription or on mitochondrial protein synthesis.[110] They may also produce effects on oxidative phosphorylation in the mitochondria.[136,137]

Nuclear receptors for thyroid hormones have been isolated and characterized.[110] They have greater affinity for T_3 than for T_4, supporting the hypothesis that conversion of T_4 to T_3 is a necessary requisite for thyroid hormone action. Mitochondrial receptor proteins have also been demonstrated,[137] and these mitochondrial receptors may be associated with observed effects on mitochondrial protein synthesis and oxidative metabolism. Unoccupied receptors for thyroid hormones have not been demonstrated in the cytosol.

The permissive actions of thyroid hormones related to that "sense of well-being" may be a consequence of effects of thyroid hormones on the nuclear-directed synthesis of adenyl cyclase or on availability of ATP through their actions on mitochondria or on both.[62] The levels of adenyl cyclase and ATP would certainly influence the effects of any of the hormones that normally produce their actions through some cyclic adenosine 3′,5′-monophosphate (cAMP)-dependent mechanism (Fig. 8-7).

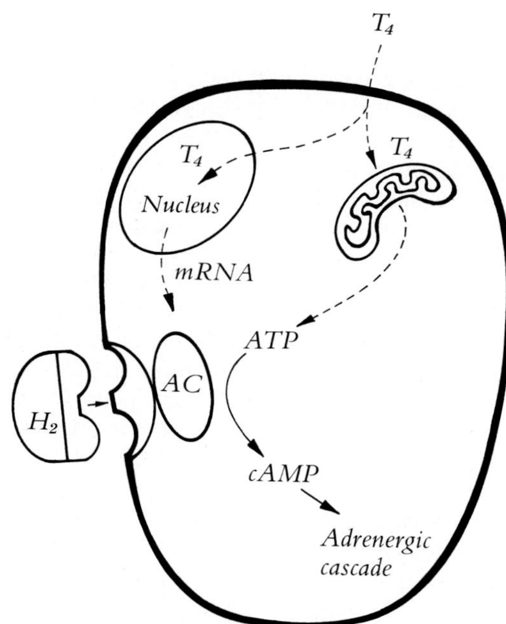

Fig. 8-7. Postulated permissive action for thyroid hormones by influencing availability of ATP, the enzyme adenyl cyclase or both, thus influencing the ability for another hormone (hormone 2 [H_2]) to produce its characteristic action. Adrenergic cascade refers to the sequence of events involving subsequent action of cAMP on other cellular events. (Modified from Hoch.[62])

Factors That Influence Thyroid Function in Mammals

A great variety of factors may influence thyroid state in mammals and thus influence many processes controlled by other hormones as well. Dietary iodide and the general level of hypothalamo-hypophysial-thyroid functioning are two very important factors. The latter is influenced by a host of different environmental factors as well as by other endocrine systems. A number of naturally occurring chemicals and synthetic drugs have been discovered that have profound effects on thyroid function. Nonendocrine factors are discussed first, including dietary factors, physical factors and internal rhythms. Under the endocrine factors affecting thyroid function are included the hypothalamic and hypophysial hormones as well as hormones produced by other endocrine glands.

Nonendocrine Factors

Dietary Iodide. Low iodide availability reduces the synthesis of thyroid hormones and leads to development of hypothyroid states. Most seriously affected by the reduction in iodide is the synthesis of DIT, which in turn reduces the proportion of T_4 that can be synthesized. Conversely, an excessive level of blood iodide inhibits uptake and accumulation of iodide by the follicular cells, presumably by poisoning the iodide-pumping mechanism. There may be little importance to this observation outside of the laboratory since in nature it would be most unusual for a mammal to be subjected to an excess of iodide.

Inhibitors of Iodide Uptake. Certain anions are effective in blocking accumulation of iodide by the follicular cells through competitive inhibition of iodide transport. Thiocyanate (SCN^-) and perchlorate ions ($HClO_3^-$) are particularly effective at blocking iodide uptake. These agents are used commonly by investigators to block thyroid function and particularly to block iodide uptake mechanisms. Some representative experimental data on the effects of anionic inhibitors are provided in Table 8-3.

Inhibitors of Formation of "Active Iodide". Compounds that interfere with thyroid hormone synthesis by inhibiting iodination of tyrosines are often termed *goitrogens.*[172] The resultant reduction in circulating hormones causes increased TSH secretion as a consequence of reduced negative feedback. Continuous stimulation of the thyroid gland by TSH results in enlargement of the thyroid and production of a goiter. Goitrogens, in addition to blocking formation of active iodide, also induce goiter formation. Many of these compounds secondarily inhibit iodide uptake by increasing the size of the intracellular inorganic iodide pool. Because agents that selectively inhibit iodide uptake also block synthesis and can lead to goiter formation, the anions, such as SCN^- and $HClO_3^-$, are often termed goitrogens.

Several synthetic drugs are capable of blocking formation of active iodide, including thiourea (TU), propylthiouracil (PTU) and other thiocarbamide derivatives.[58,172] This list is continuously being expanded as additional drugs are tested. These drugs interfere with the peroxidase system responsible for generation of H_2O_2. Treatment with such drugs can be used to "chemically thyroidectomize" an animal reversibly. Certain reduced compounds such as ascorbic acid, reduced glutathione and reduced pyrimidines remove H_2O_2 from the system and also block formation of active iodide.

Many flowering vascular plants of the family Brassicae (cabbage, brussel sprouts, rutabaga and turnips) naturally contain a compound known as *progoitrin* that can be enzymatically converted to a goitrogenic compound called *goitrin* (Fig. 8-8). If sufficient quantities of goitrin are absorbed from the intestine into the general circulation the synthesis of thyroid hormones is impaired and a hypothyroid state ensues. People or animals that consume large quantities of these plants tend to exhibit hypothyroidism, which may be accentuated if coupled with an iodide-poor diet.[52] Cooking the plants normally destroys the enzyme that converts progoitrin to goitrin, but progoitrin is not affected by the quantity of heat applied in cooking the vegetables. Bacteria in the human intestinal flora are capable of converting all ingested progoitrin into goitrin, however.

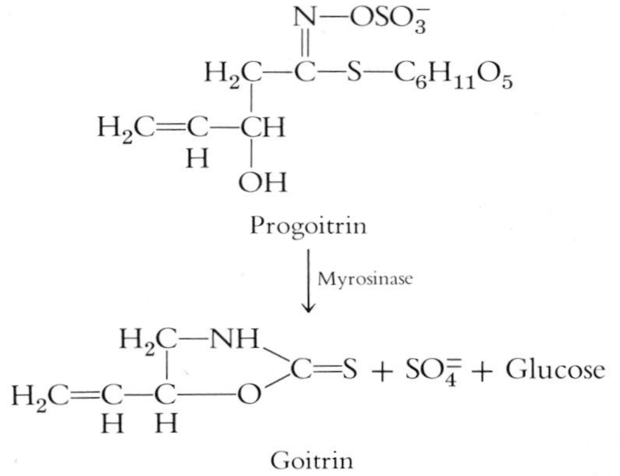

Fig. 8-8. Structure of progoitrin and the product of its enzymatic hydrolysis, goitrin. (After Yamada et al.[172])

Some vascular plants such as cauliflower contain a glycoside of thiocyanate that can be converted to free thiocyanate in the body. One would have to ingest about 10 kg of cauliflower per day to produce any serious effects on thyroid function unless dietary iodide was extremely low.[163]

Environmental Factors

Environmental factors such as photoperiod and temperature may influence thyroid hormone secretion rates through nervous or endocrine agents. Such factors may influence synthesis and release of hypothalamic and hypophysial hormones or may alter thyroid function directly through sympathetic innervation of the gland.[136]

Internal biological clocks may be related to the actions of environmental factors in regulating thyroid cycles. Cyclical variations have been reported for thyroid hormones on both a diurnal and seasonal basis. Internal secretory rhythms of hypothalamic factors might be influenced by environmental factors or might regulate the sensitivity of other effectors to the external factors.

Prolactin and Its Interactions with the Thyroid Axis

A general antagonism has been reported between prolactin (PRL) and the thyroid axis of amphibians, reptiles and birds. A number of studies have demonstrated what appears to be a goitrogenic action of PRL directly on thyroids of teleosts, amphibians, lizards and birds,[11,14,78,85,103,154] and the peripheral antagonisms of thyroxine and PRL in certain tissues of larval amphibians are well known.[30,38,102] Reports of enhancement of thyroid secretion following injections of large doses of mammalian PRL to a teleostean fish and a urodele amphibian are probably related to contamination of these preparations with TSH.[45,108,153] The reported enhancement by mammalian PRL of thyroxine-induced molting in a lizard requires further investigation (p. 192). The significance of an antagonistic interaction between thyroid hormones and PRL in fish, reptiles, birds and mammals is not clear. In amphibians the administration of anti-PRL agents (PRL antibodies or ergot derivatives) enhances responses of larval amphibians to endogenous and exogenous thyroid hormones.[35,114] These observations support an endogenous role for PRL in preventing premature metamorphosis (see Chap. 17).

In Chapter 4 it was discussed that mammalian synthetic thyrotropin-releasing hormone (TRH) causes PRL release from pituitaries of bullfrogs, turtles, birds and mammals but not from the pituitaries of red-spotted newts. These observations further complicate the picture and raise some important questions concerning the biological significance, if any, of demonstrations that PRL produces antithyroid effects.

Surgical and Chemical Thyroidectomy and Radiothyroidectomy

A basic approach employed in thyroid studies involves hypophysectomy or thyroidectomy or a combination of the two followed by classical replacement therapy. Sometimes, however, it is desirable to make an animal only slightly hypothyroid or reversibly hypothyroid or both. Chemical thyroidectomy involves administration of a chemical goitrogen (for example, PTU or TU) at a predetermined dose for a given period. Withdrawal of the goitrogen may then allow the animal to return to a euthyroid condition for comparisons. With this approach, changes in thyroid function before, during and after treatment may be examined in each individual. Caution must be exercised in that some goitrogens have been shown to produce effects on other tissues (especially the liver) that do not appear following surgical thyroidectomy.[63,175] Such "nonspecific" actions of chemical inhibitors are well known to investigators, and when possible other approaches should be used.

Large doses of ^{131}I are often employed as therapeutic agents to destroy excessive amounts of thyroid tissue in certain hyperthyroid conditions. Accumulated ^{131}I destroys cells because of the destructive effects of gamma radiation. Very large doses can be used to completely destroy thyroid tissue, especially where it is difficult to remove it surgically. Radiothyroidectomy must be interpreted with caution since radioiodide accumulation may result in destructive changes in other tissues that may not be thyroid related (Fig. 8-9).

Endocrine Factors Affecting Thyroid Gland Function

TRH Function and TSH

The hypothalamus exerts regulatory control over release of TSH from the pars distalis via secretion of TRH (see Chap. 4). Thyrotropin release is stimulated by TRH, and in turn produces an increase in circulating thyroid hormones (Fig. 8-10). Synthesis and release of TSH are regulated through a cAMP-dependent protein kinase mechanism.[136] Adenyl cyclase activity in TSH-secreting cells of the adenohypophysis is stimulated by TRH, and this activation of adenyl cyclase is related to TSH release. This cAMP-dependent mechanism is also dependent upon an influx of calcium ions following binding of TRH to the thyrotropic cell.

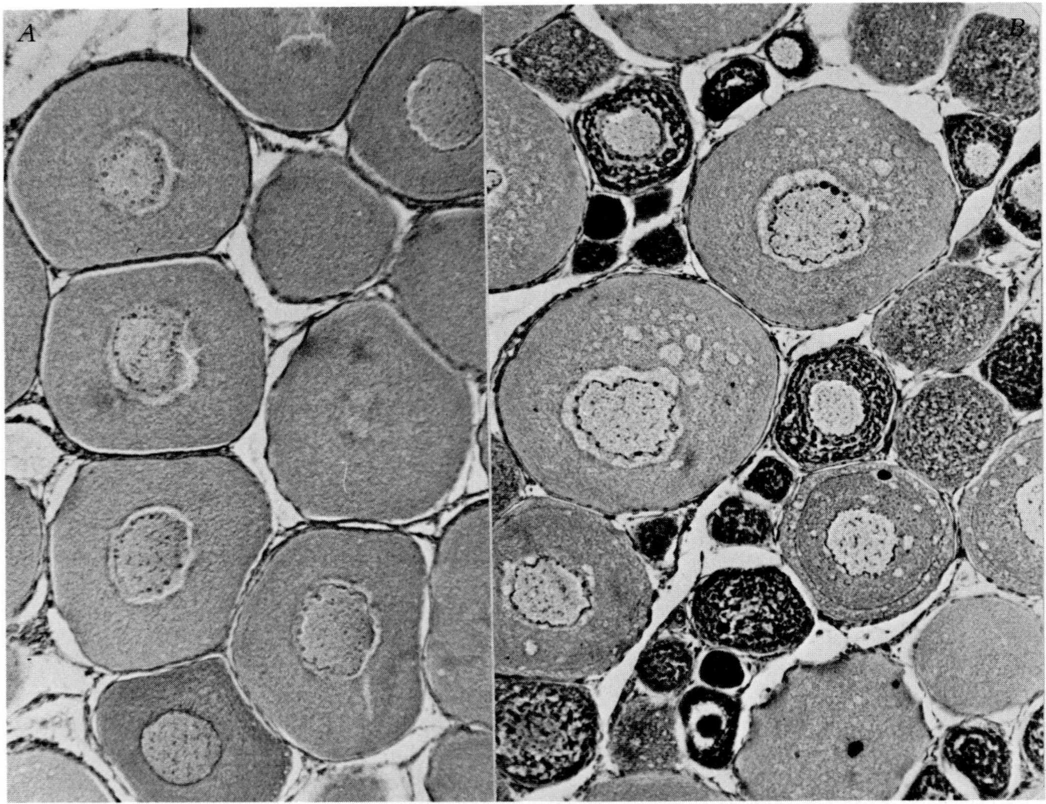

FIG. 8-9. The effect of treatment with radioiodide on ovarian structure of juvenile rainbow trout. Note the absence of smaller-sized oocytes in radiothyroidectomized trout *(A)* as compared to control *(B)*. It has not been determined whether destruction of oogonia was due to radioiodide accumulated by ovarian cells or to indirect effects of the absence of thyroid hormones. The former alternative is more likely the correct interpretation.

Thyrotropin enhances uptake of radioiodide and the synthesis of thyroglobulin and thyroid hormones. In addition, TSH induces engulfment and hydrolysis of thyroglobulin, causing thyroid hormones to be released into the blood. Continued stimulation by TSH causes structural changes in the follicular cells that are related to thyroid hormone synthesis and release. The follicular cells in an inactive or unstimulated follicle are usually flat or squamous cells. Thyrotropin can cause such flat cells to assume a cuboidal or even columnar shape, resulting in visible thickening of the follicular epithelium. Much of this enlargement of the follicular cells is due to an increase in rough endoplasmic reticulum and Golgi apparatus for thyroglobulin synthesis. This increase in follicular or cellular size due to increased cellular growth is referred to as *hypertrophy.* Chronically stimulated thyroid glands may exhibit *hyperplasia* as well, which is an increase in cellular numbers due to mitotic divisions by the stimulated cells. Mitosis is a rarely observed event in healthy thyroid glands, but highly stimulated glands may exhibit mitotic figures (Fig. 8-11). Hypertrophy or hyperplasia or both can lead to formation of a goiter.

Follicles of a stimulated gland often exhibit a reduced proportion of colloid and hence a smaller lumen because of increased endocytosis and hydrolysis of stored thyroglobulin to meet the demands for thyroid hormones. Vacuolated colloid is often observed in the follicular lumina of stimulated glands next to the epithelium, and this condition may be related to increased endocytotic activity. Colloid droplets are often seen in the apical portions of cells in

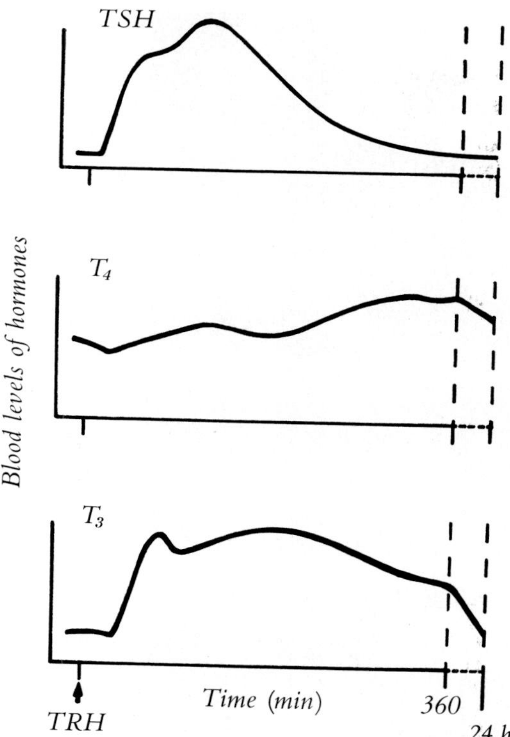

FIG. 8-10. Relative responses in serum TSH, T_4 and T_3 in euthyroid human volunteers following rapid intravenous infusion of synthetic TRH (200 mg). (Modified from Loos et al.[86])

the epithelium of a stimulated follicle. These conditions are often used as evidence for stimulation.

The increase in the cellular portion of the follicle due to hypertrophy and the reduction in colloid are reflected in a change in the diameter of the follicle with respect to the thickness of the epithelium or to the volume of the lumen. The ratio of follicle diameter to thickness of the epithelium or diameter of the follicular lumen changes predictably with TSH levels and is frequently used as a measure of the degree of stimulation by TSH. Generally a "stimulated" histology is indicative of thyroid hormone deficiencies and enhanced TSH secretion to compensate for these deficiencies. Other factors, such as cold stress, may be operating at the hypothalamus, however, to elevate TSH secretion above that normally maintained through negative feedback by the thyroid hormones.

One of the first cellular events that occurs in follicular cells following administration of TSH is activation of adenyl cyclase and resultant increase in the intracellular levels of cAMP. It is not clear which of the succeeding cellular events are mediated by cAMP (that is, iodide uptake, thyroglobulin synthesis, formation of organic iodide or engulfment and hydrolysis of colloid). Coincident with increased iodide uptake, formation of organic iodide and endocytosis of colloid is an increase in glucose oxidation that may be caused by cAMP.[147] Glucose oxidation is thought to be the "driving force" for both endocytosis and iodination, the latter involving oxidation of pyridine nucleotides and formation of H_2O_2. By controlling reactions such as glucose oxidation, cAMP could mediate several different cellular events associated with the action of TSH on the follicular cells.

T_3 and T_4 Feedback Effects

The release of TSH is regulated by negative feedback produced by thyroid hormones, and administration of exogenous thyroid hormones decreases circulating TSH and associated thyroid gland activities.[136] The major site for negative feedback is on the thyrotropic cells directly and not the hypothalamic thyrotropic center responsible for TRH production. Thyrotropes contain receptors for both T_3 and T_4,[136] and thyroid hormones are believed to interfere with the cAMP-dependent releasing mechanism by stimulating synthesis of an inhibitory protein or peptide. Thyrotropin levels seem to be maintained by direct negative feedback, and the role of TRH may be to override the system during times of increased demand for thyroid hormones. In other words, thyroid hormones determine the "set point" in the adenohypophysial TSH-secreting cells for daily regulation of thyroid gland activities.

Evidence has been reported of a stimulatory role for thyroid hormones on hypothalamic TRH release.[72] These experimental observations have not established this as a major regulatory pathway in mammals, but they do provide the basis for further investigation into the mechanism whereby hypothalamic control can override the adenohypophysial set point under conditions of increased demand for thyroid hormones.

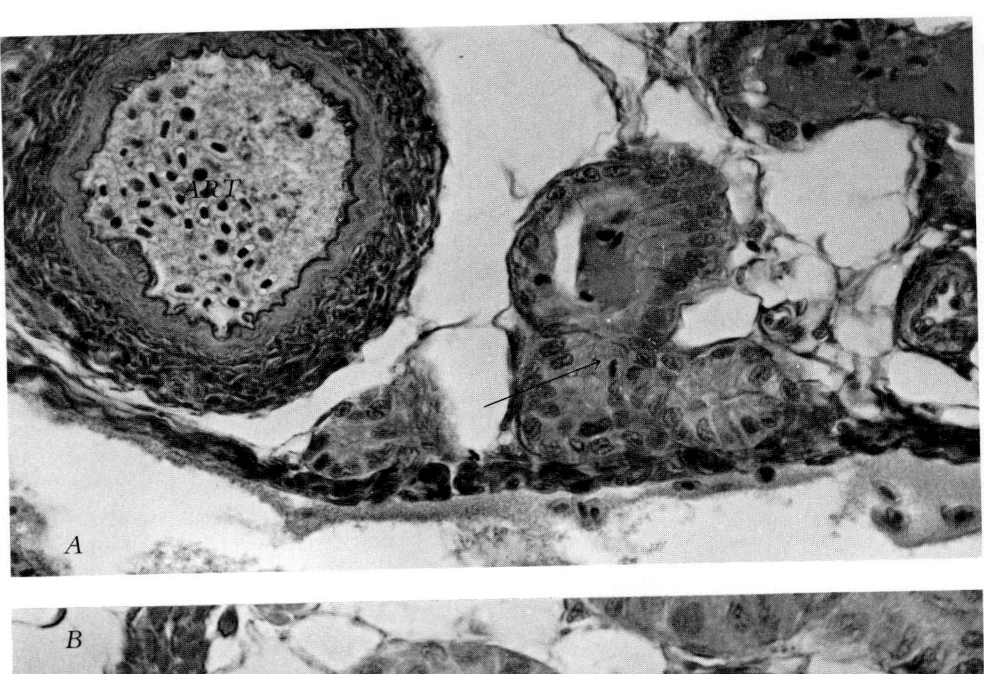

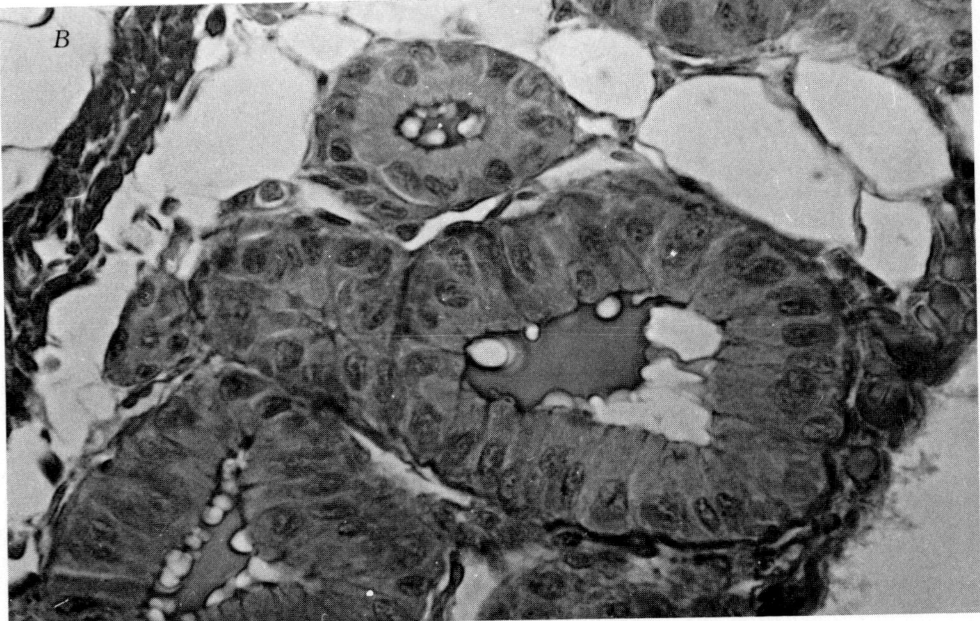

FIG. 8-11. Hyperplastic and hypertrophied follicles in the thyroid gland from a migrating adult sockeye salmon, *Oncorhynchus nerka*, prior to entering fresh water. *A*. Section from lower jaw. Note mitotic metaphase *(arrow)*, artery *(ART)*. *B*. Higher magnification of follicles showing conditions usually considered indicative of a highly stimulated gland (columnar follicular epithelium, vacuolated colloid, large ratio of epithelial thickness to diameter of follicle).

Prostaglandins

The prostaglandins are small lipids that appear to be involved in the mechanisms of action of many hormones (see Chaps. 1 and 15). Prostaglandins directly stimulate synthesis of thyroid hormones without altering circulating TSH, indicating they may be involved in the mechanism of action of TSH. Prostaglandin E_1, cAMP and TSH stimulate increased glucose oxidation, and it is possible that prostaglandins mediate the action of TSH on cAMP formation.[13,76]

The Epiphysial Complex

The pineal gland of the epiphysial complex in mammals has been implicated as a factor regulating thyroid function (see Chap. 15). This action on thyroid function is probably mediated through effects on hypothalamic TRH release. Numerous studies have demonstrated an inhibitory action for melatonin, one of the principles synthesized and released from the pineal gland. Photoperiodic influences on thyroid activity may also be mediated through the pineal. These ideas are expanded in Chapter 15.

Biological Actions of Thyroid Hormones in Mammals

Thyroid hormones affect many diverse tissues and influence major processes such as metabolism, growth, differentiation and reproduction. They are responsible for maintaining a general state of well-being for many cells so that they are capable of maximal responses to other hormones. Although other effects of thyroid hormones will be discussed here, this "permissive action" of thyroid hormones may be their single most important role.

Metabolic Actions

The effects produced by thyroid hormones on mammalian metabolism include a so-called *calorigenic* or *thermogenic action* and specific effects related to carbohydrate, lipid and protein metabolism. These actions of thyroid hormones become more meaningful when considered together with the actions of other hormones on metabolism (see Chap. 19), but an overview of these effects will be discussed here. Many of these metabolic actions are possibly permissive actions occurring in cooperation with other hormones such as epinephrine and growth hormone.

Thyroid hormones cause calorigenic or heat-generating actions in certain tissues and may be involved in certain physiological responses to cold stress. They can accelerate the rate at which glucose is oxidized and thus increase the amount of metabolic heat produced in a given time. This excess heat production could be used to warm the body. Increased glucose oxidation is reflected in an increased BMR as measured by the change in rate of oxygen consumption. In addition, thyroid hormones have been claimed to "uncouple" oxidative phosphorylation, which decreases the efficiency of ATP synthesis in the mitochondria and increases the quantity of heat released per mole of glucose oxidized. Although such uncoupling has been observed in a hyperthyroid pathological state known as thyroid storm, its role in cold stress is probably not so important as the ability to increase the total rate of glucose oxidation.[163]

Thyroid hormones may not be important in acute cold responses that are probably mediated by epinephrine from the adrenal medulla (Chap. 10). Thyroid hormones do induce increased synthesis of mitochondrial respiratory proteins, especially cytochrome C, cytochrome oxidase and succinoxidase.[10,100] This mitochondrial action would be advantageous in adapting to chronic cold stress. In general, thyroid activity in mammals is greater during prolonged periods of cold stress (winter) than during warmer periods (Fig. 8-12).[74,136]

In many nonhibernating mammals such as beaver and muskrat, thyroid activity is depressed during the winter months.[1,2] Hypothyroidism has been described for hibernating ground squirrels[165] and badgers,[98] but there does not appear to be a causal relationship between reduced thyroid function and the onset

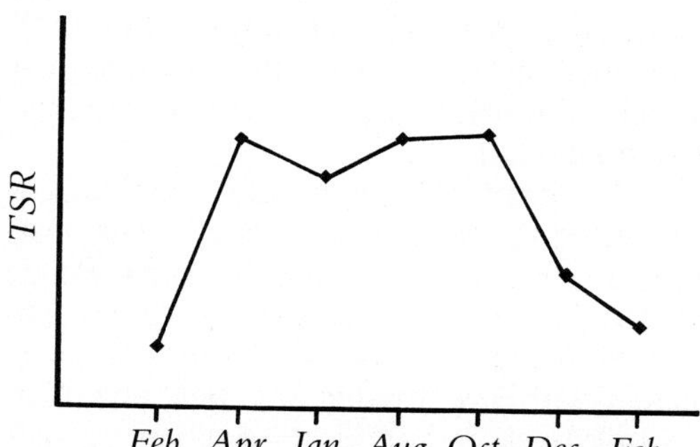

FIG. 8-12. Seasonal variations in thyroxine secretion rate *(TSR)* in the tammar wallaby *Macropus eugenii* (Protheria, Marsupialia). (After Kaethner and Good.[74]).

of hibernation.[66] Additional field studies employing sophisticated methods for assessing thyroid functions are needed before the endocrine factors related to either onset or termination of hibernation will be firmly established.

In addition to increasing glucose oxidation, thyroid hormones cause hyperglycemia and may secondarily stimulate lipid oxidation (hydrolysis of fats, or lipolysis). These actions may in part be associated with potentiation of the hyperglycemic and lipolytic actions of epinephrine (see Chaps. 10 and 19). Thyroid hormones alter nitrogen balance and are either protein anabolic or catabolic, depending on the tissue being examined and under what experimental conditions it is examined. These actions are probably related to enhancement of effects normally produced by other hormones.

Growth and Differentiation

Thyroid hormones are essential for normal growth and differentiation in mammals as evidenced in cretinism and juvenile myxedema. These growth-promoting actions of thyroid hormones are closely related to the role of pituitary growth hormone (GH),[122] and they probably represent a permissive action on GH-sensitive target cells. Thyroid hormones may also stimulate somatomedin production and hence augment the action of GH.[51]

The major tissue affected by the lack of thyroid hormones during differentiation is the nervous system. Normal development of the nervous system as well as attainment of normal mental capacities is strongly influenced by thyroid hormones. Hypothyroidism during early development seriously impairs differentiation and functioning of the nervous system. A reduction in mental capacity can occur in hypothyroid adults.

Replacement of hair in adult mammals is stimulated by thyroid hormones.[130] The postnuptial molt cycle in harbor seals *Phoca vitulina* involves thyroid hormones and cortisol from the adrenal cortex.[118] Hair loss is correlated with low thyroid function and high cortisol levels, whereas resumption of hair growth is correlated with increased T_4 and return of cortisol to basal levels. Thyroid activity also is related to molting of hair in other mammals including red fox[98] and mink.[8]

Reproduction

Another cooperative role for thyroid hormones occurs with respect to gonadal development; in general, sexual maturation is delayed in hypothyroid mammals.[6] In hypothyroid males, spermatogenesis may occur, but androgen synthesis is low. Ovarian weight is reduced and ovarian cycles irregular in hypothyroid females. These correlations to hypothyroidism have been attributed to reduced gonadotropin levels and can be alleviated by treatment with thyroid hormones.[12] Experimental studies support the notion that thyroid hormones influence gonadotropin release through an effect at the level of the hypothalamus. Reduction of gonadotropin, however, was not observed in hypothyroid female rats.[151]

Clinical Aspects of Thyroid Function

Thyrotoxicosis and Hyperthyroidism

Thyrotoxicosis is a general term referring to an excess of thyroid hormone. If this condition results from thyroid hypersecretion, it is known as hyperthyroidism. Primary hyperthyroidism may be due to *toxic multinodular goiters* consisting of multiple aggregates of small, hyperactive follicles (Marine-Lenhart Syndrome) or several large TSH-dependent hyperactive follicles (Plummer's disease). Follicular adenomas are sometimes autonomously hyperactive as well. Circulating TSH levels typically are low when autonomously hyperactive nodular goiter or adenomas are present.

Hyperthyroidism may be of a secondary nature caused by a rare pituitary adenoma of TSH-secreting cells. Certain cancerous tumors such as choriocarcinomas elaborate TRH-like or TSH-like molecules that stimulate thyroid activity. Such tumors typically are insensitive to any feedback by thyroid hormones.

Graves' disease is a secondary hyperthyroid state that may be mediated by an immunoglobulin known as LATS: *long-acting thyroid stimulator*. The basis for production of LATS is not understood.

Rarely, hyperthyroidism is due to a nonthyroid source of thyroid hormones. For example, ovarian dermoid tumors can synthesize sufficient thyroid hormones to bring about hyperthyroidism.

Juvenile thyrotoxicosis is characterized by nervousness, tremor, accelerated heart rate and thyroid enlargement (goiter). This syndrome is manifest in children beyond age 10 (80% of the cases). Exophthalmus (protrusion of the eyeballs) occurs in about half of these children. Weight gain is usually retarded.

A somewhat rare but dramatic condition is thyrotoxic crisis or *thyroid storm.* This disorder involves a sudden increase in thyroid secretion, severe hypermetabolism, fever and some other more variable symptoms. It may be precipitated in hyperthyroid patients following incomplete thyroidectomy, interruption of antithyroid therapy or even as a reaction to an infection or tooth extraction. It may also be induced by periods of excessive summer heat. The actual cause of thyroid storm is not certain and the condition could encompass a variety of different disorders.

Myxedema and Hypothyroidism

Myxedema is the condition where no thyroid hormones are secreted. In these patients there is swelling of the skin and subcutaneous tissues caused by the extracellular accumulation of a high-protein fluid. *Hypothyroidism* refers to conditions of insufficient thyroid hormones of primary (at the thyroid) or secondary (hypothalamus or pituitary) origins. It is especially serious in children because of marked effects on development. The term *juvenile hypothyroidism* refers to cases of hypothyroidism in children that do not lead to severe retardation in somatic and intellectual development. When development is markedly retarded, it is called *cretinism.* This syndrome is rather common and 1 in every 8500 births exhibits cretinism. However, if recognized early, it can be alleviated with thyroid hormone therapy so that growth and development are normal.

There are a number of symptoms characteristic of hypothyroidism including rough and dry skin, yellow pallor, coarse scalp hair, hoarse voice, slow thought and action. However, sometimes the hypothyroid person exhibits none or only a few of these symptoms. Obesity is often listed as a characteristic but it does not always accompany hypothyroidism. Persons suffering from secondary hypothyroidism are often thin. Exophthalmus which is usually correlated with hyperthyroid states may occur in primary myxedema.

Goiters

Any enlarged thyroid is referred to as a goiter regardless of the cause or nature of the enlargement. Actually there are four kinds of clinical goiters. The first kind is an hypothyroid goiter caused by failing hormone production resulting in a shortage of T_3 and T_4. Circulating TSH levels are elevated because of reduced negative feedback, and increased TSH causes enlargement of the thyroid gland and formation of a goiter.

The second and third types are hyperthyroid goiters: the hyperfunctioning goiter and the hyperfunctioning goiter of pregnancy. They are not as common as hypothyroid goiters. In the first case circulating thyroid hormones are high and TSH levels are low. Diffuse thyrotoxic goiter is often termed Graves' disease whereas toxic nodular goiters are associated with Plummer's or Marine-Lenhart syndromes. The second case of hyperthyroid goiter occurs during normal pregnancy. There is an increase in thyroxine-binding globulins and a consequent decrease in free T_4 and T_3 in maternal plasma. This results in elevated TSH and a slight thyroid enlargement in order to maintain normal functional levels of thyroid hormones. This condition usually returns to normal after pregnancy.

The last kind of goiter develops in people with otherwise normal thyroid function. Such enlargements have many different causes including infiltration of the gland with tuberculosis or syphilitic bacteria or parasites and the presence of adenomas or carcinomas. Inflammation due to autoimmune disease (thyroiditis) can also cause enlargement of the thyroid.

Thyroiditis

Thyroiditis is a general term applied to a collection of autoimmune disorders involving production of antibodies that attack thyroid proteins, especially thyroglobulins. The most common types are *Hashimoto's thyroiditis* (*struma lymphomatosa*) and *Reidel's thyroiditis* (*struma fibrosa*). Hashimoto's disease is characterized by the presence of numerous lymphoid follicles, diffuse infiltration of normal cells, extensive increase in the connective tissue components of the gland and some changes in follicular structure. One of the most common causes for goiter among adolescents is Hashiomoto's thyroiditis. In Reidel's thyroiditis the gland is progressively replaced by fibrous connective tissue. In either type of thyroiditis there is a gradual reduction in the thyroid's levels of thyroid hormones. Elevation of TSH secretion contributes to goiter formation. Antibodies produced against thyroid iodoproteins and microsomes usually are demonstrable in the blood.

Inherited Disorders

More than twenty heritable defects in thyroid gland metabolism are known and may be classified according to the type of metabolic defect. For example, there are several defects related to unresponsiveness of the thyroid cell to TSH including insufficient numbers of receptors or abnormal receptors and defects at or in the adrenergic cascade (see Chap. 1). Defects also occur in iodide transport mechanisms, iodination and coupling of iodinated tyrosines. Several defects have been identified in relation to synthesis of thyroglobulin. Deficiencies in thyroid deiodinase and total body deiodinase are known. Abnormal plasma transport proteins and tissue unresponsiveness to thyroid hormones sometimes occur as heritable errors.

Euthyroid Sick Syndrome

Many nonthyroid conditions can alter thyroid function. Even though the person is actually euthyroid, he/she will appear to be hypothyroid. For example, fasting, anorexia nervosa, protein-calorie malnutrition and untreated diabetes mellitus are all metabolic disturbances that bring about marked decreases in circulating T_3 and increases in rT_3. Thyroid hormones also are altered in a variety of liver and renal diseases, as a consequence of numerous infections and following myocardial infarctions. Some conditions may alter levels of T_4, TSH, T_3 and/or rT_3. These alterations in thyroid parameters by peripheral disorders constitute the so-called *euthyroid sick syndrome,* reflecting normal responses of the euthyroid person to the generalized disease state.

Evolution of the Thyroid Gland

The thyroid gland structurally is a conservative endocrine gland in vertebrates. It is generally found as one or two masses of highly vascularized follicles surrounded by a connective tissue capsule or as scattered follicles throughout the pharyngeal region (most fishes) (Fig. 8-13). Regardless of any gross morphological differences, follicular structure and function is mammalian-like in all the gnathostomes with respect to iodide metabolism, hormone synthesis, storage of thyroglobulin and hormone release. Biochemical differences are quantitative and not qualitative, and the same thyroid hormones, T_3 and T_4, are synthesized and released in all vertebrates.

The most primitive condition is considered to be that found in the cyclostomes in which only a few scattered follicles may be present. Extracellular storage of thyroid hormones does not occur in the cyclostome follicle, and iodoproteins are retained in the follicular cells of these primitive fishes.

The Origin of the Thyroid Gland

Although many biochemical aspects of the synthesis of thyroid hormones are well known in vertebrates, the evolutionary origin of the vertebrate thyroid and acquisition of functional significance for these iodinated compounds is uncertain. Acceptance of the simple notion that the thyroid cells evolved from specialized cells of the endostyle of protochordates, as suggested in Chapter 3, leaves some basic questions unanswered. Why were these iodinated compounds first synthesized? What was their primitive role? What selective forces were responsible for adoption of these iodinated compounds as metabolic regulators? Certainly the ability of iodide to be bound to tyrosine residues in a protein and even formation of MIT, DIT and iodinated thyronines

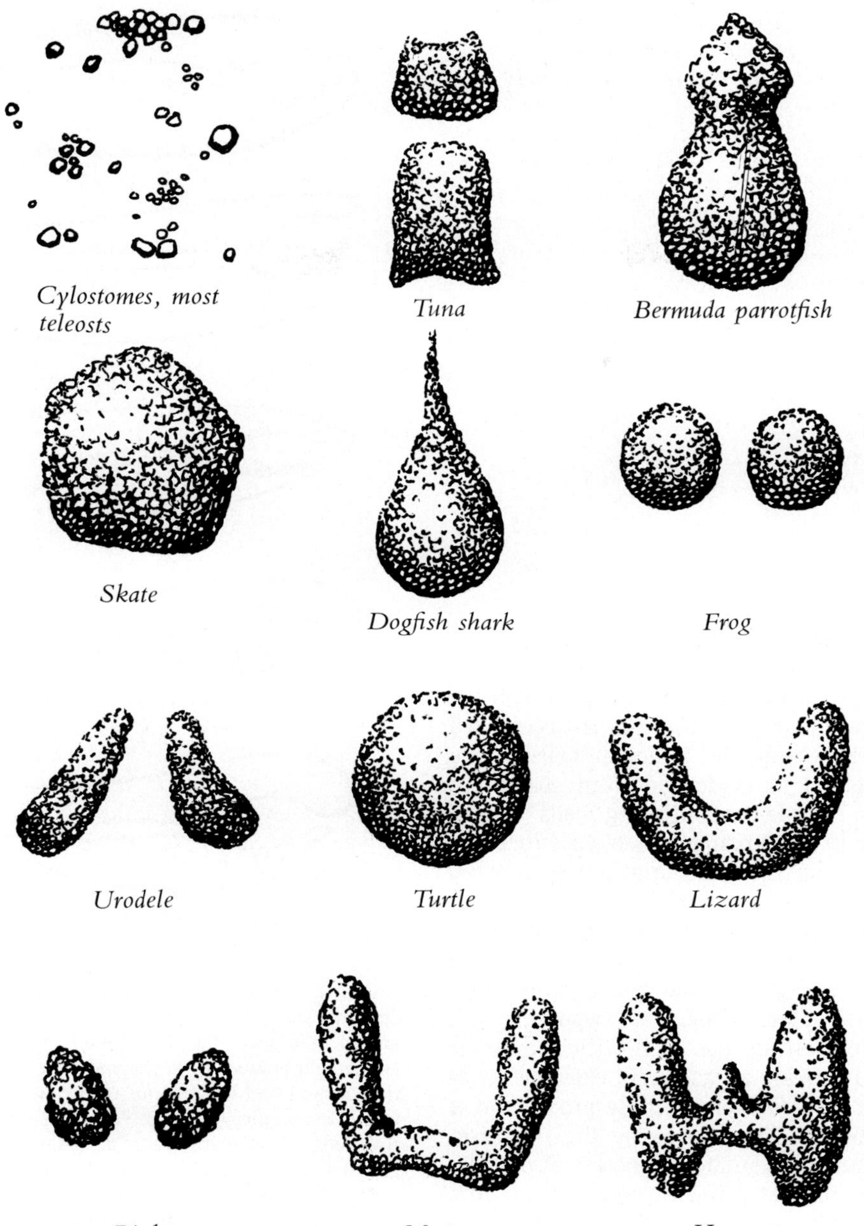

FIG. 8-13. General outline for thyroid glands in diverse vertebrate groups. (Redrawn from Gorbman and Bern.[56])

occur repeatedly among the invertebrate phyla (Table 8-9) with no suggestion of a distinct regulatory role for these iodinated molecules. One exception may be the participation of iodinated compounds in metamorphic changes of certain cnidarians.[132,135]

It has been hypothesized that these iodide-containing compounds were obtained originally from feeding activities of protochordates.[37,53] These dietary compounds supposedly were first utilized opportunistically as regulatory substances of some sort. Later the

Table 8-9. *Occurrence of Thyroid Hormones and Their Precursors in Animals and Algae*

ORGANISM	MIT	DIT	T_3	T_4
Algae	+	+		
Nereis (Annelida)	+	+	+	+
Sponge (Porifera)	+	+		
Coral (Cnidaria)	+	+		
Periplaneta (Arthropoda: cockroach)	+	+		+
Musca (Arthropoda: fly)	+	+		+
Planorbis (Mollusca)	+	+	+	+
Amphioxus (Cephalochordata)	+	+	+	+
Hagfish (Agnatha: Cyclostome)	+	+	+	+
All other vertebrates	+	+	+	+

ability to synthesize these specific compounds was acquired, culminating in the concentration of such a mechanism in certain cells of the endostyle (Fig. 8-14). These specialized cells later became the follicular cells of the thyroid gland as evidenced from studies in lampreys. Iodide-concentrating cells of the endostyle in the larval ammocete are incorporated into the thyroid gland of the lamprey during metamorphosis. The production of extracellular colloid and its resultant accumulation in the follicular lumen do not occur in modern cyclostomes and presumably were acquired at a later time. This hypothesis, although interesting, has been criticized for its failure to provide an adequate explanation as to how a food substance whose production is not controlled in any way by the organism could assume a regulatory function. A possible alternative is that primitive iodoproteins first served an enzymatic or structural function and that the basic mechanism became modified into a hormonal synthetic pathway.[38] An additional problem lies with the origin of the vertebrate thyroid and the iodide-concentrating endostyle of invertebrate chordates. If the ammocoetes endostyle is not homologous to the protochordate endostyles,[50] then accumulation of iodide and formation of iodoproteins by protochordates cannot be used to explain evolution of the vertebrate thyroid.

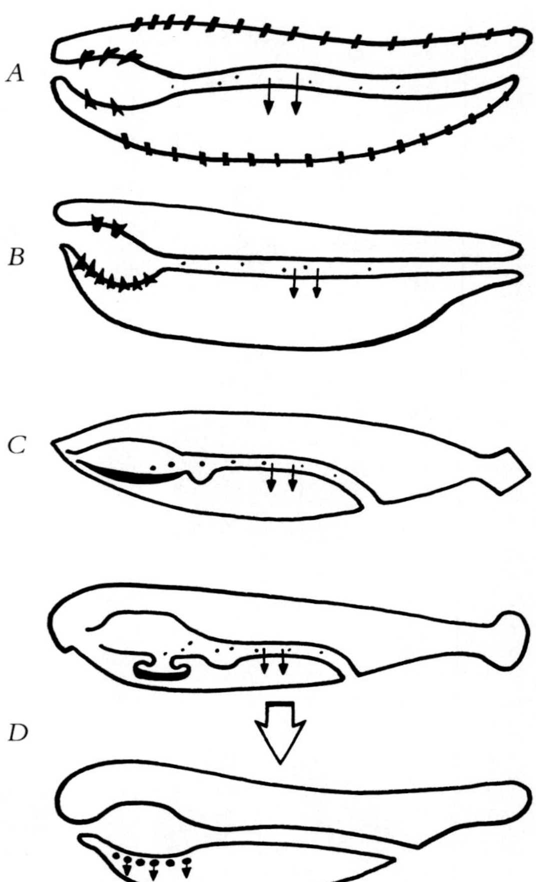

Fig. 8-14. Generalized distribution of iodinated proteins among invertebrate and vertebrate animals suggesting an evolutionary pattern from a general distribution of iodinated proteins *(A)* to a more localized relationship to the digestive tract *(B)*. Amphioxus *(C)* illustrates an even greater tendency for localization by concentrating iodoprotein production to the endostyle and with digestion of swallowed iodoproteins occurring in the intestine where enzymatically released iodinated tyrosines and thyronines could be absorbed. Finally the alteration of the endostyle of the ammocetes larva to the thyroid gland of the adult lamprey during metamorphosis is illustrated *(D)* with elimination of the enteric pathway for hydrolysis of iodoproteins and liberation of biologically active iodinated compounds. (Modified from Gorbman.[54])

There is a basic similarity among thyroid iodoproteins in all vertebrates. Thyroglobulins from birds are similar to those of rats with about 94% as 19S, about 5% as 27S and a trace of 12S thyroglobulin. Turtles, teleostean fishes and selachians exhibit lower amounts of 19S

(73%–84%), but a significant quantity of 12S thyroglobulin is present (6%–16%). Cyclostomes are the most primitive living vertebrates, and they exhibit what may be considered the most primitive condition. Lampreys produce largely a 12S component (68%), and the remainder of iodinated protein is in the form of a much smaller component (5.4S). Iodoproteins of about 7.6S have been isolated from urochordates and yield monoiodotyrosine, diiodotyrosine, T_3 and T_4 upon hydrolysis.[127] These data suggest that thyroglobulin exists as 12S monomers (or an even smaller unit) that aggregate to form 19S and 27S complexes under certain conditions. These data may also be interpreted as reflecting degrees of disruption from different vertebrates of the intact thyroglobulin during the extraction procedures.

The Origin of Thyroid Function

There appears to be no consistency in the actions of thyroid hormones when the entire subphylum Vertebrata is surveyed, although in part the inconsistency may be due to lack of thorough investigation in lower vertebrates, especially the fishes and amphibians. It has been proposed that thyroid function evolved hand in hand with endocrine control of reproduction and that the basic function for thyroid hormones is associated primitively with gonadal maturation.[44,124] This hypothesis is supported by a variety of observations, including the close parallel of thyroid activity and reproductive cycles in elasmobranch and bony fishes. Pituitary thyrotropes and TSH are apparently absent in agnathans, and these cells may have evolved later from gonadotropes. This proposed origin for thyrotropes is supported by their cytological similarity to gonadotropes, their location in the adenohypophysis of elasmobranchs (pars ventralis) and teleosts (proximal pars distalis) and by the biochemical similarity of TSH to the gonadotropins (see Chap. 5). Exogenous thyroid hormones and gonadal steroids both have inhibitory actions on thyrotropes as well as on gonadotropes in teleosts. Similar influences of thyroid hormones on gonadal function and, reciprocally, gonadal steroids on thyroid function have been reported in amphibians, reptiles and birds. Futhermore, mammalian gonadotropins stimulate thyroid function in fishes, although these same gonadotropins are ineffective when tested on mammalian thyroids. The effects of thyroid hormones that modify behavior through actions on the central nervous system presumably evolved from the general feedback effects on the hypothalamus originally associated with the gonadal axis. The actions of thyroid hormones related to growth, metabolism, development and the integument would be later evolutionary events.[124] Location of the major feedback of thyroid hormones on TSH release in the adenohypophysis rather than at the hypothalamus would be a consequence of this evolutionary sequence.

Comparative Aspects of Thyroid Function in Nonmammalian Vertebrates

The following account and Table 8-10 stress the biological actions of thyroid hormones on target tissues. The secretion of TSH and the effects of hypothalamic hormones on TSH secretion were discussed previously (Chaps. 4 and 5), and only the functions of T_3 and T_4 will be considered here.

Class Agnatha: Cyclostomata

No function for thyroid hormones has been verified in cyclostome fishes, although in lampreys the binding of iodide by the larval endostyle increases following administration of T_4,[7] and thyroid hormones may participate in metamorphosis. Circulating levels of T_4 decrease markedly as ammocetes of sea lampreys *Petromyzon marinus* undergo metamorphosis.[170]

As mentioned previously, hormone synthesis in agnathans differs from events in other vertebrates in that organic binding of iodide and storage of the iodinated proteins occurs intracellularly.[7,156] Hypophysectomy does not alter thyroid function in adult lampreys or in hagfishes,[81,96,113] and it has been concluded that TSH is absent in agnathans. These observations suggest that evolution of thyrotropes

TABLE 8-10. *Summary of Major Actions of Thyroid Hormones in Vertebrates*

VERTEBRATE CLASS	INTEGUMENT		METABOLISM		REPRODUCTION	NEURAL	
	MOLTING	OTHER	GROWTH	O_2/CAL		BEHAVIOR	DIFFERENTIATION
Agnatha							
Chondrichthyes					+	+	
Osteichthyes		+	+	+, −	+	+	
Amphibia	+[a]	+	−	+	−	+	+
Reptilia	+		+	+	+		
Aves	+		+	+	+, −	+	
Mammalia	+		+	+	+	+	+

[a]Urodeles only.
+ = stimulatory effect.
− = inhibitory effect.

and TSH occurred first in jawed fishes,[124] possibly in the placoderms. Thyroxine is present in serum from mature female sea lampreys comparable to levels reported for ammocetes of this species.[64,170] Much lower levels of T_4 are reported for mature male sea lampreys. Triiodothyronine occurs in the serum of both immature and mature sea lampreys, but the levels are higher in the mature individuals. These data suggest a relationship to reproductive maturation, but definitive data are needed before a firm relationship can be accepted.

Class Chondrichthyes

Only limited data are available with respect to thyroid function in sharks, in which the pituitary-thyroid axis appears to be well established. Most studies on sharks are related to reproduction or oxygen consumption.

REPRODUCTION. Thyroid cycles are positively correlated with reproductive cycles in sharks.[29,124] However, increased thyroid activity observed in at least one species is correlated with migratory behavior related to reproduction rather than with reproduction or gonadal maturation per se.[127]

OXYGEN CONSUMPTION. Late embryos of *Squalus suckleyi* exhibit a transient increase in oxygen consumption following treatment with T_3 or T_4, but this response cannot be maintained by continued treatment with thyroid hormones.[115] Treatment with a goitrogen, propylthiouracil, has no effect on oxygen consumption in this species. These observations do not provide strong support of a role for thyroid hormones in oxidative metabolism.

DIFFERENTIATION. Differentiation of hypothalamic neurosecretory centers is accelerated in the embryos of the oviparous shark, *S. suckleyi,* following treatment with T_3 or T_4.[57] This effect of thyroid hormones is manifest in both the preoptico-hypophysial fiber tracts and in the neurohypophysis. These data are suggestive of a role for thyroid hormones in nervous tissue differentiation and maturation of the hypothalamo-hypophysial system.

Class Osteichthyes: Chondrostei

Some limited data for sturgeons indicate peak thyroid activity coincides with spawning behavior.[38] Furthermore, thyroid treatments can reverse the degenerative changes that occur in gonads of captive sturgeon, suggesting a direct relationship between thyroid hormones and reproduction. Additional studies are needed in chondrostean fishes to examine other possible roles of thyroid hormones and to confirm this suggestive relationship with reproduction.

Class Osteichthyes: Teleostei

Thyroid function has been studied intensively in teleostean fishes and considerable information is available with respect to iodide uptake, hormone synthesis, secretion rates, clearance rates and metabolism of thyroid hormones.[33,34] Thyroid hormones are implicated in reproduction and behavior of teleostean fishes. Their role with respect to oxygen consumption is not so clear, however. Thyroid hormones are essential for normal development and growth.[28] They are also implicated in metamorphosis of young fishes and in the parr-smolt transformation of salmonid fishes.[73,104] Although thyroid hormones have been shown to influence osmoregulation (Chap. 16), carbohydrate metabolism, nitrogen metabolism and growth, other hormones are known to play more direct roles. In fact, many of the reported effects of thyroid hormones associated with these processes may be "permissive" in nature.[55]

Heterotopic Thyroid Tissue in Teleosts. The teleostean thyroid consists of scattered thyroid follicles throughout the pharyngeal region. The diffuse nature of the teleostean thyroid gland, with only a few exceptions (for example, the tuna and the Bermuda parrot fish), makes assessment of thyroid function difficult and renders surgical thyroidectomy impossible. Most of the thyroid tissue is located in the pharyngeal area where follicles are found between the second and fourth aortic arches (Fig. 8-15). Because of the absence of a covering connective tissue sheath that holds the follicles into one or more masses, thyroid follicles are frequently found outside this pharyngeal region. These extrapharyngeal thyroid follicles are termed accessory or *heterotopic* thyroid because of their location outside the normal site. Heterotopic thyroid occurs in species of some of the more recent teleostean families.[5,55,116] Relatively large numbers of thyroid follicles may be found embedded within the head kidney of some species and occasionally in other locations such as the ovary. In such species it may be important to examine the activity of heterotopic thyroid as well as of pharyngeal thyroid when attempting to assess thyroid function (Fig. 8-16).

Reproduction. There is a strong positive correlation in many teleostean species between thyroid state and reproductive cycles.[55,67,124] Thyroxine consistently stimulates precocial gonadal maturation, whereas radiothyroidectomy or treatment with goitrogens inhibits gonadal development. In several species thyroid activity is greatest at spawning.[134,173,175] In spawning Atlantic salmon, however, iodide uptake, PBI levels and T_4 secretion rates are low,[42] an observation that bears repeated investigation in lieu of more recent data and the development of newer

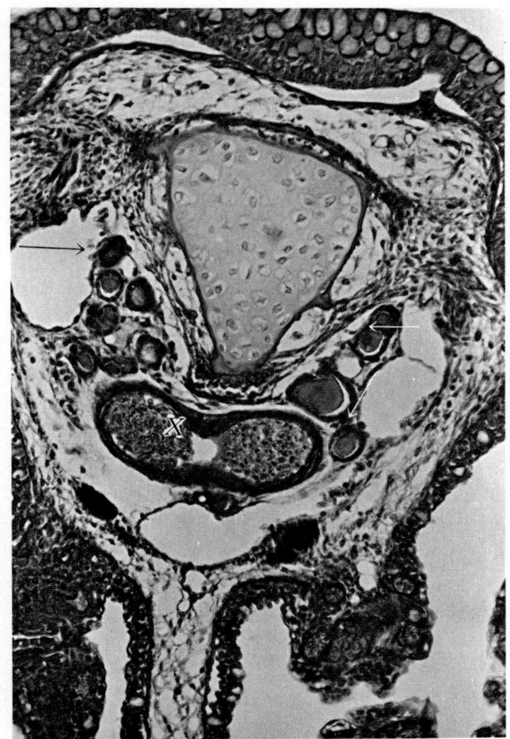

Fig. 8-15. Photomicrograph of salmon thyroid follicles. Cross-section through lower jaw of fingerling chinook salmon, *Oncorhynchus tshawytscha*, at the level of the second aortic arch *(X)*. Thyroid follicles appear dorsal to the aortic arch on both sides *(arrows)*.

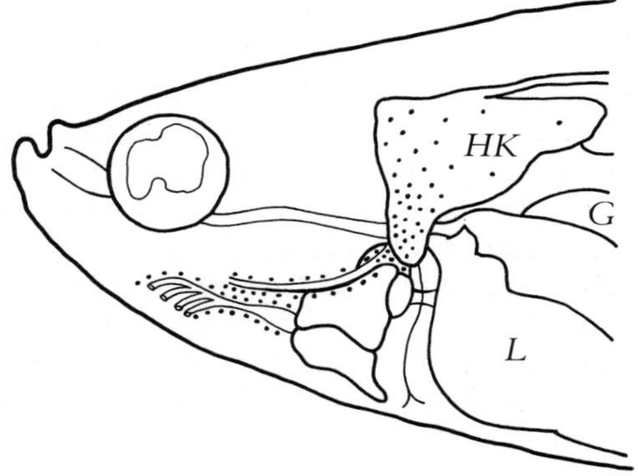

Fig. 8-16. Distribution of thyroid follicles in the pharyngeal region of a teleostean fish, *Xiphophorus maculatus*. Follicles *(black dots)* are scattered among the pharyngeal blood vessels and in the head kidney *(HK)* and may occasionally occur in gonads *(G)* or other structures. *L*, liver. (Redrawn from Baker-Cohen.[5])

techniques for assessing thyroid function. These observations may relate to other migratory species such as codfish in which increased thyroid activity is more closely correlated with the spawning migration rather than reproductive changes.[169]

Oxygen Consumption. Observations have yielded opposing results with respect to the importance of thyroid hormones in oxygen consumption by teleostean fishes. Most studies suggest that neither thyroid hormones nor goitrogens have any effects on oxygen consumption. A positive correlation has been reported for cyclic seasonal variations in thyroid activity and in oxygen consumption by *Heteropneustes fossilis.*[112] Studies of oxygen consumption are difficult to interpret because temperature, changes in behavior, and potential side effects of treatments used to render the fish hypothyroid (goitrogens, radiothyroidectomy) may have direct effects on metabolism.[55,95,122–124]

Osmoregulation. Thyroid hormones may enhance seawater adaptation and may influence migratory behavior in species that migrate between salt and fresh water. These actions may be related to a permissive type of action rather than to a causative role for thyroid hormones. The possible roles for thyroid hormones in osmoregulation and migratory behavior are discussed more fully in Chapters 16 and 18 respectively.

Behavioral Actions of Thyroid Hormones. Thyroid hormones may influence many behaviors through demonstrated actions on the nervous system.[55] Such behaviors might include spawning, premigratory and migratory behaviors. Increased thyroid function has been reported for migrating fishes, and both a preference for water of higher salinity and premigratory restless behavior have been correlated with increased thyroid function (see Chap. 18). Again the action of thyroid hormones may only enhance the sensitivities of neural components to environmental stimuli.

Class Osteichthyes: Sarcopterygii

The function of thyroid hormones in lungfishes has received only a cursory examination. Thyroid hormones have been linked to a particularly fascinating aspect of the life history of African lungfishes: the ability to survive periods of drought while encased in a "cocoon." Awakening of estivating lungfishes *Protopterus annectens* from the cocoon of dried mud when moistened may involve a neuroendocrine mechanism associated with the thyroid axis. One hypothesis, based upon limited experimental data, suggests that increasing humidity activates the hypothalamic apparatus controlling TSH release and stimulates thyroid hormone secretion.[31] Thyroid hormones in turn would increase the sensitivity of olfactory centers that evoke normal feeding behavior as well as other behaviors associated with wakening. Additional studies of thyroid function in these fishes are needed to substantiate this interesting hypothesis.

Class Amphibia

Thyroid hormones influence many processes in both anurans and urodeles, including reproduction, metamorphosis, metabolism, growth and molting. The most dramatic and best studied event among amphibians is the endocrine induction of metamorphosis from an aquatic larva to a terrestrial or semiterrestrial form.[104]

Reproduction. Experimental reduction of thyroid function, such as thyroidectomy or administration of goitrogens, accelerates gonadal development in several anurans.[23,59,65,138] In one urodele, *Ambystoma tigrinum,* circulating levels of thyroxine are inversely correlated with gonadal development,[105] although such correlations do not substantiate cause-effect relationships. Some conflicting results with respect to thyroid hormones and seasonal maturation have been reported for some adult anurans,[155,161,162] but the general relationship in amphibians appears to be an antagonistic one. All of the data reported to date are circumstantial and an absolute antagonism by endogenous thyroid hormones in natural populations is yet to be demonstrated.

Oxygen Consumption. The relationship between thyroid hormones and metabolism is not clear. Some studies have shown a positive correlation between thyroid state and oxygen consumption,[90] whereas most studies show no effects.[49,92] Oxygen consumption is not elevated during either spontaneous metamorphosis caused by elevated endogenous thyroid hormones or during induced metamorphosis caused by exogenous thyroid hormones.[46,47,84]

Liver slices prepared from T_4-treated adult frogs, *Rana pipiens,* exhibit significantly greater oxygen consumption in vitro than appropriate controls at 25°C. Oxygen consumption of treated slices is the same as controls when observed at 15°C.[111] These data suggest that the respiratory response of amphibian tissues to thyroid hormones may be temperature dependent and that the response occurs only at higher temperatures. Most studies reporting no effect for thyroid hormones on oxygen consumption were performed below 20°C. What the biological importance is for enhanced oxygen consumption at higher temperatures is open to speculation.

Metamorphosis. Thyroid hormones induce metamorphosis, a marked biochemical, physiological, morphological and behavioral transformation from an aquatic larva to a terrestrial or semiterrestrial form. These events occur in the life history of every amphibian, although the developmental sequence and duration of the various stages may be modified extensively in those species that incubate their eggs on land or are live bearing.[27]

Amphibian metamorphosis has been studied at all levels of organization and provides an excellent illustration of hormonal interactions of thyroid hormones, several additional hormones and a wide variety of tissues. Furthermore, this process is closely linked to the interaction of complex environmental factors that together with endocrine-related events constitute the metamorphosis phenomenon. Chapter 17 is devoted to a detailed examination of this fascinating process.

Thyroid hormones are also involved in a second metamorphic event, the so-called water drive associated with reproduction in newts (see Chaps. 5 and 17). Water-drive behavior is a well-known bioassay for PRL activity. Small quantities of thyroid hormones facilitate the PRL-induced water drive and associated morphological changes in the integument. Larger amounts of thyroid hormones inhibit water drive, and thyroid hormones appear to be responsible for land-drive behavior of recently metamorphosed amphibians.

Growth. The involvement of thyroid hormones in growth of amphibians, like the relationship to reproduction, deviates from the general vertebrate pattern. The surge of thyroid activity that initiates metamorphosis in larval amphibians arrests growth. Treatment of anuran tadpoles with goitrogens or mammalian PRL accelerates larval growth and blocks metamorphosis.[38,45,102] Growth in natural populations is arrested during metamorphosis. The complicated metamorphic process itself involves many drastic physiological changes and tissue rearrangements that may be responsible for arrested growth. These observations associated with larval growth do not eliminate participation of low levels of thyroid hormones in growth of the subadult or postmetamorphic juvenile forms. Such participation for thyroid hormones in the growth of metamorphosed amphibians has not been reported.

Molting and Other Integumentary Effects. Molting or shedding of skin (ecdysis) in larval and adult urodeles is under direct stimulatory control by thyroid hormones, and frequent molting accompanies and follows metamorphosis in these animals.[75] Molting in adult anurans, however, does not appear to be influenced by thyroid hormones. Here molting is stimulated by corticosteroids or indirectly by ACTH operating through its action of increasing corticosteroid secretion.[70,71] The reasons for this marked difference in hormonal control of molting between urodeles and anurans are not known.

Thyroid hormones cause a number of skin changes related to invasion of the terrestrial environment. Both a thickening of the epidermis and keratinization are induced by thyroid hormones in urodeles and anurans. In the newts, thyroid hormones antagonize the effects of PRL on the skin of the eft prior to its return to water. Prolactin reduces the keratinization and helps return the skin to a smooth, moist condition characteristic of aquatic newts.[102]

Class Reptilia

Changes in thyroid state in reptiles are correlated with reproduction, environmental temperature and activity, although cause-effect relationships have not been clearly established. Exogenous thyroid hormones also stimulate oxygen consumption, growth and molting under certain conditions.

The presence of iodinated tyrosines in the blood is a situation unique to reptiles. Blood of the striped racer *Elaphe taeniura* and the cobra *Naja naja* contains MIT and DIT.[166,167] Thyrotropin stimulates in vitro release of MIT, DIT and T_4 from chunks of thyroid tissue from a turtle *(Geochemys reevsii),* a lizard *(Gekko gecko)* and a snake *(E. rachiata)*.[22] These studies suggest that reptilian thyroid glands may lack any deiodinase to convert MIT and DIT to inorganic iodide and tyrosine. These data, however, are open to other interpretations, and additional research is needed.

Reproduction. Seasonal changes in thyroid function have been correlated positively with a number of reproductive events. An active thyroid, usually assessed histologically, is associated with spermatogenesis, ovulation and mating in a number of lizards.[60] Similar observations have been reported in snakes and in at least one turtle.[21,24,166]

Among live-bearing reptiles there is no evidence for increased thyroid function during gestation. However, thyroidectomy of pregnant lizards *Lacerta vivipara* 6 weeks prior to term caused premature discharge of some eggs, and retained eggs failed to hatch.[87]

Environmental Temperature. In general, thyroid function in reptiles varies proportionally with changes in temperature, although the cause-effect relationships are still obscure. Behaviors such as basking in lizards make it difficult to estimate body temperature when assessing thyroid state. Thyroid activity in temperate lizards is highest during the warmer seasons.[87,142,159] Lowering the environmental temperature artificially during the summer months causes reduction in thyroid activity,[142] and lizards maintained in the laboratory at high temperatures (35°C), exhibit greater thyroid function than when maintained at 15°C.[87] Thyroid function in snakes is greater during warm periods and lowest during hibernation.[125,126] The reverse is reported for lizards.[129] The greatest level of thyroid activity correlates with reproductive events in some lizards and snakes and not with temperature. Similar data have been reported for turtles.[41,131]

An exception to the relationship of thyroid activity and temperature described above is the situation found in several species of lizard inhabiting warmer climates. These lizards do not exhibit depressed thyroid function at lower temperatures. Thyroids of such lizards tend to be more active during cool periods.[40,99,160]

There appears to be a positive correlation also between thyroid state and activity in lizards and snakes.[39,78,87] Increased humidity and activity are correlated with increased thyroid function in the lizard *Agama agama savattieri,*[17] suggesting that a more complex relationship exists between thyroid state and environmental factors.

Oxygen Consumption. The relationship between thyroid state and oxygen consumption is temperature dependent. Thyroid hormones, TSH and thyroidectomy have little effect on lizards maintained at 20°C, but a positive relationship appears between oxygen consumption and thyroid state at 30°C.[89,91] Heart, brain, liver, muscle and lung tissues from lizards incubated in vitro at 30°C respond to T_4 with increased consumption of oxygen.[87,141] Homogenates of both liver and skeletal muscles from T_4-treated snakes *Natrix piscator* exhibit higher oxygen consumption at 30°C than do tissues from untreated snakes.[144] Thyroidectomy causes a decrease in oxygen consumption in these animals that is restored to normal by treatment with T_4.

Molting. Shedding of the skin is stimulated in lizards by thyroid hormones and is retarded by thyroidectomy. Implants of thyroid tissue into muscles of thyroidectomized *Lacerta* spp. restore molting that has been interrupted by thyroidectomy.[87] Apparently either mammalian TSH or PRL is capable of restoring molting in some hypophysectomized lizards,[20] and PRL enhances the effect of T_4 on intact animals.[19] Such a relationship between PRL and the thyroid axis in lizards is unlike the role for PRL in the amphibians.

In snakes thyroidectomy increases molting frequency, and cessation of molting follows administration of thyroid hormones.[87] No explanation for this marked difference between snakes and lizards has been offered. This situation is different from that found in amphibians in which thyroid hormones and corticosteroids, seem to be involved in urodeles and anurans respectively.

Growth. Although detailed studies of the relationship of thyroid state to growth are lacking for reptiles, a variety of studies employing embryonic, juvenile and adult reptiles suggest a relationship between thyroid hormones and growth that is similar to the mammalian pattern. Careful studies are still needed to substantiate this relationship.

Class Aves

The structure and function of avian thyroid glands are similar to those of mammals. Thyroid hormones have been reported to affect reproduction, growth, metabolism, temperature regulation, molting and various behaviors. Most studies on avian species have concentrated heavily on certain domestic birds (chicken, duck, pigeon), and few data are available for wild bird species. Nevertheless, with respect to most of these processes, the relationships are similar for wild and domestic species.

Reproduction. Domestic birds require thyroid hormones for normal gonadal development. For example, T_4 stimulates testicular growth, whereas thyroidectomy or goitrogen administration impairs testicular function or induces gonadal regression.[4,80,157] Thyroxine can stimulate testicular growth out of season in some wild birds as well.[99,152] Exogenous T_4 under some circumstances may exert suppressive actions on gonads.[68,82,83]

In several wild species, thyroidectomy prior to the time for normal gonadal growth results in precocious gonadal growth and maintenance at maximum condition.[16,158] Treatment with T_4 results in gonadal regression in thyroidectomized birds at any time of year.[143] In other wild species thyroidectomy simply prolongs the active gonadal phase and shortens the time during which the gonads are regressed.[145] Obviously one cannot generalize about the relationships between thyroid hormones and reproductive events in birds since each species may prove to be a special case.

Thermogenesis and Oxygen Consumption. It appears that thyroid hormones are directly involved in cold adaptation. Thermogenesis (heat production) in birds as in mammals is closely linked to oxygen consumption. Wild birds in temperate regions exhibit heightened thyroid activity in late autumn and early winter as evidenced by histological examination and changes in thyroid gland weight.[25,77,164] Thyroidectomy of adult birds depresses their ability to produce heat, and treatment with thyroid hormones increases oxygen consumption.[133,141]

Carbohydrate Metabolism and Growth. Thyroid hormones reduce glycogen stores in liver, increase free fatty acid levels and induce mild hyperglycemia. Thyroidectomy causes a decrease in blood glucose and liver fatty acid levels but an increase in blood cholesterol levels.[36,117,141] These effects may not be of primary importance since a number of other hormones, such as glucagon and epinephrine, are known to be more important than thyroid hormones with respect to controlling carbohydrate metabolism in birds. Thyroid hormones may produce a permissive effect with respect to the actions of these other "glucohormones," possibly through an effect on adenyl cyclase levels in the target tissues. These effects on carbohydrate metabolism may be related to the thermogenic action of thyroid hormones.

There is evidence that thyroid hormones act cooperatively with GH.[3] Thyroidectomy causes depression or retardation of growth in birds and seasonal changes in circulating GH and T_4 are correlated.[128]

Molting. Thyroid hormones produce stimulatory effects on the skin and feathers that are usually associated with the molting process. It is generally accepted that the gonadal axis provides the factors that directly regulate the molting process in birds.[3,38] Unlike the condition for urodele amphibians and lizards, the role for thyroid hormones in the molting process of birds may be permissive rather than causative.

Migratory Behavior. Migratory birds have been shown to possess active thyroid glands as compared to nonmigrating individuals of the same species,[3] suggesting some interaction in the migratory process. Although some of the older literature indicates that thyroid hormones may directly influence migratory behavior, the nature of this influence has not been confirmed. Thyroid hormones may alter metabolic patterns associated with energy requirements during migration. Another suggestion is that thyroid hormones "tune" the nervous system so that it is more sensitive to environmental or other endocrine cues or both. The role of environmental and endocrine factors in bird migration is discussed in Chapter 18.

Summary

The functional unit of the vertebrate thyroid gland is the thyroid follicle which is unique in gnathostomes for storing thyroid hormones (T_3 and T_4) extracellularly in the colloid of the follicular lumen. Normal thyroid gland functioning depends upon a constant supply of iodide in the diet as well as upon regulatory stimuli from the hypothalamus (TRH or possibly a TRIH in some cases) and the adenohypophysis (TSH). Iodide is accumulated by the follicular cells and is incorporated into tyrosine residues of large glycoproteins collectively referred to as thyroglobulin. Some of the iodinated tyrosines (MIT, DIT) are coupled to form iodinated thyronines (T_3 and T_4), and the iodinated thyroglobulins are secreted into the follicular lumen for storage. Engulfment of colloid (endocytosis) and intracellular hydrolysis of thyroglobulin in phagolysosomes release iodinated thyronines and allow them to diffuse into the circulation. Intracellularly released MIT and DIT are enzymatically degraded (deiodinase) to tyrosine and inorganic iodide for new synthesis of thyroglobulin and subsequent iodination of its tyrosine residues. Both synthesis and release of thyroid hormones are stimulated by TSH. Antithyroid drugs such as certain anions and the traditional goitrogens (PTU, TU, etc.) interfere with iodide uptake or the iodination process or with both, causing thyroid deficiencies. Prolactin may inhibit thyroid hormone synthesis and may also antagonize the actions of thyroid hormones at their target tissues.

The hydrophobic thyroid hormones are transported in the circulation bound to plasma proteins, and only a small proportion of free hormones is present. Thyroxine is more tightly bound to plasma proteins than T_3, and this greater affinity of T_4 for plasma proteins is probably related to its much longer biological half-life. Metabolism of T_4 to T_3, rT_3 and tetraiodothyroacetate occurs peripherally. The last two metabolic products have little biological activity. Most of the circulating T_3 arises peripherally from T_4, and it has been suggested that T_4 acts as a reservoir for T_3, which is the "active form" of the hormone. Cytoplasmic (mitochondrial) and nuclear receptors have been prepared from target tissues. These receptors have greater affinity for T_3 than for T_4, which supports the hypothesis that deiodination of T_4 to T_3 may be the important first step in its mechanism of action.

It is difficult to characterize the actions of thyroid hormones with respect to their functions in vertebrates. Generally they play a permissive role in that they tend to maintain a state of responsiveness in many cells that enables these cells to be more sensitive to other endocrine or neural stimuli. Processes that are affected in this manner include growth, metabolism, ionic and osmotic regulation and a variety of behavioral phenomena. Certain processes are directly stimulated by thyroid hormones but these processes show marked differences among and even within the different classes of vertebrates. Processes that involve direct actions of thyroid hormones in amphibians, reptiles and mammals include molting, amphibian metamorphosis and possibly some events associated with reproduction. In some cases, however, these processes may be related to the permissive action of the thyroid hormones.

The action of thyroid hormones on peripheral tissues following specific binding of the hormone to nuclear receptors is followed by activation of RNA synthesis and eventual enzyme syntheses. The permissive action of thyroid hormones may be related to the stimulation of the synthesis of the enzyme adenyl cyclase that may then be activated by other hormones to increase cAMP. Binding of thyroid hormones to mitochondrial receptors, especially in liver and kidney, may be important in the thermogenic and oxidative actions of thyroid hormones and also may influence availability of ATP for cAMP synthesis.

The thyroid follicular cell appears to originate from the iodide-concentrating cell of the protochordate endostyle. However, the origin of the functional role for thyroid hormones can only be speculated upon at this time. It has been suggested that hypothalamic-hypophysial control over thyroid function developed from the hypothalamo-gonadal axis, possibly in placoderms or even earlier in agnathans, and that the primitive role for thyroid hormones was an association with reproductive cycles. The other roles described in this chapter for thyroid hormones evolved subsequently.

References

1. Aleksiuk, M. and M.T. Cowan (1969). The winter metabolic depression in arctic beavers (*Castor canadensis* Kuhl) with comparison to California beavers. Can. J. Zool. 47:965–979.
2. Aleksiuk, M. and A. Frohlinger (1971). Seasonal metabolic organization in the muskrat *(Ondatra zibethica)*. I. Changes in growth, thyroid activity, brown adipose tissue and organ weights in nature. Can. J. Zool. 49:1143–1154.
3. Assenmacher, I. (1973). The peripheral endocrine glands. In D.S. Farner and J.R. King, eds., Avian Biology, Academic Press, New York, Vol. 3, pp. 183–286.
4. Assenmacher, I. and A. Tixier–Vidal (1962). Le réflexe photosexuel après thyroidectomie chimique chez le Canard male. C. R. Soc. Biol. 156:18–21.
5. Baker–Cohen, K.F. (1959). Renal and other heterotopic thyroid tissue in fishes. In A. Gorbman, ed., Comparative Endocrinology. John Wiley and Sons, New York, pp. 283–319.
6. Bakke, J.L., R.J. Gellert and N.L. Lawrence (1970). The persistent effects of perinatal hypothyroidism on pituitary, thyroidal and gonadal functions. J. Lab. Clin. Med. 76:25–33.
7. Barrington, E.J.W. and M. Sage (1966). On the response of the endostyle of the hypophysectomized larval lamprey to thiourea. Gen. Comp. Endocrinol. 7:463–474.
8. Boissin–Agasse, L., D. Maurel and J. Boissin (1981). Seasonal variations in the thyroxine and testosterone levels in relation to the moult in the adult male mink (*Mustela vison* Peale and Beauvois). Can. J. Zool. 59:1062–1066.
9. Boyd, J.D. (1964). Development of the human thyroid gland. In Pitt-Rivers R. and W.R. Trotters, eds., The Thyroid Gland. Butterworth and Co., Washington, Vol. 1, pp. 9–31.
10. Bronk, J.R. (1966). Thyroid hormone: Effects on electron transport. Science 153:638–639.
11. Brown, C.L. and M.H. Stetson (1983). Prolactin–thyroid interactions in *Fundulus heteroclitus*. Gen. Comp. Endocrinol. 50:167–171.
12. Bruni, J.F., S. Marshall, J.A. Dibbet and J. Meites (1975). Effects of hyper- and hypothyroidism on serum LH and FSH levels in intact and gonadectomized male and female rats. Endocrinology 97:558–563.
13. Burke, G., L–L. Change and M. Szabo (1973). Thyrotropin and cyclic nucleotide effects of prostaglandin levels in isolated thyroid cells. Science 180:872–875.
14. Campantico, F., M. Olivero, M.T. Rinando, C. Guinta and A. Guardabassi (1968). The pituitary, thyroid, liver glycogen and related enzymes, growth and metamorphosis in STH- and LTH-treated toad larvae. Monitore Zool. Ital. (NS) 2:1–13.
15. Cartouzou, G., R. Aquaron and S. Lissitzky (1964). Purification of soluble RNA from sheep thyroid gland. Absence of acceptor activity for the iodotyrosines. Biochem. Biophys. Res. Commun. 15:82–86.
16. Chandola, A. (1972). Thyroid in reproduction. Reproductive physiology of *Lonchura panctulata* in relation to iodine metabolism and hypothyroidism. Ph.D. thesis, Banaras Hindu University. Cited by Assenmacher.[3]
17. Charnier, M. and J.P. Dutarte (1956). Variations histo-physiologiques de la thyroide du lézard de la région de Dakar pendant la période de préhivernage. C. R. Soc. Biol. 150:1387–1388.
18. Chiu, K.W. and J.G. Phillips (1972). The effect of prolactin, thyroxine and thyrotropin on the sloughing cycle of the lizard *Gekko gecko* L. Gen. Comp. Endocrinol. 19:592–593.
19. Chiu, K.W., J.G. Phillips and P.F.A. Maderson (1967). The role of the thyroid in the control of the sloughing cycle in the Tokay (*Gekko gecko,* Lacertilia). J. Endocrinol. 39:463–472.

20. Chiu, K.W., J.G. Phillips and P.F.A. Maderson (1969). Seasonal changes in the thyroid gland in the male cobra, *Naja naja* L. Biol. Bull. 136:347–354.

21. Chiu, K.W., C.C. Wong, F.H. Lei and V. Tam (1975). The nature of thyroidal secretions in reptiles. Gen. Comp. Endocrinol. 25:74–82.

22. Chopra, I.J. (1972). A radioimmunoassay for measurement of thyroxine in unextracted serum. J. Clin. Endocrinol. Metab. 34:938.

23. Clerici, P. and E. Gabinino (1967). Endocrine alterations following radiothyroidectomy in *Bufo bufo* larvae. Monitore Zool. Ital. (NS) 1:91–99.

24. Combescot, C. (1956). Sur les variations thyroidiennes chez la fortue d'eau algerienne. C. R. Soc. Biol. 149:2169–2171.

25. Davis, J. and B.S. Davis (1954). The annual gonad and thyroid cycle of the English sparrow in Southern California. Condor 56:328–345.

26. Davison, T.F. (1976). Circulating thyroid hormones in the chicken before and after hatching. Gen. Comp. Endocrinol. 29:21–27.

27. Dent, J.N. (1968). Survey of amphibian metamorphosis. In W. Etkin and L.I. Gilbert, eds., Metamorphosis. Appleton–Century–Crofts, New York, pp. 271–311.

28. Dickhoff, W.W. and D.S. Darling (1983). Evolution of thyroid function and its control in lower vertebrates. Am. Zool. 23:697–707.

29. Dodd, J.M. (1983). Reproduction in cartilaginous fishes (Chondrichthyes). In W.S. Hoar, D.J. Randall and E.M. Donaldson, eds., Fish Physiology, Academic Press, New York, Vol. 9A, pp. 31–95.

30. Dodd, M.H.I. and J.M. Dodd (1976). The biology of metamorphosis. In B. Lofts, ed., Physiology of the Amphibia. Vol. 3, pp. 467–599.

31. Dupe, M. and R. Godet (1969). Conditioning of the responsiveness of the central nervous system in the life cycle of the lungfish *(Protopterus annectens)*. Gen. Comp. Endocrinol. Suppl. 2:275–283.

32. Eakin, R.M., R.E. Stebbins and D.C. Wilhoft (1959). Effects of parietalectomy and sustained temperatures on thyroid of lizard, *Sceloporus occidentalis*. Proc. Soc. Exp. Biol. Med. 101:162–164.

33. Eales, J.G. (1979). Thyroid functions in cyclostomes and fishes. In E.J.W. Barrington, ed., Hormones and Evolution, Academic Press, New York, Vol. 1, pp. 341–436.

34. Eales, J.G. (1982). Thyroid hormone and iodide metabolism in teleost fish. Gunma Symp. Endocrinol. 19:29–44.

35. Eddy, L. and H. Lipner (1975). Acceleration of thyroxine-induced metamorphosis by prolactin antiserum. Gen. Comp. Endocrinol. 25:462–466.

36. Ensor, D.M., D.M. Thomas and J.G. Phillips (1970). The possible role of the thyroid in extra-renal secretion following a hypertonic saline load in the duck *(Anas platyrhynchos)*. J. Endocrinol. 46:X.

37. Etkin, W. (1978). The thyroid—a gland in search of a function. Pers. Biol. Med. 21 (8): 19–30.

38. Etkin, W. and A.G. Gona (1974). Evolution of thyroid function in poikilothermic vertebrates. Handbook of Physiology, Sec. 7., Endocrinology. Williams & Wilkins, Baltimore, Vol. 3, pp. 5–20.

39. Evans, L.T. and M. Clapp (1940). The relation of thyroid extract to territorial behavior and to anoxemia in *Anolis carolinensis*. J. Comp. Psychol. 29:277–281.

40. Evans, L.T. and E. Hegre (1938). The effects of ovarian hormones and seasons on *Anolis carolinensis*. I. The thyroid. Anat. Rec. 72:1–9.

41. Evans, L.T. and E. Hegre (1940). Endocrine relationships in turtles. Effects of seasons and pituitary extracts on the thyroid. Endocrinology 27:144–148.

42. Fontaine, M. and J. Leloup (1962). Le fonctionnement thyroidien du saumon adulte (*Salmo salar* L.) à quelques étapes de son cycle migratoire. Gen. Comp. Endocrinol. 2:317–322.

43. Fontaine, Y.A. (1969). Studies on the heterotopic activity of preparations of mammalian gonadotropins of teleost fish. Gen. Comp. Endocrinol. Suppl. 2:417–424.

44. Fontaine, Y.A. and E. Burzawa–Gerard (1977). Esquisse de l'évolution des hormones gonadotropes et thyreotropes des vertebres. Gen. Comp. Endocrinol. 32:341–347.

45. Frye, B.E., P.S. Brown and B.W. Snyder (1972). Effects of prolactin and somatotropin on growth and metamorphosis of amphibians. Gen. Comp. Endocrinol. Suppl. 3:209–220.

46. Funkhouser, A. and K.S. Mills (1969). Oxygen consumption during spontaneous amphibian metamorphosis. Physiol. Zool. 42:15–21.

47. Funkhouser, A. and K.S. Mills (1969). Oxygen consumption during induced amphibian metamorphosis. Physiol. Zool. 42:22–28.

48. Furth, E.D., K. Rives and D.V. Becker (1966). Nonthyroidal action of prophylthiouracil in euthyroid, hypothyroid and hyperthyroid man. J. Clin. Endocrinol. Metab. 26:239–246.

49. Galton, V.A. and S.H. Ingbar (1962). Observations on the relation between the action and degradation of thyroid hormones as indicated by studies in the tadpole and the frog. Endocrinology 70:622–633.

50. Gans, C. and R.G. Northcutt (1983). Neural crest and the origin of vertebrates: A new head. Science 220:268–274.

51. Gaspard, T., R. Wondergem, M. Hamamdzic and H.M. Klitgaard (1978). Serum somatomedin stimulation in thyroxine-treated hypophysectomized rats. Endocrinology 102:606–611.

52. Gillie, R.B. (1971). Endemic goiter. Sci. Am. June, 93–101.

53. Gorbman, A. (1955). Some aspects of the comparative biochemistry of iodine utilization and evolution of thyroidal function. Physiol. Rev. 35:336–344.

54. Gorbman, A. (1959). Problems in the comparative morphology and physiology of the vertebrate thyroid gland. In A. Gorbman, ed., Comparative Endocrinology. John Wiley and Sons, New York, pp. 266–282.

55. Gorbman, A. (1969). Thyroid function and its control in fishes. In W.S. Hoar and D.J. Randall, eds., Fish Physiology. Academic Press, New York. Vol. 2, pp. 241–274.

56. Gorbman, A. and H.A. Bern (1962). A Textbook of Comparative Endocrinology. John Wiley and Sons, New York.

57. Gorbman, A. and S. Ishii (1960). Stimulation of neurosecretion in shark embryos by thyroid hormones. Proc. Soc. Exp. Biol. Med. 103:865–867.

58. Greer, M.A., J.W. Kendall and M. Smith (1964). Antithyroid compounds. In R. Pitt-Rivers and W.R. Trotter, eds., The Thyroid Gland. Butterworths, London, Vol. 1, pp. 357–389.

59. Guardabassi, A., A.M. Cocito and G. Poncetti (1969). Ectopic pituitary homotransplantations from larvae and adult donors in *Xenopus laevis* Daud. intact larvae. Monitore Zool. Ital. 3:213–224.

60. Haldar-Misra, C. and J.P. Thapliyal (1981). Thyroid in reproduction of reptiles. Gen. Comp. Endocrinol. 43:537–542.

61. Higgs, D.A. and J.G. Eales (1973). Measurement of circulating thyroxine in several freshwater teleosts by competitive binding analysis. Can. J. Zool. 51:49–53.

62. Hoch, F.L. (1974). Metabolic effects of thyroid hormones. Handbook of Physiology, Sec. 7, Endocrinology. Williams & Wilkins, Baltimore, Vol. 3, pp. 391–411.

63. Hopper, A.F. and M.B. Yatvin (1965). Protein metabolism in the liver of thiouracil-treated goldfish. Growth 29:355–360.

64. Hornsey, D.J. (1977). Triiodothyronine and thyroxine levels in the thyroid and serum of the sea lamprey *Petromyzon marinus*. Gen. Comp. Endocrinol. 31:381–383.

65. Hoskins, E.R. and M.M. Hoskins (1919). Growth and development of amphibia as affected by thyroidectomy. J. Exp. Zool. 29:1–69.

66. Hudson, J.W. and D.R. Deavers (1976). Thyroid function and basal metabolism in the ground squirrels *Ammospermophilus leucurus* and *Spermophilus* spp. Physiol. Zool. 49:425–444.

67. Hurlburt, M.E. (1977). Role of the thyroid gland in ovarian maturation of the goldfish, *Carassius auratus* L. Can. J. Zool. 55:1906–1913.

68. Jallageas, M. and I. Assenmacher (1974). Thyroid gonadal interaction in the male domestic duck in relationship with the sexual cycle. Gen. Comp. Endocrinol. 22:13–20.

69. Joasoo, A., I.P.C. Murray and J. Parkin (1975). Comparative studies of thyroid function in mammals. Gen. Comp. Endocrinol. 36:135–138.

70. Jorgensen, C.B. and L.O. Larsen (1964). Further observations on molting and its hormonal control in *Bufo bufo* L. Gen. Comp. Endocrinol. 4:389–400.

71. Jorgensen, C.B., L.O. Larsen and P. Rosenkilde (1965). Hormonal dependency of molting in amphibians: Effect of radiothyroidectomy in the toad, *Bufo bufo* (L.). Gen. Comp. Endocrinol. 5:248–251.

72. Joseph, S.A., D.E. Scott, S.S. Vaala, K.M. Knigge and G. Krobisch-Dudley (1973). Localization and content of thyrotropin releasing factor (TRF) in median eminence of the hypothalamus. Acta Endocrinol. 74:215–225.

73. Just, J.J., J. Kraus-Just, and D.A. Check (1981). Survey of chordate metamorphosis. In L.I. Gilbert and E. Frieden, eds., Metamorphosis: A Problem in Developmental Biology, Plenum Press, New York, pp. 265–326.

74. Kaethner, M.M. and B.F. Good (1975). Seasonal thyroid activity in the tammar wallaby, *Macropus eugenii* (Demarest). Aust. J. Zool. 23:363–370.

75. Kaltenbach, J.C. (1968). Nature of hormone action in amphibian metamorphosis. In W. Etkin and L.I. Gilbert, eds., Metamorphosis. Appleton-Century-Crofts, New York, pp. 399–442.

76. Kaneko, T., U. Zor and J.B. Field (1969). Thyroid-stimulating hormone and prostaglandin E, stimulation of cyclic 3′,5′-adenosine monophosphate in thyroid slices. Science 163:1062–1063.

77. Kendreigh, S.C. and H.E. Wallin (1966). Seasonal and taxonomic differences in the size and activity of the thyroid gland in birds. Ohio J. Sci. 66:369–379.

78. Kracht, J. and E.G. Weber (1978). Morphological changes in the ultrastructure of the thyroid epithelium of *Notophthalamus viridescens* after hypophysectomy and TSH- and prolactin stimulation. Cell Tissue Res. 187:305–313.

79. Krockert, G. (1941). Cited by Lynn.[87]

80. Kumaran, J.D.S. and C.W. Turner (1949). The endocrinology of spermatogenesis in birds. III. Effects of hypo- and hyperthyroidism. Poult. Sci. 28:653–665.

81. Larsen, L.O. and P. Rosenkilde (1971). Iodine metabolism in normal, hypophysectomized, and thyrotropin-treated river lampreys, *Lampetra fluviatilis* (Gray) L. (Cyclostomata). Gen. Comp. Endocrinol. 17:94–104.

82. Lehman, G.C. (1970). The effects of hypo- and hyperthyroidism on the testes and anterior pituitary gland in cockerels. Gen. Comp. Endocrinol. 14:567–577.

83. Lehman, G.C. and B.E. Frye (1976). The effect of changes in thyroid function on testis ^{32}P uptake and the response to gonadotropin in the chick. Gen. Comp. Endocrinol. 28:446–453.

84. Lewis, E.J.C. and E. Frieden (1959). Biochemistry of amphibian metamorphosis. V. Effect of triiodothyronine, thyroxine and dinitrophenol on the respiration of the tadpole. Endocrinology 65:273–282.

85. Licht, P. and R.E. Jones (1967). Effects of exogenous prolactin on reproduction and growth in adult males of the lizard *Anolis carolinensis*. Gen. Comp. Endocrinol. 8:228–244.

86. Loos, U., G. Rothenbuchner, J. Birk, E.F. Pfeiffer, G. Knapp and B.E. Schreiber (1973). Serum levels of T_3, T_4 and TSH after different modes of TRH administration. In C. Gual and E. Rosenberg, eds., Hypothalamic Hypophysiotropic Hormones. Excerpta Medica, Amsterdam, pp. 136–140.

87. Lynn, W.G. (1970). The thyroid. In A. d'A. Bellairs, C. Gans and E.E. Williams, eds., The Biology of the Reptiles. Academic Press, New York, Vol. 3, pp. 201–234.

88. Maher, M.J. (1964). Metabolic response of isolated lizard tissues to thyroxine administered in vivo. Endocrinology 74:994–995.

89. Maher, M.J. (1965). The role of the thyroid gland in the oxygen consumption of lizards. Gen. Comp. Endocrinol. 5:320–325.

90. Maher, M.J. (1967). Response to thyroxine as a function of environmental temperature in the toad, *Bufo woodhousii,* and the frog, *Rana pipiens*. Copeia 1967 2:361–365.

91. Maher, M.J. and B.H. Levedahl (1959). The effect of the thyroid gland on the oxidative metabolism of the lizard. *Anolis carolinensis.* J. Exp. Zool. 140:169–189.

92. Marusic, E., R. Martinez and J. Torretti (1966). Unresponsiveness of the adult toad to thyroxine administration. Proc. Soc. Exp. Biol. Med. 122:164–167.

93. Mason, E.B. (1977). Serum thyroxine levels in *Chrysemys picta marginata* (Reptilia, Testudines, Testudinidae) exposed to different thermal environments. J. Herpetol. 11:232–234.

94. Mathur, G.B. (1967). Anaerobic respiration in a cyprinid fish *Rasbora daniconius* (Ham). Nature 214:318–319.

95. Matty, A.J., M.A. Chaudhry and K.P. Lone (1982). The effect of thyroid hormones and temperature on protein and nucleic acid contents of liver and muscle of *Sarotherodon mossambica.* Gen. Comp. Endocrinol. 47:497–507.

96. Matty, A.J., K. Tsuneki, W.W. Dickhoff and A. Gorbman (1976). Thyroid and gonadal function in hypophysectomized hagfish, *Eptatretus stouti*. Gen. Comp. Endocrinol. 30:500–516.

97. Maurel, D. and J. Boissin (1979). Seasonal variations of thyroid activity in the adult male badger (*Meles meles* L.) Gen. Comp. Endocrinol. 38:207–214.

98. Maurel, D. and J. Boissin (1981). Plasma thyroxine and testosterone levels in the red fox (*Vulpes vulpes* L.) during the annual cycle. Gen. Comp. Endocrinol. 43:402–404.

99. Miller, M.R. (1955). Cyclic changes in the thyroid and interrenal glands of the viviparous lizard, *Xantusia vigilis*. Anat. Rec. 123:19–31.

100. Moury, D.N. and F.L. Crane (1964). Quantitative study of the effects of thyroxine on components of the electron-transfer system. Biochemistry 3:1068–1072.

101. Nadler, N.J., B.A. Young, C.P. Leblond and B. Mitmaker (1964). Elaboration of thyroglobulin in the thyroid follicle. Endocrinology 74:333–354.

102. Nicoll, C.S. (1974). Physiological actions of prolactin. Handbook of Physiology, Sec. 7, Endocrinology, Williams & Wilkins, Baltimore, Vol. 4, Part 2, pp. 253–292.

103. Norris, D.O. (1978). Hormonal and environmental factors involved in the determination of neoteny in urodeles. In P.J. Gaillard and H.H. Boer, eds., Comparative Endocrinology. Elsevier/North-Holland Biomedical Press, Amsterdam, pp. 109–112.

104. Norris, D.O. (1983). Evolution of endocrine regulation of metamorphosis in lower vertebrates. Am. Zool. 23:709–718.

105. Norris, D.O., D. Duvall, K. Greendale and W.A. Gern (1977). Thyroid function in pre- and post-spawning neotenic tiger salamanders *(Ambystoma tigrinum)*. Gen. Comp. Endocrinol. 33:512–517.

106. Norris, D.O. and J.E. Platt (1973). Effects of pituitary hormones, melatonin, and thyroidal inhibitors on radioiodide uptake by the thyroid glands of larval and adult tiger salamanders, *Ambystoma tigrinum* (Amphibia: Caudata). Gen. Comp. Endocrinol. 21:368–376.

107. Nunez, J. and J. Pommier (1982). Formation of thyroid hormones. Vit. Horm. 39:175–229.

108. Olivereau, M. (1968). Action de la prolactine chez l'anguille. IV. Metabolisme thyroidien. Z. Vergl. Physiol. 61:246–358.

109. Oppenheimer, J.H. (1983). The nuclear receptor-triiodothyronine complex: relationship to thyroid hormone distribution, metabolism, and biological origin. In J.H. Oppenheimer and H.H. Samuel, eds., Molecular Basis of Thyroid Hormone Action. Academic Press, New York, pp. 1–34.

110. Oppenheimer, J.H., H.L. Schwartz, M.I. Surks, D. Koerner and W. H. Dillmann (1976). Nuclear receptors and the initiation of thyroid hormone action. Rec. Prog. Horm. Res. 32:529–565.

111. Packard, G.C. and M.J. Packard (1975). The influence of acclimation temperature on the metabolic

response of frog tissue to thyroxine administered *in vivo*. Gen. Comp. Endocrinol. 27:162–168.

112. Pandey, B.N. and J.S.D. Munshi (1976). Role of the thyroid gland in regulation of metabolic rate in an air breathing siluroid fish, *Heteropneustes fossilis* (Bloch). J. Endocrinol. 69:421–425.

113. Pickering, A.D. (1972). Effects of hypophysectomy on the activity of the endostyle and the thyroid gland in the larval and adult river lamprey, *Lampetra fluviatilis* L. Gen. Comp. Endocrinol. 18:335–343.

114. Platt, J.E. (1976). The effects of ergocornine on tail height, spontaneous and T_4-induced metamorphosis and thyroidal uptake of radioiodide in neotenic *Ambystoma tigrinum*. Gen. Comp. Endocrinol. 28:71–81.

115. Pritchard, A.W. and A. Gorbman (1960). Thyroid hormone treatment and oxygen consumption in embryos of the spiny dogfish. Biol. Bull. 119:109–119.

116. Qureshi, T.A. (1975). Heterotopic thyroid follicles in the accessory mesonephric lobes of *Heteropneustes fossilis* (Bloch). Acta Anat. 93:506–511.

117. Riddle, O. and D.F. Opdyke (1947). The action of pituitary and other hormones on the carbohydrate and fat metabolism of young pigeons. Carnegie Inst. Wash. Publ. 569:49.

118. Riviere, J.E., F.R. Engelhardt and J. Solomon (1977). The relationship of thyroxine and cortisol to the moult of the harbor seal. *Phoca vitulina*. Gen. Comp. Endocrinol. 31:398–401.

119. Robinson, G.A. (1973). The oocytes as major competitors for radioiodide in laying Japanese quail. Gen. Comp. Endocrinol. 21:123–128.

120. Roche, J., G. Salvatore, L. Sena, S. Aloj and I. Covelli (1968). Thyroid iodoproteins in vertebrates: Ultracentrifugal pattern and iodination rate. Comp. Biochem. Physiol. 27:67–82.

121. Rosenkilde, P. and I. Jorgensen (1977). Determination of serum thyroxine in two species of toads: Variation with season. Gen. Comp. Endocrinol. 33:566–573.

122. Ruhland, M.L. (1969). Relation entre l'activité de la glande thyroide et la consommation d'oxygène chez les téleostéens, cichlides. Experientia 25:944.

123. Ruhland, M.L. (1971). La radiothyroidectomie et son effet sur la consommation d'oxygene chez les chichlides *Aequidens latifrons*. Can. J. Zool. 49:423–425.

124. Sage, M. (1973). The evolution of thyroid function in fishes. Am. Zool. 13:899–905.

125. Saint Girons, H. and R. Duguy (1962). Données histologiques sur le cycle annuel de la glande thyroide chez les vipères. Gen. Comp. Endocrinol. 2:337–346.

126. Saint Girons, H. and R. Duguy (1966). Données histophysiologiques sur les variations de la glande thyroide au cours du cycle annuel chez la couleuvre vipèrine *Natrix maura* (L.). Arch. Anat. Microsc. Morphol. Exp. 55:345–362.

127. Salvatore, G. (1969). Thyroid hormone biosynthesis in Agnatha and Protochordata. Gen. Comp. Endocrinol. Suppl. 2:535–552.

128. Scanes, C.G., M. Jallageas and I. Assenmacher (1980). Seasonal variation in the circulating concentrations of growth hormone in male Peking duck *(Anas platyrhynchos)* and teal *(Anas crecca):* correlations with thyroidal function. Gen. Comp. Endocrinol. 41:76–79.

129. Sellers, J.C., L.C. Wit, V.K. Ganjam, K.A. Etheridge and I.M. Ragland (1982). Seasonal plasma T_4 titers in the hibernating lizard *Cnemidophorus sexlineatus*. Gen. Comp. Endocrinol. 46:24–28.

130. Shellabarger, C.J. (1964). The effect of thyroid hormones on growth and differentiation. In R. Pitt-Rivers and W.R. Trotter, eds., The Thyroid Gland, Butterworths, London, Vol. I, pp. 187–198.

131. Shellabarger, C.J., A. Gorbman, F.C. Schatzlein and D. McGill (1956). Some quantitative and qualitative aspects of I^{131} metabolism in turtles. Endocrinology 59:331–339.

132. Silverstone, M., T.R. Tosteson and C.E. Cutress (1977). The effect of iodide and various iodocompounds on initiation of strobilization in *Aurelia*. Gen. Comp. Endocrinol. 32:108–113.

133. Singh, A., E.P. Reineke and R.K. Ringer (1968). Influence of thyroid states of the chick on growth and metabolism with observations on several parameters of thyroid function. Poult. Sci. 47:212–219.

134. Singh, T.P. and A.G. Sathyanesan (1968). Thyroid activity in relation to pituitary thyrotropin (TSH) level and their seasonal changes under normal and varied photoperiods in the freshwater teleost *Mysties vittalus* (Bloch). Acta Zool. 49:47–56.

135. Spangenberg, D. (1974). Thyroxine in early strobilization in *Aurelia aurita*. Am. Zool. 14:825–832.

136. Sterling, K. and J.H. Lazarus (1977). The thyroid and its control. Annu. Rev. Physiol. 39:349–372.

137. Sterling, K., P.O. Milch, M.A. Brenner and J.H. Lazarus (1977). Thyroid hormone action: The mitochondrial pathway. Science 197:996–999.

138. Swingle, W.W. (1918). The acceleration of metamorphosis in frog larvae by thyroid feeding, and the effects upon the alimentary tract and sex glands. J. Exp. Zool. 24:521–543.

139. Taurog, A. (1974). Biosynthesis of iodoamino acids. Handbook of Physiology, Sec. 7, Endocrinology. Williams & Wilkins, Baltimore, Vol. 3, pp. 101–133.

140. Tepperman, J. (1968). Metabolic and Endocrine Physiology, 2nd ed. Year Book Medical Publishers, Chicago.

141. Thapliyal, J.P. (1980). Thyroid in reptiles and birds. In S. Ishii, T. Hirano and M. Wada, eds., Hormones, Adaptations and Evolution. Jap. Sci. Soc., Tokyo/ Springer-Verlag, Berlin, pp. 241–250.

142. Thapliyal, J.P. and A. Chandola (1973). Seasonal variation in thyroid hormonogenesis in the Indian garden lizard, *Calotes versicolor*. J. Endocrinol. 56:451–462.

143. Thapliyal, J.P., R.K. Garg and S.K. Pandha (1968). Effect of thyroxine on the gonad and body weight of spotted munia, *Uroloncha punctulata*. J. Exp. Zool. 169:279–286.

144. Thapliyal, J.P., D.S. Kumar and O.V. Oommen (1975). Variations in the thyroid activity and respiratory rate during a 24-hr period and role of testosterone and thyroxine on the oxidative metabolism of the water snake, *Natrix piscator*. Gen. Comp. Endocrinol. 26:100–106.

145. Thapliyal, J.P. and S.K. Pandha (1967). Thyroidectomy and gonadal recrudescence in Lal Munia, *Estrilda amandava*. Endocrinology 81:915–918.

146. Tice, L.W. and S.H. Wollman (1974). Ultrastructural localization of peroxidase on pseudopods and other structures of the typical thyroid epithelial cell. Endocrinology 94:1555–1567.

147. Tong, W. (1974). Actions of thyroid-stimulating hormone. Handbook of Physiology, Sec. 7, Endocrinology, Vol. 3, pp. 255–283.

148. Trotter, W.R. (1964). Historical introduction. In R. Pitt-Rivers and W.R. Trotter, eds., The Thyroid Gland, Butterworths, London, Vol. 1, pp. 1–8.

149. Uhlenhuth, E. (1925). The role of the thyroid in the neoteny of the Mexican axolotl. Anat. Rec. 29:398.

150. Ui, N. (1974). Synthesis and chemistry of iodoproteins. Handbook of Physiology, Sec. 7, Endocrinology. Williams & Wilkins, Baltimore, Vol. 3, p. 55.

151. Unezu, M., J.M. Cons and P.S. Timaras (1976). Developmental patterns of follicle-stimulating, luteinizing and thyroid-stimulating hormones in the hypothyroid female rat. Ann. Biol. Anim. Biochem. Biophys. 16:385–394.

152. Vaugien, L. (1954). Influence de l'obscuration temporaire sur la durée de la phase réfractaire du cycle sexuel du Moineau domestique. Bull. Biol. Fr. Belg. 88:294–309.

153. Vellano, C., A. Peyrot and V. Mazzi (1967). Effects of prolactin on the pituito-thyroid axis, integument and behavior of the adult male crested newt. Monitore Zool. Ital. (NS) 1:207–227.

154. Wada, M., Y. Arimatsu and H. Kobayashi (1975). Effect of prolactin on thyroid function in Japanese quail *(Coturnix coturnix japonica)*. Gen. Comp. Endocrinol. 27:28–33.

155. Warren, M.R. (1940). Studies on the effect of experimental hyperthyroidism in the adult frog, *Rana pipiens* Schreber. J. Exp. Zool. 83:127–159.

156. Waterman, A.J. and A. Gorbman (1963). Thyroid tissue and some of its properties in the hagfish *Myxine glutinosa*. Gen. Comp. Endocrinol. 3:58–65.

157. Wheeler, R.S., N.E. Hoffman and C.L. Graham (1948). The value of thyroprotein in starting, growing and laying rations. I. Growth, feathering and food consumption in Rhode Island Red broilers. Poult. Sci. 27:103–111.

158. Wieselthier, A.S. and A. van Tienhoven (1972). The effect of thyroidectomy on testicular size and on the photorefractory period in the starling (*Sturnus vulgaris* L.). J. Exp. Zool. 179:331–338.

159. Wilhoft, D.C. (1958). The effect of temperature on thyroid histology and survival in the lizard, *Sceloporus occidentalis*. Copeia 1958:265–276.

160. Wilhoft, D.C. (1964). Seasonal changes in the thyroid and interrenal glands of the tropical Australian skink, *Leiolopisma rhomboidalis*. Gen. Comp. Endocrinol. 4:42–53.

161. Wille, G. (1956). Influence de l'etat fontionnel de la thyroide sur la receptivite de la *Rana temporaria* a la gonadotrophinechorionique. Ann. Endocrinol. 17:333–337.

162. Wille, G. (1957). Etude de la spermation chez *Rana esculenta ridibundi peruzi*. (Influence du poids, de la temperature, de l'etat thyroidien de l'adrenaline, de la testosterone.) Ann. Endocrinol. 18:150–157.

163. Williams, R.H. (1962). Textbook of Endocrinology, 3rd ed. W.B. Saunders Co., Philadelphia, p. 167.

164. Wilson, A.C. and D.S. Farner (1960). Effect of severe stress upon thyroid function. Ann. J. Physiol. 159:291–295.

165. Winston, B.W. and N.E. Henderson (1981). Seasonal changes in morphology of the thyroid gland of a hibernator, *Spermophilus richardsoni*. Can. J. Zool. 59:1022–1031.

166. Wong, K.L. and K.W. Chiu (1974). The snake thyroid gland. I. Seasonal variation of thyroidal and serum iodoamino acids. Gen. Comp. Endocrinol. 23:63–70.

167. Wong, K.L., K.W. Chiu and C.C. Wong (1974). The snake thyroid gland. II. Radioiodide Metabolism. Gen. Comp. Endocrinol. 23:71–81.

168. Woodhead, A.D. (1966). Thyroid activity in the ovoviviparous elasmobranch *Squalus acanthias*. J. Zool. 148:238–275.

169. Woodhead, A.D. and P.M.J. Woodhead (1965). Seasonal changes in the physiology of the Barents Sea cod, *Gadus morhua* L., in relation to its environment. I. Endocrine changes particularly affecting migration and maturation. Int. Comm. NW Atlantic Fish., Special Publ. No. 6:691–715.

170. Wright, G.M. and J.H. Youson (1977). Serum thyroxine concentrations in larval and metamorphosing anadromous sea lamprey, *Petromyzon marinus* L. J. Exp. Zool. 202:27–32.

171. Wright, G.M. and J.H. Youson (1980). Variation in serum levels of thyroxine in anadromous larval lam-

preys, *Petromyzon marinus L.* Gen. Comp. Endocrinol. 41:321–324.

172. Yamada, T., A. Kajihara, Y. Takemura and T. Onaya (1974). Antithyroid compounds. Handbook of Physiology, Sec. 7, Endocrinology. Williams & Wilkins, Baltimore, Vol. 3, pp. 345–357.

173. Yaron, Z. (1969). Correlation between spawning water temperature and thyroid activity in *Acanthobrama terrae-sanctae* (Cyprinidae) of Lake Tiberias. Gen. Comp. Endocrinol. 12:604–608.

174. Yatvin, M.B., R.W. Wannamacher and W.L. Banks, Jr. (1964). Effects of thiouracil and of thyroidectomy on liver protein metabolism. Endocrinology 74:878–884.

175. Young, G. and J.N. Ball (1983). Ultrastructural changes in the adenohypophysis during the ovarian cycle of the viviparous teleost, *Poecilia latipinna*. Gen. Comp. Endocrinol. 51:24–38.

9·The Chemistry of Steroid Hormones

Before undertaking a study of adrenals and gonads, it is necessary to first discuss the chemistry of steroid hormones. A working knowledge of the varieties of steroids and their structure, synthesis, transport and metabolism will make the roles for these glands and their hormones more comprehensible.

The chemical term steroid refers to a variety of lipoidal compounds, all of which possess the basic structure of four carbon rings known as the cyclopentanoperhydrophenanthrene nucleus (Fig. 9-1). There are many naturally occurring steroids including *cholesterol, vitamin D, 1,25-dihydroxycholecalciferol* (1,25-DHC), the *adrenocortical steroids* and the gonadal sex steroids, *androgens, estrogens* and *progestogens.* The following accounts deal specifically with the mammalian steroid hormones produced by the adrenal and gonads. The most commonly occurring steroids of these categories are provided in Table 9-1.

Androgens are defined as compounds that stimulate development of male characteristics; that is, they are masculinizing agents. The primary source for circulating androgens is the testis where luteinizing hormone (LH) from the adenohypophysis stimulates their synthesis and release into the blood. Androgens may be synthesized also by the adrenal cortex (see Chap. 10) and to some extent by the ovaries (Chap. 11).

Estrogens are compounds that are capable of stimulating cornification (deposition of the structural protein keratin) in epidermal cells lining the vagina of castrate female rats. These compounds also stimulate proliferation and vascularization of the uterine mucosa or endometrium. Luteinizing hormone and follicle-stimulating hormone (FSH) together stimulate certain ovarian cells to synthesize and release estrogens into the blood. The biological roles for estrogens are described in Chapter 11.

A progestogen is a compound that maintains pregnancy or the secretory condition of the uterine endometrium during the luteal phase of the ovarian cycle (see Chap. 11). Progestogens such as *progesterone* are produced by all steroidogenic tissues as an intermediate in the synthesis of other steroid hormones. The role of progesterone as a mammalian reproductive hormone, however, is also well established. Details concerning the actions of progesterone as a reproductive hormone are described in Chapter 11.

There are two subcategories of corticoids (corticosteroids): *glucocorticoids* and *mineralocorticoids.* Glucocorticoids can influence carbohydrate metabolism under certain conditions, and their major physiological role appears to be an influence on peripheral utilization of glucose (see Chaps. 10 and 19). Mineralocorticoids affect sodium transport mechanisms in nephrons of the kidney. It must be emphasized that these terms become rather meaningless if applied to nonmammalian vertebrates, because a given molecule that may possess glucocorticoid activity in mammals may have mineralocorticoid activity in nonmammals. *Cortisol,* for example, is a glucocor-

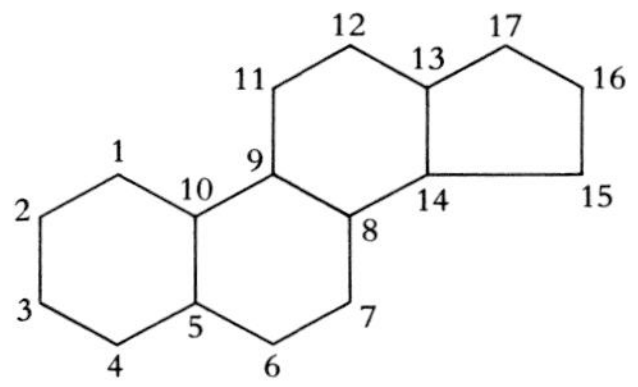

12 13 17 11 16 1 9 10 14 15 2 8 3 5 7 4 6

FIG. 9-1. Basic steroid nucleus: the cyclopentanoperhydrophenanthrene nucleus. Numbers designate each carbon in the nucleus. Additional carbons (18 and 19) may be attached to carbons 10 (18) and 13 (19) as well as to 17 (carbons 20–27).

ticoid in man, but it is apparently a mineralocorticoid in teleostean fishes. Corticoids are synthesized by the cortical (outer) portions of the adrenal gland or its homologue in nonmammals, the so-called *interrenal* tissue, following stimulation by pituitary corticotropin (ACTH). A detailed account is given in Chapter 10.

It should be obvious that these definitions for the various categories of steroid hormones are functionally derived. Although naturally occurring steroids that exhibit a particular hormonal activity in vertebrates (estrogenic, androgenic, etc.) are structurally similar to one another (Figs. 9-2 to 9-5), many structurally unrelated compounds may have similar hormonal activity when tested and would be classified accordingly. Diethylstilbestrol is a powerful estrogen by functional definition and is more potent than any of the naturally occurring estrogens. However, it is not a steroid chemically.

Steroid Nomenclature

The literature on steroid hormones is very confusing to the uninitiated in part because of the multiplicity of trivial and chemical names for a single molecule. Cortisol, for example, in addition to being designated by two different chemical names (11β,17α,21-trihydroxypregn-4-ene-3,20-dione and 11β,17α,21-trihydroxy - Δ4 - pregnene - 3,20-dione) has three trivial names: cortisol, 17-hydroxycorticosterone and hydrocortisone. Furthermore, cortisol was known as Reichstein's compound M and Kendall's compound F before its chemical structure was elucidated. In order to use the established literature it is necessary to become familiar with the various trivial names as well as to understand the bases for the chemical names. A working knowledge of the chemical nomenclature for steroids is not really necessary for the treatments provided in this textbook, although those students interested in details of synthesis and metabolism of steroids will find knowledge of the chemical nomenclature invaluable. Table 9-2 summarizes special designations used in nomenclature of steroids.

TABLE 9-1. *Some Vertebrate Steroid Hormones*

CATEGORY	TRIVIAL NAME	CHEMICAL NAME
Androgens	Testosterone	17β-hydroxy-4-androsten-3-one
	Androstenedione	4-androstene-3,17-dione
	Dehydroepiandrosterone	3β-hydroxy-5-androsten-17-one
Corticoids	Aldosterone	3,20-diketo-11β,21-dihydroxy-4-pregnene-18-ol
	Cortisol	11β,17α,21-trihydroxypregn-4-ene-3,20-dione
	Corticosterone	11β,21-dihydroxy-4-pregnene-3,20-dione
	11-Deoxycorticosterone	21-hydroxy-4-pregnene-3,20-dione
Estrogens	Estradiol-17β	1,3,5, (10) estratriene-3,17β-diol
	Estrone	3-hydroxy-1,3,5 (10)-estratrien-17-one
	Estriol	1,3,5 (10)-estratriene-3,16α,17β-triol
Progestogens	Pregnenolone	3β-hydroxy-5-pregnen-20-one
	Progesterone	4-pregnene-3,20-dione

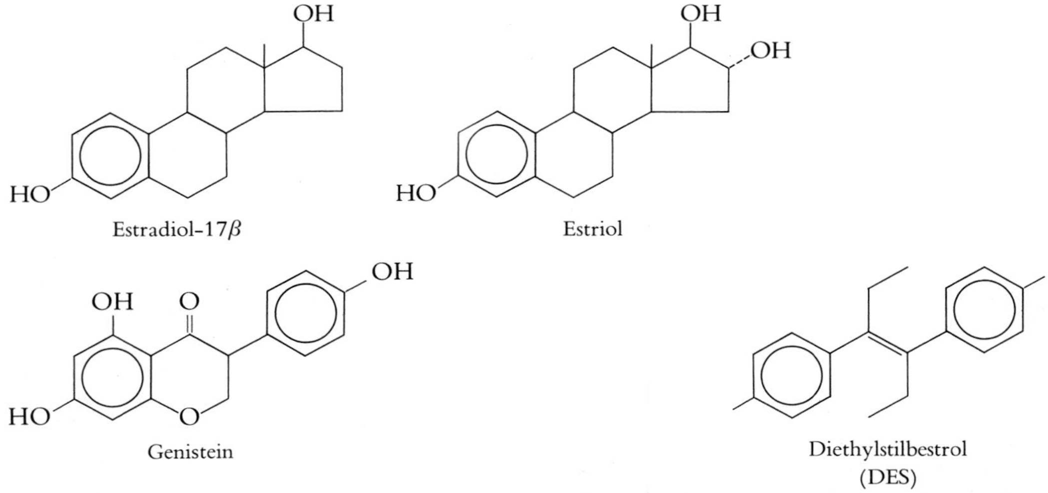

Estradiol-17β

Estriol

Genistein

Diethylstilbestrol (DES)

FIG. 9-2. Some C_{18} estrogenic steroids, the powerful synthetic estrogen, diethylstilbestrol (DES), and genistein, a substance found in certain clovers that can cause infertility in sheep.

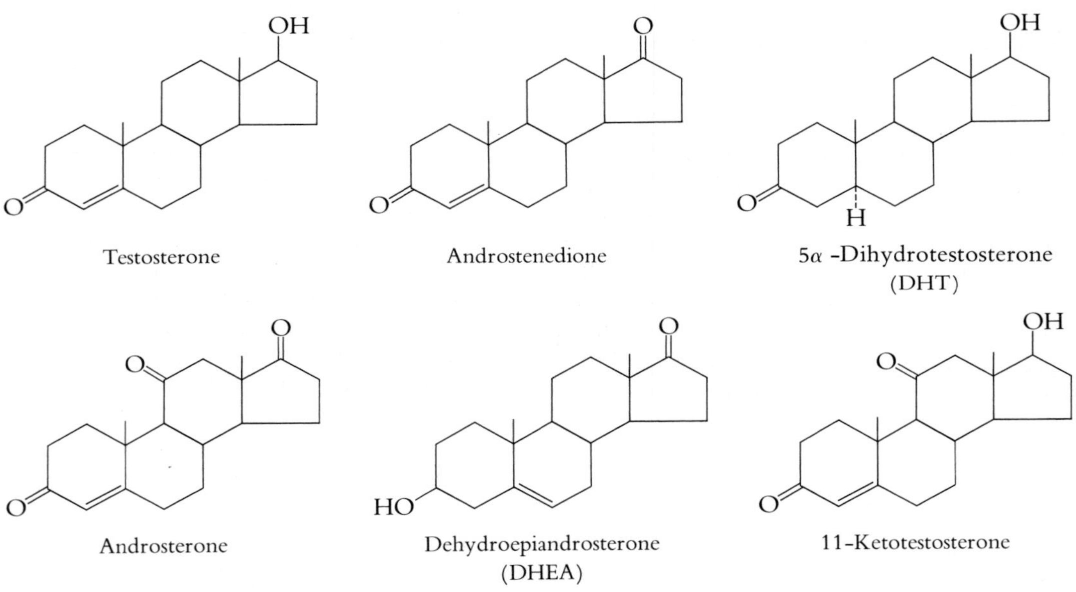

FIG. 9-3. Some C_{19} androgenic steroids.

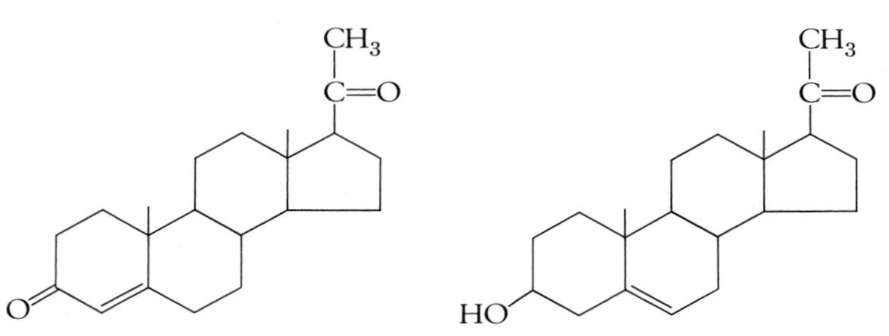

FIG. 9-4. Two important C_{21} progestogenic steroids, progesterone and its precursor, pregnenolone.

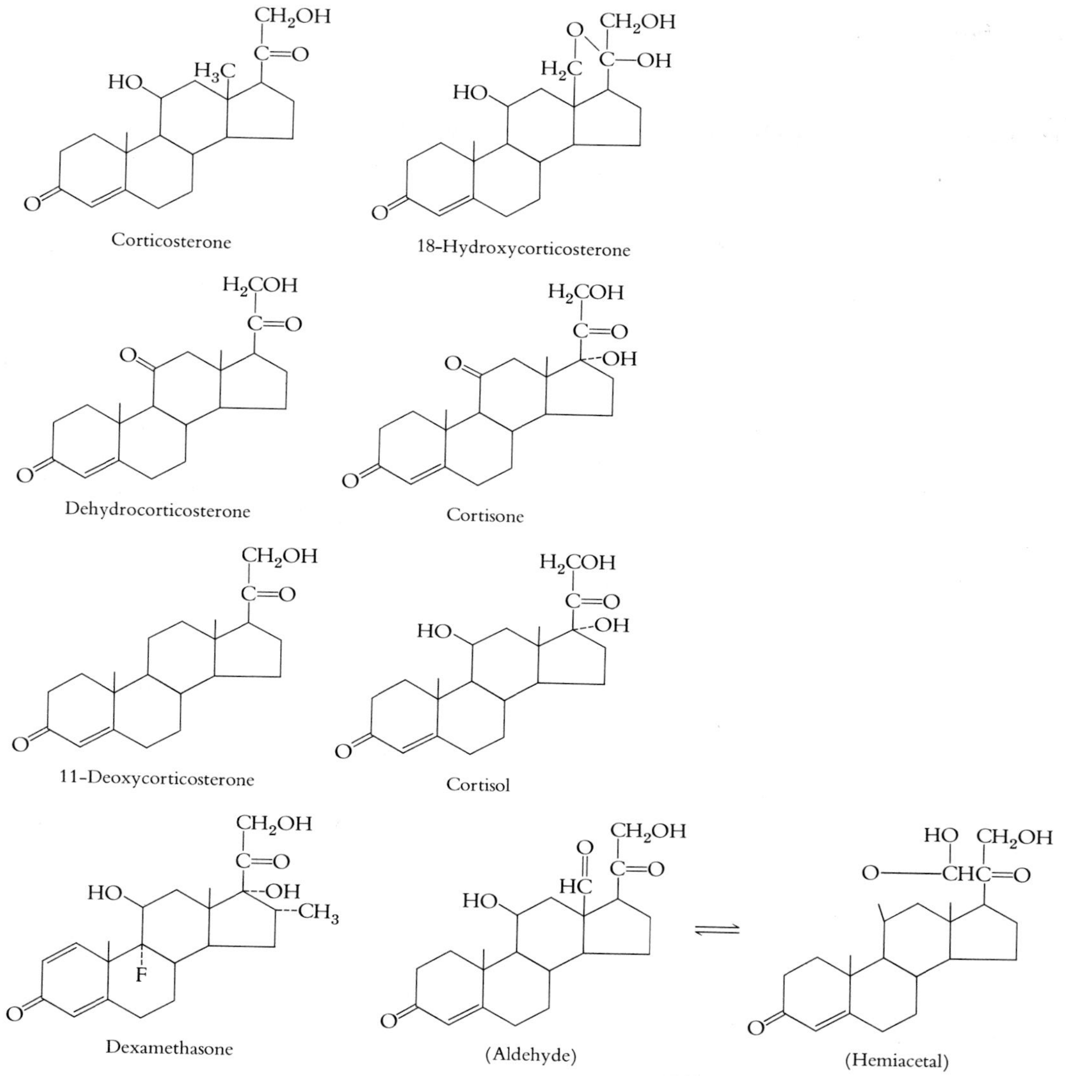

Corticosterone

18-Hydroxycorticosterone

Dehydrocorticosterone

Cortisone

11-Deoxycorticosterone

Cortisol

Dexamethasone

(Aldehyde)

(Hemiacetal)

Aldosterone

FIG. 9-5. Some C_{21} corticosteroids. Dexamethasone is a potent synthetic corticoid that mimics action of cortisol and some other corticoids.

The basic steroid nucleus contains 17 carbons, each designated by a number and arranged into four rings (Fig. 9-1). One scheme for naming steroids chemically relates each steroid to a hypothetical parent compound and modifies this name with one or more prefixes and no more than one suffix to designate the specific compound (Fig. 9-6). These hypothetical parent compounds are estrane (18 carbons or C_{18}), androstane (C_{19}) and pregnane (C_{21}). Naturally occurring estrogens and androgens possess the basic carbon skeleton of estrane and androstane respectively, whereas corticoids and progestogens are related to pregnane.

Presence of Double Bonds

The position of double bonds between carbon atoms within the steroid nucleus was formerly designated by the symbol Δ, followed by the number of the lowest-numbered steroid carbon with which the bond is involved. Thus, $\Delta 4$ would indicate a double bond between car-

TABLE 9-2. *Summary of Special Designations in Steroid Nomenclature*

DESIGNATION	EXPLANATION
Δ	location of double bond
-ene	one double bond in steroid nucleus
-diene	two double bonds in steroid nucleus
-triene	three double bonds in steroid nucleus
hydroxy-	hydroxyl (OH) substituted for hydrogen on nucleus
-ol	hydroxyl (OH) substituted for hydrogen on nucleus
oxo-	ketone (=O) substituted for hydrogen on nucleus
keto-	ketone (=O) substituted for hydrogen on nucleus
-one	ketone (=O) substituted for hydrogen on nucleus
α	atom or atoms attached to a given carbon of the steroid nucleus projects away from viewer
β	atom or atoms attached to a given carbon of the steroid nucleus projects toward viewer
Arabic number	indicates location of substitution or double bond

bons 4 and 5 in the steroid nucleus. Currently the term *ene* is used to refer to one double bond, *diene* for two double bonds, and *triene* for three double bonds in the nucleus, and the location of each bond is indicated by the number of the carbon preceding the location of the double bond (. . . 4-pregnene . . .).

Substitutions

Substituted groups applied to the steroid nucleus are designated according to the number of the carbon atom in the steroid nucleus to which they are attached. For example, *17-hydroxy* refers to the hydroxyl group (—OH) attached to carbon number 17. Hydroxyl groups are usually indicated as prefixes on the chemical name unless they are the only substitution on the parent molecule, in which case the hydroxyl group is designated by the suffix *-ol.* Ketone groups (=O) substituted on the steroid nucleus are indicated by the prefix *oxo-* or *keto-* and the suffix *-one;* 3,20-dione would refer to two ketone groups at positions 3 and 20 respectively.

Stereoisomerism

The carbon atom is capable of forming four covalent bonds. Two of these bonds are used when a given carbon is incorporated into the steroid nucleus. Because of the necessary bonding angles dictated by the tetrahedral shape of the carbon atom, the steroid nucleus itself does not exist in a flat plane as most diagrams of their chemical structures would suggest. Instead, the steroid nucleus may occur in either one of two forms termed the "boat" or the "chair," depending upon the conformation of the bonding. The chair form is believed to be the predominant form (Fig. 9-7).

The remaining two sites on the carbon atoms incorporated into the steroid nucleus can form covalent bonds with hydrogens, oxy-

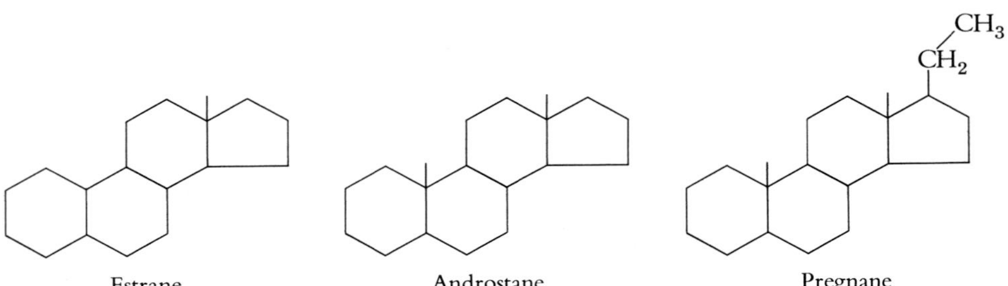

FIG. 9-6. Hypothetical steroids employed in steroid nomenclature.

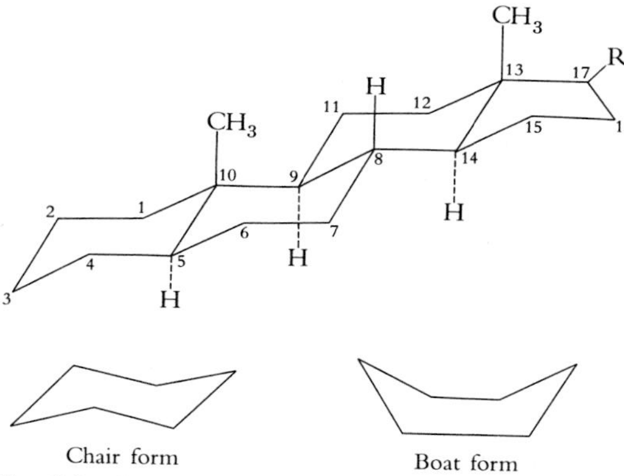

FIG. 9-7. Possible "chair" and "boat" configurations for steroid molecules. [After K.W. McKerns (1969). Steroid Hormones and Metabolism. Appleton-Century-Crofts, New York.]

gens or other carbon atoms. One of these bonds will project toward the viewer when examining the steroid as depicted in Figure 9-8, and the other will project away from the viewer, that is, into the page. Thus, two three-dimensional isomers (stereoisomers) could be formed by substituting one hydrogen on a given carbon with a hydroxyl group. The chemical formula would be the same, but the structure of the steroid would differ according to whether the —OH group projected out from or into the page. A spatial designation of α is used if the substituted group projects away from the viewer, and β is used if the group projects toward the viewer. In two-dimensional diagrams the α-position is indicated by a slashed or dotted line, whereas the β-position is designated with a solid line connecting the substituted group to its carbon (Fig. 9-8). Hydrogen atoms are usually not designated. Generally speaking, only one of the two possible isomers associated with substituted groups on the steroid nucleus will exhibit biological activity. Estradiol-17β, for example, is the most potent naturally occurring estrogen in vertebrates, whereas estradiol-17α has little or no estrogenic activity.

The chemical structures of several steroids are diagramed in Figures 9-2 to 9-5 with both chemical and trivial names indicated in Table 9-1. The reader should examine these chemical structures and determine the bases for the chemical name assigned to each steroid.

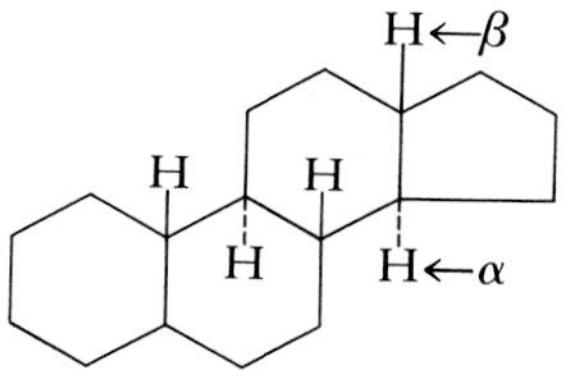

FIG. 9-8. Convention for indicating alpha and beta designations for steroids when drawn two-dimensionally.

Steroid Synthesis (Steroidogenesis)

All vertebrate steroid hormones, including vitamin D and its derivatives, are synthesized from cholesterol, a C_{27} steroid (Fig. 9-9). Cholesterol is synthesized from acetate (acetyl-coenzyme A) produced via glycolysis or via fatty acid oxidation. The synthesis of the steroid nucleus from acetate units is termed *steroidogenesis* and involves a series of enzymatically catalyzed reactions. Following synthesis of a relatively long hydrocarbon chain, a complex cyclization step results in closure of the carbon skeleton into the steroid nucleus. Some of the details of steroidogenesis are outlined in Figure 9-10. Cholesterol synthesized in this manner may be used directly in the biosynthesis of the various steroid hormones.

Most cholesterol is synthesized in the liver and is released into the blood as lipid droplets coated with protein (see Chap. 19). Adrenal cortex, ovaries and testes can utilize these lipoprotein complexes as sources of cholesterol. Synthesis of steroid hormones is accomplished from cholesterol obtained in this way or synthesized de novo in the cell.

Biosynthesis of Steroid Hormones

The first series of steps in the biosynthesis of steroid hormones from cholesterol involves side-chain hydrolysis to yield a C_{21} intermediate, *pregnenolone*. This compound may be altered further to C_{19} androgens that in turn may be modified to C_{18} estrogens. Pregnenolone may also be converted to progesterone

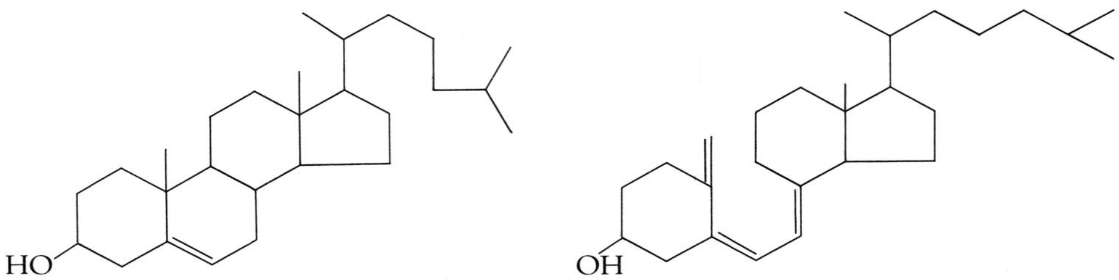

HO Cholesterol

OH Vitamin D_3 (Cholecalciferol)

FIG. 9-9. Structures of cholesterol and vitamin D_3 (cholecalciferol).

(C_{21}), from which the corticosteroids (C_{21}) may be synthesized. Corticosteroids may be synthesized directly from pregnenolone as well. Androgens and estrogens may also be synthesized from progesterone. A summary of basic pathways for steroid hormone biosynthesis is provided in Figures 9-11 to 9-14. After these schemes are examined in some detail, it should not be surprising to learn that many steroidogenic tissues produce more than one class of steroid molecule. The human adrenal cortex (adrenocortical tissue), for example, synthesizes progesterone, androgens and estrogens in addition to corticosteroids.

The mere presence of a given steroid in a tissue or the ability of a tissue to synthesize a particular steroid does not distinguish between a precursor role of that steroid for synthesis of another steroid or the possibility that the given steroid is secreted into the blood as a hormone. Furthermore, the administration of certain steroids to an animal might lead to their conversion to other steroids, and the observed effect might be due to this conversion product and not to innate activity of the applied steroids. Androgens may be converted to estrogens by a number of tissues, for example, and the observed action of the injected androgen may in reality be due to estrogens derived from the injected steroid.

Key Enzymes

Identification of certain key synthetic enzymes and quantitation of their activity levels are often used as indicators of the biosynthesis of steroid hormones. One key step is the conversion of pregnenolone. In steroidogenic tissue, catalytic activity of the enzyme responsible, *Δ5,3β-hydroxysteroid dehydrogenase* (3β-HSD), can be approximated histochemically in frozen sections, thus providing a crude measure of steroid hormone synthesis. Estimation of the rate of steroid hormone synthesis also infers a measure of the rate of release, because steroid hormones are not stored to any appreciable degree in steroidogenic cells and apparently are released into the circulation as they are synthesized. The drug *cyanoketone* is known to competitively inhibit the activity of 3β-HSD because of the structural similarity of cyanoketone to pregnenolone (Fig. 9-15). Cyanoketone blocks gonadal steroid biosynthesis and reduces circulating levels of gonadal steroids. Reduction in circulating steroids causes stimulation of gonadotropes in the adenohypophysis, and cyanoketone has proved useful in identification of gonadotropic cells.

Corticosteroidogenic tissue contains a mitochondrial enzyme, *11β-hydroxylase,* that applies a third hydroxyl group to form cortisol and corticosterone. The activity of this enzyme can be estimated with procedures similar to those described for 3β-HSD. The drug *metyrapone* selectively inhibits 11β-hydroxylase, thus blocking steroidogenesis in adrenocortical cells. Metyrapone has been used successfully to identify the illusive corticotropic cells of the adenohypophysis of many vertebrates.

Cytological Aspects of Steroid Hormone Biosynthesis

Biosynthesis of steroid hormones is, cytologically speaking, a very complex affair involving mitochondrial events as well as the

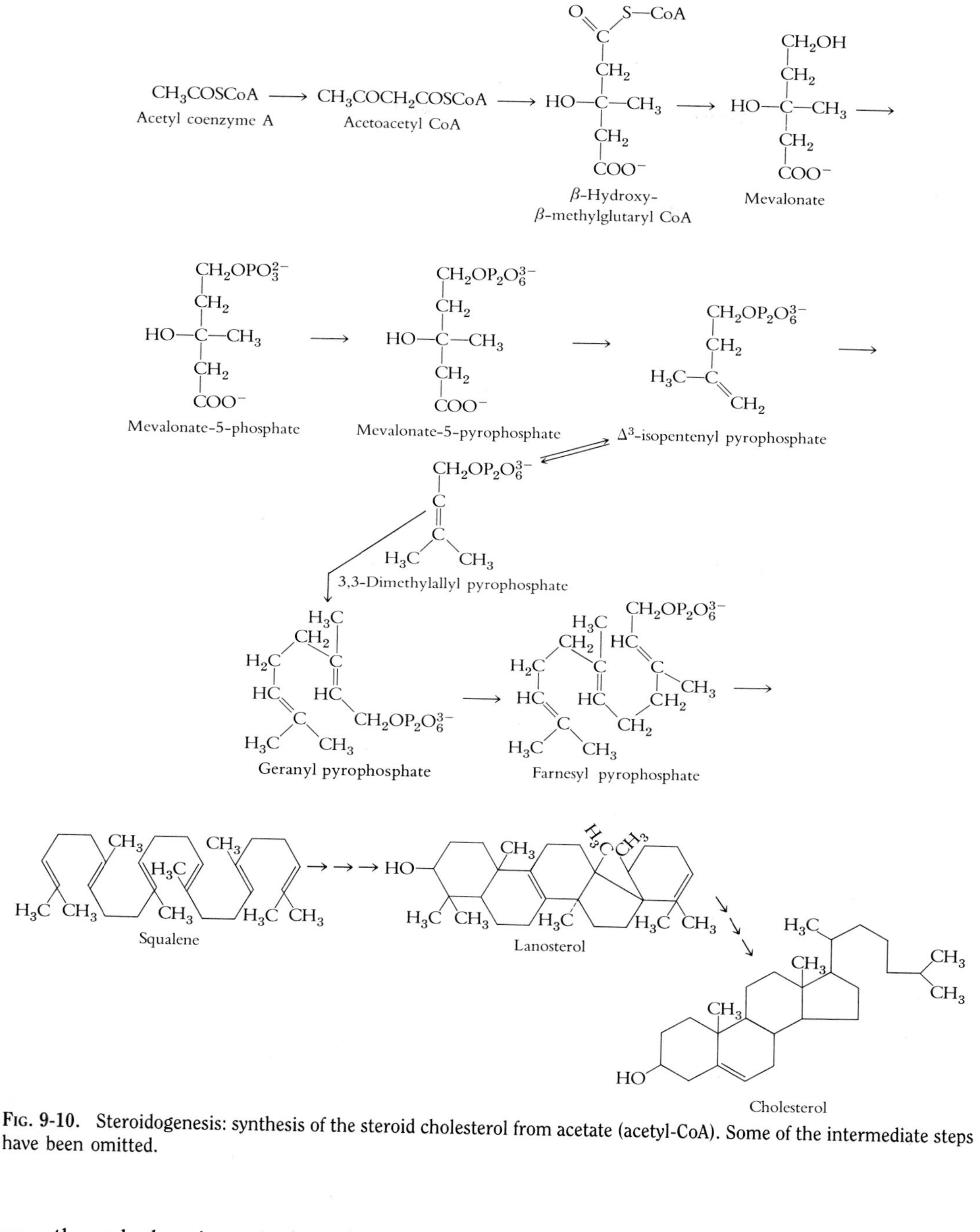

FIG. 9-10. Steroidogenesis: synthesis of the steroid cholesterol from acetate (acetyl-CoA). Some of the intermediate steps have been omitted.

smooth endoplasmic reticulum (SER). The importance of the latter is demonstrated by observations that a major cytological feature of steroidogenic cells is the abundance of SER.

The synthesis of cortisol illustrates one sequence of cellular events in steroid hormone biosynthesis (Fig. 9-16). Pregnenolone is synthesized in the mitochondria from cholesterol. The alteration of pregnenolone to progesterone, however, necessitates that pregnenolone travel to the SER for this conversion step. The addition of hydroxyl groups at the 17 and 20

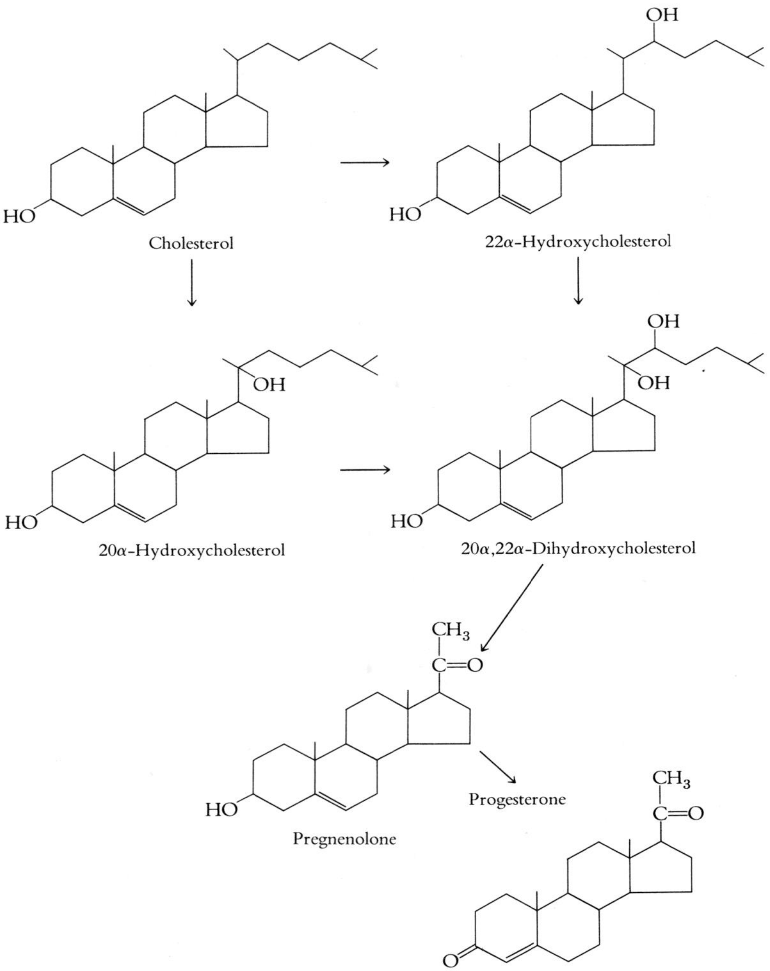

Cholesterol

22α-Hydroxycholesterol

20α-Hydroxycholesterol

20α,22α-Dihydroxycholesterol

Pregnenolone

Progesterone

FIG. 9-11. Synthesis of progesterone from cholesterol.

positions also occurs in the SER, resulting in 11-deoxycortisol. This compound must return to the mitochondria where the 11β-hydrolylase is located that converts 11-deoxycortisol to cortisol.

Transport of Steroid Hormones in Blood

Steroids are nonpolar compounds and consequently are not very soluble in aqueous solutions such as blood. Furthermore, free steroids readily pass through cellular membranes and rapidly disappear from the blood, primarily through the activities of the liver and kidneys. Therefore it is necessary that circulating steroids become associated with plasma proteins so that they can be retained longer in the circulation. Binding by plasma proteins reduces removal of active steroid hormones by the liver or kidney and their excretion via the urine. Thus, higher titers of steroid hormones can be maintained in the circulation, increasing the probability of their reaching appropriate target tissues.

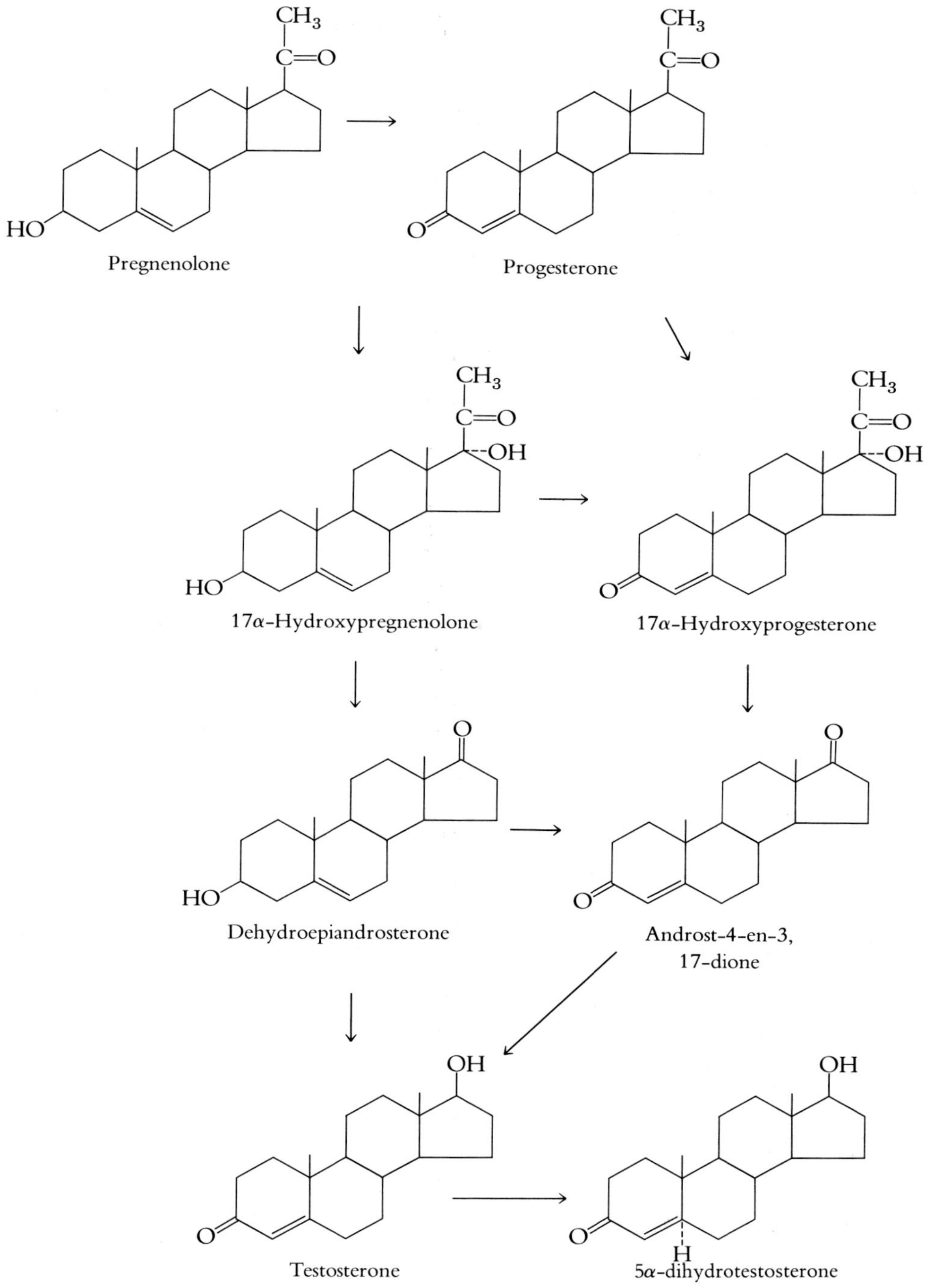
CH3
C=O
HO
Pregnenolone
CH3
C=O
O
Progesterone
CH3
C=O
OH
HO
17α-Hydroxypregnenolone
CH3
C=O
OH
O
17α-Hydroxyprogesterone
O
HO
Dehydroepiandrosterone
O
O
Androst-4-en-3,
17-dione
OH
O
Testosterone
OH
O
H
5α-dihydrotestosterone

FIG. 9-12. Synthesis of androgens.

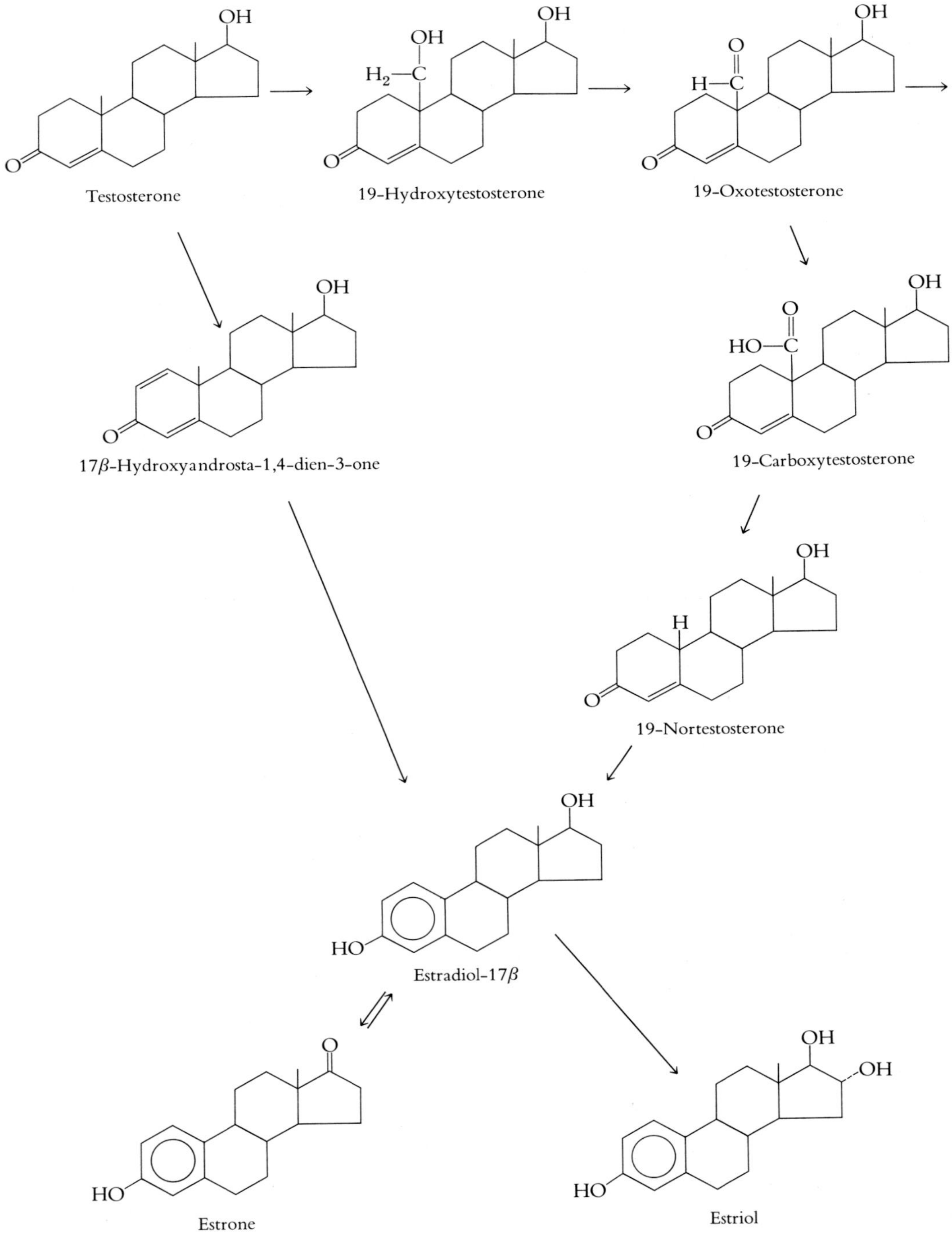

Testosterone

19-Hydroxytestosterone

19-Oxotestosterone

17β-Hydroxyandrosta-1,4-dien-3-one

19-Carboxytestosterone

19-Nortestosterone

Estradiol-17β

Estrone

Estriol

FIG. 9-13. Synthesis of estrogens.

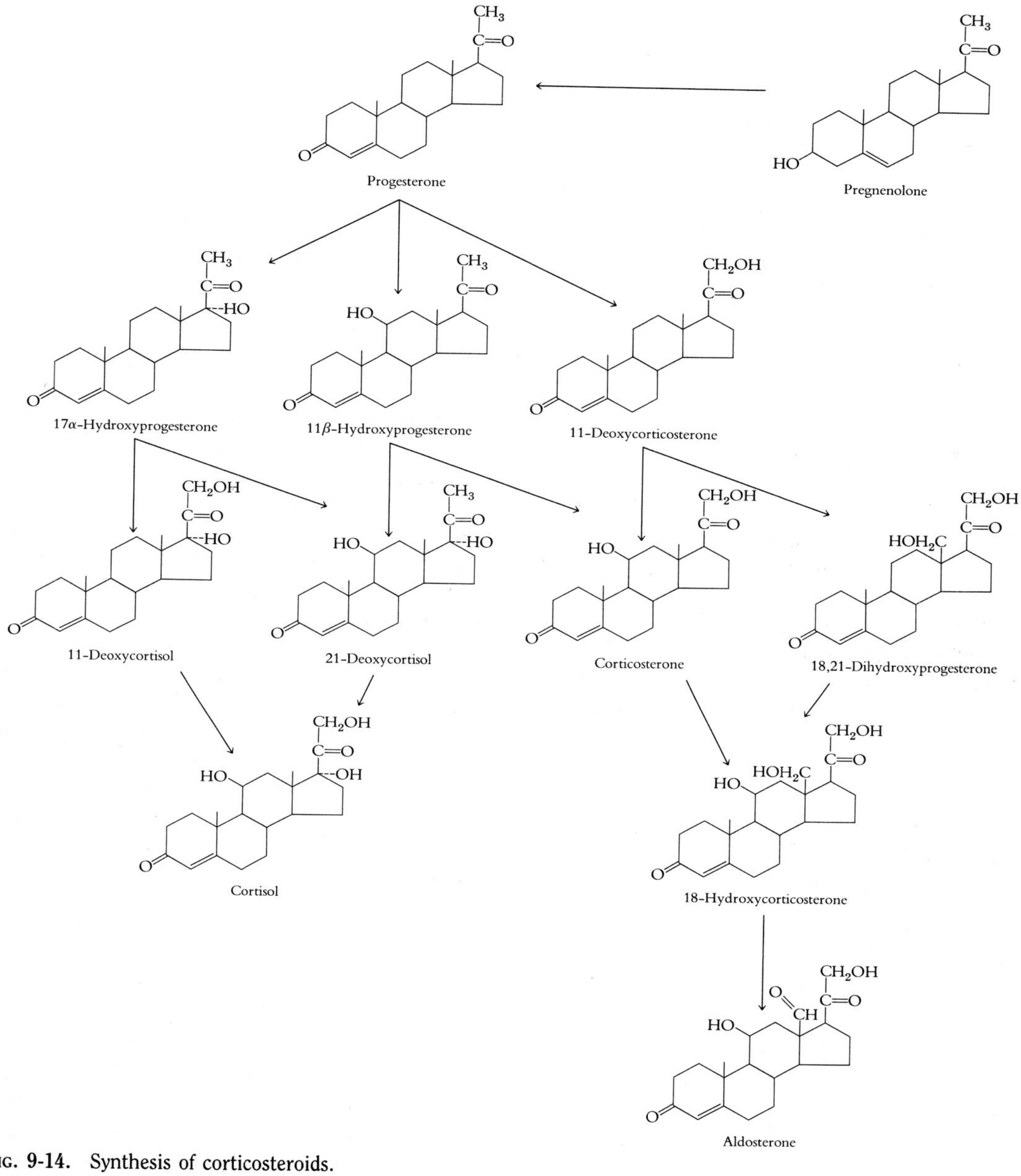

FIG. 9-14. Synthesis of corticosteroids.

Metabolism and Excretion of Steroid Hormones

Steroid hormones are metabolized primarily by the liver, which possesses a series of enzymes capable of altering the specific steroids to render them biologically inactive and water soluble. Target cells may also alter steroids metabolically, but it is the liver that performs the major task. Metabolism of steroids typically involves reduction or removal of side chains or attached groups or both, as well as conjugation of the altered molecule to glucu-

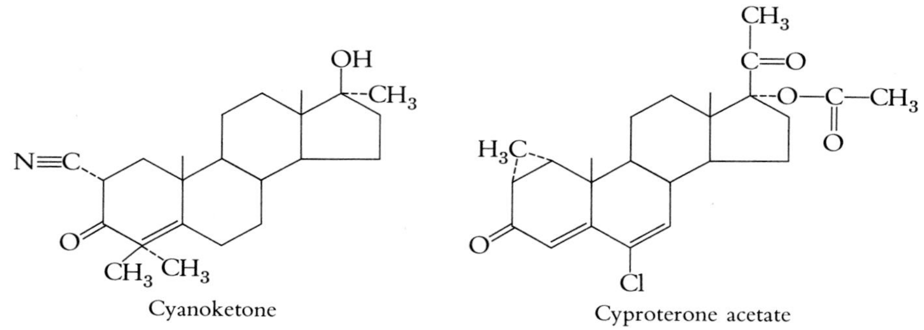

Cyanoketone

Cyproterone acetate

FIG. 9-15. Structure of cyanoketone (2α-cyano-4,4,17α-trimethyl-17-β-hydroxy-5-androsten-3-one) and the antiandrogen, cyproterone acetate (1,2α-methylene-6-chloro-Δ4,6-pregnadiene-17α-ol-3, 20-dione-17α-acetate).

ronic acid or sulfate (Fig. 9-17). The conjugates are water soluble and when released into the blood will no longer bind to serum proteins. Water soluble conjugates of steroid hormones readily appear in the urine. Some of the metabolized steroids are added to the bile and are excreted via the intestinal route.

Recently it was recognized that steroids also are metabolized via oxidative pathways as well as by reductions. These oxidized metabolites were not identified previously because they occur in a fraction of urine usually discarded when isolating urinary steroids for analysis. Oxidized steroid metabolites may represent a substantial portion of the total metabolites for a given steroid. For example, it is estimated that from 12 to 36% of circulating cortisol in humans is converted to *corotic acids* (cortolic and cortolonic acids).

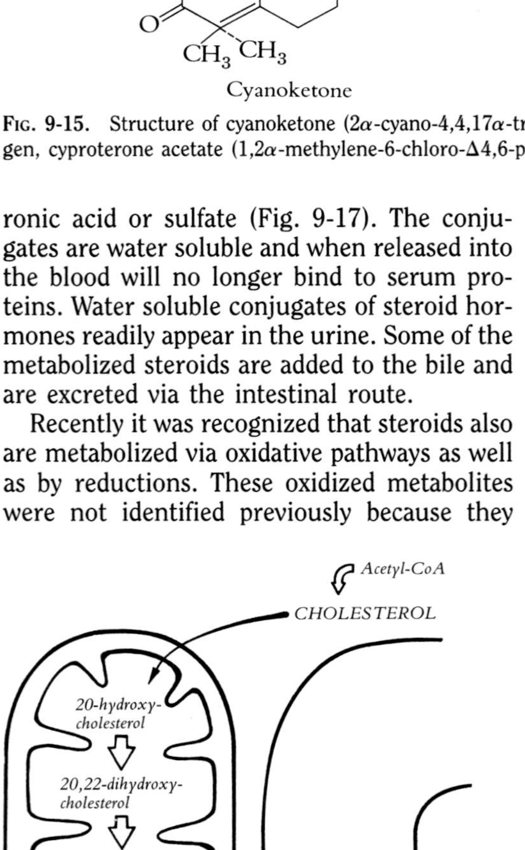

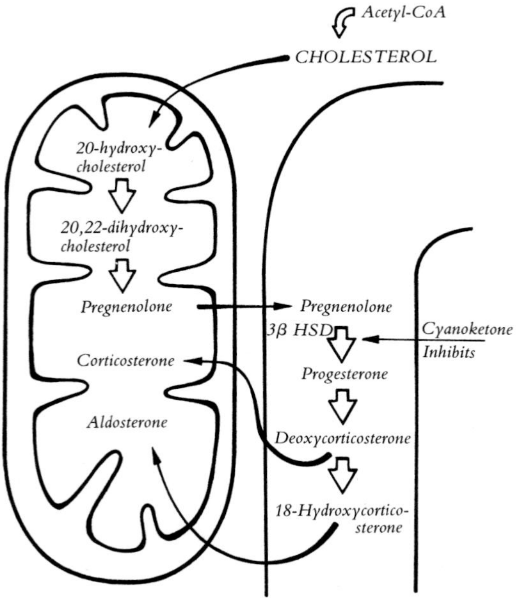

FIG. 9-16. Location of intracellular events involved in the synthesis of corticosterone. Cortisol is synthesized in a similar manner (see Fig. 9-14). [After B. Lofts and H.A. Bern (1972). The functional morphology of steroidogenic tissues. In Steroids in Nonmammalian Vertebrates. Academic Press.]

Androgens of both adrenal and gonadal origin are found in the urine primarily as sulfates and can be measured chemically as 17-ketosteroids. In addition, some androgens are found as conjugates with glucuronic acid. Estrogens may be excreted as either glucuronides or sulfates such as estriol glucosiduronate or estrone sulfate. Catechol estrogens are also common excretion products. Progestogens are excreted mainly as glucuronides of pregnanediol or pregnanetriol. However, pregnanediol may be formed from corticosteroid metabolism (that is, from deoxycorticosterone) as well as from progesterone. Pregnanetriol is formed principally from 17α-hydroxyprogesterone, but small amounts may also be produced from 11-deoxycortisol and 17α-hydroxypregnenolone. The corticosteroids are primarily excreted as 17-hydroxycorticosteroids conjugated with glucuronic acid.

A number of chemical methods have been employed to identify and quantitate various steroid metabolites in urine, the best known test probably being the Zimmermann reaction for 17-ketosteroids. However, the Zimmermann reaction does not distinguish accurately between corticoids and androgens. Pregnenolone, which is not a 17-ketosteroid and which appears in the urine during pregnancy, also gives a positive Zimmermann reaction. Preg-

Tetrahydrocortisol glucosiduronate (Cortisol)

Cortolic acid (Cortisol)

Androsterone sulfate (Testosterone)

Estrone-3-sulfate (Estradiol-17β)

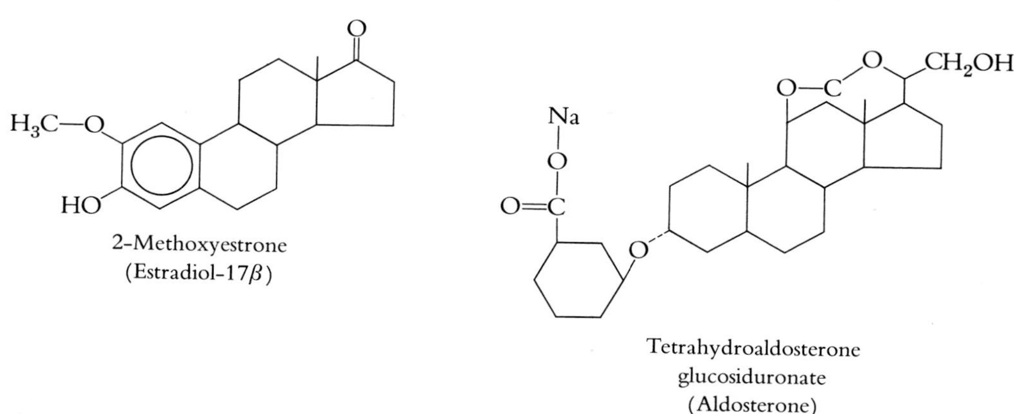

2-Methoxyestrone (Estradiol-17β)

Tetrahydroaldosterone glucosiduronate (Aldosterone)

FIG. 9-17. Steroid metabolites. The precursor hormone for each metabolite is indicated within parentheses.

nanetriol, which is characteristic of the andro-genital syndrome (masculinization or virilism in women), is also measured by this method. Because of the lack of specificity in the Zimmermann reaction and other chemical methods, as well as interference with these reactions by certain drugs and other substances that sometimes occur in urine (for example, glucose), such methods are being discarded in favor of rapid techniques such as radioimmunoassay for measuring blood levels of each specific steroid hormone. The greatest difficulty in measuring metabolic products from urine samples relates to the great variety of steroid metabolites that may appear in the urine, each of which must be determined independently. Furthermore, in the case of certain metabolites mentioned above, it is still not possible to identify which active steroid was the precursor.

Summary

Steroid hormones are synthesized from cholesterol (C_{27}), which is synthesized from acetate (steroidogenesis). In general the synthesis of steroid hormones from cholesterol is a catabolic process with respect to the carbon groups attached to the steroid nucleus. Pregnenolone (C_{21}) or progesterone (C_{21}) derived from pregnenolone, or both, may serve as intermediates in the synthesis of corticosteroids (C_{21}), androgens (C_{19}) or estrogens (C_{18}). Androgens are the immediate precursors for the synthesis of estrogens, and the glucocorticoids precede the synthesis of mineralocorticoids. The enzyme 3β-HSD is a key enzyme for pregnenolone synthesis, whereas 11β-hydroxylase is a key enzyme for corticoid synthesis. These and other enzymes may be quantified histochemically or with in-vitro assays as a measure of steroid hormone synthetic activity. Specific inhibitors of 3β-HSD and 11β-hydroxylase are cyanoketone and metyrapone respectively.

Circulating steroid hormones bind to specific plasma proteins. These hormones are removed from the blood and actively metabolized by the liver to form biologically inactive water-soluble sulfates or glucuronides. Most of these metabolites are excreted in the urine, although some steroid metabolites are eliminated via the release of bile into the intestine.

10·The Adrenal Glands: Cortical and Chromaffin Cells

The responses an animal makes to any stressful stimulus include the release of adrenal hormones. These hormones induce changes in metabolism that work to combat stress. Knowledge of this system contributes to an understanding of how animals adapt physiologically to physical and psychological traumas.

Mammals typically possess two adrenal glands, one located superior to each kidney (ad renal or supra renal) (Fig. 10-1). An adrenal gland consists of an outer portion composed largely of lipid-containing steroidogenic *adrenocortical* cells, the *adrenal cortex.* The cortex surrounds an inner mass of *chromaffin* cells, the *adrenal medulla.* The adrenocortical cells are derived from the coelomic epithelium in the pronephric region of the embryo adjacent to the genital ridge that gives rise to the gonads. These cells produce the corticosteroid hormones (see Chap. 9; Tables 10-1, 10-2) and are under the influence of corticotropin (ACTH) from the pituitary gland. In contrast, the chromaffin cells are of neural crest origin, and the medulla functions essentially like a sympathetic ganglion. The adrenal medulla is under direct neural control (cholinergic) and releases into the blood the normal neurotransmitter of most postganglionic sympathetic neurons, *norepinephrine.* In addition, the chromaffin cells secrete an important derivative of norepinephrine into the blood, *epinephrine.* (It should be noted that these substances can be considered neurotransmitters or neurohormones according to the site of release.)

There is no functional significance for the close anatomical relationship of these two distinctly different tissues (adrenocortical and chromaffin). Although there is participation of both systems with respect to adaptations to stressful stimuli, the factors controlling release of their secretions are not obviously related nor do their biological actions overlap. The anatomical closeness of the cortex and medulla in mammals as well as relationships of their homologous tissues in nonmammals may simply be a function of the physical closeness of their embryological sites of origin. There are some actions of ACTH and glucocorticoids on catecholamine synthesis by chromaffin cells, however.

The cortex and medulla are treated here as entirely separate endocrine glands, which is the case for many vertebrates. The adrenal cortex of mammals is discussed first and is followed by a comparative account of adrenocortical homologues in nonmammalian vertebrates. An account of the mammalian adrenal medulla and chromaffin tissues of nonmammals completes the chapter.

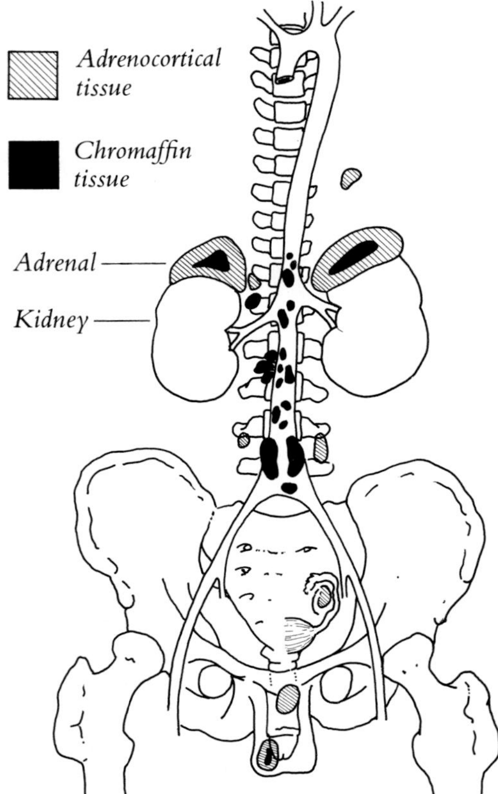

FIG. 10-1. The adrenal glands and distribution of adrenocortical and chromaffin tissues in humans. Note various locations where adrenocortical and chromaffin tissue may be found. This bisexual figure is modified from Bethune.[5]

Mammalian Adrenocortical Cells

The adrenal cortex of adult mammals may be subdivided by means of histological criteria into three well-defined regions: *zona glomerulosa, zona fasciculata* and *zona reticularis* (Fig. 10-2). In addition, a functional *fetal zone* is present in some fetal mammals and is related to maintenance of gestation.

The cells of the outermost region of the adrenal cortex, the zona glomerulosa, are smaller, more rounded and contain less lipid than those of the more central zona fasciculata. The zona glomerulosa is responsible for synthesis of the corticoid *aldosterone* as well as some other corticosteroids. There are few cytological changes in the zona glomerulosa following hypophysectomy or administration of ACTH, suggesting that the secretion of aldosterone is independent of pituitary control. Although ACTH is not necessary for steroidogenesis and release of aldosterone, the responsiveness of the glomerulosal cells to agents that normally elicit these events is reduced in hypophysectomized mammals and is enhanced with ACTH treatment.

The zona fasciculata consists of polyhedral (many-sided) cells that are sources of the so-called glucocorticoids such as *cortisol* and *corticosterone.* This region is characterized by many blood sinusoids that allow the cells to be bathed with blood. The proportion of cortisol and corticosterone secreted differs markedly, from secretion of primarily cortisol (man), through mixtures of both (cat), to primarily corticosterone (rat). The zona fasciculata is located between the zona glomerulosa and the zona reticularis and is histologically distinct from both.

The zona reticularis typically borders the adrenal medulla, and it contains numerous reticular fibers (hence its name). Some glucocorticoids and androgens are synthesized in this region,[75] but the majority of the glucocorticoids are secreted by the zona fasciculata. Unlike the zona glomerulosa both the zona reticularis and zona fasciculata atrophy following hypophysectomy, and treatment with ACTH restores them histologically and functionally to normal.

It should be noted that this "typical" anatomical pattern within the adrenal cortex and the relationship of cortex to medulla varies considerably within mammals as a group. Furthermore, ectopic nodules of functional cortical tissue are not uncommon, and this accessory adrenocortical tissue may become an important source for corticosteroids following adrenalectomy (Fig. 10-1).

The cortex of the mouse adrenal contains a unique *X-zone* between the zona reticularis and the medulla.[52] The X-zone degenerates in males at puberty and in females during the first pregnancy. The function of this region is not known.

The Fetal Zone

In many mammals, especially the human, a very conspicuous zone occupies the bulk of the

TABLE 10-1. *Circulating Levels of Corticoids in Selected Mammalian Species (Prototheria, Metatheria and Eutheria)*

SPECIES	MEAN STEROID LEVELS ± SD IN PERIPHERAL BLOOD				
	ALDOSTERONE (ng/dl)	CORTICOSTERONE (μg/dl)	CORTISOL (μg/dl)	DEOXYCORTICOSTERONE (ng/dl)	11-DEOXYCORTISOL (μg/dl)
Prototheria					
Echidna[a]	1.5	0.35	0.18	–	–
Echidna[b]	–	0.14±0.07	0.07±0.03	–	–
Echidna + ACTH[b]	–	1.06±0.56	0.42±0.23	–	–
Metatheria					
Black-tailed wallaby	8.2±4.3	0.12±0.02	1.1±0.2	3.3±0.6	0.13±0.08
Common wombat	0.9±1.4	0.06±0.02	0.04±0.04	2.0±1.3	0.14±0.08
Dingo	6.7±4.3	0.04±0.21	1.90±1.90	23.6±23.7	0.19±0.09
Koala	1.6±2.2	0.20±0.05	*	6.0±8.3	0.06±0.11
Eutheria					
Sheep	2.1±1.7	0.09±0.04	0.52±0.50	2.5±2.5	0.05±0.03
Dog	2.1±3.6	0.20±0.13	0.85±0.39	11.3±6.0	0.07±0.05
Fox	13.9±3.2	0.59±0.17	2.30±1.2	37.4±22.7	0.17±0.03
Balb/cfC3H mice[c]	–	12.00±2.16	–	–	–
Sand rat[d]	2.8±13.3	0.2±0.8	10.7±24.9	–	–

Modified from Oddie, C.J. et al.[84]
[a]Only one individual was examined.
[b]Sernia and McDonald.[102]
*Undetectable with technique employed.
[c]Hawkins et al.[43]
[d]Amirat et al.,[1] seasonal range.

adrenal gland prior to birth (Fig. 10-3). This region has been named the *fetal zone* and is responsible for the large size of the adrenal at birth. In humans the adrenal of the neonate may be as large as the total adrenal gland of a 10- to 12-year-old child.[5] During the gestation period the fetal zone synthesizes and releases

TABLE 10-2. *Corticoid and Progestogen Serum Levels in Normal Human Males*

STEROID	SERUM CONCENTRATION (ng/dl)
Progesterone	17.9
17-Hydroxyprogesterone	179.0
Deoxycorticosterone	6.6
Corticosterone[a]	421.0
Cortisol[a]	14,400.0
11-Deoxycortisol	49.0
18-Hydroxydeoxycorticosterone	20.0
Aldosterone	12.4

Modified from Schöneshöfer, M.[96]
[a]Data for corticosterone and cortisol reported for man by Oddie et al.[84] were 420±380 and 13,900±6,100 ng/dl respectively.

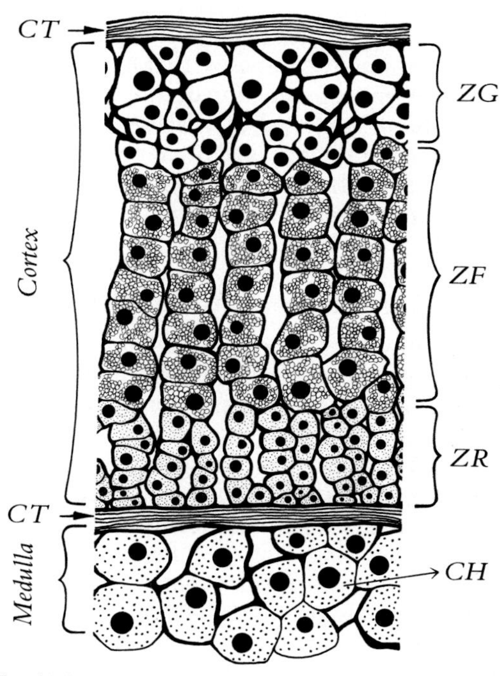

FIG. 10-2. Zonation in the mammalian adrenal: *ZG,* zona glomerulosa (cortex); *ZF,* zona fasciculata (cortex); *ZR,* zona reticularis (cortex); *CH,* chromaffin cells of the adrenal medulla, *CT,* connective tissue. (Modified from Gorbman and Bern.[40])

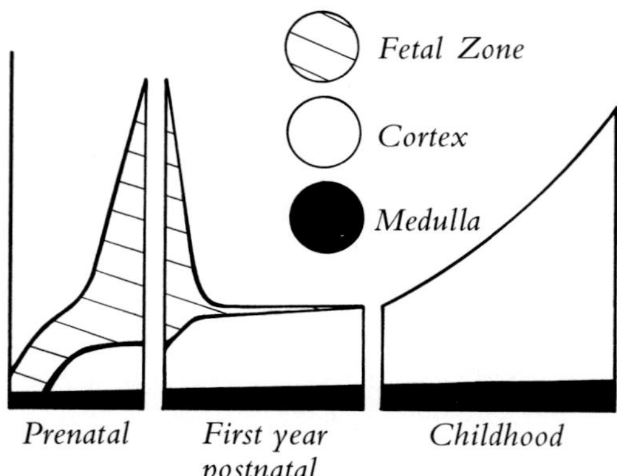

FIG. 10-3. Relative proportions of the adrenal gland represented by the fetal zone during gestation and childhood. (Modified from Bethune.[5])

relatively large quantities of the steroid *dehydroepiandrosterone sulfate* (DHEA), which serves as a precursor for synthesis of estrogens by the placenta. Failure of the fetal zone to produce adequate amounts of DHEA results in premature termination of gestation. Following birth the fetal zone ceases to function and degenerates rapidly. The zona reticularis continues to synthesize DHEA until about age 20 when its production declines. Although it has been suggested that DHEA may be an antitumor substance and/or a precursor for synthesis of other androgens or estrogens, the function of DHEA in adults is unknown.

Biological Actions of "Glucocorticoids"

Secretion of glucocorticoids from the zona fasciculata and zona reticularis is under direct control of the hypothalamo-hypophysial axis involving corticotropin-releasing hormone and ACTH respectively (see Chaps. 4 and 5). Circulating ACTH levels are depressed by elevated levels of glucocorticoids and are increased following adrenalectomy, establishing the existence of direct negative feedback of corticosteroids on ACTH release. Corticotropin is released by direct neural input to the hypothalamus as a result of such stressful events as physical trauma (injury, surgery), and this response may occur even in the presence of elevated glucocorticoid levels. Thus, stressful stimuli can bring about and maintain a severalfold increase in glucocorticoid levels. The ability of traumatic stimuli to override the normal negative feedback mechanism verifies the importance of neural control over ACTH release.

Glucocorticoids produce marked effects on energy metabolism at physiological doses as a result of changes in transport of materials into cells and induction of new enzyme syntheses. Their major effect is to supplant and conserve the energy normally derived from circulating glucose by (1) inhibiting glucose utilization by peripheral tissues (for example, muscle), (2) stimulating entry of amino acids into cells and their conversion to glucose and storage as glycogen and (3) stimulating mobilization of fat stores. It has been suggested that the normal physiological role for glucocorticoids is that of "permissive agents" that through changes in membrane permeabilities to important metabolites and the synthesis of new enzymes provide the appropriate cellular environment in which other hormones such as growth hormone and glucagon may operate. The interactions of glucocorticoids and other hormones with respect to energy metabolism are discussed in more detail in Chapter 19.

Secretion of glucocorticoids follows a circadian pattern that is thought to be entrained by the light-dark cycle. Studies in rats[65] and humans[91] suggest these cycles are regulated by food intake rather than by light-dark or wake-sleep cycles. Elevated corticoids may be related to their metabolic actions.

GLUCOCORTICOIDS AND STRESS. The responses characteristic of adaptations to chronic stress are mediated by glucocorticoids. These responses have been incorporated by Selye into a general theory of adaptation to stress termed the *general adaptation syndrome.*[100,101] According to Selye, there are three stages of adaptation by an organism to stressful stimuli. Stress is used as an all-encompassing term to include all stimuli that are harmful or potentially harmful to the organism. The first phase of the general adaptation syndrome is the *alarm reaction,* which includes a generalized increase in sympathetic stimulation involving the adrenal medulla as well as increased secretion of glucocorticoids. This phase is frequently marked by enlargement of the adrenal glands, primarily due to hypertrophy of the zona fasciculata and to some extent the zona reticularis of the cortex.

Under the influence of glucocorticoids the organism adapts to the continued presence of the stressful stimuli. This phase of adaptation is termed the stage of *resistance* and is characterized by prolonged increased secretion of glucocorticoids. (It can be argued whether this is truly adaptation or the lack of adaptation.)

Finally, under continuation of extremely stressful conditions, the ability of the organism to function normally is impaired. The continuous presence of the stressful stimuli causes the organism to enter the final stage of *exhaustion* that leads to death.

Stress of experimental animals is important when attempting to interpret data on corticosteroid levels or nutrient levels (amino acids, glucose, etc.). Laboratory conditions alone can influence the adrenal axis. Stress can also influence the levels of other hormones. For example, the order in which groups of rats were removed from a common holding facility and killed at a remote site influenced the mean levels of PRL that were measured for each group.[97] Since it is not possible to undertake experimental work on animals free from stress, detailed knowledge of how animals were maintained and all procedures involved with an experiment is essential when interpreting results.

Pharmacological Actions of Glucocorticoids. The glucocorticoids are better known for their pharmacological actions and therapeutic side effects than for their biological actions.[5] The tremendous potential for glucocorticoids in the treatment of the rare hypoadrenocorticism described by Thomas Addison in 1885 (Addison's disease) was not recognized for many years. However, the discovery of the anti-inflammatory effects of cortisone, a synthetic glucocorticoid, and its use for treatment of rheumatoid arthritis spurred a tremendous explosion in therapeutic applications of glucocorticoids. The debilitating symptoms of rheumatoid arthritis relieved by glucocorticoid therapy are the consequence of inflammation associated with an autoimmune response in which the patient produces antibody against his own connective tissue. Glucocorticoid therapy alleviates painful inflammation occurring as a result of the immune reaction but does nothing to correct the causative factors.

One of the most recent therapeutic applications of glucocorticoids is suppression of the entire immune response following tissue and organ transplantations. Although normal therapeutic doses (anti-inflammatory) of glucocorticoids do not interfere with normal antigen-antibody interactions, very high doses depress new antibody synthesis.

Glucocorticoids interfere with the elaboration of histamine or with its actions in mediating the inflammatory response, which includes local hyperemia and resultant edema, or with both. One postulated mechanism for this interference is the inhibition of the *kallikreins,* which catalyze formation of *kinins* from a plasma precursor protein.[18] Kinins also induce inflammation. The release of histamine normally observed following the combination of antigen and antibody is caused by kinins. Another suggestion for glucocorticoid anti-inflammatory activity stems from observations of their effects on lysosomes. Glucocorticoids stabilize lysosomal membranes, thereby reducing release of hydrolytic enzymes following cell injury and hence reducing the spread of the inflammatory reaction.[5] Glucocorticoids may inhibit the synthesis of leukotrienes and reduce inflammation (see Chap. 15).

Mechanism of Glucocorticoid Action. Glucocorticoid effects on target cells are described in Chapter 1. The initial requirement for glucocorticoid action on liver cells is binding to intracellular receptors and eventual stimulation of nuclear RNA synthesis (both messenger RNA and ribosomal synthesis). Approximately 2 to 4 hours following application of glucocorticoids there is an increase in new enzymes that bring about the changes in cellular metabolism characteristic of glucocorticoid action. In liver cells these new enzymes include those associated with the conversion of amino acids into glucose and the polymerization of glucose to form glycogen. Amino acid transport into the liver cell is also stimulated. In contrast, glucocorticoids inhibit the uptake of amino acids and the metabolism of glucose in peripheral tissues such as skin and adipose cells.

Excessive doses of glucocorticoids inhibit protein synthesis in certain tissues (for example, muscle, bone and lymphoid tissue), which has been related to some of the adverse side effects of glucocorticoid therapy. These protein catabolic effects are not manifest in liver cells even at very high doses. The basis for this difference is not known.

Aldosterone: The Principal Mammalian "Mineralocorticoid"

The zona glomerulosa secretes aldosterone independently of direct pituitary control, although, as mentioned earlier, ACTH appears to play a permissive role in maintaining the responsiveness of these cells to other controlling factors. The major action of aldosterone is maintenance of the normal sodium-potassium balance in body fluids, and its secondary action is to regulate extracellular fluid volume. Aldosterone stimulates sodium reabsorption by the nephrons in the kidney. The mechanism controlling secretion of aldosterone involves a most complex and seemingly round-about series of events involving both liver and kidney, the *renin-angiotensin system.*

Control of Aldosterone Secretion

The Renin-Angiotensin System. *Renin* is an enzyme produced in the kidney by the *juxtaglomerular body,* a modified group of cells in the afferent arteriole carrying blood to the glomerulus[25,88] (Fig. 10-5). This enzyme is a glycoprotein (about 40,000 daltons) possibly secreted as a larger, inactive form (mol wt 63,000) or prorenin. Conversion of prorenin to renin may be accomplished by the activity of kidney kallikrein (see Chap. 15). Development of renin activity from prorenin also occurs following mild acidification of the plasma. The juxtaglomerular body is intimately associated with a modified region of the distal convoluted portion of the nephron known as the *macula densa.* Together these two structures comprise the *juxtaglomerular apparatus.*

Blood volume (pressure in the renal arterioles) and sodium concentration in the glomerular filtrate as it enters the proximal convoluted tubule control renin release. Intrarenal arteriolar pressure is monitored by stretch receptors in the juxtaglomerular body. Renin is released in response to a decrease in this pressure. Sodium concentration in the tubular lumen is monitored by cells of the macula densa, and low sodium levels somehow trigger communication between the macula densa and the juxtaglomerular body, resulting in renin release. Changes in either or both parameters influence renin secretion.

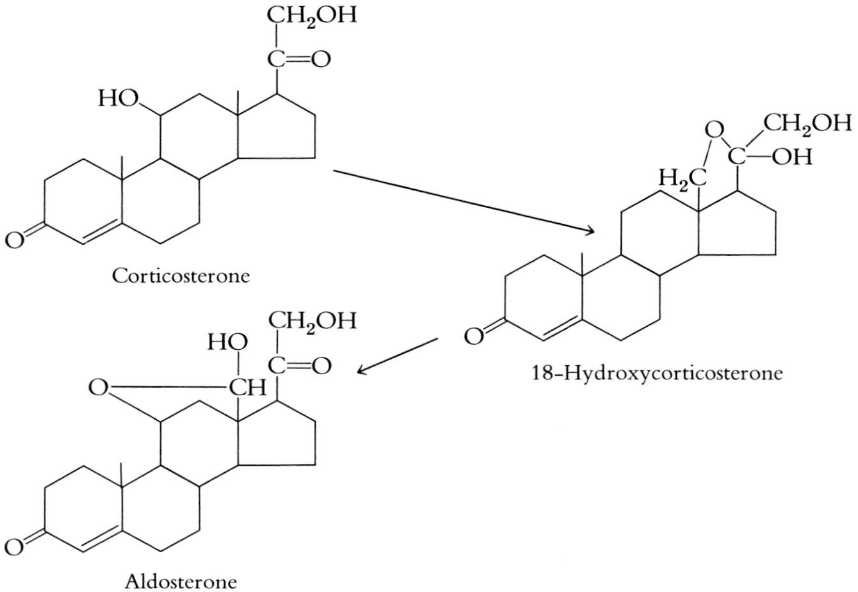

Fig. 10-4. Synthesis of aldosterone from corticosterone.

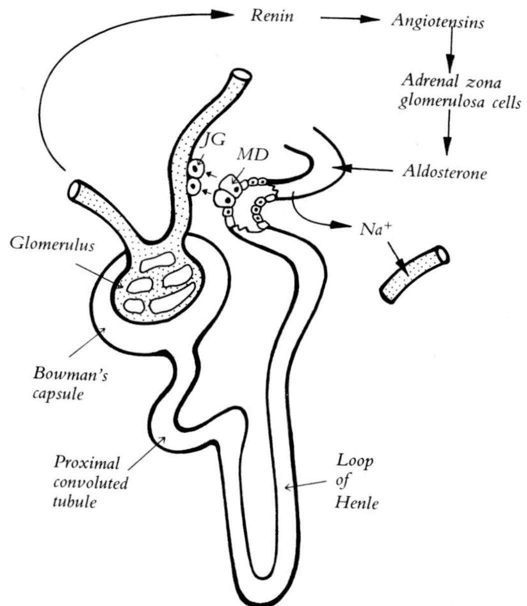

FIG. 10-5. The juxtaglomerular apparatus. The blood vascular components are stippled. Modified endothelial cells of the afferent arteriole *(JG)* produce renin; the macula densa *(MD)* consists of modified cells of the distal convoluted portion of the nephron that presumably can influence renin release from the juxtaglomerular cells *(arrows)*. Renin influences aldosterone release from the zona glomerulosa of the adrenal cortex, which in turn influences Na^+ reabsorption. See text for details and Figs. 10-6 and 10-7.

Once renin enters the blood it comes in contact with a plasma protein termed *renin substrate* that was synthesized by the liver (Fig. 10-6). Mammalian renin substrates are large glycoproteins (mol wt 58,000–110,000) and behave like α_1-globulins, α_2-globulins and albumin in humans, herbivores and rodents respectively.[88] Renin causes the enzymatic release of a small peptide (decapeptide) known as *angiotensin I* from renin substrate (angiotensinogen). Angiotensin I facilitates release of norepinephrine from the adrenal medulla and produces direct and indirect pressor effects on the cardiovascular system. One effect is the elevation of intrarenal blood pressure that is an important contributor to pathological renal hypertension. A *converting enzyme* converts angiotensin I to an octapeptide, *angiotensin II.* This octapeptide is also a potent vasoconstricting agent and helps restore blood pressure to normal by decreasing arteriole diameter.[4]

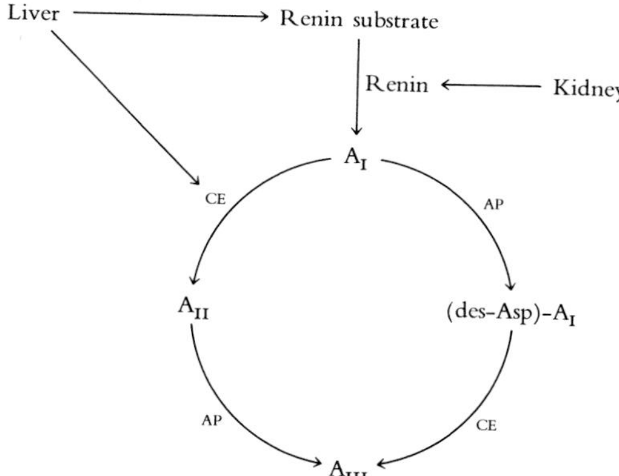

FIG. 10-6. Synthesis of angiotensins. Renin from the kidney releases angiotensins I *(A_I)* to be hydrolyzed to the octapeptide angiotensins II *(A_{II})* by the converting enzyme *(CE)*. The plasma enzyme *(AP)* forms the heptapeptide angiotensin III *(A_{III})* from A_{II}. Angiotensin III may also be formed by these same enzymes operating in reverse order through the intermediate, des-Asp-angiotensin I *(des-Asp-A_I)*.

Converting enzyme is localized to a number of capillary beds, suggesting that angiotensin II produces vascular effects in a number of tissues. The second important action of angiotensin II is the causation of increased synthesis and release of aldosterone from cells of the zona glomerulosa. Angiotensin II may be further metabolized to a heptapeptide known as *angiotensin III* (Figs. 10-5 and 10-7) that may

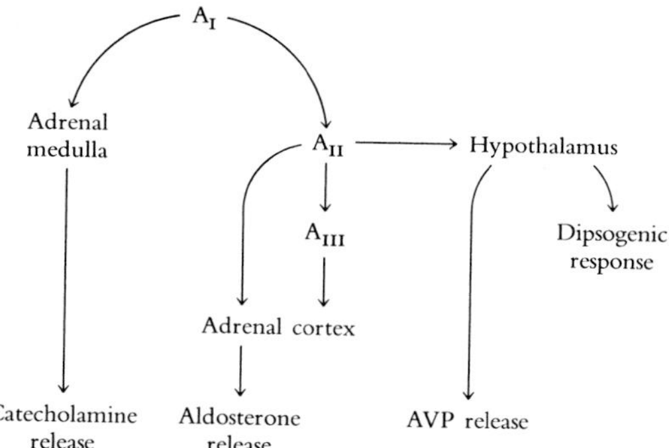

FIG. 10-7. Actions of angiotensins. Vasoactive functions are not shown. Angiotensin I *(A_I)* can directly cause release of catecholamines (epinephrine and norepinephrine) from the adrenal medulla. Angiotensin II *(A_{II})* may induce a dipsogenic response and cause release of arginine vasopressin *(AVP)* via effects on the hypothalamus. Both A_{II} and angiotensin III *(A_{III})* can stimulate aldosterone release from the adrenal cortex.

also stimulate aldosterone release. The importance of this latter conversion is not clear[88] but may be related to stepwise hydrolysis and inactivation. Aldosterone stimulates increased reabsorption of sodium and some increased excretion of potassium by cells of the distal convoluted portion of the nephron as well as increased sodium reabsorption by the proximal convoluted portion. This increased sodium reabsorption aids in water retention, reduces urine volume and helps to restore fluid volume. The renin-angiotensin-aldosterone mechanism is closely linked functionally to the role of vasopressins (arginine and lysine vasopressins) in maintaining normal blood osmotic conditions (see Chap. 7). Angiotensin II stimulates drinking (dipsogenic response) and causes release of vasopressins through actions on the hypothalamus. These two effects contribute to the maintenance of normal fluid balance.

This elegant but rather circuitous mechanism for regulation of extracellular fluid volume and sodium levels may be relatively unimportant, however, in normal homeostatic regulation of sodium concentrations and extracellular fluid volume. This suggestion is supported by observations that fixed quantities of glucocorticoids and mineralocorticoids are sufficient to maintain normal homeostatic balance in people with Addison's disease regardless of wide variations in salt and water intake. Aldosterone, like its cousins the glucocorticoids, may play a permissive role in the regulation of salt and water balance and other mechanisms may be more important for determining the magnitude and direction of salt and water movements.

Additional Factors Controlling Aldosterone Secretion. High levels of potassium in extracellular fluids directly stimulate aldosterone secretion, which, in turn, promotes renal potassium loss. In contrast, extracellular sodium variations do not directly influence aldosterone secretion unless unusually large variations are produced.

One additional extrarenal mechanism has been proposed for controlling aldosterone release. Presumably in response to low circulating sodium levels, the pineal gland secretes a peptide (?) hormone, *adrenoglomerulotropin,* that supposedly stimulates release of aldosterone.[33] However, the importance of this mechanism, not to mention its existence, is questionable.

Mechanism of Aldosterone Action. Aldosterone stimulates sodium reabsorption and potassium excretion in the distal convoluted tubule of the kidney and possibly enhances some sodium reabsorption in the proximal convoluted portion, intestinal mucosa, salivary glands and sweat glands.

Aldosterone produces the typical steroidal pattern of action on target cells. Increased nuclear RNA synthesis results in production of a specific protein, *aldosterone-induced protein,* which somehow mediates the movement of sodium across the target cells somewhat reminiscent of the mechanism for movement of calcium ions across cells of the duodenal mucosa (see Chap. 9). The actual mechanism of this sodium pump and its relationship to potassium excretion are unknown.

Pathologies of the Adrenal Axis

Glucocorticoid Hypersecretion

Cushing's Syndrome. This syndrome was described by Cushing in 1932. Hypersecretion of ACTH by basophilic pituitary adenoma is the cause of this condition. The adrenal cortices are hypertrophied and plasma cortisol levels are elevated (hypercortisolism). Excessive cortisol levels have adverse effects on metabolism of many tissues including the brain, muscles, skin, vascular tissue, kidney, liver and skeleton. Hypophysectomy alleviates the symptoms but necessitates extensive replacement therapies. Adrenalectomy requires only corticoid therapy.

Cushing's Disease. The symptoms of this disease are the same as those for Cushing's syndrome, but the cause is different. Hypercortisolism in Cushing's disease occurs from excessive secretion of cortisol by adrenal adenomas, adrenal carcinomas, gonadal-adrenal rest tumors or from endocrine or nonendocrine cancers that elaborate an ACTH-like peptide.

Corticosteroid-secreting tumors suppress CRH and ACTH which brings about atrophy of the adrenals. Adrenal hypertrophy occurs when the cause is ectopically produced ACTH-like peptides.

Glucocorticoid Hyposecretion

Addison's Disease. This disease is characterized by a shortage or absence of cortisol resulting in hypersecretion of ACTH. Hyperpigmentation (excessive darkening of the skin) occurs in most cases because of the innate MSH-activity of this ACTH. Aldosterone and adrenal androgen production are also depressed.

The person with Addison's disease is usually hypoglycemic due to lack of cortisol. Absence of aldosterone causes other symptoms including muscle weakness, water losses, hypotension and salt-craving. The loss of adrenal androgens becomes a problem only for postmenopausal or castrate women (see Chap. 11) who rely on the adrenal as their sole androgen source.

The most common cause of Addison's disease is bilateral atrophy of the adrenals resulting from tuberculosis. It may also occur as a result of drug-induced or congenital deficiencies in steroidogenetic enzymes.

Secondary Hypoadrenocorticism. Hypothalamic or pituitary lesions that block production of CRH or ACTH can produce the symptoms of hypoadrenocorticism. People with secondary hypoadrenocorticism lack the hyperpigmentation which usually accompanies Addison's disease but have the other symptoms. This condition can develop as a result of hypophysectomy, autoimmune disorders, viral illnesses, prolonged morphine administration and other causes. The most common origin of the disorder is prolonged therapy with cortisol or related steroids employed as anti-inflammatory agents or immune suppressants.

Disorders of Aldosterone Secretion

Hyperaldosteronism. This condition is characterized by low blood potassium, high blood sodium and muscle weakness. Elevated sodium levels bring about water retention and may produce hypertension. Hyperaldosteronism may result from an adenoma or carcinoma in the zona glomerulosa that autonomously secretes excessive amounts of aldosterone. These symptoms also develop when ACTH or ACTH-like peptides are elevated chronically. Treatment with aldosterone inhibitors can reduce these symptoms until the source of the excessive aldosterone is removed.

Hypoaldosteronism. Loss of the zona glomerulosa through adrenalectomy or Addison's disease, congenital or drug-induced depression of aldosterone production and defects in the renin-angiotensin system can induce hypoaldosteronism. Potassium excretion is reduced, sodium is lost in the urine and water retention is impaired. Imbalances in sodium/potassium ratios alter muscle and nerve function. These conditions can be alleviated by treatment with aldosterone.

Adrenal Excesses in Androgens

Adrenal androgen production may be elevated in several hyperadrenocorticoid conditions such as Cushing's syndrome. Adrenal tumors may secrete excessive quantities of adrenal androgens. Symptoms of excessive production of adrenal androgens in women include hirsutism, acne, seborrhea, irregular menses and reduced fertility, lowered voice pitch, atrophy of the breasts, possible thinning of hair and recession of the scalp in the temporal region, clitoral enlargement and hypertrophy of skeletal muscles. These same symptoms may be present in males but are not noticeable. Young adult women that exhibit anorexia nervosa (a disorder characterized by greatly reduced food intake) and an elevated adrenal axis may develop facial hair (hirsutism) as a result of ACTH-induced secretion of adrenal androgens.

Side Effects of Corticosteroids

Corticosteroids are administered in high doses to achieve their therapeutic effects. This is especially true of glucocorticoids. Adverse side effects occur as a consequence of prolonged therapy.

Adverse Effects of Glucocorticoid Therapy. The beneficial therapeutic effects of glucocorticoids are manifest only when applied at doses two to three times physiological levels. Consequently a number of adverse side effects occur with prolonged administration of glucocorticoids, including mild diabetes mellitus (Chap. 13), muscle weakness due to extensive protein catabolism (an effect that does not occur with physiological doses), osteoporosis due to destruction of bone substance, reduced activity of the immunological response system and mental depression.

Adverse Effects of Aldosterone Therapy. Excessive doses of mineralocorticoids (or glucocorticoids) cause sodium retention and consequent accumulation of fluids (edema), as evidenced by rapid weight gain following their administration. However, an "escape" phenomenon, due to unknown factors, occurs, and the condition is alleviated before serious complications arise and irreparable damage has occurred. In cases of cardiac failure the escape mechanism also fails.

Aldosterone therapy results in decreased blood potassium and increased urine potassium. Excessive aldosterone causes severe potassium losses that can induce muscle cramps and muscle weakness. These events occur primarily because of adverse effects on cell membrane characteristics and resultant alterations of normal muscle cell physiology.

Comparative Aspects of Adrenocortical Tissue

The anatomical organization of the adrenocortical homologues and chromaffin cells differs markedly with the only obvious uniformity being a tendency for combining both cellular types in one organ, the adrenal gland of amniotes (Fig. 10-8). Although the term chromaffin may be used to designate the catecholamine-secreting cells responsible for elaborating epinephrine and norepinephrine in all vertebrates, several terminologies have been proposed in attempting to deal with the diverse character of the adrenocortical homologues, including *interrenal cells, corticosteroidogenic cells* and *adrenocortical cells.* The last term will be used here because even though the adrenals of nonmammals lack the anatomical cortex-medulla relationship (and in many cases no adrenal gland per se is present), "adrenocortical" does denote the functional and evolutionary relationship of this cellular type to those of the mammalian adrenal cortex.

Cytologically the adrenocortical cells of nonmammals resemble the steroidogenic cells of the mammalian zona fasciculata. Adrenocortical cellular types of cyclostomes, teleosts and nonmammalian tetrapods possess a well-developed smooth endoplasmic reticulum, mitochondria with tubular cristae and numerous osmiophilic (lipoidal) inclusions. Following stimulation with ACTH, pituitary extracts or appropriate environmental stimuli, these cells exhibit increased basophilia, increased enzymatic activity (Δ^5,3β-hydroxysteroid dehydrogenase [HSD]) and decreased lipid content. Atrophy of the adrenocortical cells follows hypophysectomy.

Zonation of the adrenocortical cells is suggested cytologically in some anurans, reptiles and birds, and two separate cellular types have been claimed for the bullfrog *Rana catesbeiana* and for birds.[89,113] However, too little work has been done to establish firmly the existence of more than one type of adrenocortical cell in most nonmammals.

Adrenocortical cells of fishes differ most from the general mammalian pattern of corticosteroidogenesis with respect to some of the hormones produced. However, the general sequences for corticosteroidogenesis are similar in all the vertebrates with respect to precursor-product relationships, with many of the same enzymes being involved (Chap. 9). Among the nonmammalian tetrapods the nature of corticosteroid secretion is nearly identical, and the pattern of secretion is very similar to that described for cells of the mammalian zona glomerulosa.

Daily rhythms and seasonal variations in corticosteroid secretory patterns occur in nonmammals as well as in mammals. Peak seasonal adrenocortical activity is roughly correlated to periods of reproductive activity, although a cause-effect relationship cannot be categorically applied. Some studies suggest that "stress" may be the critical factor and that stressors associated with reproduction may be only one component involved in stimulating

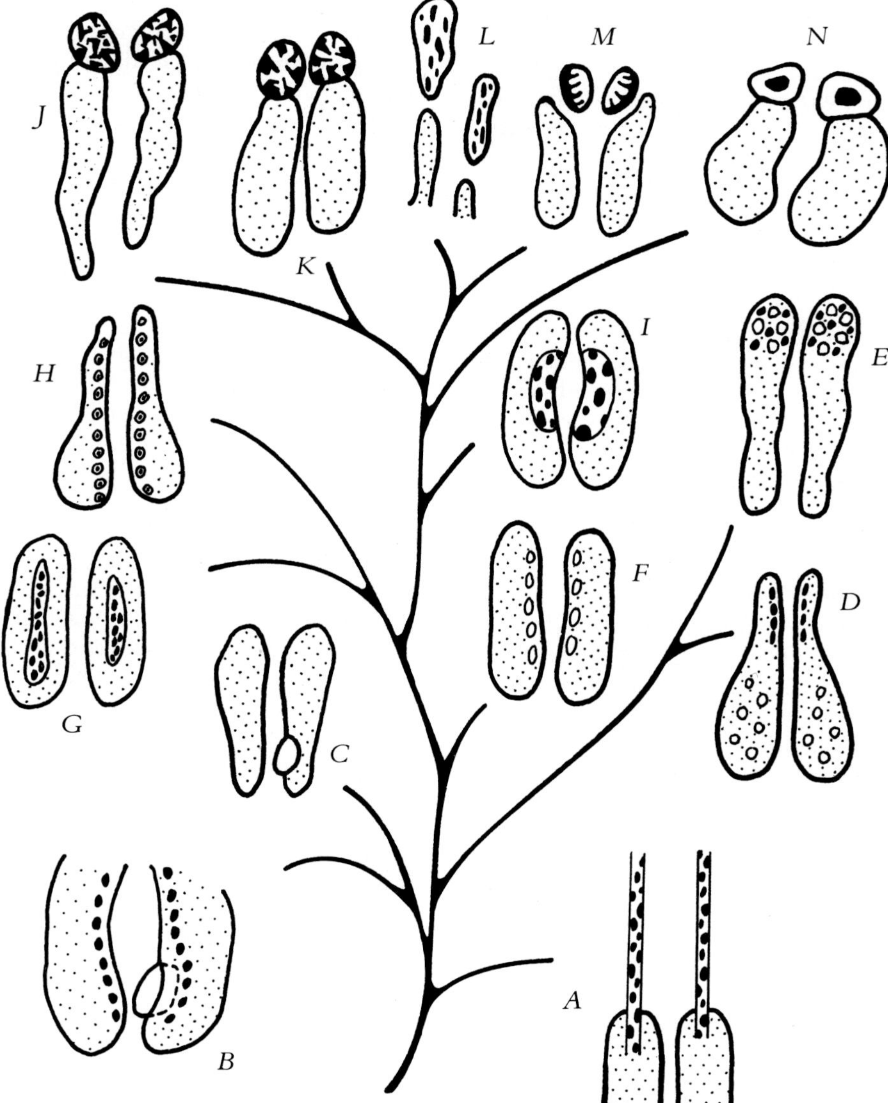

FIG. 10-8. Phylogeny and anatomy of vertebrate adrenal glands. The outlines of the much larger kidneys are shown for reference *(stipple)*. The homologous tissue to the mammalian adrenocortical cells is clear, chromaffin tissue is black. Note that in the cyclostomes the adrenal tissue follows the surface of the anteriorly projecting cardinal veins. Chromaffin tissue is not shown for the ratfish (Holocephali).
A, Cyclostomata; *B*, Elasmobranchii; *C*, Holocephali; *D*, Holostei; *E*, Teleostei; *F*, Dipnoi; *G*, Anura; *H*, Caudata; *I*, Chelonia; *J*, Aves; *K*, Crocodilia; *L*, Squamata (snakes); *M*, Squamata (lizards); *N*, Mammalia

adrenocortical function (albeit a major one). The responses of nonmammals to stresses such as surgery, forced exercise and handling are very much like those described for mammals.

Class Agnatha: Cyclostomata

In lampreys presumed adrenocortical cells have been identified as islands of cells above the pronephric funnels in the kidney as well as in the walls of the large dorsal blood vessels (postcardinal veins) in this same region.[42] Although in-vitro studies employing radioactively labeled steroidal precursors (pregnenolone, progesterone or both) have not demonstrated the ability of these presumed adrenocortical cells in lampreys or hagfishes to produce corticosteroids,[17,118] cortisol, cortisone, corticosterone and 11-deoxycortisol have been isolated from hagfish and lamprey plasma[55,118] (Table 10-3). Enzymes such as HSD have not been demonstrated in cyclostome adrenocortical cells, however.[99] The site for corticosteroidogenesis has not been established in cyclostomes, and more studies of this group are needed.

No evidence of either renin or a juxtaglomerular apparatus has been found in cyclostomes.[78,80]

Class Chondrichthyes

Elasmobranchs and holocephalans have one large unpaired gland consisting exclusively of adrenocortical cells and located between the posterior ends of the kidneys (that is, truly interrenal). In addition, small islands of adrenocortical cells may be found on the surface of the kidneys extending anteriorly.[16]

In 1934 Grollman and coworkers used extracts of the interrenal glands from three *Raja* species to maintain adrenalectomized rats, demonstrating the presence of corticosteroids in these glands.

Elasmobranchs produce a unique corticosteroid, 1α-hydroxycorticosterone.[56,109] The enzyme necessary for synthesizing this unique steroid, *1α-hydroxylase,* is found only in the elasmobranch interrenal gland. Holocephalans lack 1α-hydroxylase and cannot secrete 1α-hydroxycorticosterone. The Pacific ratfish *Hydrolagus colliei* secretes primarily cortisol.

In-vitro studies of shark interrenals *(Scyliorhinus caniculus)* using exogenous pregnenolone as a substrate result in synthesis of primarily corticosterone and 11-deoxycorticosterone with lesser amounts of 1α-hydroxycorticosterone.[103] When endogenous precursors only are involved, the primary product in vitro becomes the anticipated 1α-hydroxycorticosterone.[109] There are no 18- or 17α-hydroxylases present in the shark interrenal, and consequently aldosterone, cortisol, cortisone and 11-deoxycortisol are not synthesized (see steroid structures in Chap. 9). Data from plasma analyses, however, indicate that not only is 1α-hydroxycorticosterone secreted in elasmobranchs[57,58] but also cortisol and corticosterone[56] (Table 10-3). Such discrepancies between in-vivo plasma levels and in-vitro synthesis occur in other vertebrate classes as well, and one should be extremely cautious in extrapolating from in-vitro capabilities in which various intermediates and products accumulate to in-vivo situations in which the final products are removed (secreted into the blood). Accumulation of intermedi-

TABLE 10-3. *Circulating Corticosteroids*[a] (μg/ml) in Cyclostomes and Elasmobranch Fishes.[8]

SPECIES	TREATMENT	F	B	DOC	1α-HC	11-DOC
Cyclostomes:						
Myxine glutinosa	ACTH	0.09	0.30			0.34
	Control	0.07	0.02			
Eptatretus stouti	Untreated	—	0.008			0.027
	Saline	—	0.013			0.015
	ACTH	0.022	0.044			0.008
Petromyzon marinus	Untreated	0.005	0.002			
Elasmobranchs:						
Raja laevis			0.16	0.42	0.94	0.03
Squalus acanthias			2.50		2.80	0.16

[a]F, cortisol; B, corticosterone; DOC, deoxycorticosterone; 1α-HC, 1α-hydroxycorticosterone; 11-DOC, 11-deoxycortisol.

ates and products in the vicinity of the secretory cells under in-vitro conditions upsets chemical equilibria so that unusual ratios of steroids are observed.

Aldosterone has not been identified in vivo or in vitro in either elasmobranchs or holocephalans, and the capacity to produce this steroid may be lacking. Indeed, it would appear that the renin-angiotensin system is absent also in elasmobranchs although it may be present in holocephalans.[78–80]

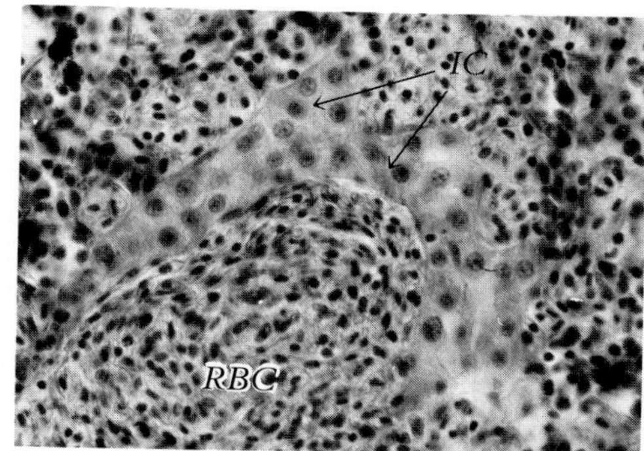

Fig. 10-9. Adrenocortical cells (interrenal) from head kidney of rainbow trout *Salmo gairdneri*. *IC*, steroidogenic cells; *RBC*, red blood cells occupying a sinusoidal space.

Class Osteichthyes: Actinopterygii

The anatomical arrangement of adrenocortical cells in the Actinopterygii differs markedly from that described for all other fish groups.[16] In the sturgeons and polypterine fishes (Chondrostei) as well as in the ganoids (Holostei) the adrenocortical cells are scattered in small clumps throughout the kidney. The identification of these cells is hampered in the ganoids *(Amia, Lepisosteus)* by the presence of large numbers of *corpuscles of Stannius,* which although not steroidogenic do resemble cytologically the adrenocortical cells. The teleostean adrenocortical cells are embedded in the most anterior portion of the kidney, known as the *head kidney.* Frequently these cells are associated with the dorsal posterior cardinal veins as described for cyclostomes. The head kidney has lost its renal function and consists mostly of lymphoid tissue, nonfunctional pronephric tubules and small islands of adrenocortical cells. The teleostean adrenocortical cells are often referred to as *interrenal tissue,* although "intrarenal" would be a more descriptive term. In a few species all of these cells surround the posterior cardinal veins, and none are associated with the kidney (Figs. 10-9, 10-10). Because of the diffuse nature of the adrenocortical tissue in teleosts it is not possible to remove these cells surgically, and one must resort to the use of selective inhibitors of corticosteroidal synthesis such as metyrapone (see Chap. 9).

The principal circulating steroid in the Chondrostei, Holostei and Teleostei is cortisol, with corticosterone, aldosterone and some others present in minor quantities in the teleosts (Table 10-4). Bony fishes lack the 1α-hydroxylase of elasmobranchs and consequently do not synthesize 1α-hydroxycorticosterone. In-vitro studies with teleostean adrenocortical cells indicate that they convert pregnenolone preferentially to cortisol. When progesterone is supplied as a precursor the

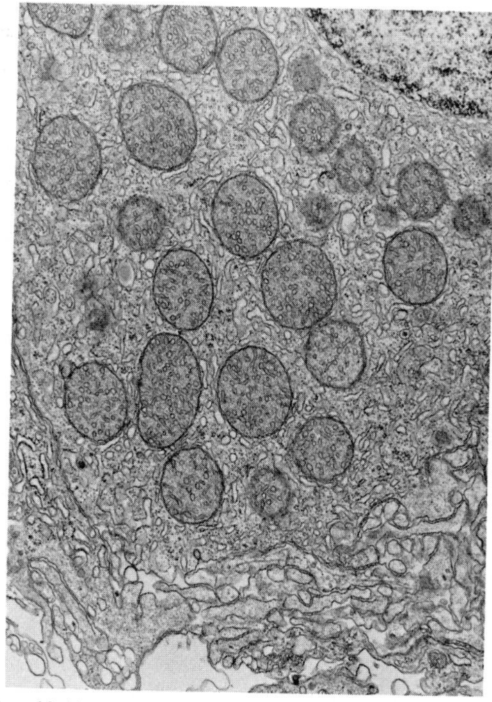

Fig. 10-10. Active adrenocortical cell of juvenile coho salmon. Prior to seaward migration the production of corticosteroids increases as reflected in this cell, which exhibits abundant smooth endoplasmic reticulum and numerous mitochondria with tubular cristae. (Courtesy of Dr. H.S. Bern and Richard Nishioka.)

TABLE 10-4. *Circulating Corticosteroids (ng/dl) in Bony Fishes*

ORDER	SPECIES	CORTISOL	CORTICO-STERONE	DOC	11-DEOXY-CORTISOL	ALDO-STERONE	REF.
Chondrostei	*Acipenser oxyrhynchus*	181	7.0	8.0	7.0		10
Holostei	*Amia calva*	760					10
Teleostei	*Salmo trutta* (M)	2,400	22.0				36
	Oncorhynchus tshawytscha	100–500					59
	Carassius auratus	44,000	7,200	800?		110?	10
	Clupea harengus	75,000	60				10
Dipnoi	*Lepidosiren paradoxa*	6,000	160		30	580	54
	Neoceratodus fosteri (M)			4.4		1.2	10
	N. fosteri (F)			3.2		5.0	10

principal product is corticosterone.[53] Nevertheless, cortisol primarily is produced in vivo.

Renin-Angiotensin System. Renin activity is present in all of the spiny-rayed fish groups. Histological and cytological identification of renal cells exhibiting renin granules has not been verified in any of the nonteleostean actinopterygian fishes, however (Table 10-5).

Corpuscles of Stannius. The corpuscles of Stannius embedded in the kidney of actinopterygian fishes were once thought to be steroidogenic. However, they lack the necessary steroidogenic enzymes, and it is unlikely that they play any significant role in the endogenous synthesis of corticosteroids.[10,59] The major function of the corpuscles of Stannius appears to be related to calcium regulation (see Chap. 12).

Class Osteichthyes: Sarcopterygii

The Dipnoi have been of special interest to comparative endocrinologists seeking to understand the evolution of corticosteroids since they represent close relatives to both the fish and tetrapod lines. In dipnoan fishes the adrenocortical cells are found as small cords located between renal and perirenal tissues adjacent to branches of the postcardinal veins. Adrenocortical cells from estivating *Protop-*

TABLE 10-5. *Distribution of Renin Activity and Presence of Renal Cells Containing Renin Granules in Fishes*

CLASSIFICATION	SPECIES	RENIN ACTIVITY	RENIN GRANULES
Osteichthyes			
Actinopterygii			
Polypteri	*Polypterus senegalis*	+	−
	Erpetoichthys calabaricus		−
Chondrostei	*Acipenser breviorostris*	+?	−
Holostei	*Amia calva*	+	−
	Lepisosteus osseus	+	−
Teleostei	*Anguilla rostrata*	+	
	Opsanus tau	+	+
Sarcopterygii			
Crossopterygii	*Latimeria chalumnae*	+	+
Dipnoi	*Lepidosiren paradoxa*	+	+
	Protopterus aethiopicus	+	+

Modified from Nishimura, H. and M. Ogawa (1973). The renin-angiotensin system in fishes. Am. Zool. 13:823–838.

terus synthesize corticosterone in vitro from progesterone.[60] However, only cortisol was identified in the plasma of the aquatic phase,[70] suggesting a tetrapod-like secretion (corticosterone) during its moist, air-breathing phase and a teleostean-like secretion (cortisol) during its aquatic phase. Although it is tempting to speculate on the evolutionary significance of these data, it would be premature to do so without further investigation.

Aldosterone, cortisol, corticosterone and a trace of 11-deoxycortisol are found in the blood of the South American lungfish *Lepidosiren paradoxa,*[54] which is more dependent on remaining in the water than its African cousin *Protopterus.* The levels of both aldosterone and cortisol were high (about 6 μg/dl for each), whereas corticosterone levels were much lower (0.16 μg/dl). The aquatic Australian lungfish *Neoceratodus fosteri* secretes aldosterone and deoxycorticosterone, but in very small amounts (1.2 and 4.4 ng/dl respectively in males and 5.0 and 31.9 ng/dl respectively in females).[6] These data would suggest that the lungfishes are intermediate between the tetrapod condition (aldosterone and corticosterone) and the actinopterygian fishes (cortisol) with respect to which corticoids are prominent. It would be interesting to know which corticosteroids are secreted by adrenocortical cells of the coelacanth fish *Latimeria* (Crossopterygii).

Renin-Angiotensin System. Renin activity and the presence of renal cells containing renin granules have been observed in the coelacanth *Latimeria chalumnae* and in two genera of lungfishes (Table 10-5). No experimental evidence for either a vascular effect or an effect on adrenocortical cells has been reported, however.

Class Amphibia

The adrenocortical cells of the Amphibia are extrarenal and extremely variable with respect to their location.[41] In anurans, adrenocortical tissue is found in irregular nodules organized loosely into a pair of interrenal glands on the ventral surface of the kidneys. However, in *Xenopus laevis* the adrenocortical tissue is organized as small islets on the ventral surface of the kidney. Each of these adrenocortical islets also contains two or three chromaffin cells. In most anurans, some chromaffin cells are associated with the interrenal glands, and in one anuran, *Rana hexadactyla,* there are more chromaffin cells than adrenocortical cells in the interrenal glands.

In addition to the adrenocortical cells and chromaffin cells, a third cellular type, the *summer* or *Stilling cell,* has been found in the interrenal glands of ranid frogs.[9] This Stilling cell appears in summer and regresses in winter frogs. It is an eosinophilic cell and resembles a mast cell (histamine-producing cell). The functional significance of the Stilling cell is unknown. It has been suggested to produce renin,[114] but this has not been confirmed.

Adrenocortical cells of both apodans and urodeles occur in scattered islands on the ventral surface of the kidney.[41] This anatomical arrangement in part explains the virtual absence of synthetic studies employing apodan or urodele adrenocortical cells in vitro.[94]

Studies with adult anuran adrenocortical tissue in vitro have shown that the major corticoids synthesized are aldosterone and corticosterone, and both hormones have been identified in adult amphibian plasma. In addition, in-vitro syntheses result in production of a large quantity of *18-hydroxycorticosterone,* which can be a precursor for aldosterone. The ratio of aldosterone:18-hydroxycorticosterone:corticosterone in vitro is 6:3:1. The high levels of this aldosterone precursor may simply be an artifact of in-vitro conditions, as mentioned previously. Ovarian production of significant quantities of 11-deoxycorticosteroids has been reported,[19] and this may be an important source for corticosteroids in sexually mature females.

Although corticosterone is the dominant corticoid reported for terrestrial amphibians, cortisol has been reported to be the major corticoid in metamorphosing ranid tadpoles and in the aquatic frog *X. laevis,* as well as in the permanently aquatic urodele *Amphiuma*[23,77] (Tables 10-6, 10-7). Aquatic-phase adult newts, *Notophthalmus viridescens,* produce substantial amounts of cortisol.[73,106] These observations would support the hypothesis that cortisol is important for maintaining sodium balance in freshwater amphibians, as reported for fishes, and that corticosterone becomes more important following metamorphosis to a terrestrial-phase amphibian. Corticosterone is

Table 10-6. *Plasma Corticosteroids Measured in Amphibians*

SPECIES	STEROIDS PRESENT	REF.
	Order Anura	
Rana catesbeiana	Corticosterone, aldosterone, deoxycorticosterone	61, 94
Rana pipiens tadpoles	Cortisol	23
Xenopus laevis	Cortisol	94
Bufo marinus	Corticosterone, aldosterone	94
	Order Caudata	
Andrias davidianus	Corticosterone, aldosterone, deoxycorticosterone	14
Amphiuma tridactyla	Corticosterone	94
Notophthalmus viridescens	Corticosterone, cortisol	73

also the major corticoid in reptiles and birds. It may be that there is a transition from cortisol to corticosterone secretion that takes place during or following metamorphosis that is possibly controlled by thyroid hormones.

Renin-angiotensin system. Renin activity is present in amphibian renal tissue,[85,104] although the secretory renin-containing granules differ morphologically from those of mammals.[67] Several studies report failure to locate a macula densa in Amphibia,[85,104] but a macula densa-like structure has been reported for a toad.[68] Substantiation of this claim is of considerable importance since a macula densa has not been reported for reptiles.

Class Reptilia

Chelonians, crocodilians and most snakes have paired suprarenally positioned adrenal glands exhibiting a variable degree of intermingling chromaffin cell cords within a mass of adrenocortical cells.[74] In lizards and some snakes the adrenocortical cells are partially encapsulated by chromaffin cells, resulting in a "cortex" homologous to the mammalian medulla. Some chromaffin cells are also found within the central mass of adrenocortical cells. The chromaffin cells of *Sphenodon* (Rhynchocephalia) surround the dorsal aspect of the gland as well as form islets within the mass of adrenocortical cells.

Although few species have been studied, all of those examined (including turtles, lizards, snakes and alligator) synthesize aldosterone and corticosterone as the major corticoids under in-vitro conditions and what appears to be 18-hydroxycorticosterone. Corticosterone synthesis predominates in vitro with the amounts of 18-hydroxycorticosterone exceeding the levels of aldosterone.

Most investigators have failed to show any effect of ACTH on in-vitro corticosteroidogenesis in snakes *(Natrix natrix, Naja*

Table 10-7. *Circulating Corticosteroids (μg/dl) in Amphibian Species (Order Anura).*

SPECIES	CORTICOSTERONE	ALDOSTERONE	REF.
Rana catesbeiana,			
Control	8.8	1.8–50.2	61,111
ACTH-treated	18.0	0.2	111
Freshly collected	0.2–1.6		72
Hypophysectomized	1.3	0.15	61
Rana esculenta	—	0.82	31
Bufo marinus			
In distilled water	380.6	54.7	37
Saline-adapted	66.2	15.2	37
Bufo americanus			
October animals	1.4	—	86

naja), turtles *(Pseudemys scripta elegans, Chrysemys p. picta)* and the alligator *(Alligator mississipiensis).* However, adrenocortical cells from turtles *(C. picta)* secrete corticosterone in vitro when mammalian ACTH or crude extracts of avian, chelonian or anuran pituitaries are added to the culture medium,[11] and ACTH stimulates adrenocorticoid synthesis in the cobra, *Naja naja.*[51] Corticosterone levels in vivo (Table 10-8) and in vitro are elevated following administration of ACTH to *Caimen crocodilus* or *C. sclerops.*[39,50] Corticotropin also elevates corticosterone levels in two lizard species but does not influence aldosterone levels.[7]

One extraadrenalocortical source of corticosteroids has been reported.[19] Isolated ovaries from the night lizard *Xantusia vigilis* synthesize 11-deoxycorticosterone, but the importance of this observation to either reptilian corticosteroidogenesis or to reproductive function is uncertain.

Renin-Angiotensin System. Renin activity has been reported for turtles, lizards and snakes, but no macula densa has been described.[78,104] This is curious considering the possibility of a macula-like structure in amphibians and evidence for a macula in birds and mammals.

Class Aves

In birds the adrenal glands are organized in the same manner as described for turtles, crocodilians and most snakes. The relative quantities of chromaffin with respect to adrenocortical cells varies, however.[38] There appears to be some zonation of cellular types on histochemical and cytological bases similar to that seen in mammals[38,48,89] (Figs. 10-11 to 10-13).

The major corticosteroids synthesized by adrenocortical cells taken from domestic species and incubated in vitro are corticosterone, aldosterone and 18-hydroxycorticosterone. This sequence of steroidogenesis (corticosterone → 18-hydroxycorticosterone → aldosterone) characteristic of birds as well as anuran amphibians and reptiles is essentially the same pattern found in cells of the mammalian zona glomerulosa (Fig. 10-4).

Studies with duck adrenal slices in vitro suggest that corticosterone is the immediate precursor for 18-hydroxycorticosterone and that the latter is converted to aldosterone.[29] However, only corticosterone and aldosterone have been found in avian plasma (Table 10-9) with the exception of 11-deoxycorticosterone in the herring gull.[48] The absence of 18-hydroxycorticosterone in plasma further supports the conclusion that it is a precursor for aldosterone synthesis, and its accumulation in vitro is an artifact. The biological half-lives for corticosteroids in avian plasma are provided in Table 10-10.

Although mammalian ACTH stimulates adrenocorticoid secretion (corticosterone) in chickens, hypophysectomy does not cause complete cessation of corticosteroidogenesis (Table 10-9). It has been proposed that melanophore-stimulating hormone produced and released by the hypothalamus maintains steroidogenesis in the hypophysectomized chicken.[94] This suggestion needs further investigation because of its implication for other studies with hypophysectomized animals.

Renin-Angiotensin System. Renin activity is present in birds, and both the juxtaglomerular

Table 10-8. *Plasma Corticosteroids in Reptiles.*

Species	Corticosterone (μg/dl)	Aldosterone (ng/dl)	Ref
Caiman crocodilus	2.2±0.47	—	37
Sceloporus cyanogenys			
Control	5.96±1.13		22
ACTH-treated	12.92±1.17		
Varanus gouldi			
Hydrated		42±7	6
Salt-loaded		18.3±6	

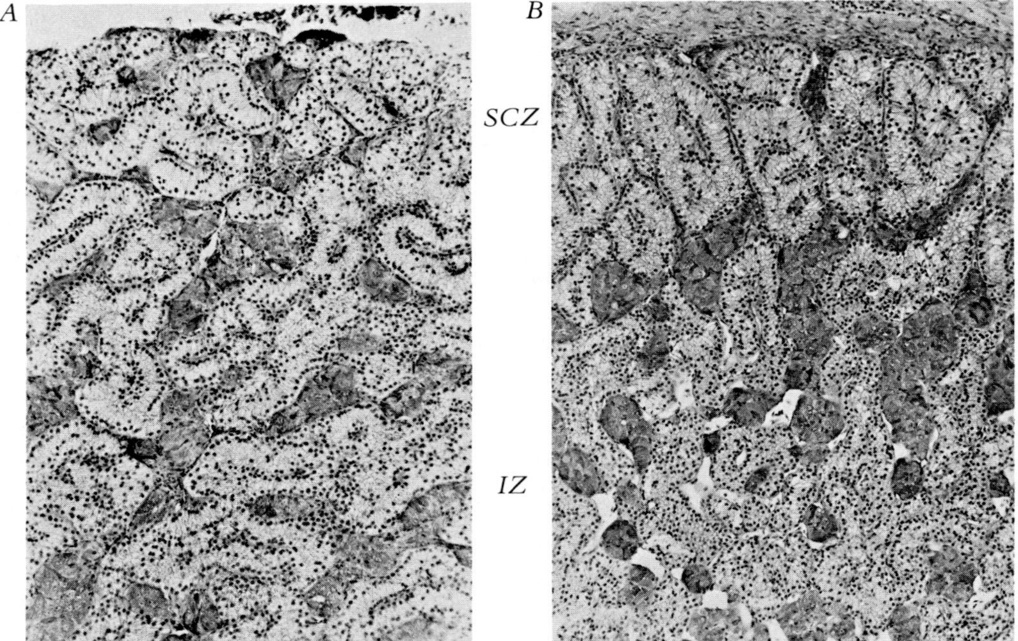

FIG. 10-11. Adrenal glands from normal *(A)* and adrenalectomized *(B)* ducks. In the outer region of adrenals from normal duck, no clear distinction is seen between cells of the subcapsular zone *(SCZ)* and of the inner portion of the gland *(IZ)*. The darker cells are chromaffin cells. Following hypophysectomy *(B)*, the adrenocortical cells of the SCZ are larger and contain numerous lipid droplets, whereas cells of the IZ are smaller and contain less lipid. (Fig. 10-11*A* is courtesy of Drs. Richard B. Pearce, James Cronshaw and W.N. Holmes. Fig. 10-11*B* is reprinted with permission from R.B. Pearce, J. Cronshaw and W.N. Holmes (1978). Evidence for the zonation of interrenal tissue in the adrenal gland of the duck *(Anas platyrhynchos)*. Cell Tissue Res. 192:363–379.)

apparatus and a macula densa have been described.[48,85,104] Cells of the avian macula densa are similar to those of mammals, with only some minor differences.[85]

Physiological Roles for Corticoids in Nonmammalian Vertebrates

The major function of corticoids investigated in nonmammals has been the effects on salt transport, particularly sodium, that is, mineralocorticoid activity. Unlike the mammalian condition, aldosterone, cortisol or corticosterone may possess mineralocorticoid activity when tested in nonmammals.

It has been hypothesized that the renin-angiotensin system evolved as a mechanism for regulating blood pressure.[78] Control over mineralocorticoid synthesis and regulation of sodium/potassium balance was acquired later.

Class Agnatha: Cyclostomata

The blood of myxinoids (hagfishes) is isosmotic to sea water, but there are some minor differences in concentrations of specific ions. Therefore, although osmotic balance per se is no problem, distribution of certain ions must be maintained actively. Injections of aldosterone or deoxycorticosterone acetate alter electrolyte composition of the body fluids with respect to sodium ions, but cortisone has no effect.[17]

Lampreys are either freshwater organisms or migrate between fresh water and the sea. While lampreys are in fresh water their body fluids are hyperosmotic to their surroundings, and they produce a large quantity of dilute urine. Sea lampreys *(Petromyzon marinus)* do not secrete corticosteroids when in sea water,[118] but when they are in fresh water corticosteroids can be identified in the circulation.[54] Aldosterone treatment can reduce renal

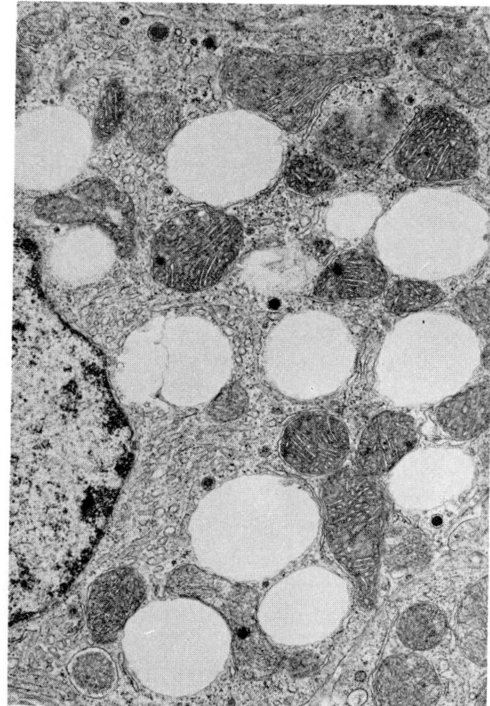

FIG. 10-12. Cytoplasmic details of a portion of an adrenocortical cell from the subcapsular zone of the duck adrenal. Mitochondria have shelf-like cristae and the ribosomes appear to be free within the cytosol. Numerous elements of smooth endoplasmic reticulum are present. (Reprinted with permission from R.B. Pearce, J. Cronshaw and W.N. Holmes (1978). Evidence for the zonation of interrenal tissue in the adrenal gland of the duck *(Anas platyrhynchos)*. Cell Tissue Res. 192:363–379.)

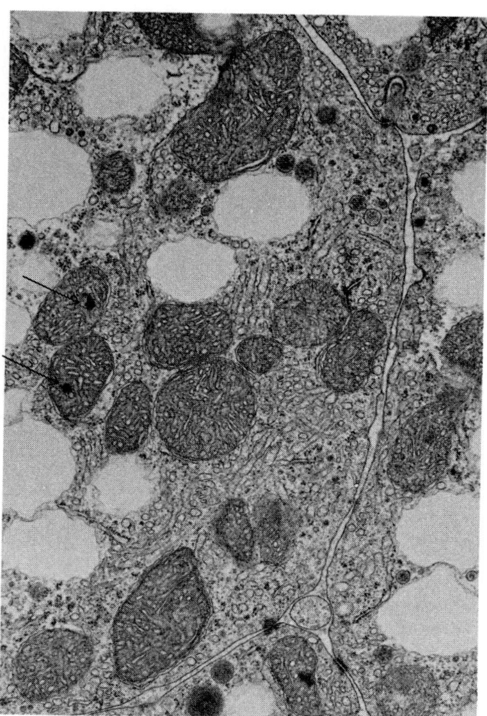

FIG. 10-13. Cytoplasmic details of a portion of an adrenocortical cell from the inner zone of the duck adrenal. These cells typically have round nuclei (not shown) and numerous lipid droplets. The mitochondria have tubular cristae and occasionally exhibit paracrystallin inclusions *(arrows)*. Numerous cisternae of smooth endoplasmic reticulum are present as are some rough endoplasmic reticulum and polyribosomal clusters. (Reprinted with permission from R.B. Pearce, J. Cronshaw and W.N. Holmes (1978). Evidence for the zonation of interrenal tissue in the adrenal gland of the duck *(Anas platyrhynchos)*. Cell Tissue Res. 192:363–379.)

and extrarenal sodium losses from lampreys held in fresh water.[4] The significance of this latter observation to osmoregulatory control in lampreys must await demonstration of aldosterone in lampreys.

Class Chondrichthyes

Elasmobranchs have plasma that is hyperosmotic to sea water and hence do not have the osmoregulatory problems exhibited by most marine fishes. This hyperosmotic condition is achieved by maintaining high circulating levels of urea and trimethylamine oxide. There is no clearly defined role for any corticosteroids, including 1α-hydroxycorticosterone, in elasmobranchs. Although corticoids stimulate salt excretion by the rectal gland,[13] this salt-secreting gland probably plays only a minor role in iono-osmotic homeostasis.[15] A possible role for corticoids in carbohydrate metabolism of elasmobranchs has been suggested.[27] There are no studies of corticoids in holocephalans.

Class Osteichthyes

Among the bony fishes, corticosteroids have been investigated with respect to function only in the teleosts. In general, corticosteroids (especially cortisol) stimulate sodium transport across gills (both influx and efflux), the mucosa of the gut and the kidney of freshwater fish. Cortisol appears to be the major corticoid

Table 10-9. *Plasma Corticosteroids (μg/dl) in Birds following Certain Experimental Manipulations*

SPECIES	TREATMENT	CORTICOSTERONE	ALDOSTERONE	REF.
Duck	Control	19.88 ± 1.66	–	48
	Hypox	9.92 ± 2.62	–	48
	Control	5.1 ± 0.49	–	28
Chicken	Hypox	1.06 ± 0.20	0.06 ± 0.01	108
	ACTH	15.16 ± 3.81	0.11 ± 0.02	108
	Surgical stress	6.58 ± 1.47	0.21 ± 0.06	108
Pigeon	Control	9.50 ± 0.63	–	48
	Hypox	5.13 ± 0.55	–	48
	Hypox with pituitary autotransplant	7.32 ± 0.79	–	48
Quail	Control	10.51 ± 1.35	–	48
	Hypox	4.68 ± 0.47	–	48
	Hypox with pituitary autotransplant	9.39 ± 1.01	–	48

in bony fishes (Table 10-4), and it appears to regulate sodium fluxes.

Freshwater-adapted eels, *Anguilla* spp, exhibit greater renin activity in sea water than in fresh water.[45,81] Furthermore, there are gradual changes in plasma renin activity during adaptation of eels to either fresh water or sea water. Administration of either ACTH or renin causes elevation of circulating cortisol levels in eels,[45] suggesting that both mechanisms for regulating corticoid levels are present in bony fishes. Infusion of isosmotic sodium chloride solution into the lungfish *Neoceratodus fosteri* causes reduction in plasma renin activity, suggesting the presence of a functional renin mechanism in the Dipnoi as well.

The problems of endocrine regulation of iono-osmotic balance in teleosts are discussed specifically in Chapter 16 with respect to adaptation of fishes to different salinities and the interactions of cortisol with various hormones, such as prolactin, on salt and water balance.

Table 10-10. *Biological Half-Life of Adrenocorticosteroids in Avian Species*

SPECIES	CORTICOSTERONE HALF-LIFE (MIN ± SE)	ALDOSTERONE HALF-LIFE (MIN ± SE)
Duck	7.5 ± 0.6	6.2 ± 0.6
Pigeon	18.4 ± 0.1	12.8 ± 1.6

Modified from Holmes, W.N. and J.G. Phillips.[48]

Seasonal and daily rhythms in circulating levels of cortisol have been reported for several species. Maximum levels of corticosteroids in rainbow trout maintained on long photoperiod are observed at night (2400 hours).[91] In the spring, plasma corticoids rise in juvenile salmonid fishes prior to their migration from fresh water to the ocean or while adapting to sea water.[105] Adult salmonids exhibit elevated corticosteroid levels during their spawning migration from the ocean to fresh water and during spawning (see Chap. 18).

Comparisons of absolute corticoid levels can not be made among different species, or in some cases even within the same species, since it is not possible to assess the role of stress in most cases. Stress produces marked elevations of corticosteroids in fishes. Just bringing wild trout into the laboratory can increase levels of plasma cortisol 2 to 5 times.[92,107] Elevated corticosteroids in migrating juvenile and adult salmonids probably reflect a response of the adrenal axis to chronic stress. Importance must be placed upon relative levels within a species under carefully described conditions.

Class Amphibia

Hypophysectomy or exposure of frogs to sea water induced atrophy of the adrenocortical tissue, presumably because of reduced requirements for corticosteroids.[95] Interrenalectomy of frogs causes a decrease in plasma sodium and an increase in plasma potassium similar to that observed in mammals.[3] Winter frogs usually survive interrenalectomy, but summer frogs die; possibly death is correlated to the yet unknown importance of the Stilling cells in summer frogs.

Aldosterone seems to be the important salt-regulating hormone acting on the skin and urinary bladder, increasing sodium influx and retention respectively. The action of aldosterone on the urinary bladder involves synthesis of new protein and would appear to be analogous to the production of aldosterone-induced protein in the mammalian distal convoluted tubule. Corticotropin elevates aldosterone, levels in *Rana esculenta,*[31] implying a direct action of ACTH on aldosterone, a condition very different from that described for mammals. Salt-depleted frogs exhibit elevated renal levels of renin, suggesting the presence of both mechanisms for regulating aldosterone production,[12] although plasma renin levels do not appear to differ between distilled-water-adapted toads and saline-adapted toads.[37]

Aldosterone treatment reversed the depression of plasma sodium caused by aminoglutethamide in the tiger salamander.[46] Higher doses of corticosterone than aldosterone were needed to bring plasma sodium back to normal, supporting a physiological role for aldosterone as a mineralocorticoid in amphibians.

Seasonal and daily rhythms of cortisol levels have been reported in plasma samples from *Rana esculenta*[30] and *Bufo americanus.*[87] The time of the daily maximum varied in *R. esculenta* from 2400 hours in May to 1900 hours in July and 0800 hours in November. Greatest secretion of corticoids coincided with reproduction in the spring. Two peaks of corticoid secretion were observed in captive and free *B. americanus.* One peak coincided with reproduction in the spring but the second peak occurred in the fall at the time of pre-hibernating migrations. Daily maxima corresponded to increased locomotor activity.

Stress causes an elevation in plasma corticosteroids. Placing freshly collected bullfrogs in sacks for up to 24 hours doubles their corticosterone levels.[72] Stress also can alter secretion of other hormones. The secretion of PRL,[82] gonadotropin and androgen[72] all decrease in amphibians following capture. The failure of some species to breed in captivity and the stimulus for some larvae to undergo metamorphosis may be consequences of stress.

Class Reptilia

A general role for corticosteroids in reptiles has not been demonstrated although one functional role has been suggested. Reptiles have nasal (orbital) salt-excreting glands similar to those found in aquatic birds. Corticosteroids appear to regulate the secretion of salt by these glands, but definitive studies are needed.[3] Injections of concentrated sodium chloride solutions (salt-loading) depress plasma aldosterone levels in several species of lizard.[7,8] Similar observations are reported for the tortoise, *Testudo hermanni.*[112] Salt-loaded lizards also have elevated levels of AVT.[8] Sodium depletion apparently does not affect renin activity in turtles.[83]

Class Aves

Corticosteroids have been implicated in salt regulation by birds. The nasal salt-excreting glands of certain aquatic birds secrete a hypertonic NaCl solution. Salt secretion is enhanced by treatment with ACTH or corticosterone,[3] and corticosterone uptake by nasal salt glands is followed by an increase in salt excretion.[15] Adrenalectomized ducks cannot excrete a salt load, but corticoid therapy restores this salt-excreting ability.[3] Metyrapone, which disrupts corticosterone synthesis, blocks nasal gland secretion.

Increases in environmental salinity are correlated with increases in Na-K-dependent adenosinetriphosphatase in salt gland cells, and this event is possibly related to increased protein synthesis caused by corticosteroids.[34] Marine birds have larger adrenal glands than do freshwater or terrestrial birds, which supports the role for corticosterone in nasal salt gland regulation.[48] Birds inhabiting brackish water have intermediate-sized adrenals.

Renin activity and angiotensin activity in blood plasma of ducks and pigeons increase following hemorrhage,[48] establishing a physiological role similar to that described for mammals. The control of corticosterone by ACTH and the importance of corticosterone in salt regulation suggest that avian corticosteroidogenesis may not be affected by the renin-angiotensin system. Studies in species that lack the dependence of nasal salt gland excretion are needed to clarify this situation.

Circadian rhythms for corticosteroids have been described in some birds. The time of the daily corticosteroids peak is believed to determine the behavioral response following injection of prolactin in white-crowned sparrows. These observations have led to hypotheses concerning the control of migratory behavior by the phase relationships between rhythms of corticosterone and PRL secretion[76] (see Chap. 18).

Stress activates the hypothalamo-adrenal axis in birds. This involves the ACTH-corticosterone axis and release of epinephrine from the adrenal medulla.[98] Activation of the endocrine stress mechanism also influences other endocrine glands. Chasing (stress) of male zebra finches for 15 minutes results in a significant depression in plasma androgens measured 2 hours later. Isolation of males in small cages for 12 hours virtually obliterates testosterone in the circulation.[90]

The Mammalian Adrenal Medulla

The medullary portion of the mammalian adrenal consists of sympathetic preganglionic neuronal endings (cholinergic) and modified cells derived from neural crest and homologous to postganglionic sympathetic neurons (adrenergic). These adrenal cells secrete either norepinephrine or epinephrine directly into the blood. In other words, the adrenal medulla is a modified sympathetic ganglion. Both epinephrine and norepinephrine (as well as small quantities of dopamine) can be extracted from the adrenal medulla, but the ratio in adult mammals strongly favors epinephrine (Table 10-1). This proportion of norepinephrine to epinephrine varies throughout life, however. Fetal and neonatal adrenals secrete predominantly norepinephrine followed by a gradual increase in the proportion of epinephrine that eventually dominates in adult mammals. Whales are an apparent exception in that the adult adrenal consists of about 83% norepinephrine.

Treatment of adrenal medullary cells with potassium dichromate or chromic acid results in formation of a yellowish or brown oxidation product, the *chromaffin reaction.* Cells that exhibit a positive chromaffin reaction are termed chromaffin cells. The catecholamine-secreting cells of the adrenal medulla show a positive chromaffin reaction, but so do other cells in the body (for example, in the intestinal epithelium and skin). Cells containing the tryptophan derivative 5-hydroxytryptamine (serotonin) also exhibit a positive chromaffin reaction. Norepinephrine-secreting cells can be distinguished from epinephrine-secreting cells by the formaldehyde treatment devised by Hillarp and Falck.[47] Formaldehyde combines chemically with norepinephrine storage granules and the resulting complex will fluoresce.

Synthesis and Metabolism of Adrenal Catecholamines

Two distinct cellular types in the mammalian adrenal medulla are related to production of norepinephrine and epinephrine respectively.[32,47] Both epinephrine and norepinephrine are synthesized from the amino acid tyrosine and employ the same biochemical pathway (Fig. 10-14). However, only one cellular type possesses the critical enzyme phenylethanolamine N-methyltransferase (PNMT) necessary for converting norepinephrine to epinephrine through addition of a methyl group donated by S-adenosylmethionine.[47]

Norepinephrine and epinephrine may be found circulating free in the plasma or as conjugates with sulfate or glucuronide. Most of the circulating epinephrine is bound to plasma proteins, especially albumin. Norepinephrine binds to plasma proteins to a much lesser degree than does epinephrine.

Circulating catecholamines have a short biological half-life and are rapidly excreted via the urine in either free or conjugated forms. The biological half-life for epinephrine is about 5 minutes.[93] The most common metabolic pathway for inactivation of catecholamines

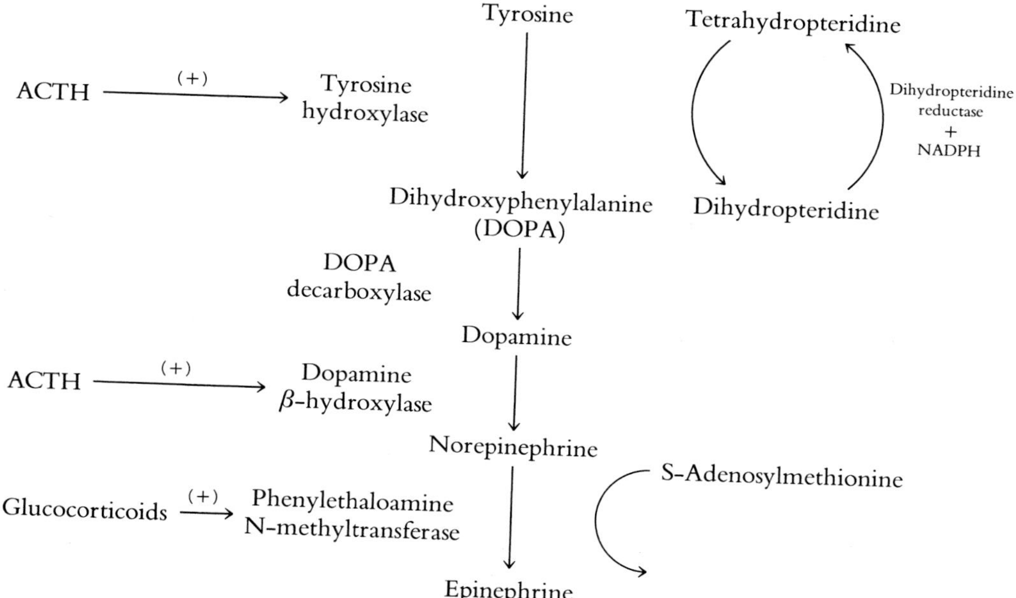

FIG. 10-14. Biosynthesis of the catecholamine adrenal hormones. Influences of ACTH and glucocorticoids on levels of specific key enzymes are indicated.

involves methylation by the enzyme catechol-O-methyltransferase and subsequent deamination and oxidation (by amine oxidase) to inactive metabolites that appear in the urine. The most common urinary metabolites are 3-methoxy-4-hydroxymandelic acid, metanephrine and normetanephrine (Fig. 10-15).

Regulation of Catecholamine Secretion

THE CENTRAL NERVOUS PATHWAY. Stimulation of the cholinergic sympathetic fibers innervating the medulla causes local release of acetylcholine (ACh), which in turn stimulates release of norepinephrine, epinephrine or both from the chromaffin cells. This action of ACh involves Ca++ uptake by the chromaffin cells. Apparently separate control centers for release of epinephrine and norepinephrine are located in the anterior and medial hypothalamus, and selective release of these medullary hormones occurs.[71] Norepinephrine and epinephrine may be released separately under differing physiological conditions, and these two catecholamines have independent physiological roles in homeostasis.

EFFECTS OF PHYSIOLOGICAL FACTORS ON CATECHOLAMINE RELEASE. Walter B. Cannon first formulated an emergency reaction hypothesis involving secretions of the adrenal medulla and activity of other portions of the sympathetic nervous system. These emergency responses include increased heart rate, vasodilation of arterioles in skeletal muscle, general venoconstriction, relaxation of bronchiolar muscles, pupillary dilatation, piloerection and mobilization of liver glycogen and free fatty acids. All of these responses contribute to increased efficiency of operation so that the organism can best respond to whatever emergency has arisen. This type of response to short-term stress may be distinguished from the response to chronic stress associated with the glucocorticoids and the general adaptation syndrome of Selye (see p. 220). However, the emergency reaction of Cannon may be thought of as being partly equivalent to the alarm reaction of the Seyle hypothesis.

The major physiological actions of adrenal medullary hormones are their effects on metabolism in response to emotional stress (anxiety, apprehension), physical stress (injury, exercise) or what might be distinguished as

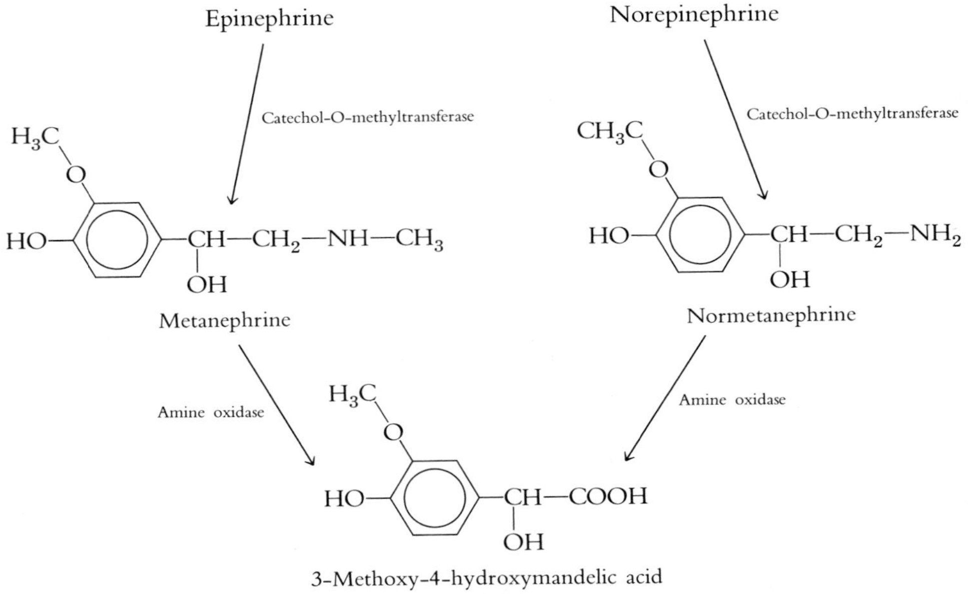

Epinephrine

Norepinephrine

Catechol-O-methyltransferase

Catechol-O-methyltransferase

H_3C–O–(HO–C_6H_3)–CH(OH)–CH_2–NH–CH_3

Metanephrine

CH_3C–O–(HO–C_6H_3)–CH(OH)–CH_2–NH_2

Normetanephrine

Amine oxidase

Amine oxidase

H_3C–O–(HO–C_6H_3)–CH(OH)–COOH

3-Methoxy-4-hydroxymandelic acid

Fig. 10-15. Interactive metabolic products of epinephrine and norepinephrine.

physiological stress (temperature, pH, oxygen availability, hypotension and hypoglycemia). The actions of adrenal catecholamines on cardiovascular events other than the acceleration of heart rate (which is actually due to metabolic effects of epinephrine on cardiac muscle) are probably secondary to the effects of norepinephrine released from postganglionic sympathetic fibers or, in the case of the skeletal muscle arterioles, the release of ACh from postganglionic sympathetic fibers. This secondary role for adrenal catecholamines is further supported by the relatively low percentages of norepinephrine in the adrenals of most adult mammals. Sympathetic control mechanisms are not well developed in fetal and neonatal mammals, and this observation could be linked to the high proportion of norepinephrine in their adrenals.

Epinephrine stimulates hydrolysis of liver glycogen to glucose and production of lactate from muscle glycogen stores. Circulating norepinephrine produces a similar effect on liver glycogen, but muscle glycogen stores are not affected by norepinephrine. This would explain the ineffectiveness of exogenous norepinephrine as a cardioacceleratory drug, whereas epinephrine is very potent. The mobilization of lipids and release of free fatty acids from adipose tissue is under neural sympathetic control and is not regulated by adrenal catecholamines. (See Chapter 19 for a more thorough discussion of hormones and metabolic events.)

Emotional and severe physical stress increases circulatory levels of catecholamines via hypothalamic adrenal pathways.[71] However, response to emotional stress such as written examinations involves an increase only in epinephrine, whereas adrenal response to anticipation involves primarily norepinephrine. Exercise causes an increase in norepinephrine levels, presumably from both adrenal and neural sources. Epinephrine secretion is not influenced by moderate exercise, but it is markedly increased during long-distance running. Several physiological factors such as cold and heat stress, alkalosis or acidosis and hypotension do not appear to involve primary actions of adrenal medullary hormones. However, responses to asphyxia or anoxia and to hypoglycemia are major factors influencing epinephrine release in adult mammals. Asphyxia causes an increase in epinephrine release, probably through direct actions of oxygen deprivation on the nervous system. In fetal or neonatal animals, asphyxia directly evokes catecholamine release from the adrenal. Insulin-induced hypoglycemia results in cardiac acceleration through stimulating epinephrine release. Hypoglycemia induces epinephrine release primarily through direct effects on glucose-sensitive centers in the hypothalamus. Epinephrine also retards the insulin-induced decrease in blood sugar through its antagonistic actions on liver glycogen.

Effects of ACTH and Glucocorticoids on Adrenal Catecholamine Secretion

Development of a close anatomical association between adrenocortical and chromaffin tissues during vertebrate evolution has suggested a concomitant development of a functional relationship as well. Studies by Wurtman and his co-workers over the past 15 years or so have demonstrated that ACTH exerts a stimulatory effect on epinephrine secretion through the former's action on circulating glucocorticoid levels. Hypophysectomy reduces adrenal epinephrine levels, and treatment with either ACTH or glucocorticoids restores adrenal levels of epinephrine to normal. Furthermore, glucocorticoids increase the activity of adrenal medullary PNMT, the enzyme responsible for conversion (methylation) of norepinephrine to epinephrine. Some studies indicate that ACTH may have a direct action on the medulla as well.[116] Levels of both tyrosine hydroxylase (tyrosine→DOPA) and dopamine-β-hydroxylase (dopamine→norepinephrine) but not PNMT are increased by ACTH treatment. These observations indicate that chronic stress may influence epinephrine secretion not only during the alarm reaction but also in the later stages of the response. It has been reported that epinephrine can cause release of ACTH through actions at either the hypothalamic or adenohypophysial level, but the physiological significance of these observations is not clear.

Mechanism of Action for Adrenal Catecholamines

The presence of specific receptors for epinephrine was first postulated in 1906 by Sir Henry Dale, who showed that ergot alkaloids (drugs such as ergocornine and ergocryptine) blocked some of the actions of epinephrine. Later studies suggested there are two kinds of *adrenergic receptors* in target cells that are capable of binding adrenal catecholamines: alpha and beta receptors (see Appendix 3). These receptors also respond to a number of epinephrine-like drugs that have been termed *sympathomimetic drugs* since they mimic actions of sympathetic catecholamines. Two common sympathomimetic drugs are isoproterenol and phenylephrine. Norepinephrine binds mainly to alpha receptors, whereas epinephrine binds to both. When both alpha and beta receptors are present on a target cell that binds epinephrine, the alpha effect predominates unless epinephrine is administered with an alpha-blocking agent (for example, phentolamine).

Detailed studies of the mechanism of adrenal catecholamine actions on target cells have concentrated on the effects of epinephrine in cardiac muscle and liver cells. In fact, it was studies in cardiac cells that led Sutherland and his co-workers to the discovery of the second-messenger role for cyclic adenosine 3′,5′ monophosphate (cAMP) and an eventual Nobel Prize in physiology and medicine (see Chap. 1). Epinephrine stimulates the breakdown of glycogen to glucose in both liver and muscle cells by first stimulating an increase in intracellular cAMP (see Figs. 1-6, 1-7 and Fig. 10-16). The glucose released from liver glycogen tends to enter the general circulation, whereas the glucose liberated from muscle glycogen is utilized for rapid ATP synthesis and production of lactate. The cellular action of epinephrine will be discussed in more detail in Chapter 19.

Evolution of Adrenal Medullary Hormones

Morphologically there has been a general trend to develop a close anatomical relationship between chromaffin tissues homologous to the mammalian adrenal medullary cells and the adrenocortical cells. Chromaffin tissue in agnathans is found in association with the posterior cardinal veins as are the separate clusters of adrenocortical cells. In the cartilagi-

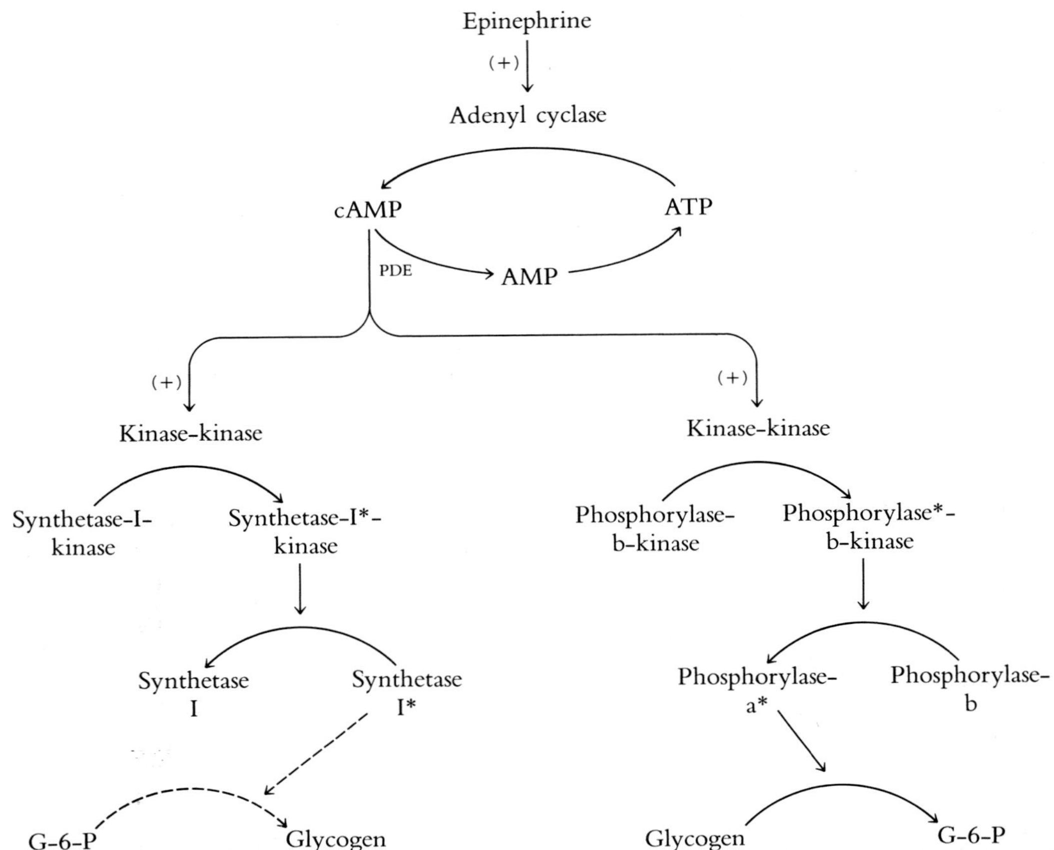

Fig. 10-16. Action of epinephrine on liver or muscle glycogen. This action employs the same mechanism whereby glucagon influences liver glycogen. This scheme shows how two separate pathways can be influenced by one hormone operating through a common mechanism of action. *=active forms of enzymes; *dotted lines* = inhibited pathways; G-6-P = glucose-6-phosphate, PDE = phosphodiesterase.

nous fishes the chromaffin tissue is more widely separated from the adrenocortical cells than in any other vertebrate group. There is considerable anatomical variation among the teleosts. Chromaffin tissue may be entirely separate from the adrenocortical cell clusters in the head kidney or may be intermingled with it, or in some species both conditions may be found. Clusters of adrenocortical cells (islets) in amphibians typically contain a few chromaffin cells. The anatomical distribution of chromaffin cells in reptiles is varied among the different groups. The adrenal glands of squamates and the tuatara *Sphenodon punctatus* have peripherally located norepinephrine-secreting chromaffin cells and central islets of epinephrine-secreting cells intermingled among the adrenocortical cells.[26,115] The avian adrenal glands consist of a mixture of cortical and chromaffin cells such that no distinction of "cortex" and "medulla" is possible.

Early studies of the proportion of adrenal catecholamines in nonmammals suggested that the mammalian fetal pattern of high norepinephrine production with increasing production of epinephrine following birth is an example of ontogeny recapitulating phylogeny. Analysis of extractable catecholamines from the shark *Squalus acanthias,* which has entirely separate chromaffin tissue, the frog *Rana temporaria,* which exhibits some mixing of chromaffin and adrenocortical cells, and the rabbit *Oryctolagus cuniculus* suggests an evo-

TABLE 10-11. *Proportion of Norepinephrine of Total Catecholamines in Adult Adrenal Extracts*

SPECIES	% NOREPINEPHRINE
Elasmobranchs	66–73[a]
Dogfish shark *Squalus acanthias*	100[b]
Amphibians	40–60[a]
Frog *Rana temporaria*	55–69[b]
Reptiles	60[a]
Snake *Xenodon merremii*	
peripheral chromaffin cells	97[c]
central chromaffin islets	15[c]
Birds	55–80[a]
Some passerine birds	0[a]
Whale	83[a]
Ungulates	15–50[a]
Carnivores	27–60[a]
Rodents	2–50[a]
Lagomorphs	0–12[a]
Rabbit *Oryctolagus cuniculus*	8–13[b]
Primates	0–20[a]

[a]Data from Gorbman and Bern.[40]
[b]Data from Coupland.[21]
[c]Data from Gabe, M.(1970). The adrenal. In C. Gans, ed., The Biology of the Reptilia. Academic Press, New York, Vol. 3, pp. 263–318.

lutionary change from reliance on norepinephrine to the progressive reliance on epinephrine (see Table 10-11). Although it seems logical to assume that the methylation step (norepinephrine→epinephrine) was a later evolutionary event, the picture is more complex (Table 10-12). Histochemical and chromatographic procedures indicate that norepinephrine predominates in some bird species whereas others produce mainly epinephrine. Still other groups show only a slight preference for one catecholamine over the other. Although norepinephrine predominates in extracts of adrenals prepared from chickens, turkeys and pigeons the major circulating catecholamine is epinephrine. These data point out the dangers of extrapolating too broadly from gland content to secretory activities.

Few comparative functional studies of adrenal catecholamines have been reported. The hyperglycemic action of epinephrine seems to be a primitive action in nonmammalian vertebrates. Norepinephrine, on the other hand, produces hypoglycemia in the ratfish[87] and in 6 to 9-week-old Japanese quail.[35] It is not clear whether these observations represent a true role for norepinephrine.

Summary

The mammalian adrenal gland consists of an outer region (cortex) of adrenocortical cells (steroidogenic) and an inner region (medulla) of chromaffin cells (adrenergic). The cortex consists of a zona glomerulosa that secretes primarily the mineralocorticoid aldosterone and two inner zones, zona fasciculata and zona reticularis, that secrete primarily glucocorticoids (typically cortisol or corticosterone). The medulla contains two chromaffin cellular types that secrete the two catecholamine hormones, norepinephrine and epinephrine respectively.

In mammals the synthesis and release of aldosterone is controlled by the renin-angiotensin system. Renin is released from the juxtaglomerular apparatus in the kidney in response to reduction in sodium levels of extracellular fluids or reduction in blood pressure. Renin acts on a protein substrate in the

TABLE 10-12. *Relative Proportions of Norepinephrine and Epinephrine in Adrenal Extracts Prepared from Some Avian Groups*

Order Galliformes	Norepinephrine predominates clearly
Order Passeriformes	Epinephrine predominates clearly
Order Cuculiformes	Slight preference for epinephrine over norepinephrine
Order Columbiformes	Slight preference for norepinephrine over epinephrine

Modified from Assenmacher, I.[2]

blood, eventually resulting in formation of angiotensin II, which in turn stimulates aldosterone release. Angiotensin II may be converted to angiotensin III, which is also active in causing aldosterone release. ACTH may play a permissive role in aldosterone secretion. Aldosterone regulates sodium levels by increasing sodium reabsorption by the kidney. This response of the cells of certain regions in the nephron to aldosterone involves the synthesis of a specific protein that is responsible for sodium reabsorption. Aldosterone plays a secondary role in regulating volume of the extracellular fluids through its action on sodium reabsorption. It also regulates potassium excretion. Angiotensins may also stimulate hypertension, drinking and vasopressin release to aid in fluid volume regulation. The renin-angiotensin system may have evolved to regulate blood pressure.

Secretion of cortisol or corticosterone is under direct pituitary control through ACTH. The main physiological actions of these glucocorticoids are related to their effects on transport of materials into cells and the induction of new cellular enzymes. They inhibit glucose utilization by peripheral tissues, stimulate amino acid uptake and conversion to glucose and storage as glycogen, and stimulate mobilization of fat stores. Their major contribution may be a permissive action in that glucocorticoids create an intracellular environment favorable to the actions of many other hormones. Glucocorticoids certainly are important in the adaptive mechanisms whereby an organism combats chronic stress (general adaptation syndrome of Selye). Some important pharmacological actions of glucocorticoids include anti-inflammatory properties, a diabetogenic action, and excessive catabolism of body proteins.

Release of epinephrine and norepinephrine in mammals is directed by separate centers in the hypothalamus through preganglionic sympathetic neurons that innervate the medulla. Glucocorticoids and ACTH may also influence the ability of the medulla to secrete catecholamines by stimulating the synthesis of key enzymes. Epinephrine is primarily a metabolic hormone, that is, it stimulates hydrolysis of glycogen to provide glucose for combating hypoglycemia (liver) or as an immediate energy source (in muscle). Epinephrine is responsible for the emergency response of Cannon and is also involved in the alarm reaction of the general adaptation syndrome of Selye. Cardiac acceleration occurs following administration of epinephrine, as a result of increased glucose, and hence ATP availability within cardiac cells. Epinephrine binds to either alpha or beta receptors in target cell membranes. Norepinephrine binds significantly only to alpha receptors, and its major physiological action is venoconstriction. Norepinephrine is not a cardiac stimulator since cardiac muscle cells possess predominantly beta receptors. In most adult mammals circulating norepinephrine appears to be of secondary importance to the sympathetic postganglionic neurons for control of vascular tone.

Nonmammals do not exhibit similar "cortex" to "medulla" relationships such as those described for mammals. However, there is a general trend throughout the vertebrates to establish a closer anatomical relationship between the steroidogenic adrenocortical cells and the chromaffin tissue. In the more primitive fishes (for example, cyclostomes and elasmobranchs) the chromaffin and adrenocortical cells are entirely separate.

The major salt-regulating corticoid in fishes is cortisol. In terrestrial tetrapods, primarily corticosterone and aldosterone are secreted by the adrenocortical cells. These adrenocortical cells are functionally like the mammalian cells of the zona glomerulosa. Corticosterone is primarily a mineralocorticoid in these groups. A glucocorticoid has not been established, but corticosterone is a candidate.

Norepinephrine predominates in the adrenals of fetal and neonatal mammals as it does in more primitive vertebrates. Tetrapods exhibit more reliance on epinephrine than norepinephrine, although the picture is variable even within a single class. Adult mammals mostly secrete a very high proportion of the total medullary catecholamines as epinephrine. The most primitive function for epinephrine appears to be its ability to elevate blood sugar levels. The role of norepinephrine from the chromaffin cells in nonmammals is not understood.

References

1. Amirat, Z., F. Khammar and R. Brudieux (1980). Seasonal changes in plasma and adrenal concentrations of cortisol, corticosterone, aldosterone, and electrolytes in the adult male sand rat (*Psammomys obesus*). Gen. Comp. Endocrinol. 40:36–43.

2. Assenmacher, I. (1973). The peripheral endocrine glands. In D.S. Farner and J.R. King, eds., Avian Biology. Academic Press, New York, Vol. 3, pp.183–286.

3. Bentley, P.J. (1971). Endocrines and Osmoregulation. Springer-Verlag, New York.

4. Bentley, P.J. and B.K. Follett (1962). The action of neurohypophysial and adrenocortical hormones on sodium balance in the cyclostome, *Lampetra fluviatilis*. Gen. Comp. Endocrinol. 2:329–335.

5. Bethune, J.E. (1974). The Adrenal Cortex: A Scope Monograph. Upjohn Co., Kalamazoo.

6. Blair-West, J.R., J.P. Coghlan, D.A. Denton, A.P. Gibson, C.J. Sawyer and B.A. Scoggins (1977). Plasma renin activity and blood corticosteroids in the Australian lungfish *Neoceratodus forsteri*. J. Endocrinol. 77:137–142.

7. Bradshaw, S.D. and C.J. Grenot (1976). Plasma aldosterone levels in two reptilian species, *Uromastix acanthinurus* and *Tiliqua rugosa*, and the effect of several experimental treatments. J. Comp. Physiol. 111:71–76.

8. Bradshaw, S.D. and G.E. Rice (1981). The effects of pituitary and adrenal hormones on renal and postrenal reabsorption of water and electrolytes in the lizard, *Varanus gouldii* (Gray). Gen. Comp. Endocrinol. 44:82–93.

9. Burgos, M.H. (1959). Histochemistry and electron microscopy of the three cell types in the adrenal gland of the frog. Anat. Record 133:163–185.

10. Butler, D.G. (1973). Structure and function of the adrenal gland of fishes. Am. Zool. 13:839–880.

11. Callard, G.V. (1975). Corticotropic effects on isolated interrenal cells of the turtle (*Chrysemys picta*). Gen. Comp. Endocrinol. 26:301–309.

12. Capelli, J.P., L.G. Wesson and G.E. Aponte (1970). A phylogenetic study of the renin-angiotensin system. Am. J. Physiol. 218:1171–1178.

13. Chan, D.K.O., J.C. Phillips and I. Chester Jones (1967). Studies on electrolyte changes in the lip shark, *Hemiscyllium plagiosum* (Bennett) with special reference to the hormonal influence on the rectal gland. Comp. Biochem. Physiol. 23:185–198.

14. Chan, S.T.H., T. Sandor and B. Lofts (1975). A histological, histochemical and biochemical study of the adrenal tissue of the Chinese giant salamander (*Andrias davidianus* Blanchard). Gen. Comp. Endocrinol. 25:509–516.

15. Chester Jones, I., D. Bellamy, D.K.O. Chan, B.K. Follett, I.W. Henderson, J.G. Phillips and R.S. Snart (1972). Biological actions of steroid hormones in nonmammalian vertebrates. In D.R. Idler, ed., Steroids in Nonmammalian Vertebrates. Academic Press, New York, pp. 414–480.

16. Chester Jones, I. and W. Mosley (1980). The interrenal gland in Pisces—Structure. In I. Chester Jones and I.W. Henderson, eds., General, Comparative and Clinical Endocrinology of the Adrenal Cortex. Academic Press, New York, Vol. 3, pp. 396–472.

17. Chester Jones, I., J.G. Phillips and D. Bellamy (1962). Studies on water and electrolytes in cyclostomes and teleosts with special reference to *Myxine glutinosa* L. (the hagfish) and *Anguilla anguilla* L. (the Atlantic eel). Gen. Comp. Endocrinol. Suppl. 1:36–47.

18. Cline, M.J. and K.L. Melmon (1966). Plasma kinins and cortisol: A possible explanation of the anti-inflammatory action of cortisol. Science 153:1135–1138.

19. Colombo, L., P.C. Belvedere, P. Prando, P. Scaffai and T. Cisotto (1977). Biosynthesis of 11-deoxycorticosteroids and androgens by the ovary of the newt *Triturus alpestris alpestris* Laur. Gen. Comp. Endocrinol. 33:480–495.

20. Colombo, L., Z. Yaron, E. Daniels and P. Belvedere (1974). Biosynthesis of 11-deoxycorticosterone by the ovary of the yucca night lizard, *Xantusia vigilis*. Gen. Comp. Endocrinol. 24:331–337.

21. Coupland, R.E. (1953). On the morphology and adrenaline-noradrenaline content of chromaffin tissue. J. Endocrinol. 9:194–203.

22. Crabbe, J. (1961). Stimulation of active sodium transport across the isolated toad bladder after injection of aldosterone to the animal. Endocrinology 69:673–682.

23. Dale, E. (1962). Steroid excretion by larval frogs. Gen. Comp. Endocrinol. 2:171–176.

24. Daugherty, D.R. and I.P. Callard (1972). Plasma corticosterone levels in the male iguanid lizard, *Sceloporus cyanogenys*, under various physiological conditions. Gen. Comp. Endocrinol. 19:69–79.

25. Davis, J.O. and R.H. Freeman (1976). Mechanisms regulating renin release. Physiol. Rev. 56:1–56.

26. DelConte, E. (1977). Contiguity of the adrenaline-storing chromaffin cells with the interrenal tissue in the adrenal of a lizard. Gen. Comp. Endocrinol. 32:1–6.

27. deRoos, R. and C.C. deRoos, (1973). Elevation of plasma glucose levels by mammalian ACTH in the spiny dogfish shark (*Squalus acanthias*). Gen. Comp. Endocrinol. 21:403–409.

28. Donaldson, E.M. and W.N. Holmes (1965). Corticosteroidogenesis in the freshwater and saline-maintained duck (*Anas platyrhynchos*). J. Endocrinol. 32:329–336.

29. Donaldson, E.M., W.N. Holmes and J. Stachenko (1965). *In vitro* corticosteroidogenesis by the duck (*Anas platyrhynchos*) adrenal. Gen. Comp. Endocrinol. 5:542–551.

30. Dupont, W., P. Bourgeois, A. Reinberg and R. Vaillant (1979). Circannual and circadian rhythms in the concentration of corticosterone in the plasma of the edible frog (*Rana esculenta* L.) J. Endocrinol. 80:117–125.

31. Dupont, W., F. LeBoulenger, H. Vaudry, and R. Vaillant (1976). Regulation of aldosterone secretion in the frog *Rana esculenta.* Gen. Comp. Endocrinol. 29:51–60.

32. Eranko, O. (1951). Histochemical evidence of the presence of acid-phosphatase-positive and -negative cell islets in the adrenal medulla of the rat. Nature 168:250–251.

33. Farrell, G. (1959). The physiological factors which influence the secretion of aldosterone. Recent Prog. Horm. Res. 15:275–310.

34. Fletcher, G.L., I.M. Stanier and W.N. Holmes (1967). Sequential changes in the adenosinetriphosphatase activity and the electrolyte excretory capacity of the nasal glands of the duck (*Anas platyrhynchos*) during the period of adaptation to hypertonic saline. J. Exp. Biol. 47:375–392.

35. Freeman, B.M. (1970). Some aspects of thermoregulation in the adult Japanese quail (*Coturnix coturnix japonica*). Comp. Biochem. Physiol. 34:871–881.

36. Fuller, J.D., P.A. Mason and R. Fraser (1976). Gas-liquid chromatography of corticosteroids in plasma of salmonidae. J. Endocrinol. 71:163–164.

37. Garland, H.W. and I.W. Henderson (1975). Influence of environmental salinity on renal and adrenocortical function in the toad, *Bufo marinus.* Gen. Comp. Endocrinol. 27:136–143.

38. Ghosh, A. (1962). A comparative study of histochemistry of the avian adrenals. Gen. Comp. Endocrinol. Suppl. 1:75–80.

39. Gist, D.H. and M.L. Kaplan (1976). Effects of stress and ACTH on plasma corticosterone levels in the caiman, *Caiman crocodilus.* Gen. Comp. Endocrinol. 28:413–419.

40. Gorbman, A. and H. Bern (1962). A Textbook of Comparative Endocrinology. John Wiley and Sons, New York.

41. Hanke, W. (1978). The adrenal cortex of the Amphibia. In I. Chester Jones and I.W. Henderson, eds., General, Comparative and Clinical Endocrinology of the Adrenal Cortex. Academic Press, New York, Vol. 2, pp. 419–495.

42. Hardisty, M.W. and M.E. Baines (1971). The ultrastructure of the interrenal tissue of the lamprey. Experientia 27:1072–1075.

43. Hawkins, E.F., P.N. Young, A.M.C. Hawkins and H.A. Bern (1975). Adrenocortical function: Corticosterone levels in female BALB/C and C34 mice under various conditions. J. Exp. Zool. 194:479–484.

44. Henderson, I.W. and H.O. Garland (1980). The Interrenal Gland in Pisces—Function. In I. Chester Jones and I.W. Henderson, eds., General, Comparative and Clinical Endocrinology of the Adrenal Cortex. Academic Press, New York, Vol. 3, pp. 473–524.

45. Henderson, I.W., V. Jotisankasa, W. Mosley and M. Oguri (1976). Endocrine and environmental influences upon plasma cortisol concentrations and plasma renin activity of the eel, *Anguilla anguilla* L. J. Endocrinol. 70:81–95.

46. Heney, H.W. and D.F. Stiffler (1983). The effects of aldosterone on sodium and potassium metabolism in larval *Ambystoma tigrinum.* Gen. Comp. Endocrinol. 49:122–127.

47. Hillarp, N.–A. and B. Hökfelt (1954). Evidence of adrenaline and noradrenaline in separate adrenal medullary cells. Acta Physiol. Scand. 30:55–68.

48. Holmes, W.N. and J.G. Phillips (1976). The adrenal cortex of birds. In I. Chester Jones and I. W. Henderson, eds., General, Comparative and Clinical Endocrinology of the Adrenal Cortex. Academic Press, New York, Vol. 1, pp. 293–420.

49. Holmes, W.N., J.G. Phillips and D.G. Butler (1961). The effect of adrenocortical steroids on the renal and extrarenal responses of the domestic duck (*Anas platyrhynchos*), after hypertonic saline loading. Endocrinology 69:483–495.

50. Honn, K.V. and W. Chavin (1977). *In vitro* ACTH stimulation of corticosterone output in relation to cyclic nucleotide alterations in the crocodilian (*Caiman sclerops*) adrenal. Gen. Comp. Endocrinol. 32:330–340.

51. Huang, D.P., G.P. Vinson and J.G. Phillips (1969). The metabolism of pregnenolone and progesterone by cobra adrenal tissue *in vitro* and the effect of ACTH on product yield-time curves. Gen. Comp. Endocrinol. 12:637–643.

52. Idelman, S. (1978). The structure of the mammalian adrenal cortex. In I. Chester Jones and I.W. Henderson, eds., General, Comparative and Clinical Endocrinology of the Adrenal Cortex. Academic Press, New York, Vol. 2, pp. 1–199.

53. Idler, D.R. and G.B. Sangalang (1971). Unpublished data. Cited by Idler and Truscott.[59]

54. Idler, D.R., G.B. Sangalang and B. Truscott (1972). Corticosteroids in the South American lungfish. Gen. Comp. Endocrinol. Suppl. 3:238–244.

55. Idler, D.R., G.B. Sangalang and M. Weisbart (1971). Are corticosteroids present in the blood of all fishes? Proc. 3rd Int. Congr. Hormonal Steroids, 1970. Excerpta Medica, Amsterdam, pp. 983–989.

56. Idler, D.R. and B. Truscott (1966). 1α-Hydroxycorticosterone from cartilaginous fish: A new adrenal steroid in blood. J. Fish. Res. Board Can. 23:615–619.

57. Idler, D.R. and B. Truscott (1967). 1α-Hydroxycorticosterone: Synthesis *in vitro* and properties of an interrenal steroid in the blood of cartilaginous fish (Genus *Raja*). Steroids 9:457–477.

58. Idler, D.R. and B. Truscott (1969). Production of 1α-hydroxycorticosterone *in vivo* and *in vitro* by elasmobranchs. Gen. Comp. Endocrinol. Suppl. 2:325–330.

59. Idler, D.R. and B. Truscott (1972). Corticosteroids in Fish. In D.R. Idler, ed., Steroids in Nonmammalian Vertebrates. Academic Press, New York, pp. 127–252.

60. Janssens, P.A., G.P. Vinson, I. Chester Jones and W. Mosley (1965). Amphibian characteristics of the adrenal cortex of the African lungfish (*Protopterus* sp.). J. Endocrinol. 32:373–382.

61. Johnston, C.I., J.O. Davis, F.S. Wright and S.S. Howards (1967). Effects of renin and ACTH on adrenal steroid secretion in the American bullfrog. Am. J. Physiol. 213:393–399.

62. Jorgensen, C.B. (1976). Sub-mammalian vertebrate hypothalamic-pituitary-adrenal interrelationships. In I. Chester Jones and I.W. Henderson, eds., General, Comparative and Clinical Endocrinology of the Adrenal Cortex. Academic Press, New York, Vol. 1, pp. 143–206.

63. Jungreis, A.M., W.H. Huibregtse, and F. Ungar (1970). Corticosteroid identification and corticosterone concentration in serum of *Rana pipiens* during dehydration in winter and summer. Comp. Biochem. Physiol. 34:683–690.

64. Kirschner, N. (1975). Biosynthesis of the catecholamines. Handbook of Physiology, Sec. 7, Endocrinology. Williams & Wilkins, Baltimore, Vol. 6. pp. 341–355.

65. Krieger, D.T. and H. Houser (1978). Comparison of synchronization of circadian corticosteroid rhythms by photoperiod and food. Proc. Nat. Acad. Sci. U.S. 75:1577–1579.

66. Kurosawa, A., A. Guidotti and E. Costa (1976). Induction of tyrosine 3-monooxygenase in adrenal medulla: Role of protein kinase activation and translocation. Science 193:691–693.

67. Lamers, A.P.M., M.E.A. Mansfeld and A.B.M. Klaassen (1976). Some morphological aspects of the renin-angiotensin system in amphibians. Gen. Comp. Endocrinol. 29:284.

68. Lamers, A.P.M., W.J. Van Dongen, J.A.M. Kemenade and G.J.A. Speijers (1974). A macula densa-like structure in the kidney of the toad *Bufo bufo*. Gen. Comp. Endocrinol. 22:355.

69. Laub, J.M., G.V. Callard and I.P. Callard (1975). The role of adrenal steroids in the negative feedback control of the amphibian adrenal gland. Gen. Comp. Endocrinol. 25:425–431.

70. Leloup-Hatey, J. (1964). Cited by Idler and Truscott.[59]

71. Lewis, G.P. (1975). Physiological mechanisms controlling secretory activity of adrenal medulla. Handbook of Physiology, Sec. 7, Endocrinology. Williams & Wilkins, Baltimore, Vol. 6, pp. 309–319.

72. Licht, P., B.R. McCreery, R. Barnes and R. Pang (1983). Seasonal and stress related changes in plasma gonadotropins, sex steroids, and corticosterone in the bullfrog, *Rana catesbeiana*. Gen. Comp. Endocrinol. 51:124–145.

73. Liversage, R.A. and B.W. Price (1973). Adrenocorticosteroid levels in adult *Diemictylus viridescens* plasma following hypophysectomy and forelimb amputation. J. Exp. Zool. 185:259–264.

74. Lofts, B. (1978). The adrenal gland of reptiles. In I. Chester Jones and I.W. Henderson, eds., General, Comparative and Clinical Endocrinology of the Adrenal Cortex. Academic Press, New York, Vol. 2, pp. 419–495.

75. Long, J.A. (1975). Zonation of the mammalian adrenal cortex. Handbook of Physiology, Sec. 7, Endocrinology. Williams & Wilkins, Baltimore, Vol. 6, pp. 13–24.

76. Meier, A.H. (1972). Temporal synergism of prolactin and adrenal steroids. Gen. Comp. Endocrinol. Suppl. 3:499–508.

77. Nandi, J. (1967). Comparative endocrinology of steroid hormones in vertebrates. Am. Zool. 7:115–133.

78. Nishimura, H. (1980). Evolution of the renin angiotensin system. In P.K.T. Pang and A. Epple, eds. Evolution of Vertebrate Endocrine Systems. Texas Tech. University, Lubbock, Texas, pp. 373–404.

79. Nishimura, H., M. Ogawa and W.H. Sawyer (1973). Renin-angiotensin system in primitive bony fishes and a holocephalian. Am. J. Physiol. 224:950–956.

80. Nishimura, H., M. Oguri, M. Ogawa, H. Sokabe and M. Imai (1970). Absence of renin in kidneys of elasmobranchs and cyclostomes. Am. J. Physiol. 218:911–915.

81. Nishimura, H., W.H. Sawyer and R.F. Nigrelli (1976). Renin, cortisol and plasma volume in marine teleost fishes adapted to dilute media. J. Endocrinol. 70:47–59.

82. Norris, D.O. (1978). Hormonal and environmental factors involved in the determination of neoteny in urodeles. In P.J. Guillard and H.H. Boers, eds., Comparative Endocrinology. Elsevier/North Holland Biomedical Press, Amsterdam, pp. 109–112.

83. Nothstine, S.A., J.O. Davis and R.M. DeRoos (1971). Kidney extracts and ACTH on adrenal steroid secretion in a turtle and a crocodilian. Am. J. Physiol. 221:726–732.

84. Oddie, C.J., E.H. Blaine, S.D. Bradshaw, J.P. Coghlan, D.A. Denton, J.F. Nelson and B.A. Scoggins (1976). Blood corticosteroids in Australian marsupial and placental mammals and one monotreme. J. Endocrinol. 69:341–348.

85. Ogawa, M., M. Oguri, H. Sokabe and N. Nishimura (1972). Juxtaglomerular apparatus in the vertebrates. Gen. Comp. Endocrinol. Suppl. 3:374–381.

86. Pancak, M.K. and D.H. Taylor (1983). Seasonal and daily plasma corticosterone rhythms in American toads, *Bufo americanus*. Gen. Comp. Endocrinol. 50:490–497.

87. Patent, G.J. (1970). Comparison of some hormonal effects on carbohydrate metabolism in an elasmobranch (*Squalus acanthias*) and a holocephalan (*Hydrolagus colliei*). Gen. Comp. Endocrinol. 14:215–242.

88. Peach, M.J. (1977). Renin-angiotensin system: Biochemistry and mechanisms of action. Physiol. Rev. 57:313–370.

89. Pearce, R.B., J. Cronshaw and W.N. Holmes (1978). Evidence for the zonation of interrenal tissue in the adrenal gland of the duck (*Anas platyrhynchos*). Cell Tissue Res. 192:363–379.

90. Prove, E. and R. Sossinka (1982). Radioimmunoassay of plasma hormones and its use in investigation of hormone and behavior correlations in birds. In C.G. Scanes, M.A. Ottinger, A.D. Kenny, J. Balthazart, J. Cronshaw and I. Chester Jones, eds., Aspects of Avian Endocrinology: Practical and Theoretical Implications. Texas Tech. Univ., Lubbock, Texas, pp. 97–103.

91. Quigley, M.E. and S.S.C. Yen (1979). A mid-day surge in cortisol levels. J. Clin. Endocrinol. Metab. 49:945–947.

92. Rance, T.A., B.I. Baker and G. Webley (1982). Variations in plasma cortisol concentrations over a 24-hour period in the rainbow trout *Salmo gairdneri*. Gen. Comp. Endocrinol. 48:269–274.

93. Randle, P.J. and R.M. Denton (1974). Hormones and Cell Metabolism. Oxford Biology Reader, Oxford University Press, London.

94. Sandor, T. (1972). Corticosteroids in Amphibia, Reptilia and Aves. In D.R. Idler, ed., Steroids in Nonmammalian Vertebrates. Academic Press, New York, pp. 253–327.

95. Scheer, B.T. and P.T. Wise (1969). Changes in the Stilling cells of frog interrenals after hypophysectomy and exposure to hypertonic saline solution. Gen. Comp. Endocrinol. 13:474–477.

96. Schöneshöfer, M. (1977). Simultaneous determination of eight adrenal steroids in human serum by radioimmunoassay. J. Steroid Biochem. 8:995–1010.

97. Seggie, J. and G.M. Brown (1976). Twenty-four hour resting prolactin levels in male rats: the effect of septal lesions and order of sacrifice. Endocrinology 98:1516–1522.

98. Siegel, H.S. (1980). Physiological stress in birds. Bioscience 30:529–534.

99. Seiler, K., R. Seiler and G. Sterba (1970). Cited by Jorgensen.[62]

100. Selye, H. (1971). Hormones and resistance. J. Pharm. Sci. 60:1–28.

101. Selye, H. (1973). The evolution of the stress concept. Am. Sci. 61:692–699.

102. Sernia, C. and I.R. McDonald (1977). Adrenocortical function in a prototherian mammal. J. Endocrinol. 72:41–52.

103. Simpson, T.H. and R.S. Wright (1970). Synthesis of corticosteroids by the interrenal gland of selachian elasmobranch fish. J. Endocrinol. 46:261–268.

104. Sokabe, H., M. Ogawa, M. Oguri and H. Nishimura (1969). Evolution of the juxtaglomerular apparatus in the vertebrate kidneys. Tex. Rep. Biol. Med. 27:868–885.

105. Specker, J.L. and C.B. Schreck (1982). Changes in plasma corticosteroids during smoltification of coho salmon, *Oncorhynchus kisutch*. Gen. Comp. Endocrinol. 46:53–58.

106. Stabler, T.A. (1969). Cited by Jungreis et al.[57]

107. Strange, R.J., C.B. Schreck and J.T. Golden (1977). Corticoid stress responses to handling and temperature in salmonids. Trans. Am. Fish. Soc. 106:213–218.

108. Taylor, A.A., J.O. Davis, R.P. Breitenbach and P.M. Hartroft (1970). Adrenal steroid secretion and a renal-pressor system in the chicken (*Gallus domesticus*). Gen. Comp. Endocrinol. 14:321–333.

109. Truscott, B. and D.R. Idler (1968). The widespread occurrence of a corticosteroid 1α-hydroxylase in the interrenals of Elasmobranchii. J. Endocrinol. 40:515–526.

110. Turner, C.D. and J.T. Bagnara (1976). General Endocrinology, 6th ed. W.B. Saunders Co., Philadelphia.

111. Ulick, S. and E. Feinholtz (1968). Metabolism and rate of secretion of aldosterone in the bullfrog. J. Clin. Invest. 47:2523–2529.

112. Uva, B., M. Vallarino, A. Mandich and G. Isola (1982). Plasma aldosterone levels in the female tortoise *Testudo hermanni* Gmelin in different experimental conditions. Gen. Comp. Endocrinol. 46:116–123.

113. Varma, M.M. (1977). Ultrastructural evidence for aldosterone- and corticosterone-secreting cells in the adrenocortical tissue of the American bullfrog, (*Rana catesbeiana*). Gen. Comp. Endocrinol. 33:61–75.

114. Volk, T.L. (1972). Morphologic observations on the summer cell of Stilling in the interrenal gland of the American bullfrog (*Rana catesbeiana*). Z. Zellforsch. 130:1–11.

115. Wasserman, G. and J. Tramezzani (1963). Separate distribution of adrenaline and noradrenaline-secreting cells in the adrenal of snakes. Gen. Comp. Endocrinol. 3:480–489.

116. Weiner, N. (1975). Control of the biosynthesis of adrenal catecholamines by the adrenal medulla. Handbook of Physiology, Sec. 7, Endocrinology. Williams & Wilkins, Baltimore, Vol. 6, pp. 357–366.

117. Weisbart, M., W.W. Dickhoff, A. Gorbman, and D.R. Idler (1980). The presence of steroids in the sera of the Pacific hagfish, *Eptatretus stouti,* and the sea lamprey, *Petromyzon marinus.* Gen. Comp. Endocrinol. 41:506–519.

118. Weisbart, M. and D.R. Idler (1970). Re-examination of the presence of corticosteroids in two cyclostomes, the Atlantic hagfish (*Myxine glutinosa* L.) and the sea lamprey (*Petromyzon marinus* L.). J. Endocrinol. 46:29–43.

119. Wurtman, R.J. and J. Axelrod (1966). Control of enzymatic synthesis of adrenaline in the adrenal medulla by adrenal cortical steroids. J. Biol. Chem. 241:2301–2305.

11·The Endocrinology of Reproduction

The Reproductive System

The oversimplified way in which even biologists sometimes view reproduction is exemplified by the following quotation from a textbook on fish biology: "the reproductive function in fishes is primarily the job of the reproductive system." In actuality, the "reproductive system" includes not only the gonads and their associated structures but also the complex hypothalamo-hypophysial axis as well as both neural and endocrine input to the hypothalamus. Furthermore, environmental factors (chemical, visual, photic, thermal and tactile stimuli) frequently determine reproductive events through their effects on sensory organs and receptors. Environmental factors contribute ultimately to both neural and endocrine input to the hypothalamus. When one thinks of reproduction, one should be considering a process of evolutionary adaptation that extends far beyond the inclusion of what is usually termed the reproductive system.

The major difficulty that arises when generalizations are made about reproduction and reproductive mechanisms stems from the central importance of these processes with respect to past and future evolutionary events. The reproductive system is possibly the central focus for selective agents since reproductive success is the major determinant of evolutionary success. Consequently the reproductive system has been highly responsive to selective forces throughout the long evolutionary history of vertebrates, and many features of extant species are more examples of specific adaptations to solve common environmental problems than they are representative of progressive "improvements" in the basic system that "culminated" in the placental mammals. A case in point would be the achievement of viviparity in all but two extant vertebrate classes, the Agnatha and Aves, as specific adaptations that, coupled with varying degrees of parental care, result in greater percentage survival of a small number of offspring. Viviparity represents only one solution, however, to similar selective pressures that confront all species. In spite of the problems of environmental adaptations that tend to confuse evolutionary relationships, there remain numerous conservative features in regulatory mechanisms of reproductive biology, and it is these that are emphasized in this chapter.

Reproduction is closely regulated through the hypothalamo-hypophysial axis, which coordinates specific gonadal events through regulation of circulating gonadotropins. Factors influencing gonadotropin release are discussed in Chapter 4 and will be summarized only briefly here.

In mammals the release of luteinizing hormone (LH) and follicle-stimulating hormone (FSH) from the adenohypophysis appears to be under the control of a single hypothalamic hormone, the gonadotropin-releasing hormone GnRH (Table 11-1). Release of this stimulatory factor is regulated by two separate regions of the hypothalamus: the *tonic center,* which maintains a relatively constant circulating level of both LH and FSH, and the *cyclic*

TABLE 11-1. *Summary of Generalized Hormone Actions in Mammalian Reproduction (Eutheria)*

HORMONE	FEMALE	MALE
GnRH	Stimulates FSH and LH secretion	Stimulates FSH and LH secretion
FSH	Initiates follicle growth; conversion of androgen to estrogen	Initiates spermatogenesis; secretion of androgen-binding protein by Sertoli cells; conversion of androgen to estrogen by Sertoli cell
LH	Androgen secretion; ovulation; formation of corpus luteum from granulosa; secretion of progesterone initiated in corpus luteum	Androgen secretion by interstitial cell (Leydig)
Prolactin	Synthesis of milk	Stimulates certain sex accessory structures (with androgen)
Oxytocin	Contraction of uterine smooth muscle: menstrual sloughing, birth, orgasm (?); milk ejection from mammary	Ejaculation of sperm; orgasm (?)
Androgens	Precursors for estrogen synthesis; stimulate sexual behavior	Complete FSH-initiated spermatogenesis; stimulate prostate gland, other sex accessory structures; stimulate secondary sexual characters, such as beard growth in man
Estrogens	Stimulate proliferation of endometrium; induce LH surge; sensitize uterus to oxytocin; negative feedback on pituitary release; may be primate luteolytic factor (estrone); may induce PRL surge	Converted from androgens; induces male hypothalamus; stimulates sexual behavior
Progesterone	Maintain secretory phase of uterus; inhibit release of gonadotropins from adenohypophysis; maintain pregnancy	None
Prostaglandins	Cause corpus luteum to degenerate at end of luteal phase (not in primate); may be involved in birth initiation (induction of labor)	Ejaculation (?)
Relaxin	Soften pelvic ligaments and cervix; possible role in lactation (?)	None
Chorionic gonadotropin	Stimulates corpus luteum to produce progesterone	None
Chorionic somatomammotropin	Stimulates mammary to synthesize milk during late pregnancy; growth hormone-like (somatotropin) actions on metabolism	None
Inhibin (Sertoli cell factor, folliculostatin)	Inhibits FSH secretion from pituitary (?)	Inhibits FSH secretion from pituitary (?)

center, responsible for the midcycle LH surge observed in sexually mature female mammals. Secretion of GnRH is under stimulatory control of adrenergic neurons and can be inhibited by endogenous opioids. One hypothesis[86] suggests that combined increases in adrenergic activity and an inhibition of opioid secreting neurons allows the ovulatory LH surge to occur.

These gonadotropins stimulate gamete maturation in both males and females as well as steroidogenesis and release of estrogens, androgens and progestogens into the general ciruclation. Gametogenesis (oogenesis, spermatogenesis) appears to be controlled primarily by FSH, whereas LH is primarily responsible for controlling steroidogenesis in both sexes as well as induction of ovulation and formation of corpora lutea in the ovaries of females. Steroidogenesis can also be influenced by FSH in both males and females. The details of these events are discussed later.

The gonadal steroids released through the action of gonadotropins control differentiation and maintenance of many primary and secondary sexual characters such as secretion by the prostate gland and beard growth in men. This was recognized in the 12th century and probably much earlier by the Chinese who used gonadal (and placental) preparations routinely to treat disorders ranging from impotence to the inability of a woman to bear sons. The interstitial cells of the testes and the cells comprising the growing follicle in the ovary are the sources of these steroids. The hypothalamic centers regulating gonadotropin release are sensitive to circulating steroids, which generally produce a negative effect on GnRH release. The notable exception to this pattern is the stimulation of LH and prolactin (PRL) release by estrogens (see p. 264). Additional evidence has been presented for a gonadal factor produced under the influence of FSH in both testes and ovaries that selectively inhibits FSH release with no effect on LH release (see p. 260). This factor is possibly a peptide, called *inhibin.*[95,117] Alternatively, the ratio of testosterone to estradiol in the circulation can influence differential release of FSH and LH and could produce the same results as claimed for inhibin.[168] The inhibin hypothesis is favored at this time.

Several other hormones are involved in mammalian reproduction in addition to those of the hypothalamo-hypophysial-gonadal axis. Prolactin and, to a lesser extent, corticotropin (ACTH) from the adenohypophysis, oxytocin from the pars nervosa, and thyroid hormones all influence reproductive events. The placenta of eutherian mammals has assumed an endocrine role in pregnant females, producing both steroids (primarily estrogens and progesterone) and polypeptide hormones (chorionic gonadotropins, chorionic somatomammotropin, chorionic corticotropin, chorionic thyrotropin). In addition, the endocrine glands of the fetus may influence reproductive events (for example, contribution of the adrenal cortex to steroidogenesis by the placenta) (see Chap. 10). The importance of the pineal gland as a modulator of photoperiod and a source of antigonadotropic factors is discussed in Chapter 15. Finally there are numerous reports of chemical agents termed *pheromones* that are produced by one sex to influence reproductive physiology, behavior or both of the opposite sex. Studies dealing with pheromones and reproduction are discussed in Chapter 15.

In the next section the generalized events of reproduction in eutherian mammals are presented, followed by a brief description of the reproductive cycle of the ewe, human female and 4-day cycling female rat. Separate discussions of the monotremes and some of the special features of marsupials complete consideration of mammalian reproduction. The final portion of this chapter is devoted to nonmammalian vertebrates.

Embryogenesis of Gonads and Their Accessory Ducts

The primordia of the mammalian gonads arise from the intermediate mesoderm as a genital ridge on either side of the midline in close association with the mesonephric kidney. Numerous derivatives of the mesonephric kidney and duct system are retained as functional portions of the vertebrate reproductive system. The gonadal primordium consists of an outer cortex derived from peritoneum and an inner medulla (Fig. 11-1). Differentiation primarily of the medullary component results

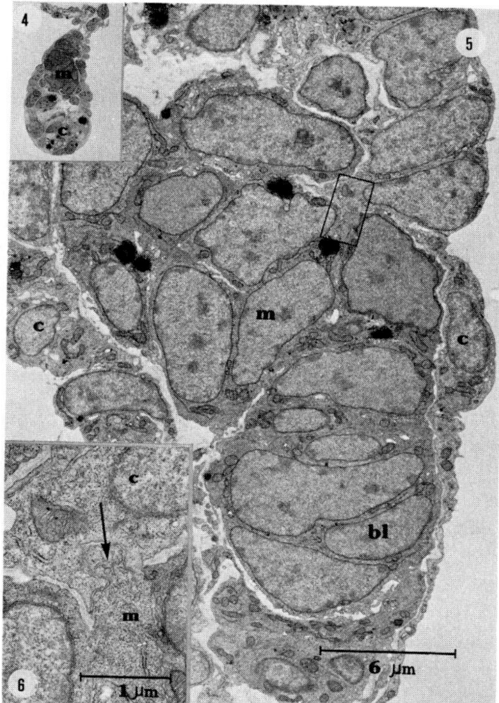

FIG. 11-1. Differentiation of the gonad. Section of gonad from 25-mm tadpole, *Rana pipiens,* showing cortical *(c)* and medullary cells *(m)* separated by a basal lamina *(bl). Upper left inset,* entire gonad. *Lower left inset,* enlargement of area in box to show direct contact of cortical and medullary cell. (Reprinted with permission from H. Merchant-Larios (1978). Ovarian differentiation. In R.E. Jones, ed., The Vertebrate Ovary. Plenum Publishing Corp., New York, pp. 47–81.)

in a testis, whereas the cortical component gives rise to an ovary. Primordial germ cells do not arise within the gonadal primordium itself but migrate from their site of origin in the yolk sac endoderm to whichever component is genetically destined to develop. Initially the medullary component in males and females differentiates into primary sex cords that in males become the seminiferous tubules of the testis. The cortical components degenerate in males. The interstitial cells arise from medullary tissue surrounding the primary sex cords. Primordial germ cells that have migrated into the primary sex cords give rise to spermatogonia. In females the primary sex cords degenerate, and secondary sex cords differentiate from the cortical region. These secondary sex cords become the definitive ovary, and the primordial germ cells give rise to oogonia.

In males the central portion of the differentiating testis forms a network of tubules, known as the *rete testis,* that do not contain seminiferous elements. The rete testis connects the seminiferous tubules with a portion of the mesonephric kidney duct called the *wolffian duct,* which under the influence of testosterone, differentiates into the *vas deferens* and conducts spermatozoa to the urethra. Some of the anterior mesonephric kidney tubules do not completely degenerate, as does most of the mesonephric kidney in mammals. In the presence of testosterone, this tissue together with a portion of the mesonephric duct forms the epididymis and seminal vesicle (Fig. 11-2).

A second pair of longitudinal ducts develops from the mesial wall of the mesonephric duct and lies parallel to the wolffian ducts. These structures are known as the *mullerian ducts.* In genetic females the mullerian ducts develop into the oviducts, uterus and part of the vagina (Fig. 11-2), usually fusing together to form a common vagina and, in some species, a single uterus as well. The wolffian ducts degenerate in females. In males it is the mullerian ducts that are suppressed in favor of wolffian duct development. *Mullerian-inhibiting substance* (MIS) was first proposed by Jost in the 1940s to explain the inhibitory effect of the testes on development of mullerian ducts in rabbit embryos. Implantation of a testis into a female embryo prevents development of the mullerian ducts. Evidence suggests that MIS is a glycoprotein. It not only blocks mullerian duct development but is capable of inhibiting growth of tumors from ovaries and mullerian duct derivatives.[44] It appears that MIS acts cooperatively with testosterone in producing its effects.[76]

Mammalian Life History Patterns

Obvious differences in life cycles can be found by examining the three major mammalian subgroupings: the egg-laying monotremes (Prototheria), the pouched marsupials (Metatheria), and the "placental" mammals (Eutheria). The monotremes have retained the

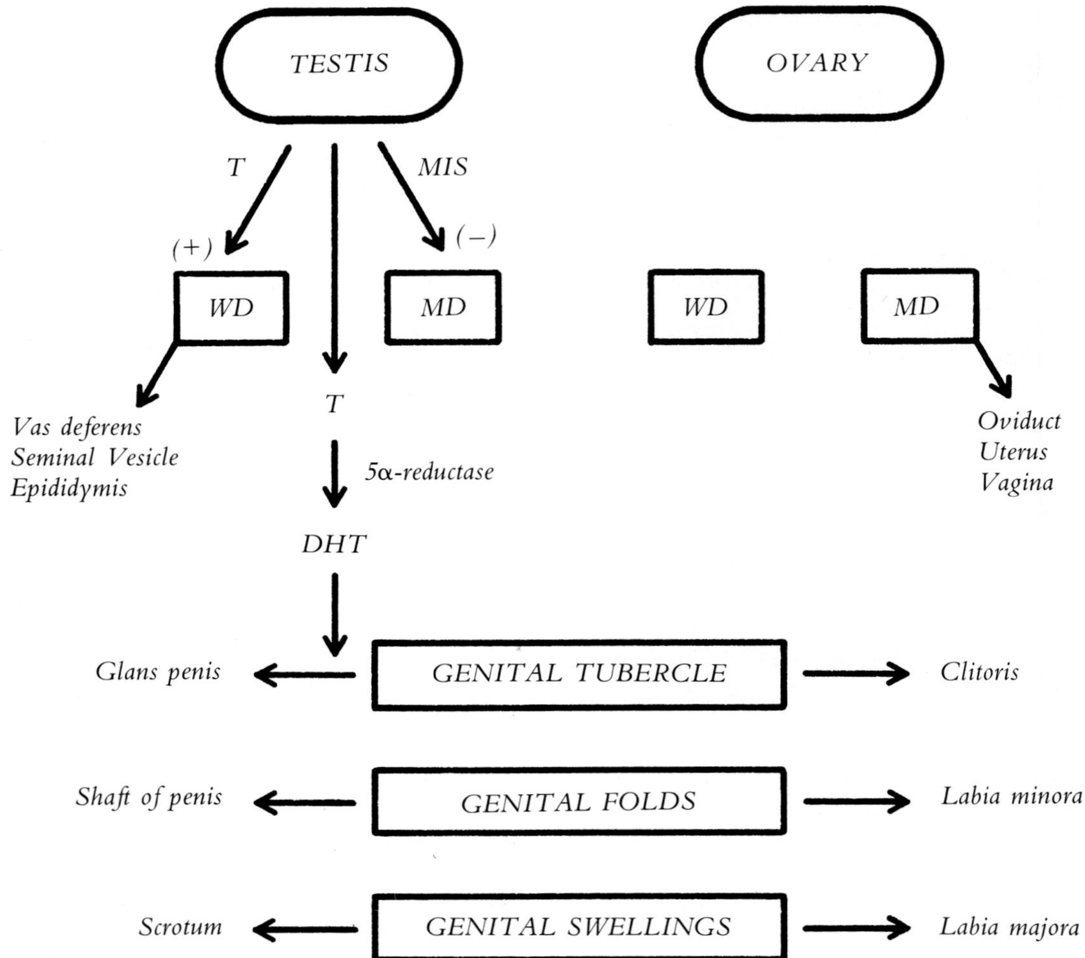

FIG. 11-2. Development of mullerian ducts, wolffian ducts and homologous external genitalia in mammals. The female pattern develops unless altered by secretions from the testes. T, testosterone; DHT, dihydrotestosterone; MIS, mullerian-inhibiting substances; WD, wolffian duct; MD, mullerian duct.

reptilian feature of laying eggs but have added the element of parental care so characteristic of mammals. The duckbill platypus lays its eggs in a nest, but the spiny anteater or echidna places the eggs in a transitory pouch where they develop to hatching. Upon hatching the monotreme appears as a tiny, fetus-like creature with only a few well-developed features that enable it to attach itself to the mother and obtain nourishment. The degree of development at hatching is similar to that of marsupials at birth.

There are about 230 species of marsupials distributed among Australia and North and South America. A primitive type of placenta does develop in marsupials, but it apparently has no endocrine function. The period of pregnancy or gestation is very short in marsupials, and the young marsupial is born in an extremely immature condition. Among the macropodids (kangaroos) the "joey" must find its way essentially unaided to the mother's pouch or *marsupium* where it permanently attaches to the nipple of a mammary gland. The joey continues its development as an "exteriorized fetus." After a long period of pouch development (about 200 days in the red kangaroo), the young marsupial disengages itself from the teat and ventures outside of the pouch, returning first at regular and later at irregular intervals for milk.

Eutherian mammals employ the placenta not only as an endocrine organ to maintain gestation but also as a replacement for the mammary glands to supply nutrition to the fetus. Consequently birth (parturition) is delayed considerably, and the newborn placental mammal (neonate) is at a comparable stage of development to the young marsupial when it first leaves the pouch. Like the juvenile marsupial the newborn placental mammal relies at first on the mammary gland as the exclusive source of nourishment but gradually abandons it for other foods.

The patterns of reproduction in eutherian mammals will be discussed in some detail, followed by separate descriptions of three representative females: ewes, women, and 4-day cycling rats. Monotremes and marsupial mammals will be considered, but only major differences with respect to eutherian mammals will be stressed.

Eutherian Reproductive Patterns

Three distinct reproductive patterns occur in sexually mature eutherians, one typically for males and two among females. Males are characterized by continuous secretion of gonadotropins and more or less continuous spermatogenesis. In many species the males are capable of siring offspring at any time of year. Most species, however, exhibit seasonal episodes of spermatogenesis, sexual activity or both such as displayed by nonmammalian vertebrates.

Females exhibit cyclic patterns of gonadotropin secretion that can be traced to a basic rhythmicity within the hypothalamus. There are two types of female cycles: the *estrous cycle* and the *menstrual cycle.* The estrous cycle is typical for most mammals and consists of a repeated series of precisely regulated endocrine events. The periods within the estrous cycle can be readily distinguished. *Proestrus* is characterized by the hormonal changes that bring about ovulation. *Estrus* immediately follows or coincides with ovulation, and it is a short period when the female is receptive to the male and during which mating can occur. It is also the time when fertilization is most likely to lead to pregnancy and successful birth of offspring. The interim between estrus and the onset of hormonal changes characteristic of proestrus in cases in which pregnancy did not result is termed *diestrus.* Carnivores may be classified as *monestrous.* If mating does not occur or if mating occurs but fertilization and implantation are unsuccessful, the female will not return to estrus until the next breeding season. Many mammalian species are *polyestrous,* however, and will return immediately to proestrus if mating does not occur or if mating is unsuccessful. In certain rodents mating without successful fertilization and implantation may result in a short period of simulated or false pregnancy, termed *pseudopregnancy,* after which the female reenters proestrus.

Some primates, including man, exhibit a different sequence of events, known as the menstrual cycle, that is characterized by sloughing of the uterine lining if fertilization does not lead to pregnancy. The sloughing of the uterine lining results in a vaginal discharge of blood and uterine epithelial cells. This stage is known as the *menses* or period of menstrual flow. The onset of menses precedes the *preovulatory* or *follicular phase* (phase of the growing follicle of the cycle) and marks the end of the *postovulatory* or *luteal phase* (the phase of the corpus luteum). Most primates exhibit estrous behavior to some degree at about the time of ovulation, including species characterized as having menstrual cycles, although a well-defined estrus is not observed in the human female. Possession of menstrual or estrous cycles should not be considered as alternative cycles.

Some mammals such as the cow and bitch discharge blood prior to ovulation and the onset of estrous behavior. This discharge is estrogen induced and is not similar to uterine breakdown and the menses of primates.

Many mammals ovulate following coitus and are termed *induced ovulators.* Several carnivores (for example, ferret, mink, raccoon, cat), rodents (for example, *Microtus californicus*), lagomorphs (for example, cottontail and domestic rabbits), one bat (lump-nosed bat) and several insectivores (for example, hedgehog, common shrew) have been proven to be induced ovulators. Some other species are suspected to be induced ovulators (the elephant seal, nutria and a marsupial, the long-nosed kangaroo rat). Induced ovulators do not exhibit a cyclic pattern of gonadotropin release, because the LH surge occurs only after copulation takes place. Most mammals are believed to be so-called *spontaneous ovulators* in that coitus does not usually cause ovulation. However, even some spontaneous ovulators can be induced to ovulate following copulation under special conditions. For example, ovulation can be induced in the rat by appropriate hormone treatment followed by copulation.[187]

Although reproductive endocrinologists consistently focus upon estrous and menstrual cycles, it is important to remember that the normal sequel to ovulation is pregnancy. In nature, it is unusual for a female to enter estrous and not become pregnant. The observation that lactating females usually do not enter estrous supports the hypothesis that elevated levels of PRL can block pulsatile LH release as well as the LH surge required for ovulation.[12]

Endocrine Regulation of Male Reproductive Events. Maleness in eutherian mammals is dependent upon secretion of androgens from the testis. In the absence of androgens the male genotype (XY) will develop as a female phenotype. Conversely, treatment of newborn females with androgens destroys the cyclic secretory pattern of the hypothalamo-hypophysial system and replaces it with a noncyclic pattern like that of males. It may be that androgen treatment destroys only the activities of the cyclic hypothalamic center whereas the tonic center of females is unaffected.

In some species postpubertal males are capable of copulating with a female whenever she is receptive. Secretion of GnRH and hence of gonadotropins is more or less continuous but with daily fluctuations occurring in circulating levels of some gonadotropins. Daily secretory patterns for gonadotropins show considerable variation among different species. Hourly fluctuations of LH have been reported in bulls, and these variations in LH are correlated with following surges in circulating testosterone (Fig. 11-3). However, in human males, FSH shows no cyclic variation in blood levels although LH and testosterone exhibit clear daily patterns with peak levels occurring

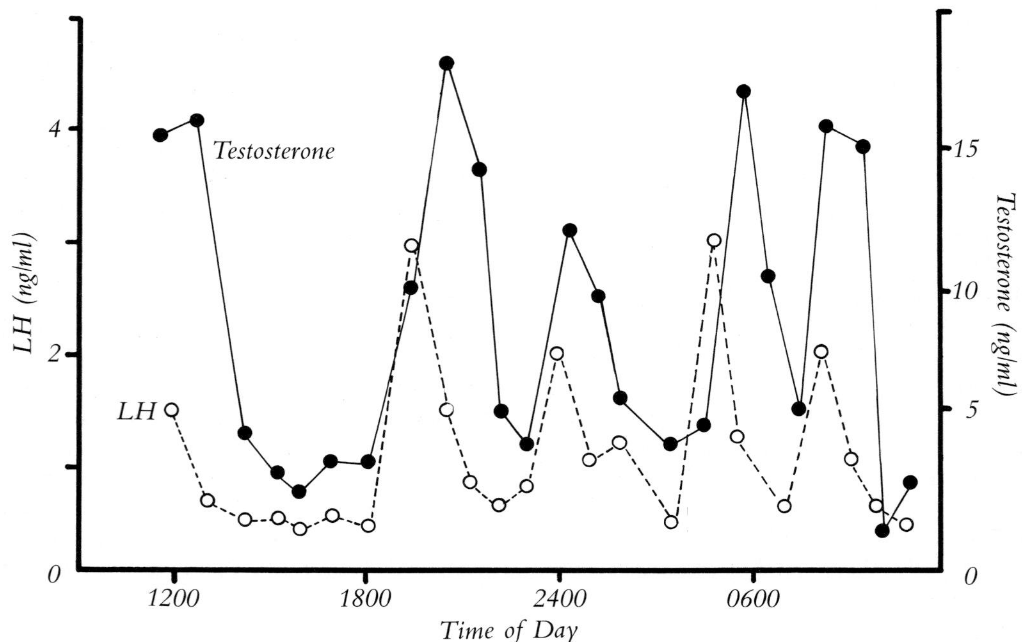

Fig. 11-3. Diurnal variations in blood levels of luteinizing hormone *(LH)* and testosterone in a bull. Release of LH precedes each peak in testosterone release from the testis. (Redrawn from Short.[169])

during early morning hours and minimum values reported for the afternoon.[149,150] Wild mammals exhibit distinct seasonal breeding, and spermatogenesis may be restricted to a few months or less.

Spermatogenesis. The testis develops primarily from the medullary portion of the embryonic gonadal blastema. Differentiation of the medullary portion with concomitant regression of the cortical components (progenitor of the ovary) appears to be controlled by embryonic androgen secretion. The medullary cords differentiate into *seminiferous tubules* and interspersed masses of *interstitial* or *Leydig cells.* These interstitial cells are steroidogenic and are located between the seminiferous tubules. Androgens are synthesized and released into the circulation by interstitial cells. The seminiferous tubules consist of large *Sertoli* or *sustentacular cells, spermatogonia* and cells derived from the latter. The seminiferous tubules are surrounded by *peritubular cells* that are believed to be responsible for contractile activity of the seminiferous tubules.[66] The Sertoli cell has an extensive cytoplasm extending from the outer edge to the lumen of the tubule. The nucleus of the Sertoli cell is located at the outer edge. In addition to the Sertoli cells, the primordial germ cells that give rise to spermatogonia are present along the outer margins of the tubules. Spermatogonial cells proliferate mitotically under the influence of FSH and eventually undergo differentiation characterized by nuclear enlargement to become *primary spermatocytes.* These cells undergo the first meiotic division to give rise to two smaller *secondary spermatocytes,* which are rarely observed in histological preparations because, once formed, they enter the second meiotic division to yield four haploid *spermatids.* Testicular androgens are somehow necessary for meiosis. These spermatids are transformed to *spermatozoa* (spermiogenesis) by concentrating the chromatin material into the spermatozoan head and by elimination of the majority of the cytoplasm. A given histological section of a seminiferous tubule may show varying numbers of spermatogonia, primary spermatocytes, spermatids and spermatozoa in sequence from the outer margin to the lumen. The tails of the spermatozoa extend into the lumen, and the heads of the spermatozoa are typically surrounded by highly folded margins of the Sertoli cells.

Millions of mature spermatozoa may be sloughed off into the lumina of the seminiferous tubules each day. This process is termed *spermiation.* These spermatozoa pass along through the tubules, which eventually coalesce into larger ducts and eventually form the *epididymis* associated with each testis. Vast numbers of mature spermatozoa are stored in the epididymis. Under the influence of androgens the epididymis secretes materials into its lumen where the spermatozoa are being held. Included in this secretion are protein-bound sialic acids (sialomucoproteins), glycerylphosphoryl-choline and carnitine. These particular substances are involved directly in maintaining spermatozoa in viable condition until ejaculation. Androgens and androgen-binding protein (ABP) produced by sustentacular cells in the seminiferous tubules are released along with spermatozoa and travel to the epididymis. Androgen freed from ABP in the lumen or androgen-ABP complexes or both are absorbed by the epididymal cells. These androgens stimulate epididymal cells to secrete materials involved in maintenance of the spermatozoa.

As a consequence of the forcible ejection (ejaculation) that occurs during copulation the spermatozoa leave the epididymis, enter the vas deferens and travel to the urethra. The spermatozoa traverse the length of the penis via the urethra and are deposited in the female's vagina during coitus. Various glands such as the prostate add their fluid secretions to the spermatozoa and epididymal secretions to form a watery mixture of spermatozoa and various organic and inorganic substances known as *semen.* The entire ejaculatory event may be induced by the release of oxytocin from the pars nervosa in response to a neural reflex initiated by mechanical stimulation of the penis.

Roles for Gonadotropins in Male Mammals. Relatively separate roles have been defined for LH and FSH in males. Spermatogenesis is initiated by FSH, which stimulates proliferation of spermatogonia and formation of primary spermatocytes (Figs. 11-4, 11-5). In addition, androgens are thought to initiate meiotic divi-

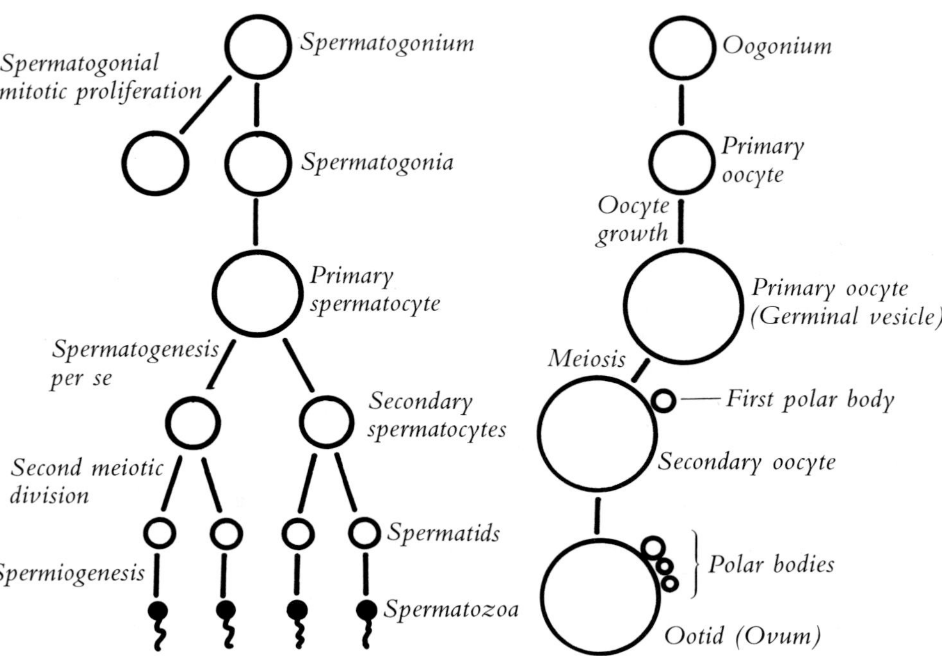

Fig. 11-4. Gametogenesis in testis and ovary. One diploid spermatogonial cell gives rise to four haploid spermatozoa via meiosis. In the ovary the oogonium gives rise to only one haploid gamete, which receives the bulk of the cytoplasm, with the remainder of the nuclear contents being partitioned into inactive polar bodies. The first polar body may not undergo the second meiotic division, and only two polar bodies may be formed.

sions of primary spermatocytes, resulting eventually in formation of spermatids.[180] The Sertoli cell of the seminiferous tubule also appears to be a target for FSH. The production of ABP by the Sertoli cell is stimulated by FSH.[66,123] This ABP is released into the testicular fluid where it binds androgens.

Spermatogenesis is apparently a temperature-sensitive process, and high temperatures such as found within the body cavity of most eutherians can impair normal spermatogenesis and produce temporary sterility. Consequently, at some time prior to the attainment of sexual maturity or prior to the annual breeding season, the testes descend into the scrotum where spermatogenesis can proceed at a slightly lower temperature. The failure of the testes to descend, a condition known as cryptorchidism, may cause irreparable damage to the seminiferous epithelium in most species. Some mammals lack a scrotum (for example, the elephant, whale, seal), and the testes are permanently located within the abdominal cavity. In such species spermatogenesis obviously does not exhibit the same temperature sensitivity characteristic for scrotal species. The male elephant, for example, is capable of producing viable sperm and copulating with a female at any time of year.

The synthesis and release of circulating androgens by the interstitial cells is controlled by LH (Fig. 11-6). Testosterone is the major circulating androgen, although other androgens such as androstenedione or 5α-hydroxytestosterone (DHT) may circulate in significant amounts.[169] Prior to attainment of puberty in bulls, androstenedione is the principal circulating androgen, but it is gradually replaced by testosterone at puberty. There is evidence for a separate FSH-sensitive site in the testis for androgen synthesis,[77] and there are data to suggest the Sertoli cell may be that site.

The interstitial cells of the testis synthesize and release estrogens as well as androgens.[144] Testicular estrogens reach dramatic levels in the stallion. Females, on the other hand, se-

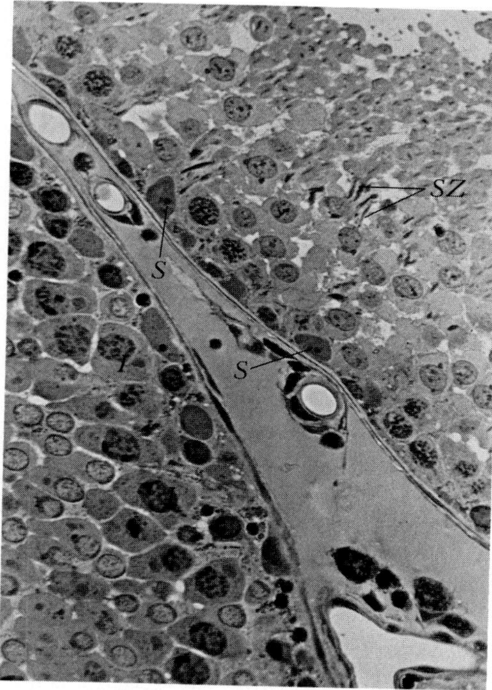

FIG. 11-5. Section of the rat testis showing adjacent seminiferous tubules. *S*, nuclei of Sertoli cells; *I*, primary spermatocytes; *Sz*, heads of spermatozoa. (Courtesy of Drs. Charles H. Muller and C. Desjardins.)

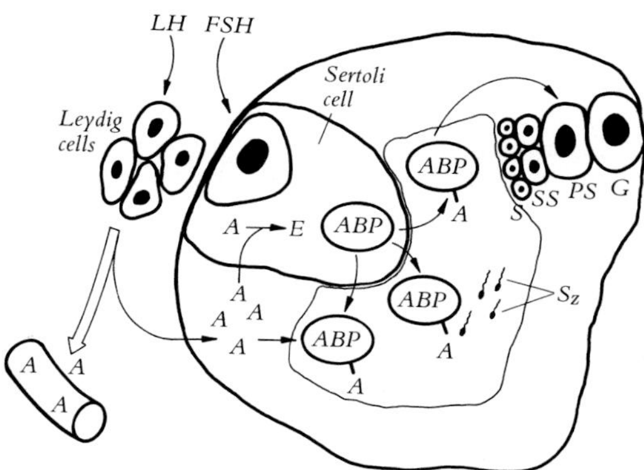

FIG. 11-6. Actions of gonadotropins on testicular cells. Under the influence of LH, Leydig cells produce androgens *(A)* that enter the general circulation. A small proportion of these androgens may enter the seminiferous tubules and may be converted to estrogens *(E)* by Sertoli cells under the influence of FSH or may be bound extracellularly to an androgen-binding protein *(ABP)* also produced by the Sertoli cells. Production of ABP is controlled by FSH. Concentration of androgens in the vicinity of the primary spermatocytes may be a consequence of the presence of ABP. The initiation of meiosis in the primary spermatocyte is caused by androgens. The production of ABP and its binding of androgens prior to its transport to the epididymis may be responsible for transport of androgens to the epididymis where they stimulate secretion. *G*, gonia; *PS*, primary spermatocyte; *SS*, secondary spermatocyte; *S*, spermatid; *Sz*, spermatozoa.

crete small quantities of androgens in addition to estrogens. Maleness or femaleness may be only an expression of the relative proportions of androgens to estrogens in the circulation, although transitory alterations in these ratios may occur normally. Estrogens may have definite physiological roles in males. Estradiol can block androgen synthesis by interstitial cells and can influence the responsiveness of these cells to gonadotropins.[135] The ratio of testosterone to estradiol in the general circulation may alter the ratios of FSH and LH being released from the pituitary.[168]

Interstitial cell function is reduced in humans as a consequence of long term treatment with GnRH. This appears to be a direct action of GnRH on the interstitial cell and not an indirect effect on the pituitary.[75] Receptors for GnRH are found on interstitial cells, and there is evidence that the testis produces a GnRH-like substance. The significance of these observations for normal testicular function is not clear.

Action and Metabolism of Androgens in Males. Circulating androgens influence development and maintenance of several glands and related structures associated with the male genital tract, such as the prostate gland and seminal vesicles, and induce development of certain secondary sexual characters such as growth of the beard in man. Androgens also exert a negative feedback effect upon the secretion of gonadotropins primarily through actions at the level of the hypothalamus (see Chap. 4).

The action of testosterone in some of its target cells is believed to involve first its conversion to 5α-dihydrotestosterone by the enzyme 5α-reductase. It is DHT which then binds to the cytoplasmic androgen receptor.[119] Development of prostate and bulbourethral glands, the penis and scrotum are dependent upon conversion of testosterone to DHT. Many androgenic responses, however, are not mediated by DHT (Table 11-2), and this conversion is not necessary for testosterone to produce its effects. In some target tissues, androgens have

TABLE 11-2. *Some Androgenic Responses Not Mediated by 5α-Dihydrotestosterone*[119]

TARGET CELL	BIOLOGICAL RESPONSE
Skeletal muscle	Anabolic response
Bone marrow	Stimulation of RNA synthesis
Chick blastoderm, "fetal" hepatocytes	(+) Heme synthesis; induction of β-amino levulinate synthetase
Brain	Sexual behavior; sex-specific characteristics
Brain[a]	Anovulatory sterility
Wolffian duct	Differentiation of epididymis, seminal vesicle and vas deferens
Mouse kidney	Induction of β-glucuronidase
Uterus	Stimulation of glandular secretions
Rat prostate	Stimulation of glandular secretions
Dog prostate	Enhanced DNA and RNA synthesis
Chick oviduct	Differentiation of magnum
Vagina (immature)	Growth and keratinization

[a] female neonate

been shown to undergo conversion to estrogens through aromatization of the A ring (see Chap. 9) and removal of the C_{19} carbon atom. This process seems to occur, for example, in nervous tissue, but it is not clear whether aromatization is essential to the mechanism of androgen action or is related to metabolism of the androgen (degradation). Development from each wolffian duct of vas deferens, epididymis, seminal vesicle and ejaculatory duct is regulated by testosterone and does not require conversion of testosterone to DHT. Sertoli cells also convert androgens to estrogens, and this aromatization of androgens is stimulated by FSH[3] (Fig. 11-6). This action of FSH on aromatization of androgen is similar to that proposed for the synthesis of estrogens in the ovarian follicle (see p. 261). The role of these testicular estrogens is uncertain, however, but may be related to the action of FSH on the synthesis of ABP by the Sertoli cell.

Aromatization of androgens such as testosterone to estrogens occurs in several areas of the brain,[21,22,120] and this conversion is necessary for some of the behavioral effects of androgens. Aromatization to an estrogen is not requisite for all behavioral effects induced by androgens, however. Induction of some male behaviors in castrates requires aromatization and cannot be induced by nonaromatizable androgens such as DHT, whereas others may be induced by either aromatizable androgens or by DHT.[1]

A separate testicular product, *inhibin,* has been proposed to regulate FSH release from the adenohypophysis.[117] This activity has been reported for rete testis fluid, seminal plasma, testicular extracts and ejaculate.[163] Sertoli cells of the rat testis produce a water-soluble, heat-labile *Sertoli cell factor* that selectively inhibits synthesis and release of pituitary FSH without affecting LH.[28,179] This Sertoli cell factor may be the inhibin molecule originally proposed by McCullagh.[117]

FEMALE CYCLES. Although marked differences can be pointed out between endocrine events related to estrous and menstrual cycles, there are probably greater differences among species exhibiting one of these types than in comparison of the two types. Nevertheless there are several distinctive similarities that characterize females, regardless of whether they exhibit estrous or menstrual cycles.

The Follicular Phase. The basis for the cyclical nature of female reproductive events resides in the hypothalamus and is a genetically determined female characteristic. During the *follicular phase* of the ovarian cycle the tonic hypothalamic center releases small quantities of GnRH into the portal circulation and relatively low but rather constant circulating levels of FSH, LH or both are maintained. In general, prior to puberty, which is characterized by increased gonadotropin levels, the ovary contains primary oocytes invested with modified stromal cells (the primary follicle). In most mammals there are no oogonia in the ovary because all of them differentiated into primary oocytes prior to or shortly after birth. The arrival of FSH at the ovary stimulates primary follicles to begin to enlarge and differentiate (Fig. 11-7). The growing oocyte becomes surrounded by two distinct layers of cells, the inner *granulosa cells* and the outer *thecal*

TABLE 11-3. *Circulating Steroid Levels per ml Plasma in Several Mammalian Species*

SPECIES[a]	TESTOSTERONE	ESTRADIOL	PROGESTERONE	REF.
Didelphis virginiana (opossum)				
pregnant marsupial F			12 ng	67
Setonix brachyurus (quokka)				
pregnant marsupial F			902 pg	67
Macaca fuscata fuscata (Japanese monkey) F follicular phase and luteal phase peaks		150–250 pg	2.0–5.3 ng	5
Loxodonta africana (African elephant)				
nonpregnant F		12, 16 pg	208, 215 pg	150
pregnant F		11, 20 pg	416, 482 pg	150
Elaphus maximus (Asian elephant)				
nonpregnant F		26, 30 pg	153, 195 pg	150
pregnant F		26 pg	263 pg	150
Chimpanzee				
nonpregnant F		0.6–1.0 ng	20 ng	154
pregnant F		5.0–8.0 ng	49–120 ng	154
Homo sapiens				
pregnant F		5.5–30 ng	45–210 ng	154
Lemur catta (ring-tailed lemur)				
nonpregnant F		120 ± 30 pg	92.5 ± 15.5 ng	186
Herpestes auropunctatus (mongoose)	2–5.5 ng			176
Rattus				
immature[b] M	1.2 ng		1.75 ng	62
basal levels F		17–21 pg	2–7 ng	19
proestrous F		88 ± 2 pg	46 ± 7 ng	19
diestrous F			24 ± 3 ng	19

NOTE: Values provided are peak levels unless indicated otherwise.
[a]F, female; M, male
[b]Extrapolated from peak diurnal variations.

cells (Fig. 11-7). Thecal cells further differentiate into an inner and an outer theca (theca interna and theca externa). The granulosa cells are separated from the thecal layers by connective tissue, and there is no penetration of capillaries into the granulosa. As the follicle grows the granulosa cells secrete fluid contributing to the *liquor folliculi* that is primarily an ultrafiltrate of blood plasma. Increasing production of liquor folliculi results in formation and progressive enlargement of a fluid-filled cavity within the follicle, the *antrum.* Most follicles degenerate to form *corpora atretica;* only a few will ever ovulate.

Under the influence of LH, FSH-primed follicular cells synthesize and release estrogens, predominantly estradiol-17β, into the general circulation. The synthesis of estrogens in the ovary appears to be a cooperative effort between cells of the theca interna and the granulosa.[48,202] Recent studies support the interpretation that LH stimulates the thecal cells to produce androgens that are aromatized by the granulosa cells to form estrogens. Furthermore, the conversion of androgens to estrogens by the granulosa cells appears to be stimulated by FSH. Consequently synthesis of ovarian estrogens may involve two gonadotropins, each producing its primary effect on a different cellular type in the growing follicle (Fig. 11-8).

Estradiol-17β stimulates differentiation and proliferation of the uterine lining or *endometrium* in preparation for implantation of the *blastocyst,* a blastula formed from the first series of cellular divisions following fertilization. The blastocyst consists of an outer extraembryonic layer of cells, the *trophoblast,* which

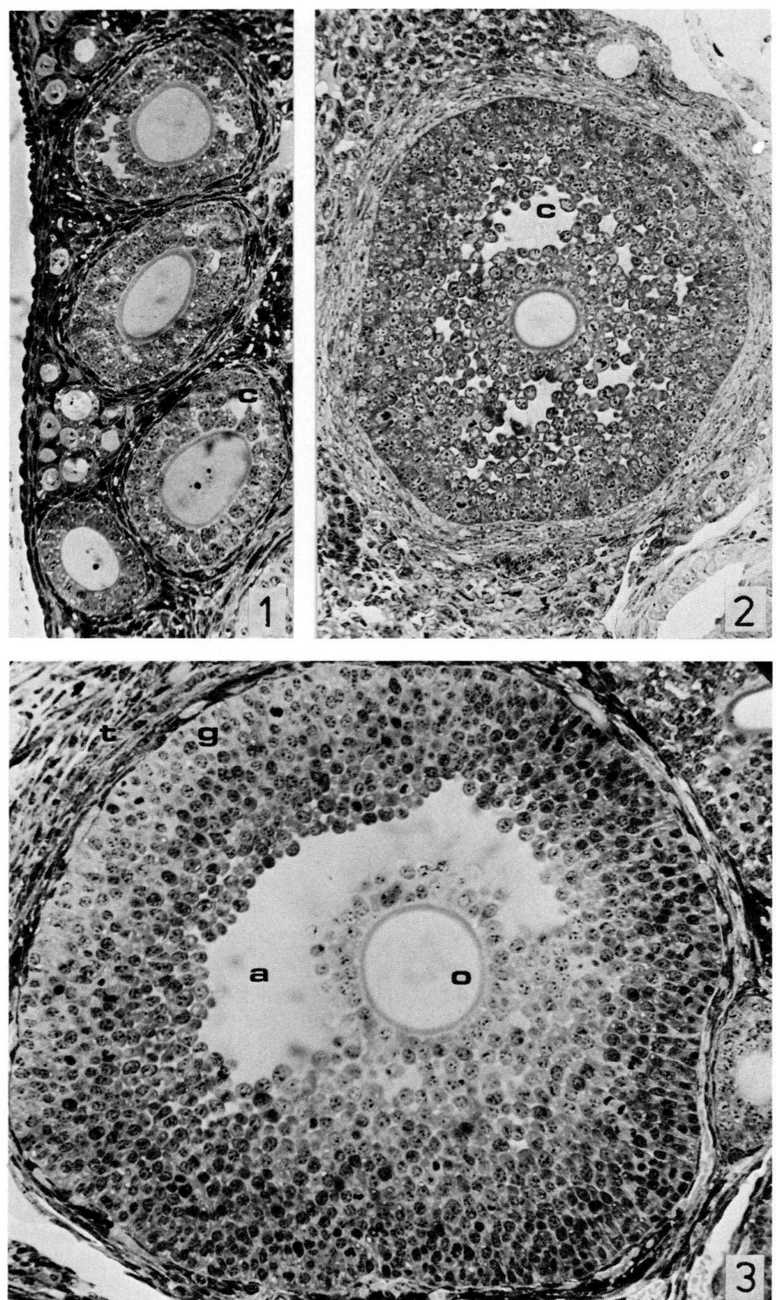

Fig. 11-7. The mammalian ovary. Section of mouse ovary showing follicles at different stages of development. *Upper left,* Naked oocytes, primary follicles and four growing follicles showing early stage of antrum formation *(c). Upper right,* A large, preantral follicle with antrum beginning to form. *Lower portion,* Young follicle with antrum *(a). g,* granulosa; *t,* theca; *o,* oocyte. (Reprinted with permission from K.P. McNatty (1978). Follicular fluid. In R.E. Jones, ed., The Vertebrate Ovary. Plenum Publishing Co., New York, pp. 215–259.)

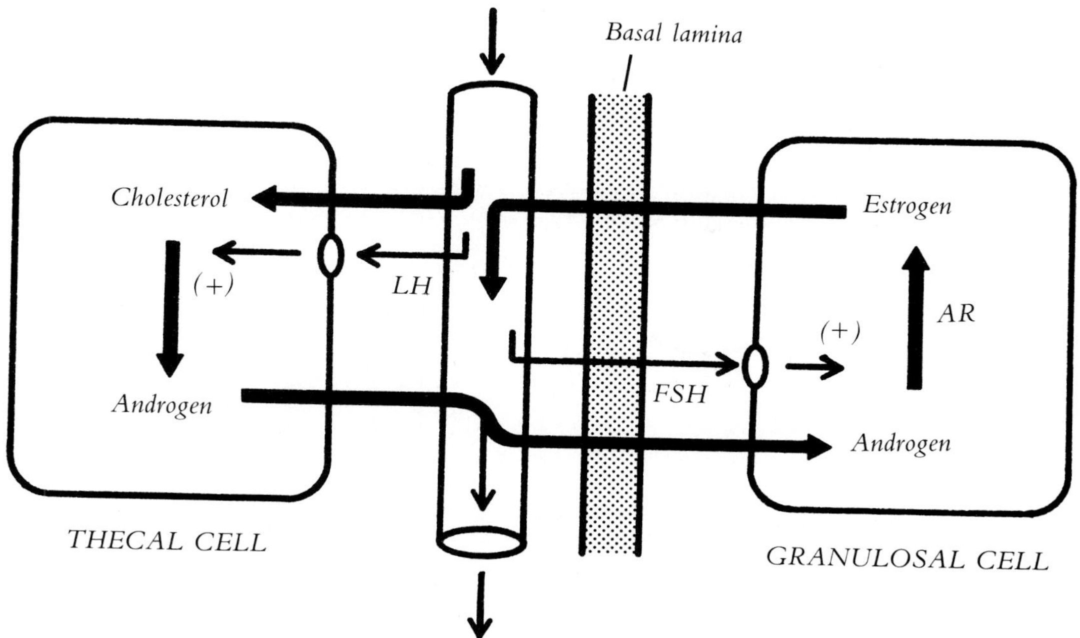

Fig. 11-8. Synthesis of steroids by the ovarian follicle. Conversion of cholesterol to androgens is stimulated in the thecal cell by LH. Androgens must diffuse through the basal lamina that separates the thecal cell and vascular supply from the granulosal cell. Under the influence of FSH the granulosal cell converts androgens to estrogens using aromatase (AR). Based on Erickson.[48]

will form the fetal component of the placenta, and an *inner cell mass,* which will become the embryo proper.

Ovulation. The levels of circulating estradiol-17β increase progressively with the growth of the follicles and the increase in thecal and granulosa cells. A maximum or critical estrogen level activates the cyclic center in the hypothalamus, which releases a large pulse of GnRH. The action of estrogens on GnRH release appears to be mediated via norepinephrine-secreting hypothalamic neurons. The pulse of GnRH released results in a dramatic increase in circulating LH with simultaneous release of FSH (Figs. 11-9 and 11-10).

This so-called LH surge causes ovulation of one or more follicles within a matter of hours. The number of follicles ovulating is species specific, varying from one in women to a dozen or more in the sow. The mechanism by which LH causes the mature follicle to rupture and release the mature oocyte is not known. The LH surge induces granulosa cells as well as some theca interna cells to differentiate into the *corpus luteum.* This process is known as *luteinization,* and the resulting corpus luteum functions as an endocrine gland, secreting both estrogens and progesterone into the general circulation. One corpus luteum will form from each ovulated follicle. In addition, other developing follicles may undergo luteinization and function as *accessory corpora lutea* during pregnancy. The importance of the smaller FSH surge may be related to initiation of follicle development in the next cycle.[155]

In lower vertebrates, meiosis in the oocyte usually is not completed until after fertilization. Prior to fertilization the ovulated cell is still termed an oocyte. If meiosis was completed prior to ovulation this cell is termed an ovum. The situation in mammals apparently varies from ovulation of oocytes to ova, but here the ovulated cell in every case will be referred to as an ovum for purposes of simplifying discussion.

The Luteal Phase. Ovulation marks the onset of the luteal phase of the ovarian cycle. The corpus luteum begins secreting large

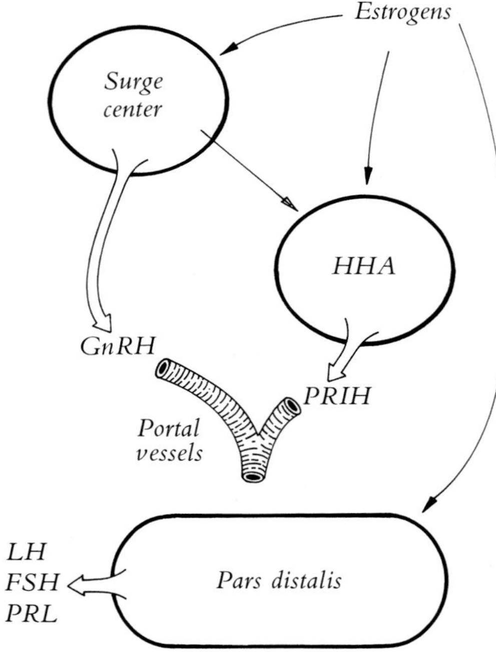

Fig. 11-9. Hypothalamic actions of estrogens in female mammals. Estrogens are known to stimulate a "surge center" in the hypothalamus controlling release of GnRH. Evidence also has been presented for an estrogen-sensitive PRL-surge center that inhibits PRIH release from the hypothalamo-hypophysiotropic area *(HHA)* in the medial basal hypothalamus. This HHA region may be directly sensitive to estrogens as well. Estrogens can directly stimulate PRL release from the pars distalis in vitro and may do so in vivo.

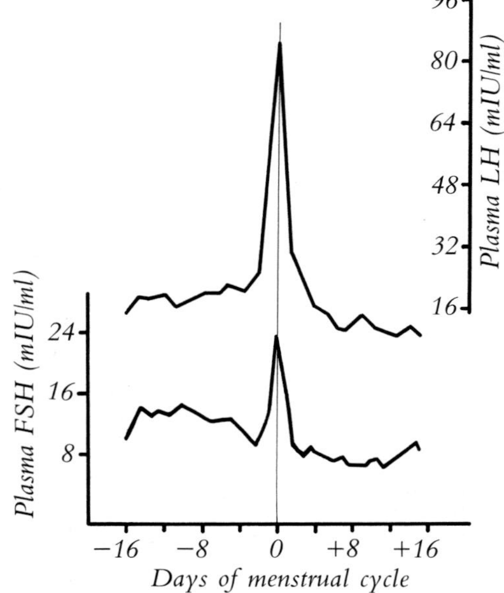

Fig. 11-10. Midcycle gonadotropin surge in normal women. The magnitude of the LH surge is accentuated by shifting the scales. (Modified from McCann.[116])

quantities of progesterone, estradiol-17β and other estrogens and progestogens. Progesterone maintains the proliferated uterine endometrium in the *secretory phase* during which the uterus secretes a fluid sometimes called *uterine milk* or *embryotroph.* Uterine milk is believed to be a source of nourishment for unimplanted blastocysts. The endometrium of marsupials produces a similar secretion. Progesterone also maintains the highly vascularized state of the uterus necessary for implantation and development of the embryo. Muscle layers of the uterus become desensitized by progesterone with respect to responding to certain stimuli with rhythmic contractions. This uterine quiescence is necessary for maintaining a successful pregnancy to term (birth or parturition). Circulating progesterone and estrogens inhibit both the tonic and cyclic hypothalamic GnRH centers during the luteal phase and during pregnancy so that follicular development is arrested and a second ovulatory episode is prevented.

Depending on the species, regulation of corpus luteum function may require LH or be independent of LH once it has formed. In sheep, prolactin (PRL) together with LH might stimulate steroid secretion by the corpus luteum. Only PRL can maintain the activity of the rat corpus luteum. Preovulatory estradiol-17β can produce a surge of PRL release in several species that might be related to corpus luteum function (Fig. 11-9).

The corpus luteum secretes steroids for only a relatively short period in most species (5 to 8 days in man) after which it begins to degenerate. As the corpus luteum undergoes degeneration, steroidogenesis declines, and the uterus enters a regressive phase unless the animal is pregnant. In some species the corpus luteum is relatively long lived, especially in monestrous species like the dog, which will not reenter estrus until the next breeding season. Corpora lutea of the bitch continue to be active for about 63 days after ovulation which is equal to the normal gestation period.

The predetermined life span for the functional corpus luteum has provided one of the most intriguing mysteries of the ovarian cycle. Apparently the corpus luteum sows the seeds of its own destruction. In female rats, mice, hamsters, rabbits, guinea pigs and ewes, progesterone from the corpus luteum stimulates the synthesis and release of molecules known as prostaglandins (PGFs) from the uterine endometrium.[59,94,169] (Prostaglandins are discussed in Chap. 15.) These PGFs, especially $PGF_{2\alpha}$, are luteolytic, that is, they cause destruction of the corpus luteum (Fig. 11-11). The mechanism of their luteolytic activity is not clear, although it may relate to an influence on the integrity of the blood vascular supply to the corpus luteum. In primates the destruction of the corpus luteum toward the end of the luteal phase is not influenced by the uterus but appears to be caused locally by a luteolytic estrogen, estrone, produced by the corpus luteum itself.[20] If fertilization has taken place, there are several possible mechanisms by which corpus luteum degeneration is prevented (see The Pregnancy Cycle later in the chapter).

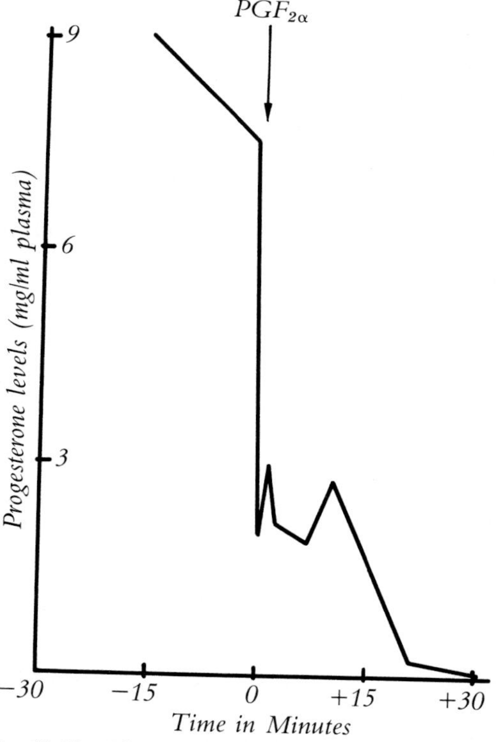

Fig. 11-11. Effect of an intrauterine infusion of prostaglandins ($PGF_{2\alpha}$) on midluteal plasma progesterone levels in the cow. Progesterone levels are shown from 15 minutes prior to the beginning of the infusion to about 30 minutes after onset of infusion. (Modified from Cumming.[38])

Should implantation not occur, the corpus luteum of most eutherian mammals will rapidly degenerate, resulting in a marked decrease in circulating levels of progesterone and estrogens. This decrease in circulating ovarian steroid brings about two major events. The endometrium undergoes regressive changes following steroid withdrawal, becoming less secretory and less capable of supporting implantation of a blastocyst should it occur. In higher primates the exposed layers of the endometrium slough so that considerable rebuilding of the endometrium must occur during the next follicular phase to prepare for implantation of blastocysts resulting from the next ovulation. The second event is the freeing of the hypothalamic GnRH centers from the inhibitory influence of estrogens and progesterone, resulting in a moderate increase in circulating gonadotropins and consequently renewal of follicular development. In fact, increased FSH release occurs during the later stages of the luteal phase in polyestrous species so that follicular growth has resumed even before regressive uterine events become obvious.

It should be emphasized that in wild sexually mature mammals, fertilization and pregnancy are normal events, and coitus occurs frequently during estrus. The character of the ovarian cycle and its rapid resumption in many species if fertilization and successful implantation do not occur ensure either rapid reentry into estrus or rapid appearance of one or more new ova or both and a second opportunity to produce offspring during that season.

The importance of the corpus luteum in maintaining pregnancy varies considerably as does the role of pituitary hormones in stimulating corpus luteum function. In rats PRL is necessary for maintaining the first half of gestation through actions on the corpus luteum, whereas in pigs the corpora lutea secrete progesterone to maintain the uterine secretory phase during the early portion of the gestation period without aid of any adenohypophysial hormones. In ewes, both LH and PRL are necessary for maintaining corpus luteum function during the first third of pregnancy, but maintenance of pregnancy actually resides in the ability of the conceptus to neutralize the uterine luteolytic factor ($PGF_{2\alpha}$).[169] Estrogens of placental origin apparently are responsible for prolonging the life span of corpora lutea in rabbits as well as promoting progesterone synthesis. If the estrogen-secreting placental cells are damaged (for example, by roentgen rays), pregnancy is abruptly terminated.

Actions of Estrogens and Progesterone on the Uterus. Estradiol-17β may have two independent targets in the uterus (see Chap. 1). One target is the epithelial cell, which responds to estrogens with new RNA and protein synthesis such as that characterized in the mechanism of action for steroids exemplified in the Jensen hypothesis. A second target may be the uterine eosinophil, which is a white blood cell that has infiltrated the uterine lining. These eosinophils supposedly possess specific cytosol receptors for estradiol-17β and appear to be responsible for the rapid uptake of water and release of histamine that characterize uterine responses to estrogens.

The mechanisms for maintenance of the secretory phase in the uterus by progesterone are not understood. However, progesterone acts as a local anesthetic to uterine smooth muscle and thus thwarts premature births, at least in some species.

Placental Types. Mammalian placental types differ considerably in terms of the degree of fetal-maternal fusion and with respect to the intimacy of the vascular relationship between the fetus and the mother. Consequently several terminologies have been devised to describe placentas structurally and functionally.

Monotremes have no placenta and are termed *aplacental.* The placenta of marsupials involves the fusion of an embryonic endodermal membrane (the yolk sac) with the chorion (a covering sac derived from the embryonic trophoblast) to form a transitory *yolk-sac placenta.* In a few marsupials, the allantois (another fetal membrane derived from the endoderm like the yolk sac) fuses with the chorion to form a chorioallantoic relationship like that of eutherian mammals.

In the true placental mammals (Eutheria), the chorion produces vascular tufts or villi that form an intimate relation with the uterine endometrium. The allantois fuses with the chorion to produce the *chorioallantoic placenta.* When the allantois is absent the unit is simply termed a *chorionic placenta.*

The true placenta, or *placenta vera,* is fused to the uterine tissues so that some of the uterine tissues are stripped off at birth, causing uterine bleeding (deciduate placentation). If there is no fusion of chorion or chorioallantois with the endometrium the unit is termed a *semiplacenta.* Animals with this type of placenta will not exhibit bleeding and shedding of uterine tissues at birth (nondeciduate placentation).

General shape is often used to classify placentas. Diffuse placentas (lemur, pig, horse) retain chorionic villi over the entire surface. Ungulates (cattle, sheep, deer) possess small tufts or rosettes, known as cotyledons, regularly spaced over the smooth chorion (cotyledonary placenta). Carnivores exhibit a zonal type in which there is a girdle-like band of villi around the middle of the chorionic sac. One or two discoid or disk-shaped masses of villi on the smooth chorionic sac are typical of insectivores, bats, rodents and most primates.

Placentas are also categorized according to the degree of intimacy between the fetal and maternal tissues. The degree of intimacy is directly proportional to the efficiency of transport of materials to and from fetal tissues. The *epitheliochorial placenta* (lemur, pig, horse) is a relationship of apposition, with chorionic tissue simply fitting into grooves and depressions of the maternal tissues. This type of placenta is nondeciduate. A second type of nondeciduate placenta is the *syndesmochorial placenta* typical of ruminant ungulates. The rosettes of chorionic villi occupy deeper pits in the uterine mucosa, resulting in localized destruction of the uterine epithelium so that the chorionic ectoderm comes in direct contact with vascular maternal tissue. At parturition the villi are merely withdrawn, and there is no tearing or bleeding the maternal tissues (nondeciduate).

Carnivores exhibit considerably more intimacy between chorionic villi and the maternal tissues than do ruminants. Erosion of the uterine tissues is more extensive and exposes the endothelium (inner lining) of maternal blood vessels to the chorionic cells. This *endotheliochorial placenta* is deciduate.

Anthropoids, insectivores, bats and lower rodents have what is termed a *hemochorial placenta* in which the endothelium of the maternal blood vessels is lost and the maternal blood directly bathes the chorionic villi. In higher rodents (rat, guinea pig) and lagomorphs (rabbits) the greatest degree of known intimacy is found in the *hemoendothelial placenta.* In this type of placenta the chorionic villi partly degenerate so that the endothelium of chorionic blood vessels is bathed directly by the maternal blood. Both hemochorial and hemoendothelial placentas result in considerable sloughing of uterine tissues and bleeding at birth (deciduate).

Generally all of these factors are taken into account in describing the type of placentation exhibited by a given species. The human, for example, exhibits deciduate placentation with a discoid-shaped placenta of the hemochorial type.

The Pregnancy Cycle. The ovum still surrounded by some of the granulosa cells (the corona radiata) enters the upper end of the fluid-filled oviduct and is propelled toward the uterus by the action of cilia lining the oviduct. The possible role of muscular contractions of the oviduct wall in transport of the ovum has been suggested but not verified. Fertilization typically occurs in the upper third of the oviduct by spermatozoa that were deposited in the vagina by the male during coitus. These spermatozoa are transported by peristalsis through the uterus and into the oviduct in which recently ovulated ova are descending. Cleavage begins soon after fertilization, and the zygote or fertilized egg becomes a minute, multicellular blastocyst that is capable of eroding and settling in the uterine endometrium for development. The gestation period may be as short as 12 days in the opossum or as long as 22 months in elephants.

Should fertilization and successful implantation occur in eutherian mammals, in which the pregnancy period exceeds the normal life of the corpus luteum, the lifespan of the corpus luteum will be prolonged until the placenta can synthesize sufficient progesterone and estrogens to maintain gestation.

A central question that has puzzled reproductive physiologists for many years is related to the mechanism whereby a mammal "knows" it is pregnant soon enough to prolong corpus luteal function. In the mare only fertilized ova ever reach the uterus, implying some sort of early chemical recognition that fertilization has occurred. The signal for prolongation of corpus luteum function in some species is the synthesis of an LH-like hormone called *chorionic gonadotropin* (CG) by the trophoblast of the blastocyst.[202] This trophoblast will develop into the fetal component of the placenta after implantation and will continue to secrete CG. In pregnant mares the chorionic hormone is known as *pregnant mare serum gonadotropin* (PMSG) because it appears in such large amounts circulating in the blood. These placental gonadotropins are structurally very similar to the pituitary gonadotropins and generally produce LH-like effects (see Chap. 5). Their synthesis and release, however, are not influenced in a negative way by steroids in the manner of the steroidal feedback on pituitary gonadotropins. Such pregnancy-recognition mechanisms are not necessary in some species such as the opossum[67] and carnivores where the length of the normal luteal phase and corpus luteum function are identical to the gestation period.

Secretion of ovarian steroids brought about by extension of the life span of the corpus luteum or during the normal luteal phase of the ovarian cycle of carnivores inhibits hypothalamic centers controlling gonadotropin release so that follicular development and ovulation are blocked in pregnant animals. The adaptive value of not having several embryos in the uterus at different stages of development should be obvious not only with respect to the sequestering of limited nutritional resources by the fetus but also to the destructive effects of parturition on the younger embryos and fetuses. The latter is probably more important since many species produce several offspring at one time and have obviously found ways to adapt to simultaneous competition among the fetuses.

During the last third of pregnancy another pituitary-like hormone, *chorionic somatomammotropin* (CS), is secreted by the placenta of a number of species (primates, mice, rats, voles, guinea pigs, sheep, chinchillas and hamsters but not bitches or rabbits). This placental hormone has both growth hormone (GH)-like and PRL-like activities, and antibodies to CS will cross-react with both GH and PRL in at least some of these species. The major roles for CS appear to be effects on metabolism (GH-like) and stimulation of the mammary gland to begin milk synthesis during the later stages of pregnancy.

The human placenta secretes PRL which is identical to pituitary PRL. Prolactin accumulates in the amniotic fluid during pregnancy where it is thought to regulate volume and ionic composition of amniotic fluid.[144] Levels of amniotic PRL are not affected by drugs that block pituitary PRL release or even by hypophysectomy of the mother.[12]

In humans two additional adenohypophysial-like hormones have been identified in placental tissues. *Chorionic thyrotropin* (hCT) and *chorionic corticotropin* (hCC) have been found, but their functions are not clear. Perhaps they too serve to provide essential adenohypophysial hormones during pregnancy when general adenohypophysial function is inhibited and these essential tropic hormones might otherwise be lacking. The placenta also synthesizes GnRH, but the significance of this is not clear.

A new pregnancy hormone, *relaxin* was named in 1932. It has several possible physiological roles.[18] Relaxin causes relaxation and softening of estrogen-primed pelvic ligaments, allowing the pelvis to stretch and expand (relax) so that the relatively large head of the mammalian fetus may pass through the pelvis during parturition. It reaches peak levels prior to birth and rapidly disappears from the maternal circulation afterward.[17] Spontaneous motility of the uterus may be inhibited by relaxin in some mammals. Relaxin working with estrogens, progesterone and prostaglandins can alter the structural collagen of the uterine cervix, increasing its distensibility at parturition. There are also data supporting an action of relaxin in combination with steroids and PRL. These hormones stimulate growth of the mammary gland and the onset of lactation.

The corpus luteum is the major source of relaxin in species where the corpus luteum is retained throughout gestation (pig, rat, carnivores).[18] Relaxin is produced by the human corpus luteum during early gestation and to some extent by the placenta. A little relaxin is found in placentae of sheep, rats, cows and rabbits, but in horses the placenta is a major source of relaxin. In humans the ovary continues to be the major site for relaxin synthesis after death of the corpus luteum.

Relaxins have been purified from pig, rat and shark. They all consist of two short A chains (22-24 amino acids) and a longer B chain (26-35 amino acids) joined together by disulfide bonds. The positioning of the disulfide bonds is the same as for insulin and the insulin-like growth factors (see Chap. 13) although there are many differences in amino acids. Rat and pig relaxins exhibit numerous amino acid substitutions although insulins from these species are similar. It has been suggested that the relaxin gene arose by duplication from the insulin gene. Among mammals there has been considerable divergence in the relaxin genes. Shark relaxin actually resembles mammalian insulins more closely than it resembles mammalian relaxins. Why has the shark relaxin gene changed so little? Perhaps the answer lies in the acquisition of new functions for relaxin in mammals and intense selection pressure on the relaxin gene products.

Delayed Implantation. Several mammals, such as mink, bats and skunks, have evolved a fascinating mechanism known as *delayed implantation* whereby development of the blastocyst is arrested and the unimplanted blastocyst remains in the oviduct or uterus for an extended period prior to implantation.[187] Among some eutherian mammals, delayed implantation appears to be an adaptation allowing copulation to occur at a particular time that is especially advantageous to the parent yet ensuring that the young are born at the most favorable time for their survival. Neither the basis for causing the blastocyst to remain in a healthy, arrested state nor the stimulus to bring about implantation is known. A similar phenomenon occurs in macropodid marsupials, however, and its continuation is related to the presence of a young suckling on a teat (see p. 276). This is clearly not the mechanism involved in eutherians.

Lactation. The development of mammary glands, their synthesis of milk and the ejection of milk to the suckling offspring are all regulated by hormones. Mammary glands in eutherian mammals usually occur as paired structures, from 2 to 18, and may be located on the thorax (man, elephant, bat), along the entire ventral thorax (sow, rabbit), in the inguinal region (horse, ruminants), along the abdomen (whale) or even dorsally (the nutria, a South American rodent). The internal structure includes supporting stromal cells and glandular epithelium that is organized into clusters of minute, sac-like structures called *alveoli.* It is the glandular epithelium that is responsible for synthesis of milk. The alveoli are continuous with ducts and various duct-derived enlargements for storing milk. In addition, there are modified epithelial cells that contain muscle-like myofilaments parallel to the long axis of the cells. The *myoepithelial cells* are capable of contracting and causing ejection of milk from the alveoli into the duct system and out of the gland in the region of the nipple.

Information obtained from the mouse and rat indicates that differentiation of mammary glands from ectoderm involves specific induction by a particular underlying mesenchyme. These glands normally develop with the aid of estrogens during the last third of the gestational period. The fetal ovary is not the source of these estrogens since mammary glands develop in the absence of fetal ovaries. Androgens suppress mammary gland development and are presumably responsible for their altered development in the male fetus.

Postnatal mammary development involves hormones from the pituitary, ovaries and adrenal cortex, at least in mice and rats. Growth of mammary ducts requires estrogens, GH and corticosterone working in concert. However, expansion of the alveoli (lobuloalveolar growth) is dependent upon the direct actions of estrogens, progesterone, PRL, GH, relaxin and corticosteroids.

Lactation can be separated into two basic processes or phases under separate endocrine control mechanisms. The first phase is *milk secretion* or *lactogenesis.* This process is under control of pituitary PRL (or CS) and corticosteroids. In primates, lactogenesis is also stimulated by GH. Lactogenesis involves synthesis of milk fat, milk protein and milk sugar, typically lactose. The synthesis of lactose ultimately depends upon protein synthesis; that is, the enzyme responsible for lactose synthesis, lactose synthetase, must be induced. Lactose synthetase is composed of two protein units, one of which is lactalbumin, which is also found in milk. Lactose, fat and milk protein (largely casein) are secreted into the lumen of the alveolus. Water and numerous water-soluble substances enter the lumen by osmosis and result in a watery liquid known as milk. Hormones are present in milk including the hypothalamic peptides, TRH and GnRH, as well as TSH, ACTH, PRL, LH, FSH, estradiol-17β, corticosteroids and thyroid hormones.[93] The composition of milk produced by the mammary gland associated with suckling the young is very different at birth from what it will be shortly thereafter. This first milk is known as *colostrum* and is characterized by having a greater concentration of protein and less carbohydrate than does later milk.[33] Colostrum contains substances that serve to protect the neonate against allergies and diseases.

The second phase of lactation is *milk ejection.* A simple reflex mechanism involving the pars nervosa controls milk ejection.[33] Mechanical stimulation of the nipple (suckling) stimulates release of oxytocin from the pars nervosa via a spinohypothalamic neuronal pathway. Release of PRL also occurs when milk is ejected and stimulates further milk synthesis. Oxytocin stimulates contraction of myoepithelial cells that causes milk to be ejected from the alveoli into the ducts and storage channels of the mammary gland. The suckling young strips milk from the gland by expressing it between the tongue and hard palate.

The milk ejection neurohormonal reflex exhibits classical conditioning responses as evidenced by stimulation of milk flow in the cow by sight and sounds of the milking parlor or in women by the cries of their hungry infant. This reflex can be influenced by other neural or chemical inputs to the hypothalamus. For example, stress or physical discomfort can inhibit ejection of milk in the presence of the stimulus that would normally elicit release of oxytocin.

Reproductive Cycles in Representative Female Eutherians. Following are detailed accounts of the reproductive cycles known for ewes, women and 4-day cycling rats.[169] These cycles emphasize both the features described previously that are characteristic of eutherian mammals and some of the marked deviations that become obvious when different species are compared. The cycles of the three species described here are among the best known, and it may be argued whether they are truly representative of all mammals. Ewes and rats are polyestrous species whereas women have no seasonal estrous behavior. Both rats and women are continuous breeders, but ewes are distinct seasonal breeders. Cows and pigs have cycles that are essentially like the ewe's although they differ somewhat in timing of the various events. None of these species exhibits delayed implantation, and all are believed to be spontaneous ovulators except under special conditions for the rat and probably the human.[29]

Ewe. Sheep estrous cycles occur seasonally, and the duration of one complete cycle is 16 days with a return to proestrus if fertilization does not occur (Fig. 11-12). Reproductive cycles can be blocked in ewes by genistein (see Fig. 9-2), an antiestrogenic compound found in certain clovers.[14] During the follicular phase (proestrus) there is marked increase in both estrogen and androgen levels, a peak being reached about 24 hours after the onset of proestrus. About 12 hours later a surge of plasma LH occurs caused by the action of estradiol-17β on the cyclic hypothalamic neurosecretory center. The high level of androgen, principally androstenedione, has been suggested to be responsible for inducing estrous behavior.[169] Usually a single ovulation follows the LH surge by about 24 hours, and a corpus luteum forms from the ruptured follicle under the influence of LH. Low levels of LH following ovulation and the estrogen-induced surge of PRL stimulate the corpus luteum to secrete progesterone. Under the influence of progesterone, the uterine endometrium synthesizes a luteolytic PGF ($PGF_{2\alpha}$) that causes degeneration of the corpus luteum and resumption of proestrus. Fertilization followed by implantation delays degeneration of the corpus luteum. Apparently the conceptus neutralizes the PGFs synthesized under the influence of progester-

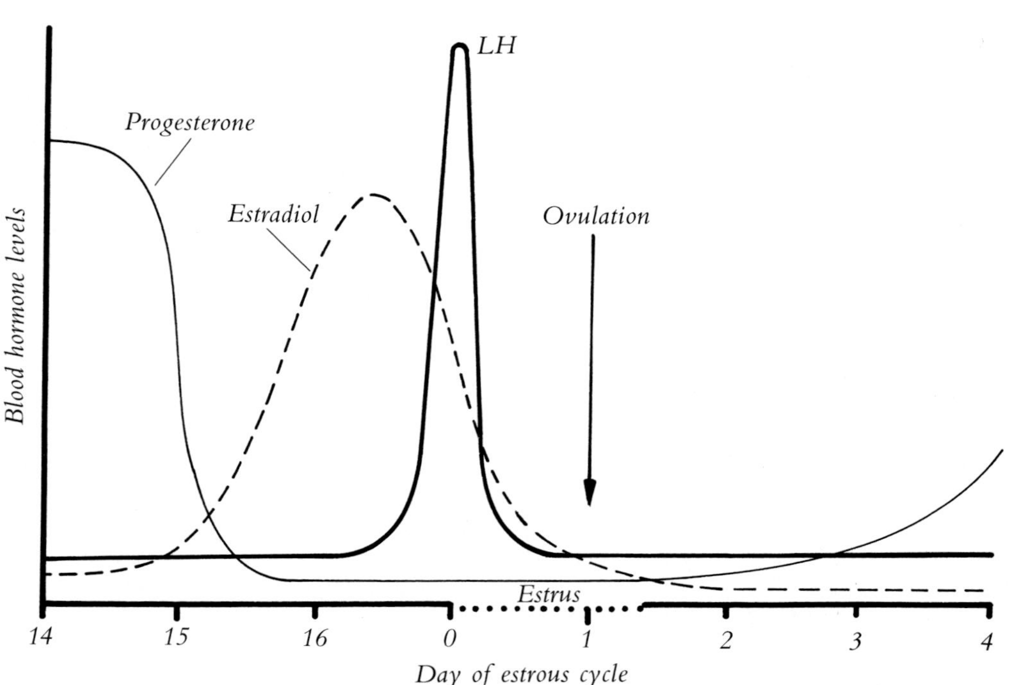

FIG. 11-12. Hormonal events during the estrous cycle of sheep (ewe). Ovulation *(arrow)* occurs during the latter half of estrus. See text for explanation. (Redrawn from Short.[169])

one. The corpus luteum continues to secrete progresterone until the placenta is capable of producing sufficient steroids to maintain gestation. The placenta also secretes both oCG and oCS.

Just prior to birth there is marked reduction in circulating steroid levels (Fig. 11-13). Presumably this marked decrease in progesterone sensitizes the uterus to oxytocin, which was unable to cause contractions in the uterus in the presence of progesterone. The contractions of the uterus initiated by oxytocin result in expulsion of the fetus as well as of the afterbirth (placenta).

It appears that follicle growth, ovulation and luteinization can be brought about by LH alone. However, both LH and PRL are necessary to induce progesterone synthesis by the corpus luteum. Although FSH has been claimed to play no role in ovarian function for the ewe,[169] several studies have reported a stimulatory effect of FSH on follicular development.[155]

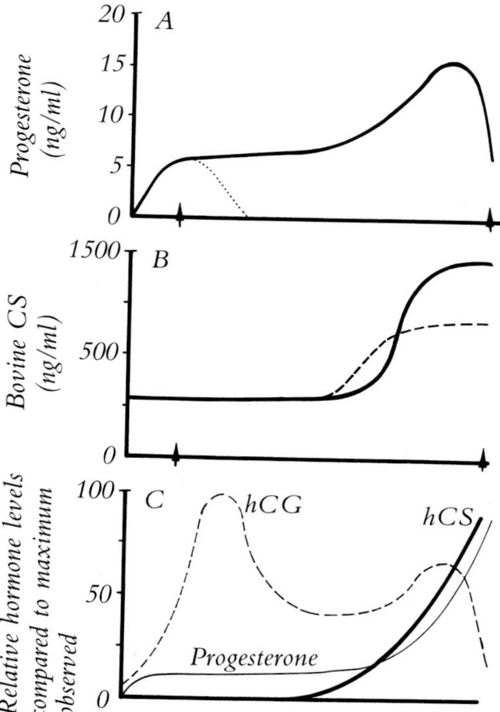

Fig. 11-13. Some hormone levels during pregnancy for ewes, cows and women.
A. Progesterone levels in ewe during nonpregnant cycle *(dotted line)* compared to pregnancy.
B. Chorionic somatomammotropin during gestation in beef *(dotted line)* and dairy cows *(solid line).*
C. Comparison of chorionic gonadotropin *(hCG),* progesterone and chorionic somatomammotropin *(hCS)* in pregnant women. The increase in estrogens parallels the curve for hCS. (Modified from several sources.)

Women. The human female exhibits continuous cycling with a mean cycle length of 28 days for most reproductively active women. The rhesus monkey also has a menstrual cycle of 28 days, and there are many parallels in the menstrual cycles of these two primates. Studies of the rhesus monkey have provided insight into factors regulating the human menstrual cycle. Although this cycle is sometimes referred to as a lunar cycle because its periodicity is equivalent to a lunar month, the human menstrual cycle is not correlated with any particular phase of the lunar month and should not be termed lunar. It could be that at one time the menstrual cycle was correlated more closely with moon phases but has become highly modified by numerous environmental and internal factors. Cycles of women can vary from as short as 14 days to as long as 360 days, depending upon both endocrine and psychological factors. Considerable variation can occur in cycle length in a given woman at different times in her life history. Short cycles and irregular cycles are associated with the onset of puberty and with the end of the reproductive life prior to menopause when the ovaries become refractory to pituitary gonadotropins, and both estrogen synthesis and ovulation cease. The absence of circulating steroids releases the hypothalamus from negative feedback, and levels of circulating gonadotropins are exceptionally high in menopausal women.

The menstrual cycle begins at the onset of the menses, which occupies the first 5 days of the cycle (Fig. 11-14). However, as soon as the corpus luteum of a previous cycle begins to regress prior to the onset of menses, there is a moderate elevation in FSH level that initiates growth of new follicles. Typically only one follicle in an ovary will reach maturity in a given cycle, with ovulation often occurring in the alternate ovary during the following cycle. The thecal cells of the growing follicles begin to secrete estrogens and progestogens, which peak on about day 14 of the normal cycle. Ste-

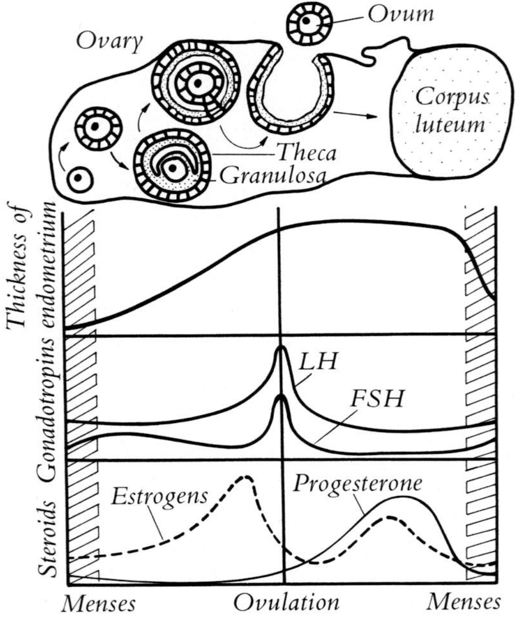

FIG. 11-14. Menstrual cycle of human female. See text for explanation. (Compiled from many sources.)

roidogenesis is regulated by FSH and LH operating on the thecal and granulosal cells. The peak in estrogen level stimulates GnRH release from the cyclic center, causing a surge of LH with release of less FSH. Ovulation follows the LH surge by about 24 hours, and the granulosa cells undergo luteinization. The resulting corpus luteum is independent of pituitary hormones and begins production of progesterone and estradiol-17β. The hypothalamic centers governing LH and FSH release are inhibited by the high levels of these circulating steroids so that neither follicular growth nor ovulation can occur during the luteal phase of the cycle. The corpus luteum functions for only a few days if the ovum is not fertilized. Unlike the sheep, in women the uterus plays no active role in degeneration of the corpus luteum. Surgical removal of the uterus (hysterectomy) does not affect the duration of the luteal phase. The human corpus luteum may produce its own luteolytic factor as does that of the rhesus monkey (see p. 265). The production of estrone by the corpus luteum of the rhesus monkey increases markedly prior to the onset of luteal degeneration. A similar mechanism may be operating in women. As the production of steroids by the corpus luteum decreases the pituitary is released from steroid-induced inhibition, and a new cycle of follicular growth begins. The outer portion of the uterine lining begins to slough off following the decline in progesterone levels, and the menses begins.

Should fertilization occur, the trophoblast of the blastocyst begins to secrete hCG prior to implantation and the production of hCG continues at an accelerated rate during early pregnancy (Fig. 11-13). Under the influence of hCG, the life span of the corpus luteum may be extended. The corpus luteum secretes both progesterone and relaxin. By about 60 days, it degenerates even in the presence of exogenous hCG. However, the placenta, with the help of the fetal adrenal cortex (see Chap. 10), is now producing sufficient estrogens and progesterone to continue the inhibition of pituitary gonadotropin release and to maintain the secretory condition of the uterus. Furthermore, the placenta appears to assume the roles for pituitary GH, PRL, ACTH and TSH through production of hCS, hCC and hCT.

The stimulus for birth is not related to a decrease in progesterone levels but to a marked increase in estrogens as well as progesterone. Apparently, high levels of estrogens nullify the anesthetic properties of progesterone on uterine smooth muscle and allow oxytocin to initiate uterine contractions and the onset of labor. This action of oxytocin seems to be a consequence of increased uterine receptors rather than a consequence of elevation in oxytocin levels. Administration of prostaglandins also can induce uterine contractions, and oxytocin may stimulate prostaglandin synthesis in the uterus. Synthetic oxytocin is normally used to induce labor in women.

Four-Day Cycling Rat. The short 4- or 5-day cycle in rats (Fig. 11-15) is believed to be a consequence of the failure of the corpora lutea to become functional during the normal luteal phase (diestrus.)[169] The rat cycle is closely cued to environmental events, ovulation, for example, occurring invariably shortly after midnight. Furthermore, there is considerable evidence for the involvement of chemical communication between male and female rats that can influence many of the reproductive events. The importance of chemical communication in mammals, especially in refer-

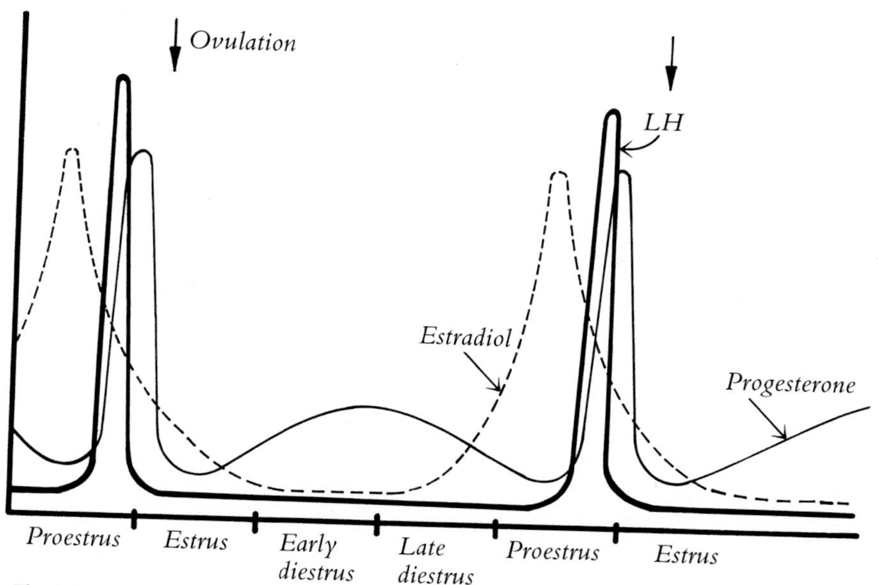

FIG. 11-15. The 4-day cycling female rat. Note that a progesterone surge follows the estradiol-induced LH surge prior to ovulation. (LH is represented by heavy black line.) This progesterone surge is necessary for normal estrous behavior. During the luteal phase secretion of progesterone is increased somewhat, but the level is considerably less than that observed prior to ovulation. (After Short.[169])

ence to reproduction, is described in Chapter 15.

On the morning of the day prior to estrus, that is, during proestrus, the levels of estrogens in the plasma reach a peak, which stimulates the typical LH surge accompanied by FSH. The surge of gonadotropins occurs on the afternoon of proestrus and is followed rapidly by a marked surge of progesterone. Ovulation occurs a few hours after midnight on the day of estrus. Several follicles usually mature simultaneously, and multiple ovulations occur. Estrus lasts about 9 to 15 hours, during which the female is receptive to the male. Ovulation occurs during estrus. Cornified cells, which were produced by the actions of estrogens, appear in the superficial layers of the vagina, and their presence in vaginal smears characterizes estrus (Fig. 11-16).

The third and fourth day of the cycle are termed diestrus I and diestrus II. Vaginal smears prepared during diestrus are characterized by the absence of cornified cells and a predominance of leukocytes in the smear. There is limited secretory function by the corpus luteum, as evidenced by a slight increase in plasma progesterone. Much of this progesterone is produced by ovarian interstitial cells, which constitute what has been called a permanent corpus luteum in the rat ovary.[169] This interstitial tissue responds to LH by secreting both progesterone and 20α-dihydroprogesterone.

Many researchers recognize a transitional period between estrus and diestrus termed *metestrus*. The female is no longer receptive to the male, but some cornified cells still appear in smears prepared from the vaginal mucosa.

Mating may stimulate gonadotropin release, and consequently the corpora lutea begin to secrete significant amounts of progestogens. This increased production of progestogens will inhibit hypothalamo-hypophysial function and delay the onset of the next cycle. If fertilization and implantation do not occur from this mating, the rat will return to proestrus within a few days. This pseudopregnancy occurs in laboratory rodents and sometimes in domestic mammals. The condition of pseudopregnancy is often accompanied by PRL-like effects on lactation and behavior presumably due to hypophysial release of PRL.

If implantation does occur the corpora lutea continue to secrete progestogens under the

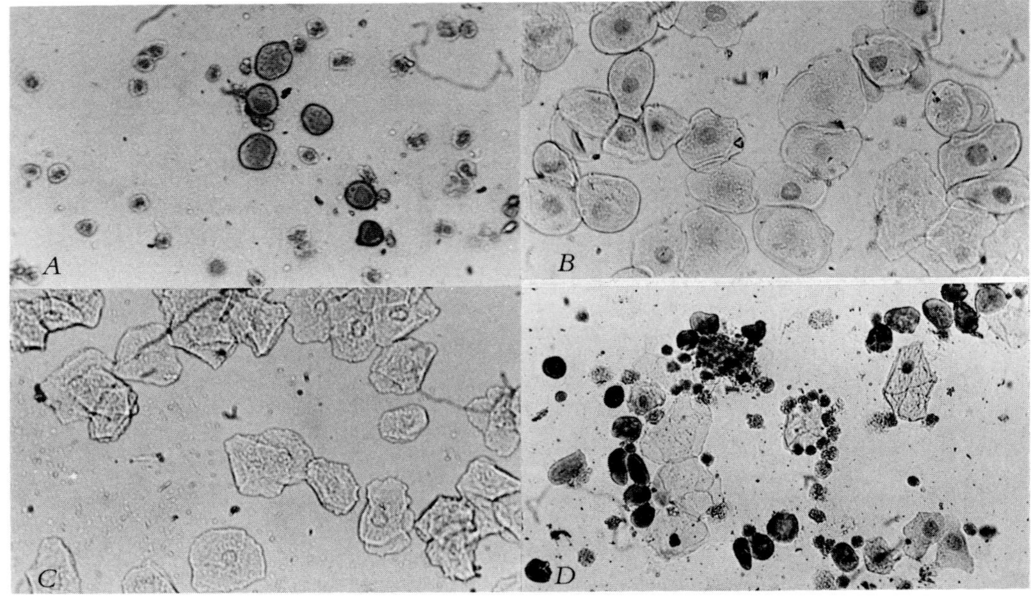

Fig. 11-16. Vaginal smears from female rats during estrous cycle.
A. Diestrus. Note the absence of cornified cells and presence of small leukocytes.
B. Proestrus. Many live epithelial cells with smooth margins.
C. Estrus. Large, cornified (keratinized) cells with irregular margins.
D. Metestrus. Many cornified cells plus infiltration of leukocytes.
(Courtesy of Dr. Richard E. Jones and Dr. David Duvall)

influence of placental CG and begin to secrete relaxin. The rat placenta also produces CS, which contributes to stimulation of mammary gland development and lactogenesis prior to birth.

Monotreme Reproductive Patterns

The egg-laying aplacental monotremes are reproductively more like reptiles than like other mammals,[126] although they do possess some strictly mammalian features.[145] The developing monotreme follicle does not form an antrum. Prior to ovulation, however, a thin layer of antral fluid is secreted by the follicular cells between the zona pellucida and the follicular cells. There is a well-developed theca interna that persists after ovulation and formation of corpora lutea. The function of the corpus luteum is not clear, but it has been suggested that it stimulates secretion of nutrient substances by the uterine glands. These nutritive substances are incorporated by the oocyte. Monotreme eggs have leathery shells like reptilian eggs. The duckbill platypus lays its eggs in a nest, but the female spiny echidna places her eggs in a brood pouch that develops seasonally. Formation of the pouch is probably dependent upon estrogens, although no experimental data are available to support this contention. The eggs develop and hatch within the pouch, and after the breeding season the pouch regresses.

Corpora atretica may form from either large or small follicles in the monotreme ovary. The contents of a large follicle typically are extruded by rupture of the follicle prior to formation of the corpus atreticum. The extruded materials enter the peritoneal cavity or the prominent intraovarian lymph spaces that characterize the monotreme ovary.

The mammary glands of monotremes lack teats. Consequently milk is secreted onto a special area, the *areola.* The newly hatched monotreme must attach itself to its mother with its forelimbs and suck or lick milk from the areola.

Marsupial Reproductive Patterns

Marsupials possess an estrous cycle with ovarian events similar to those described for eutherians,[126,145,166,167] but the period of gestation is much shorter in relation to the estrous cycle (Table 11-4). Proestrus in females is characterized by follicular enlargement and estrogen-dependent uterine proliferation and increase in size of elements of the vaginal complex. Peak uterine and vaginal development coincides with estrus and copulation. Ovulation occurs spontaneously one to several days after estrus, and postovulatory follicles transform into corpora lutea that maintain a secretory uterine condition. Progesterone continues the secretory uterine phase in castrates and is undoubtedly the hormone responsible for maintaining gestation as in eutherian mammals.

The luteal phase is the same in mated and nonmated females,[67,166,167] and no "pregnancy-recognition signal" is necessary. Pregnancy does not affect ovarian function, and both pregnant and unmated females return to proestrus at about the same time in most species. Equivalent mammary gland development occurs during postestrus in both pregnant and nonpregnant females, and newborn foster young will develop normally if attached to virgin or nonlactating females at the equivalent postestrous state to the time of parturition. Circulating progesterone and urinary pregnanediol levels are similar in pregnant, unmated and luteal phase females. There are no endocrine differences between the pregnant and nonpregnant postestrous phase, which leads to the conclusion that the marsupial placenta is not an endocrine organ.

Another unusual feature of marsupials is the ability to simultaneously produce two kinds of milk. As in eutherian mammals the first milk differs markedly in composition from that produced later during lactation. Macropodids which may have both a newborn joey and one that has already detached itself from a teat, will produce early and late milk simultaneously in the respective glands. The developmental state of a particular mammary gland would seem to be independent of endocrine conditions and strongly influenced by external conditions; that is, the joey.

A major developmental difference between eutherians and marsupials has had a profound influence on reproductive patterns in the latter group. Marsupials exhibit a primitive reptilian pattern of wolffian and mullerian duct origins. Instead of developing medially to the kidneys and ureters as in eutherians, these

TABLE 11-4. *Comparison of Length of Estrous Cycle, Gestation Period, and Ratio of Body Weight of Neonate to Body Weight of Mother in Metatherian and Eutherian Mammals*

SPECIES	LENGTH OF ESTROUS CYCLE (DAYS)	LENGTH OF GESTATION PERIOD (DAYS)	NEONATE: MOTHER BODY WEIGHT RATIO
Eutheria:			
Rat	4–5	21	—
Sheep	16	148	1:14
Metatheria:			
Virginia opossum	29	12	1:8300
Long-nosed bandicoot	26	12	1:4250
Brush possum	26	17	1:7250
Dama wallaby	30	29	1:10,000
Swamp wallaby	31	37	—
Red kangaroo	35	33	1:33,400
Western gray kangaroo	35	30	—

NOTE: The estrous cycles are similar to the gestation period in metatherians and may not require a pregnancy-recognition mechanism.[167]

ducts develop laterally. Consequently it is not possible for left and right mullerian ducts of females to fuse in the midline without placing considerable strain on the ureters. It is believed that the short gestation period of marsupials is a consequence of separate uteri and vaginas and limited space for uterine hypertrophy. A special birth canal must be formed so that parturition can occur, and in some species it forms anew each season. This development of separate vaginas has influenced evolution of the male reproductive system as well. Males of some species have a bifid penis, with left and right prongs apparently being inserted into separate vaginas during copulation.

Embryonic Diapause. Macropodid marsupials have developed a type of delayed implantation that has been termed *embryonic diapause* to distinguish it from delayed implantation, described earlier for eutherian mammals. Embryonic diapause has been reported for 14 macropodid species but does not occur in at least one species, the western gray kangaroo. One major difference from delayed implantation occurring in eutherian mammals is the condition of the resting blastocyst. The macropodid blastocyst consists of about 70 to 100 cells of a uniform type termed *protoderm*. It has not differentiated into embryonic and extraembryonic regions like that of the eutherians. The blastocyst is surrounded by a shell membrane and an albumin layer.

Presence of a joey suckling on a teat presumably evokes release of oxytocin from the pars nervosa. Oxytocin is believed to arrest corpus luteum functions while allowing lactation to occur. Removal of the suckling joey will allow the resting blastocyst to implant. Ovariectomy following ovulation induces diapause, but if ovariectomy is performed during diapause there is no effect on the duration of diapause. Progesterone administered to either intact or ovariectomized females stimulates cessation of diapause and reinstates blastocyst development.[173] Estrogen is also effective, but continued embryonic development is not as successful as following progesterone treatment.

In the red kangaroo, embryonic diapause is an adaptation to renew pregnancy immediately following the death of the joey living in the pouch. The gestation period for the red kangaroo is 33 days. After birth the newborn must find its way to the pouch virtually unaided. When it reaches the pouch the joey attaches itself permanently to a teat and continues development as an exteriorized fetus. Soon after parturition the mother kangaroo enters estrus again and mates. The presence of one joey in the pouch inhibits implantation of the blastocyst resulting from the second mating. The blastocyst remains in a suspended state of development for about 200 days, at which time the first joey disengages itself from the teat and ventures into the outside world as a juvenile kangaroo. The newly liberated kangaroo will return at intervals to the teat to which it was formerly attached for nourishment. Meanwhile the detachment of the first joey from the teat either releases an inhibition to implantation or somehow provides a stimulus for implantation of the waiting blastocyst. In about 4 weeks the gestation period terminates in birth of the second joey, which enters the pouch and attaches to a teat. The mother kangaroo again enters estrus and mates, and another blastocyst enters embryonic diapause. Thus a female red kangaroo may have a young juvenile that requires occasional nourishment, a joey attached to a teat and a blastocyst "waiting in the wings." It has been suggested that during extensive periods of drought an older joey requiring considerable amounts of milk from the mother would be allowed to die, and implantation of the waiting blastocyst soon provides another joey whose demands upon the mother's stored reserves and water reservoir would be small in comparison to the demands of the larger joey.

Major Endocrine Disorders Related to Reproduction

Precocity

Precocity is defined as the appearance of any one indicator of puberty at an age earlier than 2.5 to 3 standard deviations below the mean age at which the indicator normally appears in that population (see Table 11-5). The sequence and mean age of appearance for these indicators should be considered only as a guide. Implied precocity may not be evidence of an en-

TABLE 11-5. *Mean Age for Normal Attainment of Certain Indicators of Puberty in Humans*

	MEAN AGE IN YEARS ± SD
Female	
Budding of breasts	11.2 ± 1.1
Sparse pubic hair	11.7 ± 1.2
Peak vertical growth rate	12.1 ± 1.0
Menarche[a] (U.K.)	13.5 ± 1.0
Menarche (U.S.A.)	12.9 ± 1.2
Male	
Enlargement of testes and scrotum	11.6 ± 1.1
Lengthening of penis	12.8 ± 1.0
Sparse pubic hair	13.4 ± 2.2
Peak vertical growth rate	14.1 ± 0.9
Adult genital size and shape	14.9 ± 1.1

[a]95% reach menarche between ages 11 and 15.

docrine disorder, and variations in the sequence of these events is normal. Major deviations in a number of indicators may signal precocial endocrine activity of a pathological nature. Isosexual precocity involves early appearance of the genetically determined sex. It is termed heterosexual precocity if male features develop precocially in a female or if female features appear precocially in a male.

PRECOCITY WITH NORMAL ENDOCRINOLOGY. Idiopathic precocity (of unknown cause) may be familial. Sexual development and body growth appear normal but are accelerated. Reproduction may be possible at an early age. For example, the youngest mother on record was 5 years 8 months of age at delivery!

PRECOCITY AND PINEAL TUMORS. Pineal tumors are not common but occur most frequently in young males. Precocious sexual maturation occurs in about one third of these cases. Pineal tumors may impair release of antigonadotropic factors from the pineal and allow sexual maturation to occur prematurely. Pineal tumors have been related to delayed puberty in a few cases. These tumors may secrete more antigonadotropic factors than the normal gland.

PRECOCITY FROM ECTOPIC GONADOTROPINS OR GONADAL STEROIDS. Rare pituitary tumors may secrete excessive amounts of gonadotropins. Sometimes nonpituitary tumors secrete chorionic gonadotropin. Certain ovarian or testicular tumors produce sufficient steroids to cause external evidence of puberty. Heterosexual precocity can occur from feminizing tumors in testes or androgen-secreting tumors of the adrenals or ovaries.

Delayed Puberty

MALES. Prevalence of undescended testes or cryptorchidism is common at birth (10%) but is reduced to only 1% of males by age 1. Only about 0.3% of adult males exhibit cryptorchidism, and the case of only one undescended testis is much more common than the bilateral condition. Because of higher temperatures experienced by an undescended testis, the spermatogenetic tissue degenerates at about the time when spermatogenesis would normally begin (at about age 10). Androgen production is normal or may be reduced. The external testis of a unilateral cryptorchid develops normally, and these males are fertile.

There are several other causes for hypogonadism in males including insufficient levels of LH and FSH due to hypothalamic or pituitary dysfunction. In some cases the interstitial cells may be unresponsive to gonadotropins.

FEMALES. *Primary amenorrhea* is the failure for menarche to occur at the normal time (Table 11-5). This condition can be related to many different causes including disorders of the hypothalamus, pituitary and ovaries. Poor nutrition, stress or rigorous athletic training programs can delay puberty through inhibitory actions on the hypothalamo-hypophysial-gonadal axis. For example, levels of LH and FSH are depressed in women suffering from anorexia nervosa, a disorder in which food intake is greatly reduced. Simple weight loss can depress FSH levels for a time but does not inhibit LH secretion.

Secondary amenorrhea occurs after menarche and can result from many endocrine disorders including thyrotoxicosis, drug therapy, premature menopause and a variety of hypothalamic, pituitary and gonadal disorders. Two of the more common gonadal disorders associated with secondary amenorrhea are *polycystic ovarian syndrome* (POS) and *luteinization of atretic follicles* (LAF). The name for POS is derived from the general thickening and luteinization of ovarian follicles resulting in formation of numerous cysts in the ovaries. These cysts develop from thecal cells, and there is a loss of granulosa cells. Progesterone and estrogen production are diminished and gonadotropin secretion consequently is elevated. Androgenic steroids are produced but can not be aromatized to estrogens. Uterine abnormalities and infertility result. Hirsuitism, occasional balding and obesity may accompany POS.

The LAF syndrome results from premature luteinization of ovarian follicles prior to formation of the cumulus oophorus. Gonadotropin levels are elevated, but masculinization usually does not happen. Numerous small ovarian cysts may be present, but these are easily distinguished from the large cysts that characterize POS.

Hereditary Disorders

Hermaphroditism and Pseudohermaphroditism. Occasionally people are born with a combination of ovarian and testicular tissue. Most of these people possess an ovotestis on one or both sides of the body. Rarely, an individual is found who has an ovary and attendant mullerian derivatives on one side and a testis with its wolffian duct derivatives on the other. Pseudohermaphrodites have gonads of one sex but externally resemble the other sex. For example, a person with *testicular feminization syndrome* is a genetic male. Although the testis is normal, the external appearance is that of a woman because of the congenital absence of androgen receptors in the tissues.

A most unusual example of pseudohermaphroditism is the apparent shift of sex at puberty that occurs in a few people from several small villages of the Dominican Republic. This disorder is the result of a genetic deficiency for the ability to synthesize 5α-reductase. Males with this defect are born with undescended testes that synthesize testosterone like normal testes. However, these males can not convert testosterone to DHT without 5α-reductase. Testosterone-dependent structures develop normally (such as the vasa deferentia, epididymi) but DHT-dependent structures such as the prostate gland, penis and scrotum do not develop. These males understandably are raised as girls until they begin to synthesize DHT at puberty. The presence of 5α-reductase allows the penis to enlarge and facial hair to appear. Although these men change social roles after puberty, they are infertile.

Klinefelter's Syndrome. Person's with Klinefelter's syndrome are born with an abnormal number of sex chromosomes: XXY. This familial disorder occurs at fertilization and is present in about 0.2 to 0.3% of males. Klinefelter's syndrome can exist without obvious somatic abnormalities, although these persons are infertile and exhibit differing degrees of mental retardation. Similar syndromes have been described with additional sex chromosomes (XXYY, XXXY, etc.). Severity of the symptoms increases with the number of X chromosomes present.

Turner's Syndrome. Another disorder arising at fertilization is the loss of one sex chromosome so that the resulting genotype is XO (one X chromosome and no Y or no second X chromosome). Sometimes this condition occurs when a twin is found to exhibit Klinefelter's syndrome. Individuals with Turner's syndrome have a female phenotype but are infertile. They also exhibit a number of anatomical defects as well as cardiovascular and kidney disorders.

Galactorrhea

Secretion of a lactescent (milky) fluid from the breasts of either sex is called *galactorrhea.*

It is usually caused by excessive secretion of PRL. Breast enlargement is not prerequisite for its appearance. Galactorrhea frequently occurs in severe hypothyroidism characterized by elevated circulating levels of TSH and TRH. Prolactin release is evoked by the high TRH levels.

Comparative Aspects of Reproduction in Nonmammalian Vertebrates

It is difficult to generalize about nonmammalian vertebrate reproductive patterns, as was demonstrated for mammals in the preceding pages. Attainment of sexual maturity occurs at a definite time characteristic for individual species and is followed by a series of reproductive cycles closely attuned to certain environmental factors. Depending on the species, sexual maturity may occur during the first year of life (many teleosts), after more than 15 years of juvenile existence (Atlantic eel, sturgeon) or at some intermediate period. Some animals have no reproductive cycle in that they breed only once after attaining sexual maturity and die soon afterward (for example, Pacific salmon, *Oncorhynchus* spp; see Chap. 18), whereas most species exhibit many reproductive cycles over many years. Some of these may produce successive broods in a given year or season or may exhibit only one or two cycles per year.

Environmental factors, such as temperature and photoperiod and presence of suitable breeding or nesting sites, operate through the central nervous system and the hypothalamo-hypophysial axis to regulate gonadal maturation and secretion of sex hormones. Steroid hormones, adenohypophysial hormones or both determine development of various sex-dependent characters and influence courtship, breeding and possibly parental behaviors.

Like mammals, nonmammalian species may be viviparous or oviparous, with the exception of the cyclostomes and birds, which are exclusively oviparous. The term viviparity is used here to designate situations in which fertilized eggs are incubated in utero, and nourishment for development is supplied at least in part by the maternal organism. Young are born alive. Ovoviviparous species retain eggs for variable periods of time during which development procedes. The eggs are usually laid in a more advanced stage of development. In some cases the egg may hatch in utero. If young are born alive, they have received no additional nourishment (other than yolk) from the maternal organism. Use of the term "viviparous" here will indicate live-bearing species and actually may include some ovoviviparous species. Ovoviviparous species that lay eggs will be included in "oviparous". Oviparous species all lay eggs with protective coverings from which the larval or juvenile form will later hatch.

Ovarian structures and events occurring in the gonads of nonmammalian vertebrates are related to the mammalian condition. Oocyte development is regulated by pituitary gonadotropins. The process of yolk formation is called *vitellogenesis.* Synthesis of yolk precursors or *vitellogenins* occurs in the liver and is stimulated by estrogens.[141] When released into the blood, these lipoproteins bind calcium ions and are responsible for an elevation of total blood calcium in females undergoing vitellogenesis (see Chap. 12). Thus, marked increases in blood calcium can be used as an indicator of vitellogenesis. Incorporation of vitellogenins by growing oocytes and their conversion to yolk proteins are controlled by gonadotropins.

There is a major difference in the structure of testes in most anamniotes and amniote vertebrates. Whereas testes of mammals, birds, reptiles and anurans exhibit the tubular pattern of seminiferous elements with interspersed clumps of interstitial cells, the testes of urodele amphibians and fishes consist of *lobes* or *lobules,* each of which is composed of large *cellular cysts.* Each cyst is derived from a *spermatogonial nest,* and all of the cells within a cyst and usually all the cysts within a lobule will be in the same stage of spermatogenesis. (Seminiferous tubules of anurans also exhibit a pattern of cystic spermatogenesis.) Sustentacular (Sertoli) cells are present in each cyst. The more posterior lobules may be in a more advanced stage of spermatogenesis in repeating breeders than are the more anterior lobules. Spermiation in these anamniotes is usually followed by complete evacuation of spermatozoa from the mature lobules (more posterior ones) and regression of remaining cellular elements. Differentiation of lobules containing new cell nests occurs anteriorly from connective tissue elements and residual germ cells in the covering of the testis (tunica albuginea). In some fish species, however, all lobules develop and discharge sperm more or less simultaneously, and if breeding recurs there must be extensive regeneration of spermatogonial nests and new cysts prior to the next breeding season. True interstitial tissue is lacking in most anamniotes, and the synthesis of androgenic hormones occurs in cells associated with lobule walls. These steroidogenic cells are termed *lobule boundary cells.*

An additional steroidogenic tissue, the *interstitial gland,* may develop in the ovaries of gnathostomes.[64,157] Interstitial glands develop from thecal cells derived from atretic previtellogenic follicles. It has been suggested that much of the estrogen synthesized during reproductive cycles is from the interstitial gland.

The endocrine factors in nonmammalian vertebrates are similar to and in many cases identical to those already described for mammals. There appear to be two distinct gonadotropins, FSH and LH, in all tetrapods (except teleosts and squamate reptiles), and their release is under stimulatory hypothalamic control. Follicle development in females and spermatogonial mitoses in males are stimulated by FSH, with meiotic events in males being influenced locally by androgens produced in sustentacular cells. Spermiation and ovulation are generally controlled by LH-like gonadotropin. However, in teleostean fishes only an LH-like gonadotropin has been purified, and mammalian LH can regulate all aspects of reproduction in these fishes. Mammalian FSH is ineffective.[160] Even spermatogonial mitoses are under control of LH in teleosts. In contrast, reproduction in squamate reptiles requires only an FSH-like gonadotropin.

The major circulating estrogen in nonmammals is estradiol-17β, and testosterone or a closely related androgen is characteristic for males. Androgen and estrogen levels are higher than in mammals (compare Table 11-3 and 11-6) due to high circulating levels of steroid-binding globulin. Furthermore, relative levels of androgens and estrogens are not correlated with sex. For example, females may exhibit levels of androgens at certain times that exceed estrogen levels. The actions of gonadal steroids, including negative feedback effects on the hypothalamo-hypophysial axis, are similar in nonmammals to those described for mammals. Gonaduct differentiation and function, differentiation and maintenance of sex accessory structures and induction of certain behaviors are regulated by gonadal steroids.

As in mammals, PRL exhibits in certain species some specialized functions that are closely linked to reproductive events. The specific involvements of PRL will be discussed in some of the accounts that follow.

The relationships between thyroid hormones and reproductive events were discussed in Chapter 8 and will not be considered in this chapter. In summary, thyroid hormones appear to enhance the onset of gametogenesis, especially in males. It is only in the Amphibia and certain avian species that a negative correlation has been reported between thyroid activity and the onset of sexual maturation.

Internal fertilization requires evolution of a technique for transferring spermatozoa from the male to the female. Some viviparous anurans (for example, *Nectophrynoides*) and birds transfer spermatozoa through cloacal aposition or what has been termed the cloacal kiss.

Aquatic fishes and urodele amphibians, which practice internal fertilization, rely on spermatophores for transfer of spermatozoa. The spermatophore consists of a bundle of spermatozoa that are aggregated and enclosed in a gelatinous substance that will not rapidly dissolve in water. This structure allows the male to directly or indirectly transfer spermatozoa without excessive dilution of the "semen." Elasmobranchs, viviparous teleosts, apodan amphibians, one anuran and many reptiles possess intromittent organs that allow direct transfer of spermatozoa from male to female. In contrast, an aquatic male urodele deposits his spermatophore on the substrate and through a complicated behavioral ritual induces the female to pick it up with her cloaca. Frequently the female receiving a spermatophore has a special storage site *(spermatotheca)* that is capable in some species of storing viable spermatozoa for months. The spermatotheca thus may also possess special

TABLE 11-6. *Circulating Steroid Levels (per ml Plasma or Serum) in Selected Nonmammalian Vertebrates*

CLASS AND SPECIES[a]	TESTOSTERONE	ESTRADIOL	PROGESTERONE	REF
Agnatha				
Petromyzon marinus	UND[c]			88
Eptatretus stouti	23.9 pg			121
Chondrichthyes				
Torpedo marmorata M	15.6–35 ng			115
Raja radiata M	28–102 ng			139
R. radiata F	0.2–6 ng			139
Scyliorhinus canicula	2–6 ng			100,140
Osteichthyes				
Oncorhynchus nerka M	17 ng			139
O. nerka F	78 ng			139
Salmo trutta M	2–33 ng			90
S. trutta F	20–77 ng			90
Salmo gairdneri, prespawning F	52–235 ng	24–48 ng	8–15[d] ng	162
S. gairdneri, spawning F	65–84 ng	2–3 ng	354–416[d] ng	162
S. gairdneri, spent F	2–5 ng	1–2 ng	8–19[d] ng	162
Amphibia				
Taricha granulosa, seasonal M	1–55 ng			177
Cynops pyrrhogaster, seasonal M	0.7–23 ng			183
Pleurodeles waltlii	40 ng	0.6 ng		139,140
Bufo marinus F	0.2–7.5 ng			99
Rana esculenta, seasonal M	1–20 ng			41
R. esculenta, seasonal F	1–14 ng	1–4 ng		41
R. catesbeiana, ovipositing F	11–120 ng	0.22–2.7 ng	5.6 ng	106
Reptilia				
Chrysemys picta M	15–40 ng			101
C. picta, preovulatory F	3.2–5.7 ng	0.79–1.37 ng	1.2–1.5 ng	23
C. picta, postovulatory F	0.2 ng	UND[c]	0.3–0.5 ng	23
Stenotherus ordonatus F	250–1500 pg	500–5000 pg	700–4000 pg	118
S. ordonatus M	10–75 ng			
Lacerta vivipara	27–390 ng			32
Uromastix hardwicki, preovulatory F	0.37 ng	0.18 ng	1.6 ng	4
U. hardwicki, gravid F	1.57 ng	0.46 ng	13.41 ng	4
Iguana iguana M	100 pg	79 pg		85
I. iguana F	3 pg	270 pg		85
Natrix fasciata F	50–1065 pg	10–540 pg	90–1445 pg	99
Naja naja M	60–2300 pg			
N. naja F	30–700 pg	10–310 pg	1.4–25 ng	13
Nerodia sipedon M	2–21 ng			191
Aves				
Anas platyrhynchos, domestic		125–275 pg	2–9 ng	182
A. platyrhynchos, wild M	2.42 ng			142
Gallus domesticus, preovulatory F	2.5 ng	0.32 ng[b]	200 ng	165
Streptopelia risoria				
courting F			3 ng	171
incubating F			1.1 ng	171
incubating M			1.3 ng	171

[a] M, male; F, female
[b] Total estrogens
[c] UND, undetectable
[d] 17β,20α-dihydroxy-4-pregnen-3-one

mechanisms (enzymatic?) to disperse the bundle of spermatozoa so that they can perform their destined functions.

Class Agnatha: Cyclostomata

Lampreys (Petromyzontidae) are characterized by having no breeding cycle, and all individuals die after spawning only once. In contrast, hagfishes (Myxinoidea) apparently breed more than once. Little is known about the reproductive biology of the hagfishes, and the following account of agnathan reproduction by necessity must emphasize the lampreys.

It appears that the cyclostome gonad arises entirely from the embryonic cortex whether it is destined to be a testis or an ovary.[60] This singular embryonic origin may account for the common observations of what appear to be hermaphroditic gonads among the hagfishes. Males exhibit a single median testis with cystic spermatogenesis. Because of fusion of the paired primordia early in development the female lamprey has a single ovary. The single ovary of myxinoids is due to the failure of one primordium to develop. Steroid-binding proteins are not present in cyclostome blood, and circulating levels of steroids are very low[60] (Table 11-6). Gonaducts are absent in cyclostomes, and the gametes are shed into the coelom from which they exit via abdominal pores.

Petromyzontidae

Male Lampreys. The mature lamprey testis exhibits the typical piscine pattern of lobules with germinal cysts. When the cysts have completed formation of spermatozoa, they simultaneously rupture and release spermatozoa into the body cavity. The testis of parasitic forms such as *Lampetra fluviatilis* contains only primary spermatocytes at the time of migration to the breeding grounds. These spermatocytes are transformed rapidly near the time of spawning into spermatozoal masses. Typical interstitial cell masses can be identified cytologically between the lobules in testes of migrating lampreys. These cells accumulate cholesterol-positive lipids and have become densely lipoidal by spawning time.[69] Cytologically, interstitial cells appear to be steroidogenic and exhibit maximum hydroxysteroid dehydrogenase (3β-HSD) activity in February and March prior to the time of spawning.[68] Development of lobule boundary cells during the later stages of spermatogenesis has been observed in *L. fluviatilis.*[103] These cells are sensitive to hypophysectomy, and they may be homologous to sustentacular cells,[68] although 3β-HSD activity has not been reported.

Female Lampreys. Oogenesis has been carefully examined in the parasitic sea lamprey *Petromyzon marinus* and in the river lamprey *L. fluviatilis.*[68,103–105] In *P. marinus,* oogonia proliferate mitotically in the larvae to form the primary oocytes. By the time of metamorphosis of the larva to the juvenile, there are no oogonia remaining in the ovary. The primary ovarian follicles become more vascularized at this time. During the prolonged parasitic phase of body growth (about 10 to 20 months), the oocytes continue to enlarge slowly. The single follicular cell layer becomes thinner and less vascularized as spawning approaches, and the oocyte enters a period of rapid enlargement to reach the preovulatory condition. The mature follicles rupture immediately before spawning, and the eggs enter the coelom. Follicular atresia occurs throughout the history of ovarian development, and most oocytes undergo atresia, establishing this basic pattern early in the phylogeny of vertebrates. Phagocytes derived from the follicular cells ingest the yolk, and the follicle layers and surrounding stroma collapse into the area formerly occupied by the oocyte.

Oocyte growth in parasitic *L. fluviatilis* accelerates markedly just prior to spawning. The granulosa, which covers only the vegetal pole in close contact with the oocyte, reaches maximal development about 1 month sooner. The thecal cells are greatly reduced and with the aid of the electron microscope can be seen covering the granulosa layer and the animal pole. The theca interna consists of a single layer of cells in which there is a marked increase in smooth endoplasmic reticulum and mitochondrial differentiation during vitellogenesis. These cells show maximum cytological activity prior to the time of most intensive vitellogenesis, following which they undergo progressive regression until the time of ovulation. The theca externa consists of fibroblasts, collagen fibers and capillaries. Hydroxysteroid dehydrogenase activity is apparently confined to the thecal cells where peak activity is observed about 1 month prior to the appearance of secondary sex characters and the acceleration of follicular development.

Vitellogenesis appears to be an estrogen-dependent event in lampreys involving cooperative action of the liver, which produces proteins that are secreted into the blood and are sequestered by the ovary to be incorporated in the developing oocyte. Estrogens stimulate liver hypertrophy and elevate plasma protein-bound calcium,[147,148] suggesting the presence of a mechanism such as the one that has been documented so carefully in birds and other nonmammals (see below).

In the free-living lampreys that do not feed after metamorphosis the ovarian events occur over a much shorter time and are consequently more dramatic.[68] In brook lampreys the immediate postmetamorphic period is marked by the onset of both vitellogenesis and massive atresia. As many as 70% of the follicles present at metamorphosis may become atretic, and phagocytosis of the yolk may provide an essential nutritional source for growth of the remaining oocytes to maturity.

Endocrine Function in Lampreys. The endocrine control of reproduction in lampreys has been studied by several investigators. The importance of gonadal steroids to development of sex accessory structures has been demonstrated through classical experiments involving hypophysectomy, gonadectomy and appropriate hormone therapy to either hypophysectomized or castrate animals.[49,50] Pituitary gonadotropins stimulate gonadal hormone secretions, which in turn stimulate formation of secondary sex characters. The gonads of hypophysectomized *L. fluviatilis* were found to be less developed than those of sham-operated controls, although treatment of immature lampreys with mammalian gonadotropins has no effect on the gonads.[42]

Myxinoidea. The reproductive biology of deep water myxinoids is poorly known, and there is little literature available.[60,100] The hagfishes are apparently seasonal breeders and, unlike the lampreys, exhibit continuous reproductive cycles. Only *Eptatretus burgeri,* which lives in the shallow coastal waters of Japan, shows a seasonal cycle of gonadal activity. There is a single gonad in adults similar to that described in lampreys. Although a few cytological observations have been reported with respect to follicular development and formation of both preovulatory "corpora lutea" (atretic follicles) and postovulatory "corpora lutea," the possible endocrine functions of such structures are unknown. Male hagfishes apparently lack true interstitial cells, and it is not clear whether steroidogenic lobule boundary cells are present.

Although almost no experimental work is available with respect to the function of the hypothalamo-hypophysial system in hagfishes, hypophysectomy of the Pacific hagfish *Eptatretus stouti* results in testicular degeneration in males,[61] but hypophysectomy of females has no effect on either ovarian structure or circulating steroid hormone levels.[121] Vitellogenesis is stimulated by treatment of *E. stouti* with estradiol.[203]

Class Chondrichthyes

The elasmobranchs have been studied extensively, probably because of the incidence of viviparity in these species (present in ten families of sharks and four families of rays).[71,111] Unfortunately no data are available on reproduction in ratfishes. Elasmobranchs are characterized by internal fertilization regardless of whether they are viviparous or oviparous.[187] Several different reproductive patterns have been described, extending from species that lay a precise number of eggs in a particular sequence, such as the oviparous clear-nosed skate *Raja eglanteria,* to the viviparous spotted dogfish *Scyliorhinus canicula* that is sexually active throughout the year and may have embryos in different stages of development in utero at the same time.[187]

Male Elasmobranchs. Spermatogenesis in paired testes is of the cystic type. Sustentacular cells have been identified, and they possess 3β-HSD activity. These cells become densely lipoidal and cholesterol positive following spermiation and are eventually resorbed. Sustentacular cells for the next cycle differentiate from connective tissue cells (fibroblasts) in the wall of the testis. Nests of spermatogonia proliferate from germ cells in the same regions, and they are responsible for producing spermatozoa utilized during the next breeding period.

Spermatophores produced by elasmobranchs are the result of secretory activities of male accessory ducts. After spermiation, spermatozoa pass through vasa efferentia and enter the coiled tubules of the so-called *Leydig gland,* which is derived from the anterior portion of the mesonephric kidney. Spermatozoa and secretions of the Leydig gland pass on to an expanded region of the vas deferens known as the *ampulla.* Here the spermatozoa are consolidated and receive additional secretory material to form complex spermatophores typical for each species. Fertilization is internal, and spermatophores are transferred to the female by specialized structures termed claspers.

Endocrine Factors in Male Elasmobranchs. The importance of the ventral lobe of the elasmobranch pituitary as the source of gonadotropin controlling spermatogonial proliferation (mitotis) has been demonstrated in the spotted dogfish.[42] Degenerative changes in the testes appear 6 weeks after removal of only the ventral lobe, and 22 months later the testes contain only spermatogonia and mature spermatozoa, indicating that removal of the ventral lobe blocks further differentiation of spermatogonia to spermatocytes, whereas all spermatocytes present at the time of surgery are able to complete meiosis and spermiogenesis. Removal of the rostral or neurointermediate lobes of the pituitary is without observable effect on the testes.

Female Elasmobranchs. The elasmobranch ovary is covered by germinal epithelium and may contain a cavity derived from large lymph spaces within the stroma. Elasmobranch follicles are similar to those of mammals in possessing several distinct layers of cells. The connective tissue near a nest of oogonia will differentiate into the theca. As each follicle begins to develop, some epithelial cells undergo hypertrophy and hyperplasia to become the granulosa. In some species the granulosa may consist of only a single layer of cells. These cells are responsible for yolk deposition during oocyte growth as well as for yolk resorption should a given follicle become atretic. Granulosa cells are also thought to be the source of estrogens since they exhibit more 3β-HSD activity than do thecal cells. Most estrogen synthesis occurs in the mature follicle, which has a well developed granulosa. During follicular development a theca interna and theca externa can be discerned. However, both layers largely consist of connective tissue elements, and only a small amount of 3β-HSD activity has been observed in the theca interna cells.

The granulosa cells provide the source of both preovulatory (atretic) and postovulatory corpora lutea. The connective tissue layers surrounding these structures are derived from the theca. Corpora lutea of several species have been shown to possess 3β-HSD activity, and corpora lutea persist during gestation in *Squalus acanthias,* the spiny dogfish. Furthermore, the corpora lutea from pregnant *S. acanthias* produce twice as much progesterone in vitro as do those from nonpregnant females, which possess only preovulatory corpora lutea formed from atretic follicles.[24] These observations strongly support an endocrine role for postovulatory corpora lutea in the viviparous elasmobranchs. Atresia is a common occurrence in elasmobranch ovaries. Depending upon the species being examined, either thecal or granulosa cells may contribute to formation of the preovulatory corpora lutea. Conflicting data have been published with respect to the question whether these atretic follicles are steroidogenic or not, and final resolution awaits further study.[111]

Elasmobranch females have well-developed mullerian ducts that give rise to the oviducts as well as to the uterus of viviparous species. Oviducts have been examined in oviparous species that secrete horny shells to protect the eggs laid in the ocean as well as in viviparous species, and they possess a number of specialized features. *Oviducal* or *nidamental glands* secrete albumen and mucus in oviparious species. Villus-like structures may develop in the uterine portion of the oviducts of certain viviparous females, and they provide nourishment for their young. The oviductal glands of oviparous species are often differentiated into an anterior albumin-secreting area and a posterior shell-secreting region. An intermediate mucus-secreting zone may be found in some species. In one dogfish species the shell-secreting portion of the oviduct serves as a spermatotheca.

Endocrine Factors in Female Elasmobranchs. Removal of the ventral lobe of the adenohypophysis blocks oviposition in female *S. canicula,* and all follicles containing oocytes larger than 4 mm diameter undergo atresia.[42] As in the male, removal of rostral or neurointermediate lobes has no effects on reproduction. The roles for steroids in reproduction have not been elucidated, although the possible role of progesterone from corpora lutea during gestation was suggested earlier. Additional studies with immature elasmobranchs, employing both gonadectomy and removal of the ventral lobe together with hormonal replacement therapy, are necessary to develop a complete understanding of endocrine factors responsible for reproduction in elasmobranchs.

Class Osteichthyes

The bony fishes, or more specifically the teleosts, exhibit almost every reproductive pattern and strategy known for vertebrates, including some that are unique to these fishes. Most of the account here is based on teleosts, but there are many similarities between teleosts and the other orders of bony fishes. Like that of cyclostomes the teleostean gonad develops only from a cortical primordium. Bony fishes may be dioecious or hermaphroditic. Among the hermaphrodites there are examples of protandry (function first as males and later transform to females) and protogyny (function first as females and later transform to males), and there are simultaneous hermaphrodites that may even exhibit self-fertilization. Fertilization may be external or internal as in the viviparous teleosts and in the viviparous coelacanth, *Latimeria.* In some viviparous teleosts the fertilized egg is known to develop within the ovary. Elaborate patterns of courtship, nest building, parental care and other specific reproductive behaviors have been reported among diverse groups. An incredible account of reproductive variations has been compiled by Breder and Rosen;[15] many endocrine aspects of reproduction have been described.[39,45,71,109,111]

Breeding is cyclic, with each species exhibiting a well-defined spawning period regulated by environmental factors (seasonal changes in photoperiod, temperature, etc.). Although some species spawn only once and die, others may spawn several times during a single breeding season (for example, *Reprohanus melanochir,* an Australian garfish).

There are many viviparous species of teleostean fishes that may utilize any of several known patterns, not to mention some patterns that may still be unknown to scientists. Some species, such as the guppy *Poecilia reticulata,* have short cycles. Soon after birth of the young, a new batch of oocytes is ready to be fertilized and another brood may be reared. Other species may require a longer "interbrood period" for oocyte maturation and vitellogenesis *(Mollienesia* and *Gambusia).* However, in *Quintana atrizoma,* oocyte development occurs during gestation so that a new batch of eggs can be fertilized as soon as the young are born. It would be most interesting to know the details of the patterns of hormone secretion in these different species, but they have not been studied.

Endogenous seasonal or annual rhythms have not been demonstrated in fishes although seasonal reproductive cycles are clearly evident even in tropical species.[161] The effects of artificial lengthening and decreasing of the photophase may accelerate spawning in spring and fall spawners respectively. A classic demonstration of environmental phasing of reproduction has been demonstrated by transporting a poecilid, *Jenynsia lineata,* from South America, where it normally spawned in January and February, to the northern hemisphere.[185] In the new pond location where photoperiod and seasons were reversed, the fish switched to spawning in July and August. However, the possible importance of the temperature regimen, which was also switched, should not be overlooked. In some species, temperature has been shown to be the critical factor in controlling recrudescence regardless of the light regimen imposed on the fish. In the tropics where photoperiod and temperature show little or no fluctuations, the reproductive cycles of freshwater and brackish water fishes appear to be tuned to the wet and dry seasons, which profoundly influence the aquatic environments. Periodic flooding and drying cause marked changes in water availability and also influence salinity and chemical composition of the aquatic environment. Some tropical fishes, such as many of the cichlid species that live in permanent bodies of water, may exhibit successive breeding over most of the year. It would be most interesting to examine the involvement of endocrines in these species with respect to timing and initiation of each breeding cycle.

Male Bony Fishes. Spermatogenesis in bony fishes is of the cystic lobular type, except for testes of atheriniform teleosts, such as the guppy, which have a tubular organization.[127] Spermatogenesis in cyclic spawners resumes soon after breeding. Nests of spermatogonia proliferate from germ cells near the margins of the testicular lobules. Sustentacular cells have been described in a number of species, apparently arising from connective tissue elements of the spent lobule walls. Hydroxysteroid dehydrogenase activity has been shown in sustentacular cells,[9,192] implying a role for these cells in the synthesis of steroids.

The major circulating androgens in teleosts are testosterone and 11-ketotestosterone (see Chap. 9). In many teleosts the androgen-secreting cells are located in the lobule walls (lobule boundary cells), and true interstitial (interlobular) cells are absent. These lobule boundary cells are believed to differentiate from fibroblasts in the lobule wall. Interstitial cells have been described in some species, and these cells possess 3β-HSD activity in teleosts, lungfishes and in the coelacanth *Latimeria.*

A seasonal cycle of lipid accumulation and depletion has been described in detail for lobule boundary cells of pike, *Esox lucius,* and similar cells have been observed for other teleostean species.[111] Viviparous teleosts, like their distant elasmobranch relatives, produce spermatophores, employing secretions by the male gonaducts. These structures and the endocrine control of their secretory activities have not been examined sufficiently.

Spermatogenesis, 3β-HSD activity in interlobular or lobule boundary cells and spermiation are stimulated by treatment with LH but not FSH. Numerous studies have demonstrated that teleosts would appear to possess only one pituitary gonadotropin and that it is basically LH-like in its action (see Chaps. 4 and 5). This is a particularly interesting observation since spermatogenesis in amphibians and amniotes is undoubtedly influenced strongly by FSH rather than LH.

Many species show marked seasonal development in sperm ducts, accessory glands and secondary sexual characters that are presumed to be under androgenic control. For example, testosterone induces formation of nuptial tubercles on the head of fathead minnows (Fig. 11-17), a distinctive male sexual characteristic in several cyprinid species.[174] Sperm ducts are derived from the coelomic walls. There are no wolffian ducts, and the sperm ducts of bony fishes are not homologous to the vasa deferentia of tetrapods or of elasmobranchs.[127]

Female Bony Fishes. The teleostean ovary has been studied in considerable detail with respect to gonadal differentiation, oogenesis and vitellogenesis and ovulation, both in oviparous and viviparous species. The ovary of most teleosts is hollow, whereas solid ovaries have been reported in most Dipnoi and Chondrostei. Some teleosts also have solid ovaries. Unlike the hollow ovary of elasmobranchs and amphibians, in the ovary of teleosts the cavity as well as the outer surface is lined with germinal epithelium. Each hollow ovary is continuous with an oviduct which

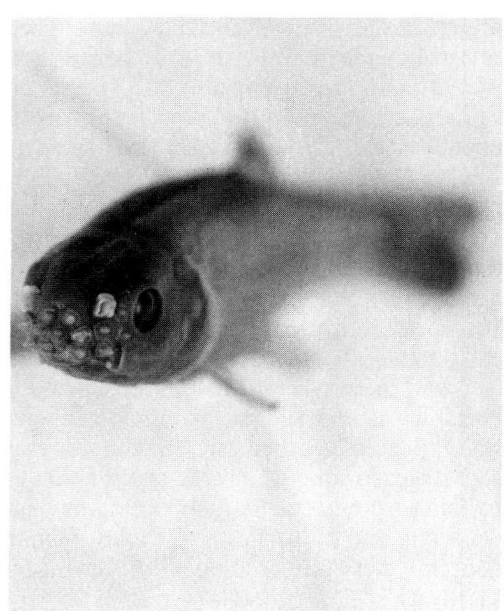

Fig. 11-17. Nuptial tubercles on the snout of the minnow *Pimephales.* These secondary sexual characters of a number of cyprinid males are androgen dependent.

is not homologous to mullerian duct derivatives of other vertebrates. Eggs are discharged directly into the oviduct. In species with solid ovaries the eggs are discharged into the body cavity from which they pass to the exterior via oviducts or directly through openings in the body wall.

Salmon gonadotropin, mammalian LH, hCG or PMSG (in large doses) induces vitellogenesis, ovulation and oviposition in several species, including the Indian catfish *Heteropneustes fossilis,* the goldfish *Carassius auratus* and pink salmon *Oncorhynchus gorbuscha.*[2,56,181,200] Synthetic mammalian GnRH also induces ovulation in goldfish.[96] Mammalian FSH has not been effective in stimulating reproductive events in female teleosts. In the carp a peak in plasma gonadotropin occurs during ovulation,[16] and the highest circulating gonadotropin levels in salmonids have been reported for prespawning females.[36]

Evidence has been presented for non-glycoprotein gonadotropin in teleosts.[146] This gonadotropin stimulates uptake by oocytes of yolk precursors from the blood. This function is controlled by LH in other vertebrate groups. Basically the teleostean ovary consists of masses of follicles embedded in a rather sparse stroma. Each follicle begins as a single-layered epithelium surrounding the oocyte. As the follicle grows these epithelial cells undergo hyperplasia and hypertrophy to form the granulosa. Connective elements in the stroma near the follicular nest will differentiate into a theca, which may further differentiate into a theca externa and a theca interna. The granulosa cells are responsible for yolk deposition in the oocyte during follicular growth and resorption of yolk during atresia.[71] Steroidogenesis may occur in granulosa cells based upon measurements of 3β-HSD and 17β-HSD activity, although in some species the theca may exhibit more 3β-HSD activity than does the granulosa. In tilapia, 3β-HSD activity has been reported for both thecal and granulosa cells.[111]

Three types of ovaries can be identified in teleosts.[127] In the *synchronous ovary* all oocytes are in the same stage of development. Species with a synchronous ovary spawn only once (for example, *Oncorhynchus* spp., *Anguilla* spp.). Species such as rainbow trout and flounder have a *group-synchronous ovary* with at least two populations of oocytes. These species generally spawn once a year during a short breeding season. The last type is the *asynchronous ovary* which has oocytes in all stages of development. These species spawn frequently each year during a prolonged breeding season.

Teleostean ovarian tissue synthesizes estrogens in vitro from radioactive precursors and also synthesizes testosterone, 11-ketotestosterone and deoxycorticosterone.[31] Adrenal androgens may serve as precursors for the synthesis of 11-ketotestosterone.[54] These three steroids have been identified in the peripheral plasma of teleostean species.[25,89,194] In several species the levels of testosterone are greater in prespawning females than in males.[25,54] Ovarian androgens may be precursors for estrogen synthesis. A possible role for DOC in ovulation has been claimed for *H. fossilis.*[181]

All groups of bony fishes develop preovulatory corpora lutea as a result of atresia of developing follicles and develop postovulatory corpora lutea following ovulation. However, a convincing endocrine function of corpora lutea is not yet established among bony fishes. Atretic follicles do not have detectable 3β-HSD activity.

Vitellogenesis by the liver is apparently stimulated by estradiol. When released into the blood, these proteins bind free calcium and cause more calcium to be released from calcium reservoirs to replace the free calcium. Consequently total plasma calcium levels are elevated[8] (see Chap. 12 for details of calcium metabolism). Reproductively active oviparous females exhibit significantly greater plasma calcium levels than do males or immature females (Table 11-7), presumably because of elevated estradiol levels and vitellogenesis.

Reproductive Behavior in Bony Fishes. Many aspects of reproductive behavior have been studied in teleosts, including migration, courtship, nest building, spawning, copulation and parental care.[109] Most of this work has concentrated on roles of testis, testosterone and synthetic androgens in males. Castration of males blocks breeding behavior and causes reversal to nonbreeding condition of androgen-dependent characters. Some variations have been reported for agonistic (territorial)

TABLE 11-7. *Reproductive State and Serum Calcium Levels during the Spring in Steelhead Trout* Salmo gairdneri *from a Natural Population*

	N	MEAN BODY WEIGHT (g)	MEAN SERUM CALCIUM (mg/dl + SE)
Immature males and females	12	38.4	11.6 ± 0.43
Sexually mature male prior to spawning	11	213.6	11.5 ± 0.74
Sexually mature females after ovulation but prior to spawning	9	204.9	15.5 ± 1.44

NOTE: Sexually mature female trout differ significantly ($p < 0.01$) from sexually mature males and immature trout.

behavior, which often accompanies breeding, depending upon the time of castration. In *Gasterosteus aculeatus,* form *trachurus,* castration more than a week before building of the first nest abolishes all related behaviors.[7] If castration is performed within the week prior to building of the first nest, however, agonistic behavior remains at a high level for 3 to 4 weeks. In some species, castration does not result in a decrease in agonistic behavior. Androgens may not be required to maintain the behavior once it has been induced.

The roles of estrogens and androgens in relation to the breeding behaviors of females have been studied less than the roles of androgens in males. Castration of females may result in complete abolition of all reproductive behavior, loss of only some or only a decrease in intensity. In one case, ovariectomized *G. aculeatus,* form *leiurus,* show more aggressive behavior than intact females, implying that steroids normally depress aggressive behavior in females. Estrogens have proven ineffective in inducing female behavior in females. Possible roles for androgens have not been studied. Spawning behavior in females appears to be under control of gonadotropins, although in *Fundulus heteroclitus* neurohypophysial preparations or synthetic oxytocin induces reflexive spawning movements in hypophysectomized or castrated females (see Chap. 7). This spawning reflex is a behavior not dependent upon shedding of ova. Similar observations have been reported for a few additional species.[109,193] Spawning behavior in females may be stimulated by prostaglandins.[173] Possible roles of pheromones in spawning are discussed in Chapter 15.

Mammalian PRL has been shown to influence certain aspects of parental behavior and implies a role for endogenous PRL. Fanning behavior associated with aeration of the eggs can be stimulated in *Symphysodon aequifasciata* and *Pterophyllum scalare* by PRL treatment,[11] whereas similar treatment inhibits fanning behavior in sticklebacks.[175] Stimulation of a mucous secretion that is fed to young *S. aequifasciata* is a PRL-dependent event. Mucous secretions are also stimulated by PRL in other species. It is not clear whether this behavior of feeding mucus to the young in *S. aequifasciata* is caused by PRL treatment.

The implication of hormones in migratory behavior is largely circumstantial (see Chap. 18). The gonads and their secretions probably do not play a causative role, since gonadal maturation usually occurs during migration. Thyroid hormones have been claimed to be causative factors of migratory behavior, and increased thyroid activity coincides with migratory behavior. It is possible that the increased activity of the thyroid gland is correlated to "permissive" effects related to metabolism and osmoregulation. Thyroid hormones may only enhance the physiological states favorable to migration, whereas the behavioral changes are neurally controlled through actions of environmental factors such as photoperiod and temperature or possibly by endogenous rhythmic neural cycles that are regulated by these environmental factors.

Class Amphibia

The origin of modern amphibians from their amphibian progenitors suggests that the primitive reproductive pattern for amphibians involved production of a small number of large, heavily yolked eggs.[132] If direct development is primitive to amphibians, then it follows that the possession of an aquatic larval intermediate is a secondarily derived condition. The importance of the larval stage would seem to be that it allows for an intercalated feeding stage where growth can be optimized without using energy stores or food resources of the parents.[43] If this interpretation is correct the presence of aquatic larvae should not be assumed to be a primitive feature and does not support the notion that study of species exhibiting this life history pattern will provide evolutionary clues. Nevertheless, during metamorphosis of these fish-like larvae to terrestrial-type tetrapods, the same problems are encountered and solved that allowed for the evolution of terrestrial vertebrates.

Within the modern Amphibia several trends in reproductive evolution are evident.[110,111,189] All three extant orders show a reduction in the use of the aquatic habitat with a tendency toward terrestrial development. This trend is accompanied by greater reliance on internal fertilization, a secondary reduction in clutch size (number of eggs produced per breeding) and development of simple parental care of eggs and young. Mate selection and courtship patterns have become very elaborate in some species. Finally, oviparity has given rise to viviparity, especially in the anurans and apodans.

Oviparity. Many anuran amphibians are oviparous animals with external fertilization, although internal fertilization occurs in several species. Breeding in oviparous species is tied closely to a seasonal cycle involving photoperiod, temperature or availability of moisture or a combination of these, although a few species are continuous breeders (the Indian frogs *Rana tigrina* and *R. erytrea* and the South American toads *Bufo arenarum* and *B. paracmenis*).

One predominant reproductive pattern is found in oviparous anurans. Spermatogenesis and ovarian follicular development are completed in the fall, and the animals simply "hibernate" until suitable breeding conditions occur in the spring. Many oviparous species lay their eggs in temporary or permanent ponds with the egg developing into a free-swimming larval form. Tadpole larvae are the characteristic fish-like larval form of anurans and differ markedly from the larvae of urodeles, which possess external gills and four limbs. Anurans have internal gills like fishes and obtain their limbs later during metamorphosis (see Chap. 17). One anuran *(Ascaphus)* is known to lay its eggs in streams, and the tadpole larvae that result have special modifications to keep from being swept downstream. Some anuran and urodele species lay their eggs on land, usually in moist places such as under logs or in the axil of tree branches. Terrestrial eggs that are heavily yolked develop directly into miniature adults. No aquatic larval stage exists except within the egg.

Oviparous urodeles exhibit several reproductive patterns. In some species the pattern is similar to that of anurans *(Triturus cristatus, Notophthalmus viridescens)*. Spermatogenesis in the hellbender *Cryptobranchus alleganiensis* occurs in July shortly before breeding in August and September. Other species such as the mudpuppy, *Necturus* spp., transfer spermatozoa to the females in the fall, and oviposition occurs the next spring when males are not present.

A number of oviparous apodans have been described, all of which lay terrestrial eggs. In *Ichthyophis* the eggs are laid in a burrow near a stream, and the newly hatched larva must emerge from the burrow and find its way to the stream. Apodans generally produce larger eggs than do the other amphibian groups, and clutch sizes are small.

Viviparity. Two European land salamanders *Salamandra salamandra* and *S. atra,* give birth to live offspring that develop in the posterior portion of the oviducts. In *S. atra,* one young develops and undergoes metamorphosis in each oviduct during a 4-year gestation period. Gestation is shorter in *S. salamandra,* which gives birth to larval salamanders.

Viviparity in anurans typically involves a modification of a pouch that allows the eggs to develop into tadpoles on the body of the maternal animal. The South American tree frogs carry their eggs in a single mass on their back. A fold of skin may develop that completely covers the eggs in a pouch such as that found in the so-called marsupial frogs, *Gastrotheca* spp., of South America. In others, such as the African frog *Pipa pipa,* each egg develops in its own dermal chamber. Oviductal incubation of eggs occurs in *Nectophyrnoides* and *Elutherodactylus,* and at least one species broods its young in its gut.

Viviparity may occur in the majority of apodan species.[189] The contribution of maternal energy through oviductal secretion to support the developing young is considerable. In *Typhlonectes* one female may produce as many as nine larvae, each of which weighs about 40% of the mother's body weight at birth.

Male Amphibians: Caudata. Spermatogenesis is of the cystic type in urodeles, and testicular structure and function are very similar to those of fishes.[110,111] The urodele testis consists of one or more *lobes,* each containing several *ampullae,* which in turn are comprised of several germinal cysts (Fig. 11-18). Germ cells associated with a germinal cyst divide mitotically to produce a cluster of secondary spermatogonia. These cells undergo synchronous differentiation to primary spermatocytes and enter meiosis. All of the cysts within an ampulla develop synchronously although it is typically only the more posterior ampullae that exhibit spermatogenesis prior to a given breeding season. Sustentacular cells develop from fibroblasts in the cyst walls while the spermatogonial divisions are taking place. As

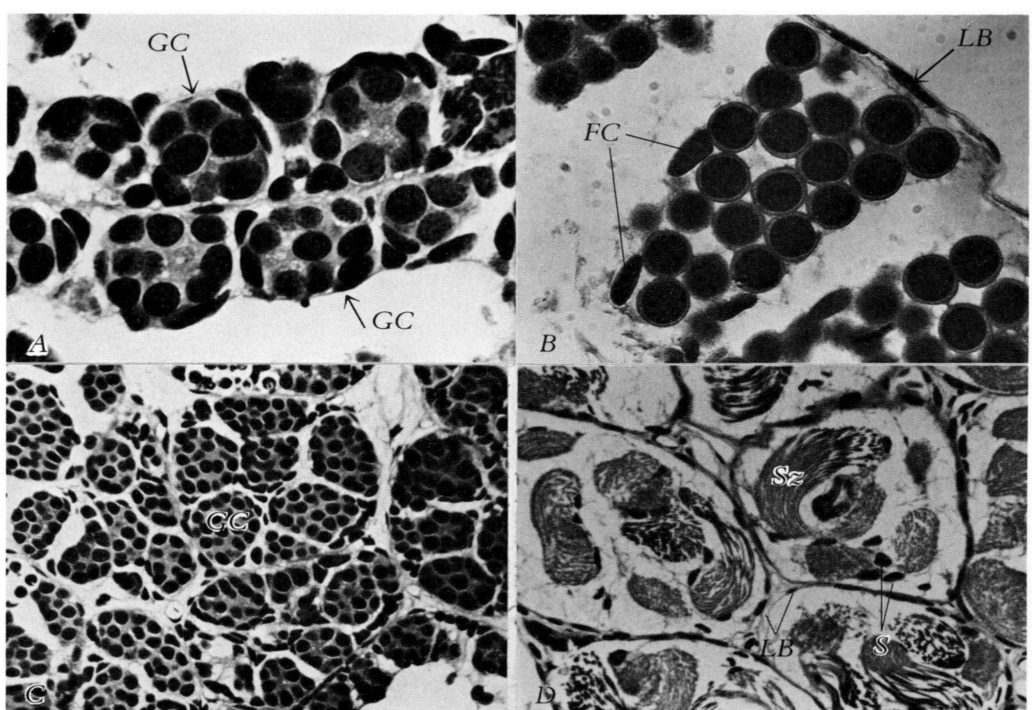

Fig. 11-18. Testis of the newt, *Taricha granulosa.* (Courtesy of Dr. Frank L. Moore.)
A. Early germinal cysts *(GC).* Note mitotic figures in all cells of one cyst, indicating synchronous divisions *(upper right).*
B. Enlargement of an older cyst containing secondary spermatogonia. Both follicle cells *(FC)* and quiescent lobule boundary cells *(LB)* are present.
C. Low magnification of section showing several ampullae containing six to eight germinal cysts *(GC)* comprised of secondary spermatogonia (rounded nuclei) derived mitotically from primary spermatogonia. The flattened, irregular nuclei are of follicle cells that will differentiate into either Sertoli cells or lobule boundary cells. Note that all ampullae in this lobe of the testis are at the same stage of differentiation.
D. Section from lobe of testis containing cysts with whorls of spermatozoa *(Sz).* The lobule boundary cells are quiescent, and nuclei of Sertoli cells *(S)* are prominent.

the ampullae mature the posterior portion of the testis becomes swollen with spermatozoa, whereas ampullae of the anteriormost portion consist primarily of spermatogonia. The posterior portion of the testis becomes dense and whitish because of masses of spermatozoa. After spermiation occurs the collapsed ampullae that have discharged their spermatozoa into the male ducts are resorbed, and after breeding, spermatogenesis is initiated in the anterior portion of the testis. If spermiation occurs in the fall, spermatogenesis will not be resumed until the next summer. New ampullae differentiate from connective tissue elements and germ cells in the tunica albuginea.

The urodele testis possesses lobule boundary cells in the ampulla walls. These cells exhibit a marked seasonal pattern of lipid accumulation, steroidogenesis and lipid depletion. Lipid accumulation begins when the secondary sexual characters develop or hypertrophy. The lobule boundary cells become intensely lipoidal and cholesterol-positive following breeding when androgen-dependent accessory structures are regressing. Both lobule boundary cells and sustentacular cells possess 3β-HSD activity, and it is likely that both are influenced by pituitary gonadotropins.

Androgen levels generally are greater in urodeles than in anurans (Table 11-5). Seasonal patterns of androgen secretion have been reported for *Taricha granulosa*[177] and *Cynops pyrrhogaster*.[183] In both species androgen levels appear to be low during breeding. Failure to find seasonal variations in captive animals of other species may be a response to stress which shuts down androgen secretion.[106]

Testosterone or estrogens can stimulate hypertrophy of the vas deferens, but only testosterone stimulates development of the male-type cloaca in urodeles. This cloacal gland complex is responsible for secretion of various components of the spermatophore. Spermatozoa are stored in the vasa deferentia. Contraction of the vasa deferentia and discharge of spermatozoa are caused by AVT.[204]

Testosterone also stimulates development of nuptial pads in the newt *N. viridescens*, but maximal development is obtained by simultaneous treatment with PRL and testosterone. In urodeles such as *N. viridescens*, *T. cristatus* and *A. tigrinum*, PRL is known to influence the movement of land-phase animals to water for breeding (see Chaps. 17 and 18) and also induces heightening of the tail fin, which is a male secondary sex character.

Internal fertilization in both aquatic and terrestrial urodeles occurs through the production of an elaborate spermatophore produced through the actions of the cloacal glands of the male.[164] The spermatophore consists of a glycoprotein matrix to which a packet of spermatozoa is attached, the glycoprotein matrix acting as a base upon which the spermatozoan packet rests. Following an elaborate courtship procedure,[157] a female is induced to pick off the spermatozoan packets by her cloacal lips. The spermatozoan packet may then be stored in a specialized portion of the cloaca (spermatotheca) until ovulation occurs.

Male Amphibians: Anura. The anuran testis is similar in structure to that of amniotes and consists of a mass of seminiferous tubules with permanent germinal epithelium and conspicuous interstitial tissue[110] (Fig. 11-19). The cells

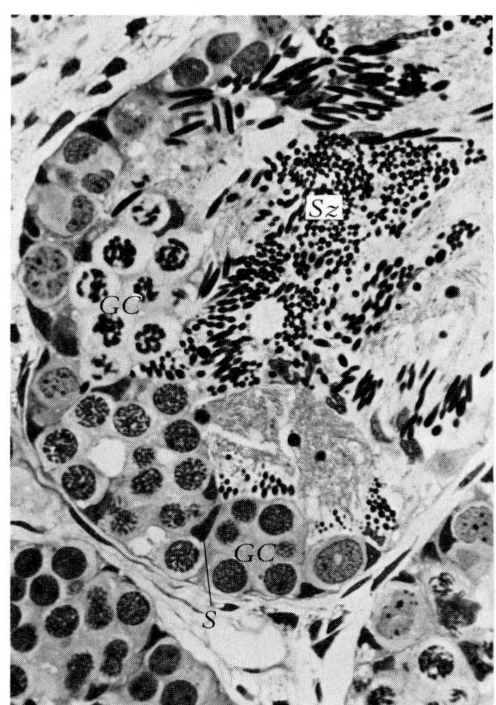

Fig. 11-19. Testis of the bullfrog *Rana catesbeiana*. *Sz*, spermatozoa; *GC*, germinal cysts; *S*, Sertoli cells. (Courtesy of Dr. Charles H. Muller.)

of the latter tissue are ultrastructurally like mammalian interstitial cells and possess 3β-HSD activity. The lipid cycle within the interstitial cells and the degree of 3β-HSD activity closely parallel the development of androgen-dependent sex accessory structures such as the enlarged thumb pads of ranids. Interstitial cells of postspawning anurans exhibit considerable lipoidal accumulation but very low 3β-HSD activity. Thumb pads regress in ranids at this time.

During winter months, sustentacular cells of ranid testes lack lipid, but these cells elongate and exhibit small lipoidal granules as the breeding season approaches. Sustentacular cells of breeding animals have a well-developed smooth endoplasmic reticulum, and 3β-HSD activity is detectable. After spermiation the sustentacular cells detach from the tubule wall and degenerate. New cells for the next reproductive period differentiate from fibroblasts in the tubule walls.

Circulating testosterone, FSH and LH vary seasonally, but estradiol levels are very low. Highest values of hormones occur during mating in *Rana catesbeiana*[106] but not in *Rana esculenta.*[41]

Male Amphibians: Apoda. Male caecilians differ from urodeles and almost all anurans by possessing an elaborate intromittent organ, the *phallodeum,* associated with the posterior part of the cloaca.[189] Consequently fertilization is internal in all apodans. Another unique feature is the retention of the posterior portion of the mullerian ducts that form the *mullerian glands.* These tubular apocrine glands are believed to produce the seminal fluid and would be analogous to the prostate of mammals.[189]

The structure of the lobed testes is similar to that of urodeles, but the cell nests within an ampulla are not all in the same stage of spermatogenesis.

Female Amphibians: Anura and Caudata. Amphibian ovaries are hollow, sac-like structures derived from the embryonic cortex and covered by germinal epithelium (Fig. 11-20). A derivative of embryonic medullary tissues forms the inner lining of the ovary. Oogonia are present in the germinal epithelium, and they give rise to nests of oocytes. The follicular epithelium consists of a single layer of granulosa cells throughout the maturation period. A thecal layer does form around the follicle, but it is not easily seen with the light microscope (Fig. 11-21).

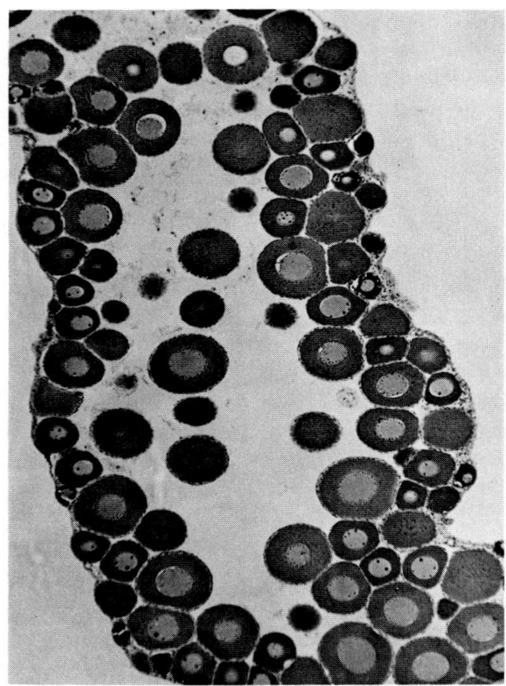

Fig. 11-20. Ovary of the toad *Bufo marinus.* (From an immature specimen.) Note the attachment of oocytes to the germinal epithelium. (Courtesy Dr. Charles H. Muller.)

Hydroxysteroid dehydrogenase has been demonstrated in granulosa cells as well as in thecal cells, but no 3β-HSD activity was observed in the interstitial cells of the ovary. Follicular cells of vitellogenic and mature oocytes in *Xenopus laevis* have been shown to possess increased 3β-, 17α- and 17β-HSD activity following PMSG treatment.[154] Both thecal and granulosa cells may be sources of circulating ovarian steroids, but cytological evidence favors the granulosa as the major source.[98]

At the end of a breeding season the ovary contains young follicles that will become the next crop of mature oocytes, numerous cell nests that will become the young follicles of the next vitellogenic period and primary germ cells that will give rise to new cell nests. Progression from primary germ cells to mature oocytes may require three breeding seasons for completion.[172]

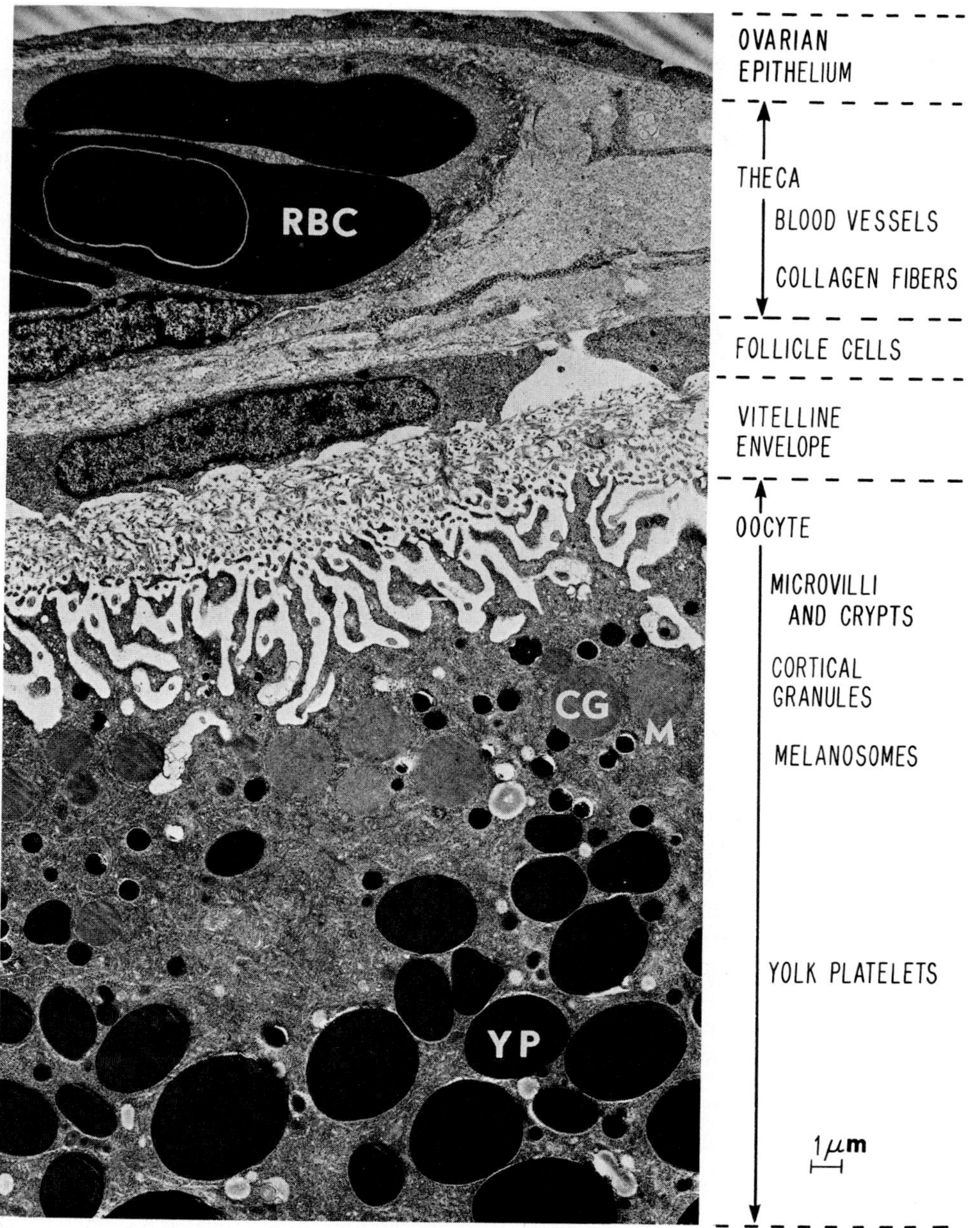

FIG. 11-21. Vitellogenic follicle of *Xenopus laevis.* This electron micrograph shows the vascular theca and its relation to microvillous processes projecting from the developing oocyte. The smaller dark bodies are melanosomes, and the larger ones are yolk platelets. (Dumont, J.N. and A.R. Brummett (1978). Oogenesis in *Xenopus laevis* (Daudin). V. Relationships between developing oocytes and their investing follicular tissues. J. Morphol. 155:73–97. Reprinted with permission of the authors, publisher and the Oak Ridge National Laboratory operated by Union Carbide Corporation for the Department of Energy.)

Ovarian estrogens control development of sex accessory structures such as the hypertrophy of oviducts prior to ovulation.[110] In the marsupial frog *Gastrotheca riobambae,* the development of the brood pouch is also dependent upon estrogens from the preovulatory follicles.[83]

Postnuptial ovaries frequently contain postovulatory corpora lutea, which are shortlived in oviparous species. Granulosa cells hypertrophy after ovulation and accumulate cholesterol-positive lipids. The follicle collapses and becomes a central mass of lipoidal cells surrounded by a fibrous capsule derived from the thecal layer. Postovulatory corpora lutea of *T. cristatus* and *Rana esculenta* possess 3β-HSD activity and may be sources for steroids.[111] No functional endocrine role for postovulatory corpora lutea has been demonstrated in oviparous species.

In viviparous amphibians such as the anuran *Nectophrynoides occidentalis,* postovulatory corpora lutea are more persistent and appear to be functional throughout gestation.[97] Furthermore, postovulatory corpora lutea from this species are capable of converting pregnenolone to progesterone, suggesting they may be endocrine structures.[199] The granulosa-lutein cells of the postovulatory corpora lutea in viviparous *S. salamandra* possess 3β-HSD activity and appear cytologically to be steroidogenic.[78] Thirty or more corpora lutea persist in each ovary during the first 2 years of gestation and gradually decrease in both size and number over the next 2 years until the young are born.[188] In *Nectophrynoides occidentalis* as well as in oviparous *Taricha torosa,* the succeeding crop of follicles begins development only after degeneration of the postovulatory corpora lutea.[97,124] These latter data suggest an inhibitory action of progesterone produced in the postovulatory corpora lutea on release of gonadotropins from the adenohypophysis.

Atresia occurs frequently during follicular development in amphibians. Granulosa cells are responsible for phagocytosis of yolk and formation of the preovulatory corpora lutea (corpora atretica). Since no 3β-HSD activity has been identified in these structures, they should be termed corpora atretica.

The process of vitellogenesis and yolk deposition in oocytes of oviparous amphibians has been reviewed.[52,57] In *X. laevis,* gonadotropin stimulates micropinocytosis of vitellogenin by oocytes. Micropinocytotic vesicles of vitellogenin are hydrolyzed enzymatically in the yolk platelets to produce the yolk proteins *phosvitin* and *lipovitellin.* The yolk platelets containing these yolk proteins are utilized as an energy source during early embryogenesis. Estrogens will induce vitellogenin synthesis in both female and male livers when administered in vivo.[190] Circulating vitellogenin binds free calcium ions, resulting in elevated total plasma calcium levels through release of calcium from storage sites (see Chap. 12).

Hypophysectomy results in atresia of all vitellogenic follicles in excess of about 0.4 mm diameter, indicating the importance of endogenous pituitary gonadotropins in the process of vitellogenesis. Mammalian FSH will augment the growth of vitellogenic follicles and prevent atresia following hypophysectomy. The failure of mammalian gonadotropins to stimulate formation and growth of previtellogenic follicles (less than 0.4 mm diameter) coupled with their apparent insensitivity to hypophysectomy has led to the suggestion that these processes are completely independent of pituitary control. However, experimental studies have not ruled out completely a role for gonadotropin in the development of previtellogenic follicles, and it is possible that low endogenous levels of amphibian gonadotropin are necessary for even the earliest events in gametogenesis.

Amphibian ovaries in vitro produce progesterone, estradiol, estrone, testosterone, deoxycorticosterone and dihydrotestosterone.[98] The high levels of circulating testosterone reported for some anurans[41,106] may be related to a precursor role for peripheral aromatization to estrogens. The follicular wall and/or interstitial gland is/are the source of these hormones.[64,110,157]

Ovulation is under control of an LH-like gonadotropin and progesterone.[57] In-vitro studies of the ovary were initiated by Wright[197,198] and subsequently elaborated by others. These studies have examined the actions of various pituitary hormones as well as a wide variety of steroids in inducing ovulation and oocyte maturation (completion of meiosis and breakdown of the germinal vesicle) in vitro. Although many hormones are effective in vitro if sufficiently large doses are employed, LH and progesterone are the most potent, and it is reasonable to presume they play a role in normal ovulatory events. Prolactin enhanced the sensitivity of oocytes to gonadotropin or progesterone both in vivo and in vitro.[133] This enhancement can be blocked by simultaneous in vivo treatment with thyroxine prior to examining oocyte maturation and ovulation in vitro. The synthesis of progesterone is under control of LH, and the action of progesterone is believed to be indirect, operating through stimulation of a "maturation-promoting factor."[57] The source of the progesterone "surge" believed to occur just prior to ovulation is not clear,[98] and it has been proposed that progesterone is produced by interrenal cells.[111]

Ovarian maturation typically is completed in autumn, and ovulation is delayed over winter until favorable conditions occur in the spring. The endocrine basis for this diapause is not clear but may involve direct inhibition of ovulation by one or more pituitary hormones. Hypophysectomy of both gravid anurans and at least one urodele results in ovulation and oviposition.[128,133] Furthermore, hypophysectomy of gravid neotenic tiger salamanders increases their sensitivity to induced ovulation in response to a single injection of hCG.[133] This "reflexive" ovulation could be due to inadvertent release of gonadotropins by the operation itself or to removal of an active inhibitory substance of pituitary origin or to both.

Growth of oviducts is stimulated by estrogens or androgens.[110] In mature females contraction of oviducts is caused by AVT[102] and presumably is the hormonal stimulus in oviposition. Oviducts of breeding animals are more sensitive to AVT than are those of nonbreeding adults.[70] Progesterone induces responsiveness to AVT in immature oviducts, but estrogens are not effective.[134] Possibly the pre- or postovulatory follicle releases sufficient progesterone to alter receptor levels for AVT in the muscles of the oviducts.

Bidder's Organ. Among both sexes of bufonids (toads) are found rudimentary ovaries or *Bidder's organs* that form from cortical remnants of the embryonic genital ridge (Fig. 11-22). Histologically Bidder's organ consists of a compact mass of very small oocytes. After castration, Bidder's organ hypertrophies and forms a functional ovary in either males or females. Even prior to castration it is capable of synthesizing steroids.[26] It is not clear whether these structures have functional roles or whether they represent only a curious occurrence.

Fat Bodies. Conspicuous masses of adipose tissue called *fat bodies* are located adjacent to the gonads of amphibians. In female anurans and urodeles the size of the fat body is inversely correlated with gonadal weight, and it has been proposed that the lipoidal substances stored in the fat bodies are utilized for oocyte growth. Fat bodies of both male and female newts *(Triturus cristatus)* may be steroidogenic tissues and therefore may influence gonadal function, accessory sex structures or both.[114] In *Rana esculenta,* function of fat bodies appears to be regulated by pituitary gonadotropins.[27]

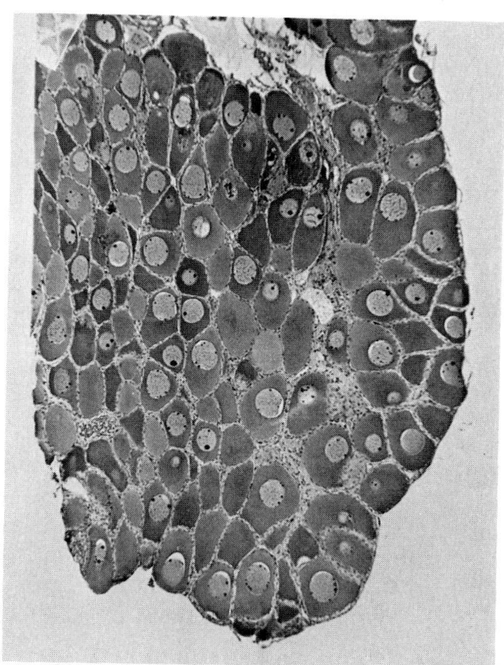

FIG. 11-22. Bidder's organ from the toad *Bufo marinus.* This cortical remnant consists mainly of closely packed, partially developed oocytes. (Courtesy of Dr. Charles H. Muller.)

Female Amphibians; Apoda. Fertilization normally occurs in the upper portion of the oviduct, and the fertilized eggs are either laid in burrows or, as may prove to be the case for most species, are retained in the oviducts until the developing larvae have completed metamorphosis.[189]

Ovarian development is very similar to that described for anurans and urodeles, but in apodans the eggs tend to be larger and fewer.[189] Postovulatory corpora lutea develop in the ovaries, and they appear to be important for maintaining oviductal secretion (even in oviparous species) and pregnancy. Oviductal secretions provide nutrition for the developing young, and these secretions may be controlled by hormones released from the corpora lutea.

Sufficient numbers of specimens have not been examined to determine the seasonalness of breeding and ovarian cycles in caecilians. The endocrine factors involved in reproductive events can only be inferred at this time from studies on anurans and urodeles.

Reproductive Behavior in Amphibians. Numerous aspects of reproductive behavior have been described for many amphibians,[158] but little is known about its endocrine control.[125] Reproductive behavior includes migration (see Chap. 18), calling, courtship, clasping, spawning and parental care. Studies involving castration, hypophysectomy and/or injections of pituitary hormones support the conclusion that testicular hormones are involved in calling, courtship and clasping. However, attempts to stimulate reproductive behavior with androgens have not been successful. Recent studies support a role for neural peptides (AVT, GnRH, ACTH) in triggering mating behavior in androgen-primed animals.[125] For example, when a female frog that is not ready to spawn is clasped by a courting male, she croaks to signal her nonreceptivity. A receptive female will not emit this release call. This female has accumulated water that will be used in ovulation and oviposition. Water retention is caused by AVT (see Chap. 7). Administration of AVT inhibits the release call possibly through effects on the brain.[40]

Class Reptilia

Living reptiles are members of diverse orders, and it is not surprising that considerable differences occur, making it difficult to generalize about reptilian reproduction. In many respects the squamate reptiles possess features unique to their order, whereas the other orders may be more typical of reptiles with respect to exhibition of primitive features. Most reptilian species are oviparous and exhibit well-defined annual reproductive cycles and breeding seasons.[111,187] In addition, many examples of viviparity are known among snakes and lizards. Only a few, heavily yolked eggs are produced by most species. Clutch sizes may be large in some turtles, crocodilians and snakes. Fertilization is internal in all reptiles. Males have copulatory organs for placing spermatozoa into the cloaca of a female. Mating frequently follows complicated behavioral patterns including male-male interactions. Females of many species can store spermatozoa in the cloaca for months.

Reptiles may produce two distinct gonadotropins, although squamates rely on an FSH-like gonadotropin. There is disagreement with respect to relative roles of LH and FSH in reptilian reproduction, making a definite statement impossible at this time.[98,107] The hypothalamus regulates gonadotropin release in response to environmental stimuli such as photoperiod and temperature.

Reptiles have been characterized by their lack of parental behavior and, in some cases, even lack of recognition of their offspring. In recent years, studies have demonstrated that there may be considerable investment in parental care even among oviparous species. Although members of the oldest extant order, the chelonians, typically abandon their nests once the eggs are laid, crocodilian parents participate in the hatching process and in protecting the young.[151] Evidence of nestbuilding and parental care has been unearthed for some extinct dinosaurs as well.[74] Thus, complex parental care did not appear de novo in birds and mammals but evolved in primitive reptiles.

Male Reptiles. The reptilian testis is typical of amniotes and consists of convoluted seminiferous tubules (Fig. 11-23), each surrounded by a connective tissue sheath, the *tunica propria.*[111] The entire testis is enclosed by a connective tissue layer, the *tunica albuginea.* Spermatogenesis recurs soon after the breeding season and is completed in most species prior to the onset of winter. Pituitary gonado-

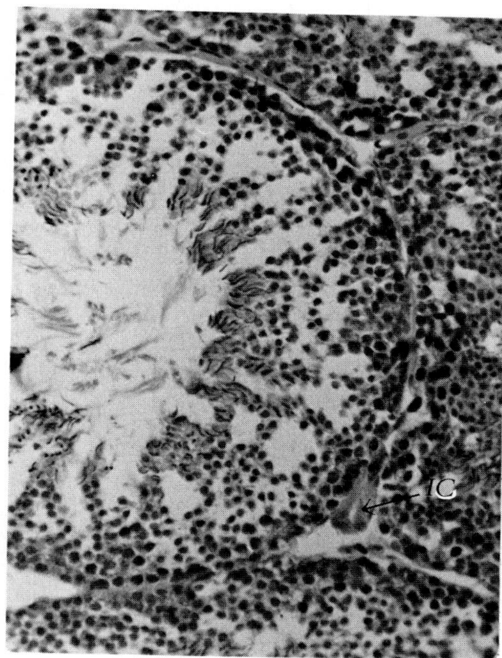

FIG. 11-23. Testis of the lizard *Scincella (Leiolopisma, Lygosoma) lateralis.* This section shows most of a seminiferous tubule with spermatozoa. Compare with Figs. 11-5, 11-18 and 11-19. *IC,* interstitial cells. (Courtesy of Dr. Richard E. Jones)

tropins stimulate spermatogenesis in a variety of reptilian species. Spermatozoa may be stored for up to several months prior to mating during the breeding season. Sustentacular cells are common, and they have been shown to be steroidogenic. After spermiation and testicular collapse, the sustentacular cells fill with cholesterol-positive lipids. Soon there occurs a clearing of the lipid from the cells at the time mitosis resumes in the spermatogonia. Follicle-stimulating hormone causes clearing of these cells and the resumption of spermatogenesis.

Typical interstitial cells have been described in the reptilian testis (Fig. 11-23), and they undergo cyclical changes associated with particular reproductive events.[111] Seasonal changes in lipid content and 3β-HSD activity are correlated with androgen secretion and sexual changes in androgen-dependent sex accessory structures[111] (Fig. 11-24).

In sexually active squamates a portion of the kidney tubules hypertrophy under the influence of androgens.[152] This modified kidney structure is known as the *sexual segment* of the kidney, and it appears to secrete materials that help maintain spermatozoa that are stored in this region prior to ejaculation.[37] It has been suggested that the sexual segment is homologous to the seminal vesicles of male mammals.[152]

FEMALE REPTILES. Reptiles have paired hollow ovaries with little stromal tissue. Oogonia are present in the mature ovary as described for anamniotes and give rise to primary oocytes throughout reproductive life. The developing oocyte (Fig. 11-25) becomes invested with granulosa cells, which are separated from the surrounding thecal cells by a connective tissue layer (membrana propria). The theca is differentiated into an inner, granular theca interna surrounded by a fibrous theca externa. The cells of the granulosa are considered the primary source of follicular estrogen during ovarian recrudescence,[98] although some histochemical evidence implies that thecal cells also may be steroidogenic.[111] Histochemical changes in cholesterol-positive lipid inclusions and 3β-HSD activity parallel estrogen-dependent oviductal growth and changes in other sex accessory structures as well as changes in the gonadotropes in the adenohypophysis. As the oocyte enlarges it begins to project into the ovarian cavity.

The squamate granulosa contains a unique flask-shaped cell, the *pyriform cell* (Fig. 11-25), that is in direct contact with the developing oocyte.[130] These cells apparently are involved with early steps in oocyte development as they either degenerate or transform into typical granulosa cells at the onset of vitellogenesis.

As ovulation approaches the granulosa cells begin to accumulate cholesterol-positive lipids, and, following ovulation, they proliferate and luteinize to form corpora lutea. These corpora lutea are well vascularized, exhibit 3β-HSD activity and synthesize progesterone.[98,201] They persist throughout egg laying in oviparous species or throughout gestation in viviparous forms. Corpora lutea of viviparous species synthesize greater amounts of progesterone than do those of oviparous species.[24] Plasma progesterone levels are greatest following ovulation and are maintained at elevated levels throughout gestation in viviparous lizards and snakes, whereas preovulatory peaks

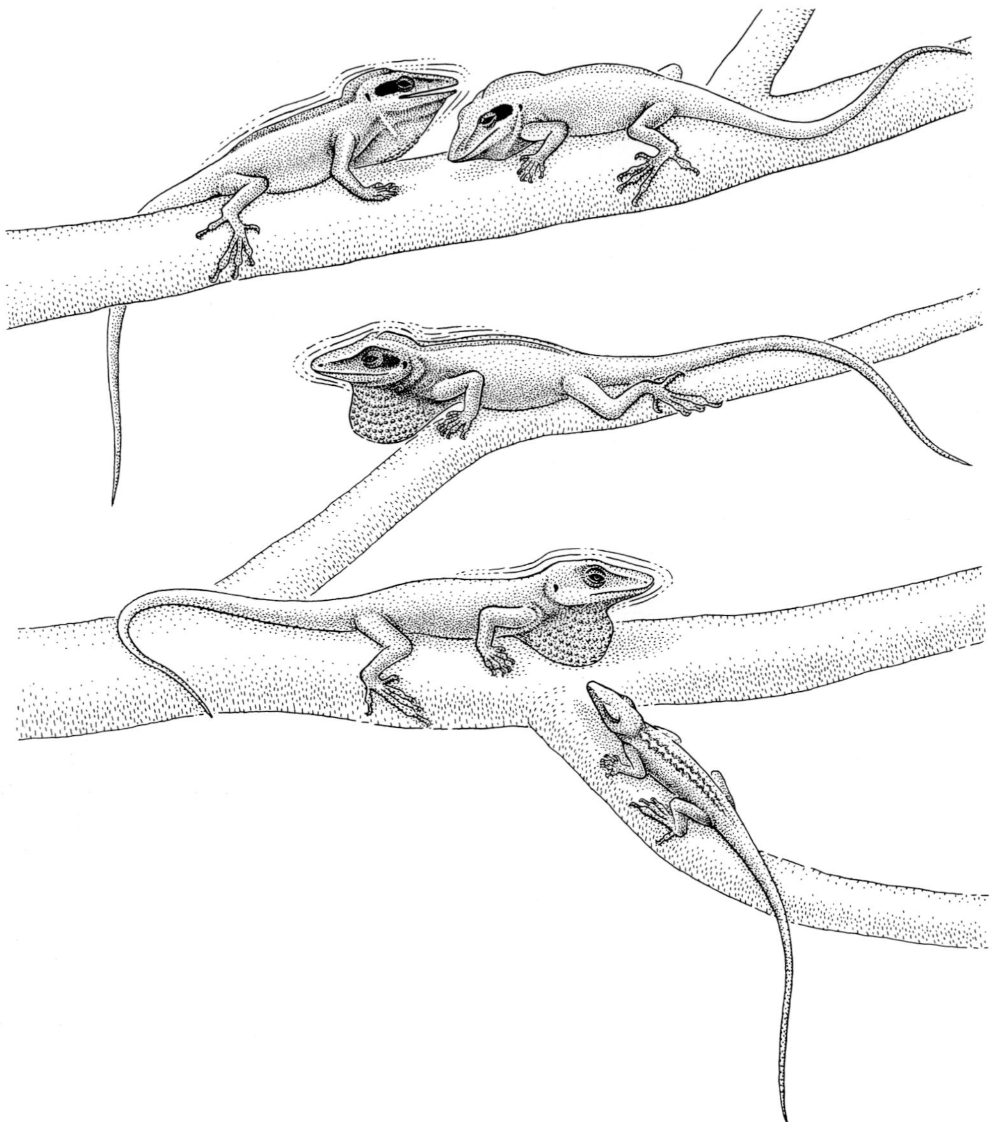

Fig. 11-24. Displays exhibited by male *Anolis carolinensis.* The dewlap is an androgen-dependent structure that may be extended from the throat region. On the top limb, two males are displaying during an aggressive bout. The male on the middle limb is exhibiting an assertion-challenge display that is performed by the dominant animal following an aggressive bout. Beneath him, another male provides a courtship display for a female. These displays in male *A. carolinensis* are also androgen-dependent. (Reprinted with permission from D. Crews (1978): Integration of internal and external stimuli in the regulation of lizard reproduction. In N. Greenberg and P.D. MacLean (eds.): The Behavior and Neurology of Lizards. NIMH, Rockville, Md., pp. 149–171.)

of progesterone are found in oviparous turtles (Table 11-8).

Generally speaking only a few follicles reach maturity at a given time; the majority undergo atresia. Follicular atresia is a common occurrence in reptilian ovaries as in other vertebrates, and formation of corpora atretica is also common. The importance of the latter structures is unknown, but the absence of 3β-HSD activity in corpora atretica makes it

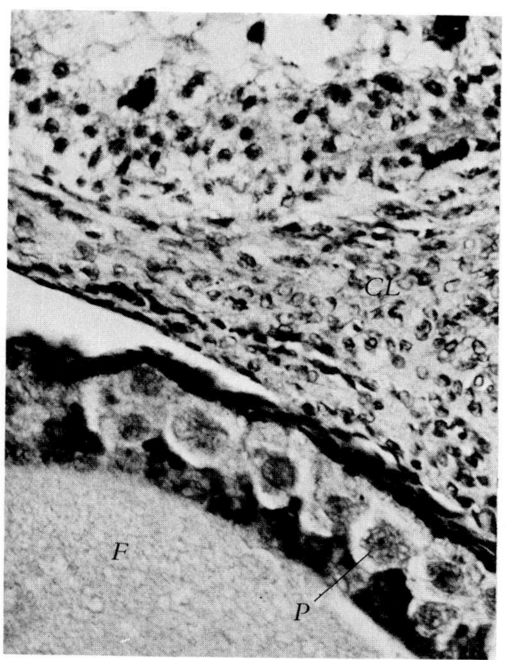

FIG. 11-25. Ovary of the viviparous lizard *Sceloporus jarrovi.* This section shows a portion of a large, previtellogenic follicle *(F)* and a developing corpus luteum *(CL).* Note the large pyriform cells *(P)* in the granulosa of the growing follicle. (Courtesy of Dr. Louis J. Guillette, Jr.)

unlikely they would have an endocrine function.[111,129] However, steroidogenic cells from atretic follicles may give rise to an "interstitial gland" that is believed to be a major source of ovarian estrogens.[64,157]

Ovaries of reptiles show different patterns of follicular maturation and ovulation.[80] Some produce several eggs simultaneously from each ovary (most reptiles). Others may alternate production of a single egg from each ovary (anoline lizards). Still others (turtles) may produce most eggs in one ovary during one season and most from the other ovary the next season. Differences in follicular atresia rather than in the number of oocytes beginning development may be responsible for these patterns.[81]

Oviductal development apparently is under the influence of ovarian estrogens, and progesterone is without effect.[122] In oviparous species, estrogens probably influence the secretion around the egg of albumin and shell from the anterior end of each oviduct. Estrogens also stimulate synthesis of vitellogenic proteins by the liver and cause increases in serum calcium of snakes, lizards and turtles (Table 11-9). Crocodiles produce yolk proteins that are biochemically similar to those of birds.[30] Measurement of calcium may be used as an indirect quantitative measurement of plasma

TABLE 11-8. *Circulating Progesterone Levels (ng/ml plasma) during Reproductive Cycles of Turtles, Lizards and Snakes*

SPECIES	PERIOD OF EARLY FOLLICLE GROWTH	PREOVU-LATORY STAGE	EARLY POSTOVU-LATORY	MID-PREGNANCY	LATE PREGNANCY
Turtles					
Chrysemys picta (oviparous)	0.2 ± 0.06	5.0 ± 1.02	0.5 ± 0.01	—	—
Chelonia mydas (oviparous)	0.2 ± 0.08	1.8 ± 0.13	0.7 ± 0.88	—	—
Lizards					
Sceloporus cyanogenys	0.7 ± 0.15	0.9 ± 0.38	3.3 ± 0.48	—	3.5 ± 0.34
Chamaelo pumilis	0.9	1.0 ± 0.71	5.0 ± 3.90	2.3 ± 0.34	—
Snakes					
Natrix taxispilota	0.4 ± 0.04	0.9 ± 0.08	1.9 ± 0.24	—	—
Nerodia sipedon	1.3 ± 0.19	3.9 ± 0.83	5.0 ± 1.41	6.9 ± 0.78	2.8 ± 0.44
Thamnophis elegans	—	—	1.7 ± 0.30	6.2 ± 1.00	—

Modified from Lance and Callard.[99]

TABLE 11-9. *Effect of Estradiol-17β on Serum Calcium Levels of Ovariectomized Female Lizards* Anolis carolinensis

	N	SERUM CALCIUM (mg/dl ± SE)
Ovariectomized saline-injected females	5	14.8 ± 1.05
Reproductively active, sham-operated females	4	21.2 ± 3.47
Ovariectomized females injected with 1.0 μg estradiol per day for 7 days	5	213.2 ± 9.88
Ovariectomized females injected with 10 μg estradiol per day for 7 days	7	256.0 ± 22.13

Unpublished data of K. Faber and D. Norris.

vitellogenin.[98] Undoubtedly the details of this process are very similar to those described for amphibians and for birds, although vitellogenesis has not been investigated as extensively in reptiles.

Oviposition or birth of live young is controlled by AVT in turtles, lizards and snakes.[63,102] In the American chameleon, *Anolis carolinensis,* the sensitivity of the uterus to AVT is determined by presence or absence of a corpus luteum in the adjacent ovary.[84]

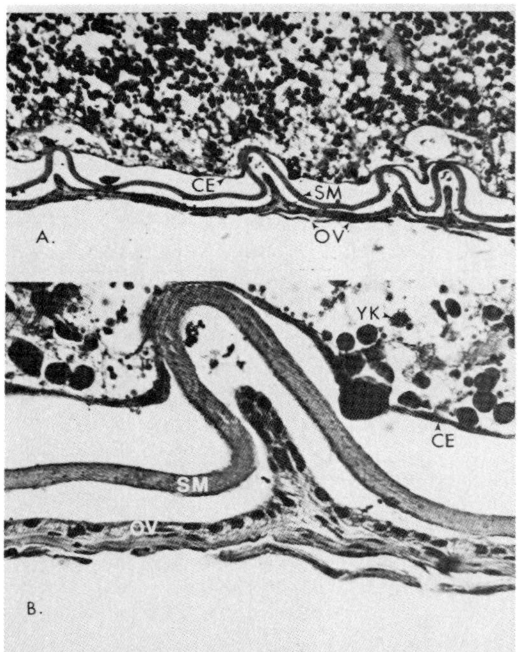

FIG. 11-26. The yolk sac placenta of the viviparous lizard *Sceloporus jarrovi* (A, 100X; B, 400X). Materials can be passed from the oviduct (OV) through the shell membrane (SM) and chorionic epithelium (CE) and into the yolk (YK). This species also produces a vascularized chorioallantoic placenta through which exchange of materials occurs. The spaces shown between the cellular layers are artifacts caused by the procedures employed to prepare these sections. (Reprinted with permission from L.J. Guillette, Jr., S. Spielvogel and F.L. Moore (1981). Luteal development, placentation, and plasma progesterone concentration in the viviparous lizard *Sceloporus jarrovi.* Gen. Comp. Endocrinol. 43:20–29.)

ENVIRONMENT, BEHAVIOR AND REPRODUCTION OF REPTILES. The role that physical and biological components of the environment play in sexual behavior and reproduction has been extensively studied in reptiles.[34,35,46] Species living in temperate climates exhibit distinct seasonal patterns. Reproduction in tropical reptilian species varies from cyclic patterns to continuous breeding. There is a strong tendency for an observed increase in the incidence of viviparity among species inhabiting colder climates (altitude or latitude), but it is not clear which is cause or consequence.

Among temperate lizards, temperature is the dominant environmental factor influencing reproduction. Photoperiod, humidity, and nutritional status play decisive roles in some species. Other groups of reptiles have not been studied as extensively as lizards.

Class Aves

Avian reproductive organs reflect a general anatomical adaptation to flight. In females of most species only the left ovary and its attendant oviduct develop, whereas the right-hand components remain in a rudimentary state. This asymmetry noted in the female is reflected in the male where the left testis usually is larger than the right although both are functional. Should the left ovary be removed surgically or destroyed by disease, the right rudiment may develop, but it will usually form an ovotestis or a testis.

Avian gonads develop from a pair of undifferentiated primordia associated with the embryonic nephrotome. These primordia are invaded by primordial germ cells that migrate through the blood from the splanchnopleure and develop into the germinal epithelium. The embryonic gonad goes through a bipotential state in which both cortical and medullary components are present. Differentiation of cortical tissue is necessary for ovarian development and the medullary portion is suppressed. The reverse condition prevails in male birds. In contrast to mammals it is the male bird that is the homogametic sex (similar sex chromosomes), and it is the female that has unlike sex chromosomes. Developing a female phenotype requires estrogens. Castration of a young female causes development of male plumage. Development or suppression of the mullerian and wolffian ducts eventually depends on the direction of gonadal development as it does in other vertebrates. In females in which only the left half of the reproductive system usually develops, the left ovary receives the larger proportion of germ cells that migrate to the gonads. The mechanism behind this disproportionate distribution of germ cells is not known.

All birds are oviparous but display significantly more parental behavior than any other nonmammalian group of vertebrates. Birds are endothermiclike mammals and use their body heat to support development of the embryo within the egg much as the mammal does in utero. Consequently birds can breed successfully under conditions that are too cold for their reptilian relatives. The adaptation of long-distance flight allows utilization of polar and subpolar regions where winter conditions are too severe for survival but where during the summer months there is adequate warmth and food to breed and rear young birds to a size sufficient to migrate to warmer latitudes for winter.

Reproduction is decisively cyclic in adult birds and is closely attuned to environmental factors.[112,187] Migratory and nonmigratory polar and temperate species typically exhibit seasonal cycles with breeding occurring in the spring and possibly continuing through much of the summer. On the other hand, species occupying arid regions may show irregular cycles cued to the availability of water, which may not occur with any seasonal regularity. One tropical species, *Zonotrichia capensis,* has been reported to breed every 6 months regardless of rainfall as long as food is available.

Both ovaries and testes remain small in nonbreeding birds but may undergo tremendous hypertrophy in a very short time. This is especially advantageous for migratory species or species relying on particular stimuli for breeding where gonadal recrudescence can await arrival on the breeding grounds or appearance of suitable conditions such as abundant food.

Male Birds. The testes are permanently located in the body cavity, and each testis consists of a mass of convoluted seminiferous tubules lined with a germinal epithelium and surrounded by connective tissue.[111] Both developing germ cells and sustentacular cells can be seen in the germinal epithelium as well as numerous fibroblasts. As in mammals and other vertebrates the cytoplasm of the sustentacular cells completely envelops the germ cells and cytologically and histochemically appear to be steroidogenic. Typical steroidogenic interstitial cells occur between the seminiferous tubules.

In nonbreeding birds, testes are very small, and histologically these quiescent testes appear to be composed largely of interstitial cells. However, this is only an artifact produced by a marked postbreeding regression of spermatogenetic tissue. The onset of spermatogenesis (recrudescence) results in rapid and marked increase in testicular size. Such rapid and extreme growth (to as much as 500 times the resting gonad weight) results in considerable strain and damage to the tunica albuginea surrounding the testis, and it must be replaced each year during the postnuptial phase of the testicular cycle. Replacement is accomplished through differentiation of fibroblasts and formation of a new tunica directly beneath the damaged one. It is often possible to distinguish between juvenile birds and postnuptial birds by the presence of two connective tissue capsules around the testis in the latter.[111]

Testicular recrudescence may involve a single synchronous spermatogenetic event or separate spermatogenetic waves, depending whether a given species produces successive clutches during a particular breeding season. In either event, following spermiation spermatozoa migrate to expanded distal ends of the vasa deferentia known as *seminal sacs.* Spermatozoa will be ejaculated from the seminal sacs during mating.

The annual testicular cycle of temperate birds has three more or less distinct phases: (1) the regeneration or *preparatory phase,* (2) the acceleration or *progressive phase,* and (3) the *culmination phase.* Similar phases can be identified in all birds regardless of the seasonal nature of their reproductive cycles or what environmental factors control testicular events. The preparatory phase begins immediately after the reproductive period and is characterized by marked collapse of the testis. The most common environmental factor influencing the avian testis is photoperiod. Placing quiescent, temperate birds on long photoperiods will typically stimulate testicular recrudescence, whereas maintenance of birds on short photoperiods into the normal breeding season represses anticipated testicular events. Animals in the preparatory phase are insensitive to effects of long photoperiod and are termed *refractory.* The end of the preparatory phase is heralded by restoration of photosensitivity. The endocrinological basis for the photorefractory period in birds is not clear and more than one mechanism may be involved in different species.[82] Some studies suggest that feedback of testosterone is responsible for induction of the photorefractory period and for low levels of LH during the photorefractory period. Other investigations point to changes in hypothalamic sensitivity and/or steroid metabolism.

During the progressive phase there is an increase in gonadotropin secretion brought about by actions of lengthening photoperiod on the hypothalamo-hypophysial axis. Increased circulating gonadotropins stimulate both spermatogensis and androgen secretion by the interstitial cells. An increasingly intensive period of sexual activity and song occurs, and males of some species may begin exhibiting territorial behavior and mate selection. This effect of long photoperiod can be blocked by low temperatures.

The culmination phase coincides with the time of ovulation in females and includes the time of insemination. The male typically is ready for breeding before the female, and his testes will be bulging with spermatozoa. Successful breeding involves a complex, hormonally dependent series of events involving precise male-female interactions.

Interstitial Cells. A characteristic lipid cycle occurs in avian interstitial cells similar to that described for other vertebrates.[111,112] There is accumulation of lipid in young birds followed by rapid depletion coincident with onset of the first breeding season and spermatogenesis. The interstitial cells of adult birds are small and sparsely lipoidal in winter although they occupy a large proportion of the testis because of the regressed nature of the seminiferous tubules. There is gradual accumulation of lipids, including cholesterol, throughout the progressive phase as well as an increase in 3β-HSD activity. At the time of maximum sexual display there is rapid depletion of interstitial cell lipid. Cholesterol disappears completely, but 3β-HSD activity remains strong, indicating lipid depletion is a consequence of rapid synthesis and secretion of androgens. The activity of 17α-hydroxylase is also high at this time. A massive disintegration of interstitial cells occurs during the preparatory phase, and new interstitial cells differentiate from fibroblasts.

Sustentacular Cells. Cyclical changes in lipid content are characteristic of avian sustentacular cells that ultrastructurally resemble steroidogenic cells.[111] Both 3β-HSD and 17β-HSD activities have been reported for these cells. They become densely lipoidal following the breeding season, and no detectable 3β-HSD activity remains. The lipid is depleted with the onset of the next period of spermatogenesis.

Endocrine Control of Testicular Function. The hypothalamus contains two gonadotropic centers that separately control release of LH and FSH from the adenohypophysis.[91,112] Hyperplasia of interstitial cells is caused by LH, and they become lipoidal and exhibit increased 3β-HSD activity. Avian testes are much more sensitive to avian LH than to mammalian LH.[100] Androgens secreted by these cells stimulate sex accessory structures and secondary sexual characters. Purified mammalian FSH is less effective than avian FSH in stimulating spermatogenesis. Local effects of androgens from sustentacular cells are responsible for stimulating meiosis. Androgens are known to maintain spermatogenesis even in hypophysectomized birds.

Prolactin is present in the male pituitary and has been reported to inhibit FSH release and block spermatogenesis in some species. The formation of incubation patches on males of certain species is induced in part by PRL working cooperatively with testicular steroids.[79]

Sex Accessory Structures in Male Birds. Wolffian ducts give rise to paired vasa deferentia, vasa efferentia and the epididymides, all of which exhibit hypertrophy with the onset of sexual activity. These events are all prevented by castration. A testis is connected to the vasa efferentia by small rete tubules in the tunica albuginea that become enlarged during the breeding season. The vasa efferentia show increased secretory activity during the breeding season and coalesce to form a long, coiled tube and epididymis. Hypertrophy of the epididymis is accompanied by secretion of seminal fluid. Spermatozoa are not stored in the epididymis but enter the enlarged vas deferens. The distal end of each vas deferens (seminal sac) fills with spermatozoa. The posterior walls of the seminal sacs protrude into the cloaca as erectile papillae that facilitate transfer of spermatozoa. During copulation the cloaca is everted and these papillae are brought into contact with the vagina of the female. In some species the cloaca is modified into a penis-like intromittent organ.

The Avian Ovary. Few studies of avian reproduction have employed wild species, and much of our knowledge of ovarian reproductive events has been gleaned from domestic species, in particular the hen.[112,187] However, these studies have provided relatively complete assessment of ovarian function in domestic species and provide a basis for comparison to wild species. In many respects, ovarian function in birds is like that of their oviparous ancestors, the reptiles.

The domestic hen differs most importantly from wild birds by being a continuous breeder. Prior to hatching there is a proliferation of oogonia to produce thousands of primary oocytes that will serve the hen throughout her long and busy reproductive life. No new oocytes will be formed after hatching, unlike the situation for many anamniotes. Most of these oocytes will undergo atresia during early maturational stages. The primary follicle consists of an oocyte surrounded by a layer of granulosa cells. As the follicles grow, thecal layers are added, and the follicles become highly vascularized. Both granulosa and thecal cells are steroidogenic and possess 3β-HSD activity. Estrogens secreted from the follicle cells cause the liver to produce large quantities of plasma phosphoprotein (vitellogenin) that are sequestered from the blood by growing oocytes.[10] Vitellogenin binds free calcium ions in the blood, and the complex is incorporated into growing oocytes. The additional demand for calcium to construct the shell stimulates appropriate endocrine mechanisms to meet this need (see Chap. 12). Vitellogenin is enzymatically hydrolyzed to produce phosvitin and lipovitellin. The liver also synthesizes large quantities of triglycerides that are transported in the blood as β-lipoproteins. Micropinocytosis by the oocytes of these phosphoproteins and triglycerides is stimulated by FSH. The growing avian oocyte completely fills the follicle, and antrum formation does not occur.

Developing follicles bulge conspicuously from the surface of the avian ovary, giving it the appearance of a bunch of grapes. The largest follicles become suspended from the ovary only by a narrow band of tissue. At this stage the follicle is highly vascularized except for a rough, avascular spot, the *stigma,* where the follicle will rupture at ovulation.

Atresia of developing follicles may occur at any time during follicular development. These atretic follicles can be easily recognized by an influx of fibroblasts that phagocytize the yolk materials. Granulosa and thecal cells are lipoidal and contain cholesterol. There are many corpora atretica at all times in the ovary, but their importance, if any, is not recognized. As they disintegrate, some of the cells of the corpora atretica may become stromal interstitial cells and secrete estrogens.[64,157]

Birds are characterized by the absence of persistent corpora lutea following ovulation. Collapsed follicles consist largely of granulosa cells containing progesterone, abundant smooth endoplasmic reticulum and considerable 3β-HSD activity. The only evidence for a functional role, however, is the observation that surgical removal of these ruptured follicles increases the time that the ovulated egg is retained in the oviduct.

Endocrine Control of Ovarian Function in Birds. There is a close correlation between pituitary gonadotropin content and ovarian function in both domestic and wild birds.[100,112] Hypophysectomy causes ovarian regression and extensive follicular atresia, which can be prevented by gonadotropin replacement therapy. Follicular development is stimulated by FSH, and FSH will maintain oviducts in hypophysectomized birds. Estrogen secretion is controlled by both LH and FSH. Mammalian gonadotropins, however, are not always as effective in birds as are avian pituitary or gonadotropin preparations.[100] Furthermore, avian FSH is very effective at stimulating follicle development in lizards,[108] emphasizing the close similarity between reptilian and avian pituitary hormones and the cautions necessary when interpreting the effects of mammalian hormones in birds.

As is the case for certain reptiles, growth of follicles and ovulation is a continual process throughout the breeding season. Ovarian function is regulated so that typically only one egg is discharged at a time. This condition is reminiscent of the human and the lizard *Anolis carolinensis,* in which only one ovum is discharged, and the ovaries alternate in providing the ovum. A hierarchy of graded follicle size is maintained. The endocrinological basis for establishment of such a hierarchy, however, is not known for either reptiles or birds, and it represents one of the major unanswered questions in reproductive biology.[81]

The synthesis of vitellogenin by the liver is induced by estrogens.[159] Total serum calcium concomitantly increases, which is related to the binding of calcium by vitellogenin (Table 11-10). In addition to incorporation of vitellin proteins into the oocyte, circulating calcium is sequestered by the shell glands of the "uterus" (expanded region of the oviduct) for construction of the egg shell. Thus estrogens provide for transfer of calcium from storage sites (bone) to the egg shell as well as for stimulation of vitellogenin production.

Pituitary LH is responsible for triggering ovulation of the fully mature follicle. Plasma LH peaks about 6 to 8 hours before ovulation in domestic hens as well as in Japanese quail,[53,87] but the magnitude of the avian LH surge is considerably smaller than that observed in mammals. This lower surge of LH might be an adaptation to ensure only sufficient LH for ovulating the largest follicle.[112]

Calcium availability may be a potent factor regulating reproduction in female birds.[113] Production of shelled eggs in domestic species directs as much as 10% of the body calcium stores per day into eggs. If large amounts of calcium are not available in the diet, the reproductive axis is shut down before damage to the skeleton occurs. When sufficient calcium becomes available, the birds resume laying. It is possible that calcium depletion in wild birds contributes to cessation of breeding and induction of the refractory period.

Another pituitary hormone, PRL, plays an essential role in development of a specialized, defeathered region in some species known as an incubation patch, which aids in incubating eggs.[79] As described in Chapters 1 and 5, the action of PRL on secretion of crop milk by the pigeon crop sac for use in feeding young birds has resulted in development of a most useful biological assay for PRL activity in all tetrapod pituitaries. Prolactin does not affect steroidogenesis in cultured chick granulosa cells and probably has no effect on progesterone synthesis.[65]

Oviduct. Estrogens are secreted by the growing follicle as a result of the actions of FSH on thecal cells and probably on granulosa cells as well. Their primary influences are on liver (vitellogenesis) and on the oviduct. Estrogens stimulate hypertrophy of the oviduct and differentiation of secretory regions. Five differentiated regions can be identified in the mature oviduct: *infundibulum, magnum, isth-*

TABLE 11-10. *Effect of Mammalian Parathyroid Extract and the Influence of the Egg-Laying Cycle on Total Serum Calcium of Chicken*[6]

	CONTROL mg/dl ± SE	TREATED WITH PARATHYROID EXTRACT mg/dl ± SE
Rooster	10.1 ± 0.2	19.5 ± 3
Nonlaying hen	13.4 ± 2	19.5 ± 4
Laying hen	29.8 ± 11	47.7 ± 9

mus, shell gland and *vagina.* After ovulation the ovum enters the infundibulum and is fertilized in the upper end of the oviduct before albumen is added. The middle portion of the oviduct or magnum becomes highly glandular under the influence of estrogens, forming tubular glands and goblet cells.[92] Estrogens stimulate synthesis of *ovalbumen* protein by the tubular glands,[138] whereas progesterone stimulates the goblet cells to produce the other major egg white protein, *avidin.*[136,137] After accumulation of several coatings of albumen the egg passes to the muscular isthmus where two shell membranes are applied. These membranes are composed of protein fibers cemented together with albumen. The shell consists largely of calcium salts supported by a fibrous protein matrix deposited on the outermost shell membrane by the shell gland or "uterus." After the shell has been applied, contraction of a powerful sphincter muscle causes the egg to rotate in the vagina and enter the cloaca pointed-end first. Movement of the egg into the cloaca as well as its extrusion into the nest (oviposition) is controlled by a neurohypophysial hormone. An increase in plasma arginine vasotocin together with a concomitant decrease in neurohypophysial arginine vasotocin coincides with oviposition, and treatment with either arginine vasopressin or oxytocin can cause premature oviposition.[112]

INCUBATION PATCHES. In many avian species a ventral region (apterium) becomes defeathered, highly vascularized and edematous just prior to or during egg laying.[79] In addition, the epidermis of this region may become hyperplastic. This specialized region is termed an *incubation* or *brood patch,* and when in contact with the eggs provides an efficient transfer of warmth from the parent bird to the eggs. Incubation patches may form in females, males or both, depending upon the species and which sex is responsible for incubating eggs. However, mere possession of an incubation patch is not proof of incubating behavior. Male house sparrows *(Passer domesticus)* have no incubation patch yet exhibit incubating behavior, whereas male flycatchers (genus *Empidonax*) develop an incubation patch but do not show incubating behavior.

Formation of incubation patches involves cooperative actions of both estrogens and PRL.[79] Estrogens seem to stimulate vascularization of the patch region, and PRL stimulates defeathering and epidermal hyperplasia. Both hormones are necessary for normal patch development. Furthermore, the response of epidermis in forming a patch is both site specific and tissue specific. After transplant to the dorsal surface ventral skin will still respond to PRL but not to estrogen. Vascularization of the ventral skin occurs only when it is in its normal location. On the other hand, dorsal skin transplanted to the normal patch site will not respond to either estrogens or PRL.

ANDROGEN-DEPENDENT SECONDARY SEX CHARACTERS IN MALES AND FEMALES. Androgens play important roles in both male and female birds. In a number of species a change in bill color is associated with breeding. Such changes are induced in both sexes by androgens but not by estrogens or progesterone.[195] However, there is at least one case in which bill color change occurs only in the female, and the color change is induced by estrogens.

Plumage color changes may also be controlled by androgens. This is the case for phalaropes in which the females possess the more colorful plumage.[72,73] One cannot presume this to be the case unless specific studies have been performed, because androgens are not always responsible for nuptial plumage. For example, development of nuptial plumage in castrated male weaver finches, *Euplectes orix,* has long been known as the classical bioassay for LH (see Chap. 5). Estrogens apparently inhibit formation of nuptial dress, and castrated females will develop male plumage. Assumption of nuptial dress in males can also be blocked with estrogens.[112]

In some strains of chicken both sexes have female type plumage and castration causes development of male plumage. Treatment of castrated males with testosterone causes a return to female type plumage, but growth of the comb and wattle are stimulated (a normal male trait). If castrated males are treated with DHT, the growth of the comb and wattle are stimulated but there is no reversion to female plumage. In these strains of chicken, the skin aromatizes testosterone to estrogens and stimulates female plumage. In the comb and wattle, 5α-reductase converts testosterone to DHT. Since DHT can not be aromatized, the plumage of DHT-treated castrated males does not revert to the female type.[58]

Reproductive Behavior in Birds. Each avian species exhibits a precise sequence of endocrine-dependent behaviors such as migration, acquisition of territory, advertisement by song, attraction of mate, pairing, nest building, egg laying, incubating and rearing young birds. The actual sequence of events and their endocrinological bases are species specific and cannot easily be generalized.[47,170] Successful breeding involves a complex interaction of male and female birds in precise sequences (that is, if male does A, then female does B, which stimulates male to do C, etc.) as well as presence of suitable environmental cues such as proper nesting material, availability of water, etc. Little experimental work has been done with wild birds since it is difficult to get them to perform under laboratory conditions although several descriptive studies on hormone levels and behavior are available.[170]

Androgens appear to be responsible for territorial display and aggression in wild birds.[170] Aggressive behavior can be stimulated also by FSH but not LH in males. Courtship appears to involve negative feedback of testosterone on FSH levels, which results in reduction in circulating androgens and allows for subsequent, less aggressive behaviors. Androgen levels are low during mating. Androgens antagonize incubation patch development, and a reduction in circulating testosterone may be necessary for patch development in males of certain species. In domestic chickens and ring doves, testosterone does stimulate courtship and copulation.[170]

Bowing behavior in feral pigeons coincides with maximum androgen synthesis but decreases prior to egg laying, coincident with an increase in progesterone levels. Progesterone is a well-known stimulus for incubation behavior in laying pigeons. Removal of the postovulatory follicle from chickens blocks nesting behavior.[196] Prolactin can induce incubation behavior, but this action is presumed to be due to increased release of progesterone.[112]

Summary

Reproduction involves a precise integration of environmental factors (photoperiod, temperature, availability of nesting sites, etc.), physiological factors (nutritional state, general endocrine state with respect to thyroid hormones, adrenocortical functions, etc.) and specific endocrine secretions (FSH, LH, androgens, estrogens, progestogens, PRL, etc.). Reproductive patterns are finely tuned to environmental conditions in order to maximize evolutionary success, and this results in frequent observations of greater similarities in reproductive patterns between phylogenetically divergent species facing similar environmental problems than between closely related species living in diverse environments.

Environmental factors operate through the nervous system and specifically the hypothalamus to control release of gonadotropins and in certain cases PRL. Prolactin molecules or PRL activity as well as FSH and LH molecules have been identified in all tetrapods. Fishes have a PRL-like hormone, but they may have only one gonadotropin that appears to be LH-like. Piscine gonadotropin performs functions characteristically associated with both LH and FSH in other groups. Follicle-stimulating hormone initiates spermatogenesis in males and follicular development in females. Local androgens secreted from testicular cells under the influence of FSH appear to be necessary for initiating reductional division (meiosis) of primary spermatocytes. Luteinizing hormone induces androgen synthesis by interstitial (Leydig) or lobule-boundary cells in males and estrogen synthesis and ovulation in females. Androgen synthesis in female mammals may also be stimulated in thecal cells by LH. Thecal androgens are thought to be converted to estrogens by granulosa cells. Comparative studies in other vertebrates may help to clarify this dual system for estrogen synthesis. Follicular atresia associated with formation of corpora atretica is a common occurrence in females. Atresia appears to be a mechanism for effectively reducing the biotic potential and placing reliance in production of a smaller number of offspring with better individual survival for evolutionary success. Corpora lutea form in many vertebrates primarily from granulosa cells of ruptured follicles, and corpora lutea synthesize progesterone that is related to gestation in many viviparous vertebrates.

Courtship and breeding behavior appear to be controlled primarily by gonadal steroids although evidence is accumulating for participation of peptides. In addition, estrogens produce dramatic effects on vitellogenesis in nonmammalian liver and bring about a consequent disturbance in calcium metabolism. The basic oviparous mode of reproduction has become modified with respect to the development of viviparity in all nonmammalian classes except Aves and Agnatha.

Numerous peculiarities occur in different species or species groups that are not easily generalized, and the interested reader must attend to the voluminous literature on the reproductive biology of vertebrates to obtain an appreciation of the endocrinology of vertebrate reproduction.

References

1. Adkins, E.K. (1978). Androgen aromatization and the sexual behavior of male quail *(Coturnix coturnix japonica)*. Am. Zool. 18:603.

2. Anand, T.C. and B.I. Sundararaj (1974). Ovarian maintenance in the hypophysectomized catfish. *Heteropneustes fossilis* (Bloch), with mammalian hypophyseal and placental hormones, and gonadal and adrenocortical steroids. Gen. Comp. Endocrinol. 22:154–168.

3. Armstrong, D.T., Y.S. Moon, I.B. Fritz and J.H. Dorrington (1975). Synthesis of estradiol-17β by Sertoli cells in culture: Stimulation by FSH and dibutyryl cyclic AMP. In F.S. French, V. Hansson, E.M. Ritzen and S.N. Nayfeh, eds., Hormonal regulation of Spermatogenesis. Plenum Press, New York, pp. 85–96.

4. Arslan, M., P. Zaidi, J. Lobo, A.A. Zaidi and M.H. Qazi (1978). Steroid levels in preovulatory and gravid lizards *(Uromastix hardwicki)*. Gen. Comp. Endocrinol. 34:300–303.

5. Aso, T., T. Tominaga, K. Oshima and K. Matsubayashi (1977). Seasonal changes of plasma estradiol and progesterone in the Japanese monkey *(Macaca fuscata fuscata)*. Endocrinology 100:745–750.

6. Assenmacher, I. (1973). The peripheral endocrine glands. In D.S. Farner and J.R. King, eds., Avian Biology. Academic Press, New York, Vol. 3, pp. 183–286.

7. Baggerman, B. (1966). On the endocrine control of reproductive behavior in the male three-spined stickleback (*Gasterosteus aculeatus* L.). Symp. Soc. Exp. Biol. 20:427–456.

8. Bailey, R.E. (1957). The effect of estradiol on serum calcium, phosphorus and protein of goldfish. J. Exp. Zool. 136:455–470.

9. Bara, G. (1969). Histochemical demonstration of 3β-, 3α, 11β- and 17β-hydroxysteroid dehydrogenases in the testis of *Fundulus heteroclitus*. Gen. Comp. Endocrinol. 13:189–200.

10. Bergink, E.W., R.A. Wallace, J.A. Van de Berg, E.S. Bos, M. Gruber and G. Ab (1974). Estrogen-induced synthesis of yolk proteins in roosters. Am. Zool. 14:1177–1193.

11. Blum, V. and K. Fiedler (1965). Hormonal control of reproductive behavior in some cichlid fish. Gen. Comp. Endocrinol. 5:186–196.

12. Bohnet, H.G. and A.S. McNeily (1979). Prolactin—Assessment of its role in the human female. Horm. Metab. Res. 11:533–546.

13. Bona-Gallo, A., P. Licht, D.S. MacKenzie and B. Lofts (1980). Annual cycles in levels of pituitary and plasma gonadotropin, gonadal steroids, and thyroid activity in the Chinese cobra *(Naja naja)*. Gen. Comp. Endocrinol. 42:477–493.

14. Braden, A.W.H. and I.W. McDonald (1970). Disorders of grazing animals due to plant constituents. In R.A. Moore, ed., Australian Grasslands. Australian National University Press, Canberra, pp. 381–392.

15. Breder, C.M., Jr. and D.E. Rosen (1966). Modes of Reproduction in Fishes. Natural History Press, Garden City, N.Y.

16. Breton, B., R. Billard and B. Jalabert (1973). Specificite d'action et relations immunologiques des hormones gonadotropes de quelques teleosteens. Ann. Biol. Anim. Biochem. Biophys. 13:347–362.

17. Bryant, G.D. and W.A. Chamley (1976). Plasma relaxin and prolactin immunoreactivities in pregnancy and at parturition in ewe. J. Reprod. Fertil. 48:201–204.

18. Bryant-Greenwood, G.D. (1982). Relaxin as a new hormone. Endocr. Revs. 3:62–90.

19. Butcher, R.L., W.E. Collins and N.W. Fugo (1974). Plasma concentration of LH, FSH, prolactin, progesterone and estradiol-17β throughout the 4-day estrous cycle of the rat. Endocrinology 94:1704–1708.

20. Butler, W.R., J. Hotchkiss and E. Knobil (1975). Functional luteolysis in the rhesus monkey: Ovarian estrogen and progesterone during the luteal phase of the menstrual cycle. Endocrinology 96:1509–1512.

21. Callard, G. (1983). Androgen and estrogen actions in the vertebrate brain. Am. Zool. 23:607–620.

22. Callard, G.V., Z. Petro and K.J. Ryan (1978). Conversion of androgen to estrogen and other steroids in the vertebrate brain. Am. Zool. 18:511–523.

23. Callard, I.P., V. Lance, A.R. Salhanick and D. Barad (1978). The annual ovarian cycle of *Chrysemys picta:* Correlated changes in plasma steroids and parameters of vitellogenesis. Gen. Comp. Endocrinol. 35:245–257.

24. Callard, I.P. and J.H. Leathem (1965). *In vitro* steroid synthesis by the ovaries of elasmobranchs and snakes. Arch. Anat. Microsc. Morphol. Exp. 54:35–48.

25. Campbell, C.M. and D.R. Idler (1976). Hormonal control of vitellogenesis in hypophysectomized winter flounder (*Pseudopleuronectes americanus* Walbaum). Gen. Comp. Endocrinol. 28:143–150.

26. Chieffi, G. and C. Lupo (1961). Identificazione degli ormoni steroidi nel testicoli e negli organi di Bidder di *Bufo vulgaris.* Atti. Accad. Naz. Lincei Rend. Cl. Sci. Fis. Mat. Nat. (Roma) 30:339–402.

27. Chieffi, G., R.K. Rastogi, L. Iela, and M. Milone (1975). The function of fat bodies in relation to the hypothalamo-hypophyseal-gonadal axis in the frog, *Rana esculenta.* Cell Tissue Res. 161:157–165.

28. Chowdhury, M.A., A. Steinberger and E. Steinberger (1978). Inhibition of *de novo* synthesis of FSH by the Sertoli cell factor (SCF). Endocrinology 103:644–647.

29. Clark, J.H. and M.X. Zarrow (1971). Influence of copulation on time of ovulation in women. Am. J. Obstet. Gynecol. 109:1083–1085.

30. Clark, R.C. and I. van Zyl (1976). The composition of phosvitin from crocodile eggs. Int. J. Biochem. 7:229–233.

31. Colombo, L., S. Pesavento and D.W. Johnson (1972). Patterns of steroid metabolism in teleost and ganoid fishes. Gen. Comp. Endocrinol. Suppl. 3:245–253.

32. Courty, Y. and J.P. Dufaure (1980). Levels of testosterone, dihydrotestosterone, and androstenedione in the plasma and testis of a lizard (*Lacerta vivipara* Jacquin) during the annual cycle. Gen. Comp. Endocrinol. 42:325–333.

33. Cowie, A.T. (1972). Lactation and its hormonal control. In C.R. Austin and R.V. Short, eds., Hormones in Reproduction, Cambridge University Press, Book 3, pp. 106–144.

34. Crews, D. (1978). Integration of internal and external stimuli in the regulation of lizard reproduction. In N. Greenberg and P.D. MacLean, eds., The Behavior and Neurology of Lizards. NIMH, Rockville, MD., pp. 149–171.

35. Crews, D. (1983). Alternative reproductive tactics in reptiles. Bioscience 33:562–566.

36. Crim, L.W., E.G. Watts and D.M. Evans (1975). The plasma gonadotropin profile during sexual maturation in a variety of salmonid fishes. Gen. Comp. Endocrinol. 27:62–70.

37. Cuellar, H.S., J.J. Roth, J.D. Fawcett and R.E. Jones (1972). Evidence for sperm sustenance by secretions of the renal sexual segment of male lizards, *Anolis carolinensis.* Herpetologica 28:53–57.

38. Cumming, I.A. (1975). The ovine and bovine oestrous cycle. J. Reprod. Fertil. 43:583–596.

39. deVlaming, V.L. (1974). Environmental and endocrine control of teleost reproduction. In C.B. Schreck, ed., Control of Sex in Fishes. Virginia Polytechnic Institute and State University, Blacksburg, pp. 13–83.

40. Diakow, C. (1978). Hormonal basis for breeding behavior in female frogs: Vasotocin inhibits the release call of *Rana pipiens.* Science 199:1456–1457.

41. D'Istria, M., G. Delrio, V. Botte and G. Chieffi (1974). Radioimmunoassay of testosterone, 17β-oestradiol, and oestrone in the male and female plasma of *Rana esculenta* during sexual cycle. Steroids Lipids Res. 5:42–48.

42. Dodd, J.M., P.J. Evennett and C.K. Goddard (1960). Reproductive endocrinology in cyclostomes and elasmobranchs. Symp. Zool. Soc. Lond. 1:77–103.

43. Dodd, M.H.I. and J.M. Dodd (1976). The biology of metamorphosis. In B. Lofts, ed., Physiology of the Amphibia. Academic Press, New York, Vol. 3, pp. 467–599.

44. Donahoe, P.K., G.P. Budzik, R. Trelstad, M. Mudgett-Hunter, A. Fuller, Jr., J.M. Hutson, H. Ikawa, A. Hayashi and D. MacLaughlin (1982). Mullerian-inhibiting substance: an update. Rec. Prog. Horm. Res. 38:279–330.

45. Donaldson, E.M. (1973). Reproductive endocrinology of fishes. Am. Zool. 13:909–928.

46. Duvall, D., L.J. Guillette, Jr. and R.E. Jones (1982). Environmental control of reptilian reproductive cycles. In C. Gans and H. Pough, eds., Biology of the Reptilia. Academic Press, New York, Vol. 13, pp. 201–231.

47. Eisner, E. (1960). The relationship of hormones to the reproductive behaviour of birds, referring especially to parental behaviour: A review. Anim. Behav. 8:155–179.

48. Erickson, G.F. (1983). Primary cultures of ovarian cells in serum-free medium as models of hormone-dependent differentiation. Mol. Cell. Endocrinol. 29:21–49.

49. Evennett, P.J. and J.M. Dodd (1963). Endocrinology of reproduction in the river lamprey. Nature 197:715–716.

50. Evennett, P.J. and J.M. Dodd (1963). The pituitary gland and reproduction in the lamprey (*Lampetra fluviatilis* L.). J. Endocrinol. 26:14–15.

51. Follett, B.K., T.J. Nicholls and M.R. Redshaw (1968). The vitellogenic response in the South African clawed toad (*Xenopus laevis* Daudin). J. Cell Physiol. 72, Suppl. 1:91–102.

52. Follett, B.K., and M.R. Redshaw (1974). The physiology of vitellogenesis. In B. Lofts, ed., Physiology of the Amphibia. Academic Press, New York. Vol. 2, pp. 219–309.

53. Follett, B.K., C.G. Scanes and T.J. Nicholls (1972). The chemistry and physiology of the avian gonadotropins. In Hormones Glycoproteiques Hypophysaires. Colloque Inserm, Paris, pp. 193–211.

54. Fostier, A., B. Jalabert, R. Billard, B. Breton and Y. Zohar (1983). The gonadal steroids. In W.S. Hoar, D.J. Randall and E.M. Donaldson, eds., Fish Physiology. Academic Press, New York, Vol. IX, pp. 277–372.

55. Fuchs, A.-R., F. Fuchs and P. Husslein (1982). Oxytocin receptors and human parturition: a dual role for oxytocin in the initiation of labor. Science 215:1396–1398.

56. Funk, J.D., E.M. Donaldson and H.M. Dye (1973). Induction of precocious sexual development in female pink salmon *(Oncorhynchus gorbuscha)*. Can. J. Zool. 51:493–500.

57. Gallien, L. (1975). Sequential endocrine activities controlling oogenesis: A general survey. Am. Zool. 15, Suppl. 1:197–214.

58. George, F.W., J.F. Noble and J.D. Wilson (1981). Female feathering in Seabright cocks is due to conversion of testosterone to estradiol in skin. Science 213:557–559.

59. Goding, J.R., I.A. Cumming, W.A. Chamley, J.M. Brown, M.D. Cain, J.C. Cerini, M.E.D. Cerini, J.K. Findlay, J.D. O'Shea and D.H. Pemberton (1971/1972). Prostaglandin $F_{2\alpha}$, 'the' luteolysin in the mammal? Gynecol. Invest. 2:73–97.

60. Gorbman, A. (1983). Reproduction in cyclostome fishes and its regulation. In W.S. Hoar, D.J. Randall and E.M. Donaldson, eds., Fish Physiology. Academic Press, New York, Vol. IX, pp. 1–29.

61. Gorbman, A. and K. Tsuneki (1975). A technique for hypophysectomy of the Pacific hagfish: First observations. Gen. Comp. Endocrinol. 26:420–422.

62. Grotjan, H.E. and D.C. Johnson (1976). Temporal variations in reproductive hormones in the immature male rat. Proc. Soc. Exp. Biol. Med. 152:381–384.

63. Guillette, L.J. (1979). Stimulation of parturition in a viviparous lizard *(Sceloporus jarrovi)* by arginine vasotocin. Gen Comp. Endocrinol. 38:457–460.

64. Guraya, S.S. (1976). Recent advances in the morphology, histochemistry, and biochemistry of steroid-synthesizing cellular sites in the nonmammalian vertebrate ovary. Intern. Rev. Cytol. 44:365–409.

65. Hammond, R.W., W.H. Burke and F. Hertelendy (1982). Prolactin does not affect steroidogenesis in isolated chicken granulosa cells. Gen. Comp. Endocrinol. 48:285–287.

66. Hansson, V., R. Calandra, K. Purvis, M. Ritzen and F.S. French (1976). Hormonal regulation of spermatogenesis. Vitam. Horm. 34:187–214.

67. Harder, J.D. and M.W. Fleming (1981). Estradiol and progesterone profiles indicate a lack of endocrine recognition of pregnancy in the opossum. Science 212:1400–1402.

68. Hardisty, M.W. (1971). Gonadogenesis, sex differentiation and gametogenesis. In M.W. Hardisty and I.C. Potter, eds., The Biology of Lampreys. Academic Press, New York, Vol. 1, pp. 295–359.

69. Hardisty, M.W., B.R. Rothwell and K. Steele (1967). The interstitial tissue of the testis of the river lamprey, *Lampetra fluviatilis*. J. Zool. Lond. 152:9–18.

70. Heller, H. (1972). The effect of neurohypophysial hormones on the female reproductive tract of lower vertebrates. Gen. Comp. Endocrinol. Suppl. 3:703–714.

71. Hoar, W.S. (1969). Reproduction. In W.S. Hoar and D.J. Randall, eds., Fish Physiology. Academic Press, New York, Vol. 3, pp. 1–72.

72. Höhn, E.O. (1970). Gonadal hormone concentration in northern phalaropes in relation to nuptial plumage. Can. J. Zool. 48:400–401.

73. Höhn, E.O. and S.C. Cheng (1967). Gonadal hormones on Wilson's phalarope *(Steganopus tricolor)*

and other birds in relation to plumage and sex behaviour. Gen. Comp. Endocrinol. 8: 1–11.

74. Horner, J.R. (1982). Evidence of colonial nesting and "site fidelity" among ornithischian dinosaurs. Nature 297:675–676.

75. Hsueh, A.J.W. (1982). Direct effect of gonadotropin releasing hormone on testicular Leydig cell functions. Ann. N.Y. Acad. Sci. 383:249–269.

76. Hutson, J.H., M.E. Fallat, S. Kamagata, P.K. Donahoe and G.P. Budzik (1984). Phosphorylation events during mullerian duct regression. Science 223:586–589.

77. Johnson, B.H. and L.L. Ewing (1971). Follicle-stimulating hormone and the regulation of testosterone secretion in rabbit testes. Science 173:635–637.

78. Joly, J. and B. Picheral (1972). Ultrastructure, hìstochimie et physiologie du follicule préovulatoire et du corps jaune de l'urodele ovovìpare *Salamandra salamandra* (L.). Gen. Comp. Endocrinol. 18:235–259.

79. Jones, R.E. (1971). The incubation patch of birds. Biol. Rev. 46:315–339.

80. Jones, R.E. (1978). Ovarian cycles in nonmammalian vertebrates. In R.E. Jones, ed., The Vertebrate Ovary. Plenum Publishing Corp., New York, pp. 731–762.

81. Jones, R.E. (1978). Control of follicular selection. In R.E. Jones, ed., The Vertebrate Ovary. Plenum Publishing Corp, New York, pp. 763–788.

82. Jones, R.E. (1981). Mechanisms controlling seasonal ovarian quiescence. In N.B. Schwartz and M. Hunzicker-Dunn, eds., Dynamics of Ovarian Function. Raven Press, New York, pp. 205–234.

83. Jones, R.E., A.M. Gerrard, and J.J. Roth (1973). Estrogen and brood pouch formation in the marsupial frog, *Gastrotheca riobambae.* J. Exp. Zool. 184:177–184.

84. Jones, R.E., L.J. Guillette, Jr., M.F. Norman and J.J. Roth (1982). Corpus luteum-uterine relationships in the control of uterine contraction in the lizard *Anolis carolinensis.* Gen. Comp. Endocrinol. 48:104–112.

85. Judd, H. L., G.A. Laughlin, J.P. Bacon and K. Benirschke (1976). Circulating androgen and estrogen concentrations in lizards *(Iguana iguana).* Gen. Comp. Endocrinol. 30:391–395.

86. Kalra, S.P. (1983). Opioid peptides—Inhibitory neuronal systems in regulation of gonadotropin secretion. In S.M. McCann and D.S. Dhindsa, eds., Role of Peptides and Proteins in Control of Reproduction. Elsevier Science, New York, pp. 63–87.

87. Kappauf, B. and A. van Tienhoven (1972). Progesterone concentrations in peripheral plasma of laying hens in relation to the time of ovulation. Endocrinology 90:1350–1355.

88. Katz, Y., L. Dashow and A. Epple (1982). Circulating steroid hormones of anadromous sea lampreys under various experimental conditions. Gen. Comp. Endocrinol. 48:261–268.

89. Katz, Y. and B. Eckstein (1974). Changes in steroid concentration in blood of female *Tilapia aurea* (Teleostei, Cichlidae) during initiation of spawning. Endocrinology 95:963–967.

90. Kime, D.E. and N.J. Manning (1982). Seasonal patterns of free and conjugated androgens in the brown trout *Salmo trutta.* Gen. Comp. Endocrinol. 48:221–231.

91. Kobayashi, H. and M. Wada (1973). Neuroendocrinology in birds. In D.S. Farner and J.R. King, eds., Avian Biology, Academic Press, New York, Vol. 3, pp. 287–347.

92. Kohler, P.O., P.M. Grimley and B.W. O'Malley (1969). Estrogen-induced cytodifferentiation of the ovalbumin-secreting glands of the chick oviduct. J. Cell Biol. 40:8–27.

93. Koldovsky, O. (1980). Hormones in milk. Life Sci. 26:1833–1836.

94. Labhsetwar, A.P. (1972). Luteolytic and ovulation-inducing properties of prostaglandin $F_{2\alpha}$ in pregnant mice. J. Reprod. Fertil. 28:451–452.

95. Labrie, F., P. Borgeat, J. Drouin, M. Bealieu, L. Lagacé, L. Ferland and V. Raymond (1979). Mechanism of action of hypothalamic hormones in the adenohypophysis. Annu. Rev. Physiol. 41:555–569.

96. Lam, T.J., S. Pandey and W.S. Hoar (1975). Induction of ovulation in goldfish by synthetic luteinizing hormone-releasing hormone (LH-RH). Can. J. Zool. 53:1189–1192.

97. Lamotte, M. and P. Rey (1954). Existence de corpora lutea chez un Batracien anoure vivipare, *Nectophyrnoides occidentalis* Angel; leur évolution morphologique. C.R. Acad. Sci. Paris 238:393–395.

98. Lance, V. and I.P. Callard (1978). Hormonal control of ovarian steroidogenesis. In R.E. Jones, ed., The Vertebrate Ovary. Plenum Press, New York, pp. 361–407.

99. Lance, V. and I.P. Callard (1978). *In vivo* responses of female snakes *(Natrix fasciata)* and female turtles *(Chrysemys picta)* to ovine gonadotropins (FSH and LH) as measured by plasma progesterone, testosterone and estradiol levels. Gen. Comp. Endocrinol. 35:295–301.

100. Lance, V. and I.P. Callard (1980). Phylogenetic trends in hormonal control of gonadal steroidogenesis. In P.K.T. Pang and A. Epple, eds., Evolution of Vertebrate Endocrine Systems. Texas Tech Press, Lubbock, Texas, pp. 167–231.

101. Lance, V., C. Scanes and I.P. Callard (1977). Plasma testosterone levels in male turtles, *Chrysemys picta,* following single injections of mammalian, avian and teleostean gonadotropins. Gen. Comp. Endocrinol. 31:435–441.

102. LaPointe, J. (1977). Comparative physiology of neurohypophysial hormone action on the vertebrate oviduct-uterus. Am. Zool. 17:763–773.

103. Larsen, L.O. (1965). Effects of hypophysectomy in a cyclostome, *Lampetra fluviatilis* (L.) Gray. Gen. Comp. Endocrinol. 5:16–30.

104. Larsen, L.O. (1970). The lamprey egg at ovulation. (*Lampetra fluviatilis* L. Gray). Biol. Reprod. 2:37–47.

105. Lewis, J.C. and D.B. McMillan (1965). The development of the ovary of the sea lamprey (*Petromyzon marinus* L). J. Morphol. 117:425–466.

106. Licht, P., B.R. McCreery, R. Barnes and R. Pang (1983). Seasonal and stress related changes in plasma gonadotropins, sex steroids, and corticosterone in the bullfrog, *Rana catesbeiana*. Gen. Comp. Endocrinol. 50:124–145.

107. Licht, P., H. Papkoff, S.W. Farmer, C.H. Muller, H.W. Tsui and D. Crews (1977). Evolution of gonadotropin structure and function. Recent Prog. Horm. Res. 33:169–248.

108. Licht, P. and A. Stockell-Hartree (1971). Actions of mammalian, avian and piscine gonadotropins in the lizard. J. Endocrinol. 49:113–124.

109. Liley, N.R. (1969). Hormones and reproductive behavior in fishes. In W.S. Hoar and D.J. Randall, eds., Fish Physiology, Academic Press, New York, Vol. 3, pp. 73–116.

110. Lofts, B. (1974). Reproduction. In Lofts, B., ed., Physiology of the Amphibia. Academic Press, New York, Vol. 2, pp. 107–218.

111. Lofts, B. and H.A. Bern (1972). The functional morphology of steroidogenic tissues. In D.R. Idler, ed., Steroids in Non-mammalian Vertebrates. Academic Press, New York, pp. 37–125.

112. Lofts, B. and R.K. Murton (1973). Reproduction in birds. In D.S. Farner and J.R. King, eds., Avian Biology. Academic Press, New York, Vol. 3, pp. 1–107.

113. Luck, M.R. and C.G. Scanes (1982). Calcium homeostasis and the control of ovulation. In C.G. Scanes, M.A. Ottinger, A.D. Kenny, J. Balthazart, J. Cronshaw and I. Chester Jones, eds., Aspects of Avian Endocrinology: Practical and Theoretical Aspects. Texas Tech Press, Lubbock, Texas, pp. 263–282.

114. Lupo Di Prisco, C., L.B. Cardinelli, A. Polzonetti, A.P. Magni, C. Basile and G. Rochhi (1973). The metabolic fate of pregnenolone-7-^{3}H and progesterone-4-^{14}C in the ovaries and fat bodies of female *Triturus cristatus carnifex*. Comp. Biochem. Physiol. 44B:567–576.

115. Lupo di Prisco, C., C. Vellano and C. Chieffi (1967). Steroid hormones in the plasma of the elasmobranch *Torpedo marmorata* at various stages of the sexual cycle. Gen Comp. Endocrinol. 8:325–331.

116. McCann, S.M. (1974). Regulation of secretion of follicle-stimulating hormone and luteinizing hormone. Handbook of Physiology, Sec. 7, Endocrinology. Williams & Wilkins, Baltimore, Vol. 4, Part 2, pp. 489–518.

117. McCullagh, D.R. (1932). Dual endocrine activity of the testis. Science 76:19–20.

118. McPherson, R.J., L.R. Boots, R. MacGregor III, and K.R. Marion (1982). Plasma steroids associated with seasonal reproductive changes in a multiclutched freshwater turtle, *Sternotherus odoratus*. Gen Comp Endocrinol 48:440–451.

119. Mainwaring, W.I.P. (1977). The Mechanism of Action of Androgens. Monogr. Endocrinol. 10, Springer-Verlag, New York.

120. Martini, L. (1982). The 5α-reduction of testosterone in the neuroendocrine structures. Biochemical and physiological implications. Endocr. Rev. 3:1–25.

121. Matty, A.J., K. Tsuneki, W.W. Dickhoff and A. Gorbman (1976). Thyroid and gonadal function in hypophysectomized hagfish, *Eptatretus stouti*. Gen. Comp. Endocrinol. 30:500–516.

122. Mead, R.A., V.P. Eroschenko and D.R. Highfill (1981). Effects of progesterone and estrogen on the histology of the oviduct of the garter snake, *Thamnophis elegans*. Gen. Comp. Endocrinol. 45:345–354.

123. Means, A.R., J. L. Fakunding, C. Huckins, D.J. Tindall and R. Vitale (1976). Follicle-stimulating hormone, the Sertoli cell and spermatogenesis. Recent Prog. Horm. Res. 32:477–522.

124. Miller, M.R. and M.E. Robbins (1954). The reproductive cycle in *Taricha torosa (Triturus torosus)*. J. Exp. Zool. 125:415–445.

125. Moore, F.L. (1983). Behavioral endocrinology of amphibian reproduction. Bioscience 33:557–561.

126. Mossman, H.W. and K.L. Duke (1973). Comparative Morphology of the Mammalian Ovary. University of Wisconsin Press, Madison.

127. Nagahama, Y. (1983). The functional morphology of teleost gonads. In W.S. Hoar, D.J. Randall and E.M. Donaldson, eds., Fish Physiology. Academic Press, New York, Vol. IX, pp. 223–275.

128. Nalbandov, A.V. (1961). Mechanisms controlling ovulation of avian and mammalian follicles. In C.A. Villee, ed., Control of Ovulation. Pergamon Press, New York, pp. 122–131.

129. Nandi, J. (1967). Comparative endocrinology of steroid hormones in vertebrates. Ann. Zool. 7:115–133.

130. Neaves, W.B. (1971). Intercellular bridges between follicle cells and oocyte in the lizard, *Anolis carolinensis*. Anat. Rec. 170:285–302.

131. Neill, J.D. (1974). Prolactin and its secretion and control. Handbook of Physiology, Sec. 7, Endocrinology. Williams & Wilkins, Baltimore. Vol. 4, Part 2, pp. 469–488.

132. Noble, G.K. (1931). The Biology of the Amphibia. Mcgraw-Hill, New York.

133. Norris, D.O. and D. Duvall (1981). Hormone-induced ovulation in *Ambystoma tigrinum:* influence of prolactin and thyroxine. J. Exp. Zool. 216:175–180.

134. Norris, D.O., L.J. Guillette, and M.F. Norman (1980). Response of urodele oviduct to arginine vasotocin (AVT) in vitro: influence of steroids. Am. Zool. 20:831.

135. Nozu, K., A. Dehejia, L. Zawistowich, K.J. Catt and M.L. Dufau (1982). Gonadotropin-induced desensitization of Leydig cells *in vivo* and *in vitro:* estrogen-action in the testis. Ann. N.Y. Acad. Sci. 383:212–229.

136. O'Malley, B.W. (1967). *In vitro* hormonal induction of a specific protein (avidin) in chick oviduct. Biochemistry 6:2546–2551.

137. O'Malley, B.W., W.L. McGuire and S.G. Korenman (1967). Estrogen stimulation of synthesis of specific proteins and RNA polymerase activity in the immature chicken oviduct. Biochim. Biophys. Acta 145:204–207.

138. O'Malley, B.W., S.L. Woo, S.E. Harris, J.M. Rosen, J.P. Comstock, L. Chan, C.B. Bordelon, J.W. Holder, P. Sperry and A.R. Means (1975). Steroid action in animal cells. Am. Zool. 15, Suppl. 1:215–225.

139. Ozon, R. (1972). Androgens in fishes, amphibians, reptiles and birds. In D.R. Idler, ed., Steroids in Nonmammalian Vertebrates. Academic Press, New York, pp. 329–389.

140. Ozon, R. (1972). Estrogens in fishes, amphibians, reptiles and birds. In D.R. Idler, ed., Steroids in Nonmammalian Vertebrates. Academic Press, New York, pp. 390–414.

141. Pan, M.L., W.J. Bell and W.H. Telfer (1969). Vitellogenic blood protein synthesis by insect fat body. Science 165:393–394.

142. Paulke, E. and E. Haase (1978). A comparison of seasonal changes in the concentrations of androgens in the peripheral blood of wild and domestic ducks. Gen. Comp. Endocrinol. 34:381–390.

143. Payne, A.H. and R.P. Kelch (1975). Comparison of steroid metabolism in testicular compartments of human and rat testes. In F.S. French, V. Hansson, E.M. Ritzen and S.N. Nayfeh, eds., Hormonal Regulation of Spermatogenesis. Plenum Press, New York, pp. 97–108.

144. Perks, A.M. (1977). Developmental and evolutionary aspects of the neurohypophysis. Am. Zool. 17:833–849.

145. Perry, J.S. (1972). The Ovarian Cycle of Mammals. Hafner Publishing Co., New York.

146. Peter, R.E. and L.W. Crim (1979). Reproductive endocrinology of fishes: Gonadal cycles and gonadotropin in teleosts. Annu. Rev. Physiol. 41:323–335.

147. Pickering, A.D. (1976). Effects of gonadectomy, oestradiol and testosterone on the migrating river lamprey, *Lampetra fluviatilis* (L.). Gen. Comp. Endocrinol. 28:473–480.

148. Pickering, A.D. (1976). Stimulation of intestinal degeneration by oestradiol and testosterone implantation in the migrating river lamprey, *Lampetra fluviatilis* L. Gen. Comp. Endocrinol. 30:340–346.

149. Piro, C., F. Fraioli, F. Sciarra and C. Conti (1973). Circadian rhythm of plasma testosterone, cortisone and gonadotropins in normal male subjects. J. Steroid Biochem. 4:321.

150. Plotka, E.D., U.S. Seal, E.E. Schobert and G.C. Schmoller (1975). Serum progesterone and estrogens in elephants. Endocrinology 97:485–487.

151. Pooley, A.C. and C. Gans. (1976). The Nile Crocodile. Sci. Amer. 234(4):114–124.

152. Prasad, M.R.N. and P.R.K. Reddy (1972). Physiology of the sexual segment of the kidney in reptiles. Gen. Comp. Endocrinol. Suppl. 3:649–662.

153. Redshaw, M.R. and T.J. Nicholls (1971). Oestrogen biosynthesis by ovarian tissue of the South African clawed toad, *Xenopus laevis* Daudin. Gen. Comp. Endocrinol. 16:85–96.

154. Reyes, F.I., J.S.D. Winter, C. Faiman and W.C. Hobson (1975). Serial serum levels of gonadotropins, prolactin and sex steroids in the nonpregnant and pregnant chimpanzee. Endocrinology 96:1447–1455.

155. Richards, J.S. (1978). Hormonal control of follicular growth and maturation in mammals. In R.E. Jones, ed., The Vertebrate Ovary. Plenum Press, New York, pp. 331–360.

156. Rowe, P.H., P.A. Racey, G.A. Lincoln, M. Ellwood, J. Lehane and J.C. Shenton (1975). The temporal relationship between the secretion of luteinizing hormone and testosterone in man. J. Endocrinol. 64:17–26.

157. Saidapur, S.K. (1978). Follicular atresia in ovaries of nonmammalian vertebrates. Intern. Rev. Cytol. 54:225–244.

158. Salthe, S.N. and J.S. Mecham (1974). Reproductive and courtship patterns. In B. Lofts, ed., Physiology of the Amphibia. Academic Press, New York, Vol. 2, pp. 310–522.

159. Schjeide, O.A., M. Wilkens, R. McCandless, R. Munn, M. Peterson, and G. Carlson (1963). Liver synthesis, plasma transport and structural alterations accompanying passage of yolk protein. Am. Zool. 3:167–184.

160. Schreibman, M.P., J.F. Leatherland and B.A. McKeown (1973). Functional morphology of the teleost pituitary gland. Am. Zool. 13:719–742.

161. Schwassman, H.O. (1971). Biological rhythms. In W.S. Hoar and D.J. Randall, eds., Fish Physiology. Academic Press, New York, Vol. 6, pp. 371–428.

162. Scott, A.P., E.L. Sheldrick and A.P.F. Flint (1982). Measurement of $17\alpha,20\beta$-dihydroxy-4-pregnen-3-one in plasma of trout (*Salmo gairdneri* Richardson): Seasonal changes and response to salmon pituitary extract. Gen. Comp. Endocrinol. 46:444–451.

163. Setchell, B.P., R.V. Davies and S.J. Main (1977). Inhibin. In Johnson, A.D. and W.R. Gomes, eds., The Testis. Academic Press, New York, Vol. 4, p. 189.

164. Sever, D.M. (1978). Male cloacal glands of *Plethodon*

cinereus and *Plethodon dorsalis* (Amphibia: Plethodontidae). Herpetologica 34:1–19.

165. Shahabi, N.A., H.W. Norton, and A.V. Nalbandov (1975). Steroid levels in follicles and plasma of hens during the ovulatory cycle. Endocrinology 96:962–968.

166. Sharman, G.B. (1970). Reproductive physiology of marsupials. Science 167:1221–1228.

167. Sharman, G.B. (1976). Evolution of viviparity in mammals. In C.R. Austin and R.V. Short, eds., Reproduction in Mammals. Cambridge University Press, Book 6, pp. 32–70.

168. Sherins, R.J., A.P. Patterson, D. Brightwell, R. Udelsman and J. Sartor (1982). Alteration in the plasma testosterone:estradiol ratio: an alternative to the inhibin hypothesis. Ann. N.Y. Acad. Sci. 383:295–306.

169. Short, R.V. (1972). Role of hormones in sex cycles. In C.R. Austin and R.V. Short, eds., Reproduction in Mammals. Cambridge University Press, Book 3, pp. 42–72.

170. Silver, R. and M. Cooper (1983). Avian behavioral endocrinology. Bioscience 33:567–572.

171. Silver, R., C. Reboulleau, D.S. Lehrman and H.H. Feder (1974). Radioimmunoassay of plasma progesterone during the reproductive cycle of male and female ring doves *(Streptopelia risoria)*. Endocrinology 94:1547–1554.

172. Smith, C.L. (1955). Reproduction in female Amphibia. Mem. Soc. Endocrinol. 4:39–56.

173. Smith, M.J. and G.B. Sharman (1969). Development of dormant blastocysts induced by oestrogen in the ovariectomized marsupial, *Macropus eugenie*. Aust. J. Biol. Sci. 22:171–180.

174. Smith, R.J.F. (1974). Effects of 17β-methyltestosterone on the dorsal pad and tubercles of fathead minnows *(Pimephales promelas)*. Can. J. Zool. 52:1031–1038.

175. Smith, R.J.F. and W.S. Hoar (1967). The effects of prolactin and testosterone on the parental behaviour of the male stickleback *Gasterosteus aculeatus*. Anim. Behav. 15:342–352.

176. Soares, M.J. and J.C. Hoffmann (1981). Seasonal reproduction in the mongoose. *Herpestes auropunctatus*. I Androgen, luteinizing hormone and follicle-stimulating hormone in the male. Gen. Comp. Endocrinol. 44:350–358.

177. Specker, J.L. and F.L. Moore (1980). Annual cycle of plasma androgens and testicular composition in the rough-skinned newt, *Taricha granulosa*. Gen. Comp. Endocrinol. 42:297–303.

178. Stacey, N. (1983). Hormones and pheromones in fish sexual behavior. Bioscience 33:552–556.

179. Steinberger, A. and E. Steinberger (1976). Secretion of an FSH-inhibiting factor by cultured Sertoli cells. Endocrinology 99:918–921.

180. Steinberger, E. (1971). Hormonal control of mammalian spermatogenesis. Physiol. Rev. 51:1–21.

181. Sundararaj, B.I. and S.V. Goswami (1966). Effects of mammalian hypophysial hormones, placental gonadotropins, gonadal hormones, and adrenal corticosteroids on ovulation and spawning in hypophysectomized catfish, *Heteropneustes fossilis* (Bloch). J. Exp. Zool. 161:287–296.

182. Tanabe, Y., T. Nakamura, Y. Omiya, and T. Yano (1980). Changes in the plasma LH, progesterone, and estradiol during the ovulatory cycle of the duck *(Anas platyrhynchos domestica)* exposed to different photoperiods. Gen. Comp. Endocrinol. 41:378–383.

183. Tanaka, S. and H. Takikawa (1983). Seasonal changes in plasma testosterone and 5α-dihydrotestosterone levels in the adult male newt, *Cynops pyrrhogaster pyrrhogaster*. Endocrinol. Japon. 30:1–6.

184. Truscott, B., D.R. Idler, B.I. Sundararaj, and S.V. Goswami (1978). Effects of gonadotropins and adrenocorticotropin on plasmatic steroids of the catfish. *Heteropneustes fossilis* (Bloch). Gen. Comp. Endocrinol. 34:149–157.

185. Turner, C.L. (1957). The breeding cycle of the South American fish, *Jenynsia lineata*, in the Northern Hemisphere. Copeia 1957: 195–203.

186. Van Horn, R.N. and J.A. Resko (1977). The reproductive cycle of the ring-tailed lemur (Lemur catta): Sex steroid levels and sexual receptivity under controlled photoperiods. Endocrinology 101:1579–1586.

187. Van Tienhoven, A. (1968). Reproductive Physiology of Vertebrates. W.B. Saunders Co., Philadelphia.

188. Vilter, V. and A. Vilter (1964). Sur l'evolution des corps jaunes ovariens chez *Salamandra atra* Laur. des Alpes vaudoises. C.R. Soc. Biol. 48:457–461.

189. Wake, M.H. (1977). The reproductive biology of caecilians: An evolutionary perspective. In D.H. Taylor and S.I. Guttman, eds., The Reproductive Biology of Amphibians. Plenum Press, New York, pp. 73–101.

190. Wallace, R.A. and E.W. Bergink (1974). Amphibian vitellogenin: Properties, hormonal regulation of hepatic synthesis and ovarian uptake, and conversion to yolk proteins. Am. Zool. 14:1159–1176.

191. Weil, M.R. and R.D. Aldridge (1981). Seasonal androgenesis in the male water snake, *Nerodia sipedon*. Gen. Comp. Endocrinol. 44:44–53.

192. Wiebe, J.P. (1969). Steroid dehydrogenases and steroids in gonads of the sea perch *Cymatogaster aggregata* Gibbons. Gen. Comp. Endocrinol. 12:256–266.

193. Wilhelmi, A.E., G.E. Pickford and W.H. Sawyer (1955). Initiation of the spawning reflex response in *Fundulus* by the administration of fish and mammalian neurohypophyseal preparations and synthetic oxytocin. Endocrinology 57:243–252.

194. Wingfield, J.C. and A.S. Grimm (1976). Preliminary identification of plasma steroids in the plaice,

Pleuronectes platessa L. Gen. Comp. Endocrinol. 29:78–83.

195. Witschi, E. (1961). Sex and secondary sexual characters. In A.J. Marshall, ed., Biology and Comparative Physiology of Birds. Academic Press, Vol. 2, New York, pp. 115–168.

196. Wood-Gush, D.G.M. and A.B. Gilbert (1975). The physiological basis of a behaviour pattern in the domestic hen. Symp. Zool. Soc. Lond. 35:261–276.

197. Wright, P. (1945). Factors affecting *in vitro* ovulation in the frog. J. Exp. Zool. 100:565–575.

198. Wright, P.A. (1961). Induction of ovulation in vitro in *Rana pipiens* with steroids. Gen. Comp. Endocrinol. 1:20–23.

199. Xavier, F. and R. Ozon (1971). Recherches sur l'activité endocrine de l'ovaire de *Nectophrynoides occidentalis* Angel (Amphibien Anoure vivipare). II. Synthèse *in vitro* des steroids. Gen. Comp. Endocrinol. 16:30–40.

200. Yamazaki, F. and E.M. Donaldson (1968). The effects of partially purfied salmon pituitary gonadotropin on spermatogenesis, vitellogenesis, and ovulation in hypophysectomized goldfish *(Carassius auratus).* Gen. Comp. Endocrinol. 11:292–299.

201. Yaron, Z. (1972). Endocrine aspects of gestation in viviparous reptiles. Gen. Comp. Endocrinol. Suppl. 33:663–674.

202. Yoshinaga, K. (1978). Cyclic hormone secretion by the mammalian ovary. In R.E. Jones, ed., The Vertebrate Ovary. Plenum Press, New York, pp. 691–729.

203. Yu, J.Y.-L., W. Dickhoff, P. Swanson, and A. Gorbman (1981). Vitellogenesis and its hormonal regulation in the Pacific hagfish, *Eptatretus stouti* L. Gen. Comp. Endocrinol. 43:492–502.

204. Zoeller, R.T., L.T. Lais, and F.L. Moore (1983). Contractions of amphibian wolffian duct in response to acetylcholine, norepinephrine, and arginine vasotocin. J. Exp. Zool. 226:53–57.

PART III

12·Calcium and Phosphate Homeostasis

Calcium and phosphate are as important as sodium and potassium in the regulation of basic body functions. Inorganic calcium and phosphate are not related closely with respect to most of their essential roles in vertebrate physiology, but these ions are "inseparable" with respect to their involvement in the structure of bone and teeth. Calcium phosphate incorporated into bone matrix serves as the major reservoir for these ions. Consequently a discussion of the endocrine regulation of calcium homeostasis cannot be divorced entirely from the regulation of phosphate. The succeeding discussion of the mammalian pattern of calcium and phosphate homeostasis in mammals will provide a basis for making comparisons to other vertebrates.

Importance of Calcium and Phosphate

Calcium Homeostasis

During embryonic development and in growing mammals calcium is required for formation and growth of bone and teeth, which consist largely of calcium salts, especially calcium phosphate. Calcium ions (Ca^{++}) are essential components of blood plasma, where Ca^{++} functions as a cofactor for certain enzymes involved in the normal blood-clotting process. In addition, many intracellular enzymes require Ca^{++} as a cofactor.

Plasma Ca^{++} levels determine the Ca^{++} concentration of interstitial fluids (usually about 70% of plasma values) and influence the excitability of neurons and muscle cells. The formation of the actinomyosin complex in contracting muscle cells following neural stimulation is initiated by Ca^{++}. The quantity of acetylcholine released from motor end plates is proportional to the concentration of Ca^{++} in the interstitial fluids. Low extracellular Ca^{++} levels, however, may cause stimulation of a motor neuron as a result of the effects of Ca^{++} on cell membrane permeability to other ions such as Na^{+} and K^{+}. Furthermore, low extracellular Ca^{++} levels may stimulate myosin ATP-ase activity within muscle cells, resulting in uncontrolled contractions.

Recent studies of hormone actions, especially those hormones causing release of other hormones, have shown that the Ca^{++} content of the medium is important to their mechanisms of action. Normal release of hormones and certain other cellular products seems to be dependent upon Ca^{++}, and many neural and endocrine factors that influence hormone secretion may operate through controlling the availability of Ca^{++} (see Chap. 1).

Calcium Regulation. The calcium level in adult mammalian blood plasma is maintained at about 10 mg/dl or approximately 2.5 mM/liter. Somewhat less than half of this calcium is free in the plasma (that is, in ionic form), and the remainder is bound to circulating proteins, primarily albumin. It is this free ionic calcium that is essential to so many important life processes. Table 12-1 shows the variation in total body calcium with size and age.

After birth, calcium is obtained in the diet, absorbed through the small intestine, deposited in bone and teeth or excreted via urine or

TABLE 12-1. *Calcium Content of Human Body*[33]

AGE (YR)	BODY WEIGHT (kg)	CALCIUM CONTENT (g)
1	10.6	100
5	19.1	219
10	33.3	396
15	55.0	806
20	67.0	1078

feces. Urinary excretion of calcium is directly proportional to plasma levels, and little calcium is excreted unless plasma calcium levels exceed normal. Calcium deposited in bone serves as a reservoir to provide adequate plasma Ca^{++} for minute-to-minute regulation of body needs and during acute or chronic periods of dietary deprivation.

Phosphate Homeostasis

Phosphate, like calcium, is an essential component of bone and teeth. Approximately 80% of the total body phosphate is locked into the skeleton as calcium phosphate. In addition, many essential molecules contain phosphate, including structural phospholipids in cellular membranes, nucleic acids, nucleotides and hexose phosphates. Furthermore, phosphate is indispensable for energy storage within cells in the form of ATP or creatine phosphate. Hydrolysis of ATP or guanosine triphosphate (GTP) to form cyclic adenosine 3′, 5′-monophosphate (cAMP) or cyclic guanosine 3′, 5′-monophosphate (cGMP) respectively, is necessary for mediating the actions of many hormones, for neural transmission and for many other cellular processes. The presence or absence of phosphate may determine whether an enzyme has biological activity or not. Finally, phosphate ions play only a minor role as buffers of hydrogen ions in the body fluids, but they are the major buffer system in urine. It is rare that phosphate becomes a limiting factor for an organism, and the usual phosphate disturbances in mammals are a result of excessive levels of phosphate.

Inorganic phosphate (P_i) in mammalian plasma is generally found to be about 3.1 mg/dl (about 1.0 mM/liter). Most of this phosphate (about 80%) is in the form of HPO_4^{-2} with almost 20% occurring as $H_2PO_4^{-1}$ and only a trace as PO_4^{-3}. Henceforth the chemical formula HPO_4^{-2} will be used to represent all of the phosphate ions.

In normal plasma about 90% of the P_i is free ionic (filterable) phosphate, and about 10% is bound to the plasma proteins. In addition to P_i, plasma contains considerable amounts of lipid-bound phosphate and esterified phosphate so that total plasma phosphate is actually about 12.5 mg/dl. Phosphate values vary considerably with diet, age and metabolic state, however, and it is difficult to provide a "normal" value without specifying the conditions under which this "normal" occurs.

Interrelationship of Ca^{++} and HPO_4^{-2}

Calcium and phosphate are regulated in such a way that the product of the plasma concentrations of Ca^{++} and HPO_4^{-2} always equals some constant $[(Ca^{++}) \cdot (HPO_4^{-2}) = k]$. This constant however, may change according to differing physiological states or pathological conditions. For example, k is greater in growing mammals than it is in adults. This relationship between Ca^{++} and HPO_4^{-2} implies that if there is an increase in Ca^{++} a corresponding decrease in HPO_4^{-2} should follow. Likewise, an increase in HPO_4^{-2} should cause a decrease in Ca^{++}. Although plasma HPO_4^{-2} levels may change without observed alterations in plasma Ca^{++}, this generalization concerning relative amounts of these ions in plasma is useful to illustrate some of the relationships that exist between the regulatory mechanisms governing these ions.

Minute-to-minute adjustments of Ca^{++} and HPO_4^{-2} levels in extracellular fluids are accomplished primarily through a combination of bone destruction (resorption) or formation, absorption of dietary calcium by the small intestine and renal excretion of phosphate.

Bone Formation and Resorption in Mammals

Bone is the major body reservoir for both Ca^{++} and HPO_4^{-2}. Calcium phosphate occurs in the form of small submicroscopic crystals deposited upon an organic matrix composed primarily of collagen fibers. These crystals assume a uniform structural and chemical form known as *hydroxyapatite crystals.* Construction of bone through formation of calcium phosphate is not completely understood, but some of the major features are well accepted.

Bone formation may involve deposition of new hydroxyapatite crystals, *apatite formation,* or simply the additional growth of existing crystals, *mineral accumulation.* Exchange of Ca^{++}, HPO_4^{-2} and water can occur between the surface of these crystals and the extracellular fluids. This exchange is inversely proportional to the size of the crystal. Thus, larger crystals contain considerable amounts of calcium phosphate that cannot engage in free exchange with the extracellular fluids. About 99% of bone calcium phosphate is found in these larger, nonexchangeable stable or "diffusion-locked" crystals. The specific process of bone formation and growth also involves a number of local chemical factors that are responsible for collagen matrix formation, cartilage matrix deposition and formation of hydroxyapatite crystals as well as cellular replication and differentiation.[5,70]

Cells known as *osteoblasts* (literally, bone forming) are responsible for bone formation. The homologous cell in teeth is termed an odontoblast. The osteoblasts comprise the *endosteal membrane* that lines the cavities within bone, and they synthesize the collagen matrix upon which apatite formation occurs. The factors controlling osteoblast activities are poorly understood. Some osteoblasts give rise to osteocytes that become completely surrounded by bone except for minute channels through which the osteocytes communicate with one another. There seems to be little agreement on the role for osteocytes in calcium-phosphate metabolism, but they may be targets for hormonal regulation.

Resorption of bone may involve either removal of the collagen matrix and/or solubilization of hydroxyapatite crystals with consequent release of Ca^{++} and HPO_4^{-2}. Apparently both processes usually occur during bone resorption. Another bone cell, the *osteoclast* (literally, bone destroying) is primarily responsible for bone resorption. The osteoclast is a large, multinucleate cell and is easy to distinguish from uninucleate osteoblasts (Fig. 12-1). Osteoclasts may arise from either osteoblasts or bone marrow cells, but the details of their formation are not clear.

Endocrine Regulation of Calcium and Phosphate in Mammals

In mammals the regulation of calcium is accomplished primarily by the actions of two hormones: *parathyroid hormone* (PTH), produced by the parathyroid glands, and *calcitonin* (CT), produced by the parafollicular or C cells of the thyroid gland. Parathyroid hormone is a hypercalcemic factor, that is, it causes an elevation in the level of plasma calcium. Release of PTH is increased by low plasma calcium levels and is decreased by elevated plasma calcium levels, but PTH release is not directly influenced by fluctuations in phosphate levels.[65] Calcitonin is a hypocalcemic agent, and its release is directly related to changes in plasma calcium.

A major site of action for PTH is bone, where it may stimulate calcium deposition in bone or bone resorption and release both calcium and phosphate ions into the circulation. Parathyroid hormone also controls phosphate levels by increasing tubular excretion of phosphate by the kidney. Increased calcium reabsorption by the nephron may occur in association with the excretion of phosphate. The net result of bone, renal and possible intestinal actions of PTH is an increase in plasma calcium with a decrease in plasma phosphate levels and a concomitant increase in urinary phosphate. These actions of PTH on bone and

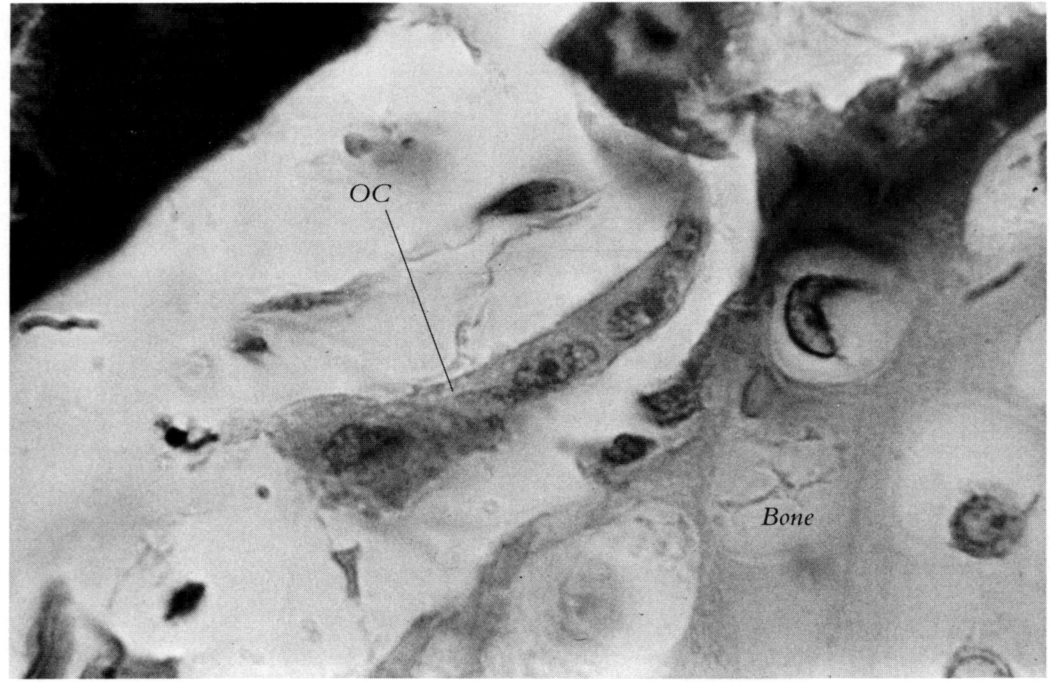

FIG. 12-1. Multinucleate osteoclast from a turtle bone, *OC,* osteoclast. (Photomicrograph courtesy of Nancy B. Clark.)

possibly on the kidney appear to require the presence of certain derivatives of vitamin D. Dietary calcium uptake through the intestional muscosa is also vitamin D-dependent and may be indirectly influenced by PTH.

The Parathyroid Glands

Although the parathyroid glands had been observed previously, Sandstrom rediscovered and named them in 1880. Frequently the parathyroids, which develop like the thyroid from pharyngeal tissues (Fig. 12-2), are embedded within the thyroid glands (Fig. 12-3), for example, in the mouse, cat and man. In other mammals, such as goats and rabbits, they are separate glands located near the thyroid. Some mammals may have as many as four separate parathyroid glands. In addition to the definitive parathyroid glands, accessory parathyroid tissue exists in some species. These anatomical peculiarities among different species are reflected in observations that thyroidectomy may result in lowered Ca^{++} plasma levels in some species because of concomitant removal of the parathyroids, whereas parathyroidectomy in another species may not alter plasma Ca^{++} markedly because of the continued presence of accessory parathyroid tissue.

Historically the parathyroid glands have been reported to be derived from pharyngeal endoderm. Parathyroid cells, however, have been reported to arise from neuroectoderm,[56] in the frog *Rana temporaria* suggesting they are also part of the amine precursor uptake and decarboxylation (APUD) series of polypeptide-secreting cells (Chap. 1). Indirect evidence also supports a similar origin for PTH-secreting cells in birds and mammals.[25,56]

Two cellular types have been described in mammalian parathyroid glands: *chief cells* and *oxyphils.* Chief cells are cuboidal with no unique cytological features (other than the presence of granules containing immunoreactive PTH). They are the dominant cellular type and comprise about 99% of the cellular population in most species. In a few species, such as deer, the parathyroids are composed exclusively of chief cells. The oxyphils are rare (sometimes absent) eosinophilic cells rich in

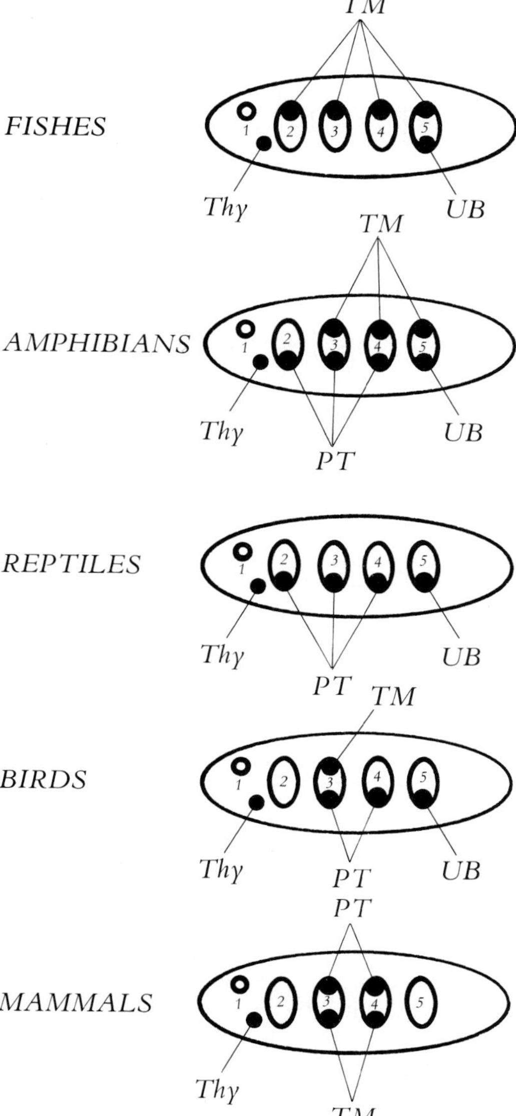

FIG. 12-2. Embryonic origins from pharyngeal pouches for thymus *(Tm)*, thyroid *(Thy)*, parathyroid *(PT)* and ultimobranchial *(UB)* tissues in vertebrates. The numbers refer to pharyngeal pouches. Pouch 1 remains only as a spiracle or as the eustachian tube. Thymus in reptiles develops from pouches 2,3 (lizards), 3,4 (turtles) and 4,5 (snakes). Based in part on Copp.[17]

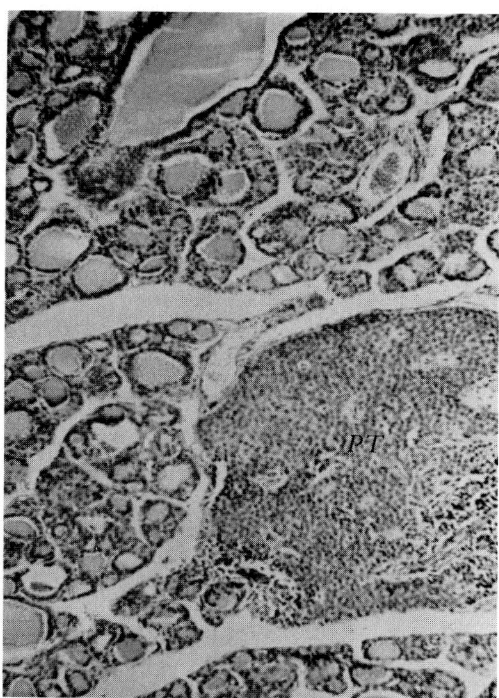

FIG. 12-3. A mammalian parathyroid gland *(PT)* embedded in follicular thyroid tissue.

mitochondria (hence their name). The function of the oxyphil and the significance of the large number of mitochondria are unknown.

PARATHYROID HORMONE. Parathyroid hormone is a hypercalcemic agent, and its primary role is to increase circulating Ca^{++} and to augment renal phosphate excretion. Mammalian PTH has been isolated and characterized from several species. It is a large polypeptide consisting of 84 amino acids (Fig. 12-4). Apparently all of the biological activity resides in the first 34 amino acids. Parathyroid hormone is synthesized in the chief cells as a larger polypeptide that is later cleaved to release the smaller PTH unit.[31] This synthetic mechanism is essentially like that described for other polypeptide hormones, including growth hormone, prolactin (Chap. 5) and insulin (Chap. 13).

Synthesis of PTH occurs in two steps. A large polypeptide of 115 amino acid residues (pre-proparathyroid hormone [PreProPTH]) is synthesized on the ribosomes of the rough endoplasmic reticulum (RER) but is rapidly cleaved at the amine terminus to a smaller peptide, proparathyroid hormone (ProPTH), of 90 amino acids as it enters the cisterna of the RER. ProPTH travels through the cisterna to the Golgi apparatus where the remaining 6

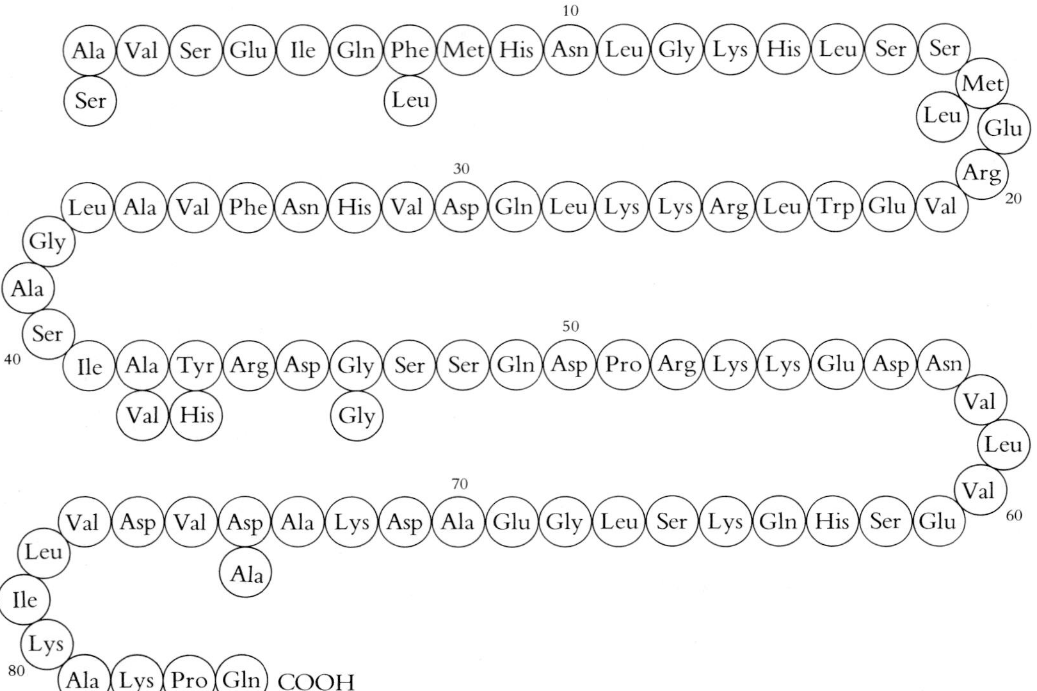

FIG. 12-4. Amino acid sequence for bovine parathyroid hormone. Porcine PTH differs at seven positions (attached circles). (After Habener et al.[31])

amine terminal residues of the prohormone are removed. The resulting 84-amino acid sequence of PTH is then packaged into storage vesicles to await release.

The classical bioassay for PTH is the increase in plasma calcium following administration of parathyroid gland extracts or PTH to normal or parathyroidectomized dogs.[30] More recent bioassays employ parathyroidectomized rats maintained on a calcium-deficient diet.[75]

Parathyroid hormone may occur as peptide fragments in the circulation, varying from 4500 to 9000 daltons. In terms of biological activity, the biological half-life for PTH is about 20 minutes in cattle or rats.[21] The native 84-amino acid PTH peptide is cleared from the blood much more rapidly (2 to 4 minutes) indicating that the remainder of the bioassayable activity is due to persistence of fragments produced by partial hydrolysis of native PTH.

PARATHYROIDECTOMY. The effects of removing the parathyroid glands (parathyroidectomy) are variable from species to species. In all cases, parathyroidectomy causes a reduction in plasma Ca^{++} and consequent detrimental muscular effects. As Ca^{++} levels decrease, hyperexcitability of motor neurons and skeletal muscles occurs, resulting in twitches, spasms and, in extreme cases, violent convulsions. This condition is known as *low-calcium-induced tetany.* If prolonged contractions (tetany) of the respiratory muscles occur, death due to asphyxiation may result. The severity of these neuromuscular effects however, differs markedly with respect to species involved and various physiological conditions. For example, exercise raises the body temperature and increases the breathing rate, causing a reduction of blood CO_2. Reduced blood CO_2 in turn alters blood pH (alkalosis) and retards ionization of Ca^{++}. This further reduction in Ca^{++} in a parathyroidectomized animal may precipitate a tetanic seizure. Animals on diets low in Ca^{++} and high in HPO_4^{-2} exhibit tetany following parathyroidectomy more readily than do animals on normal diets.

The Parafollicular Cells

The parafollicular (C cells) cells of the mammalian thyroid gland have been identified unequivocally as the source of CT in mammals. However, the actual origin of these cells is unclear. The most generally accepted origin is that proposed by Godwin suggesting that these cells originated from the ultimobranchial body that develops from the sixth pharyngeal pouch (endoderm).[29] These ultimobranchial cells become incorporated into the thyroid gland of mammals as parathyroids frequently do. The ultimobranchial body remains as a distinct separate structure in other vertebrate groups (Fig. 12-6).

The parafollicular cells of the mammalian thyroid exhibit APUD characteristics. Some elegant studies employing cellular chimeras of

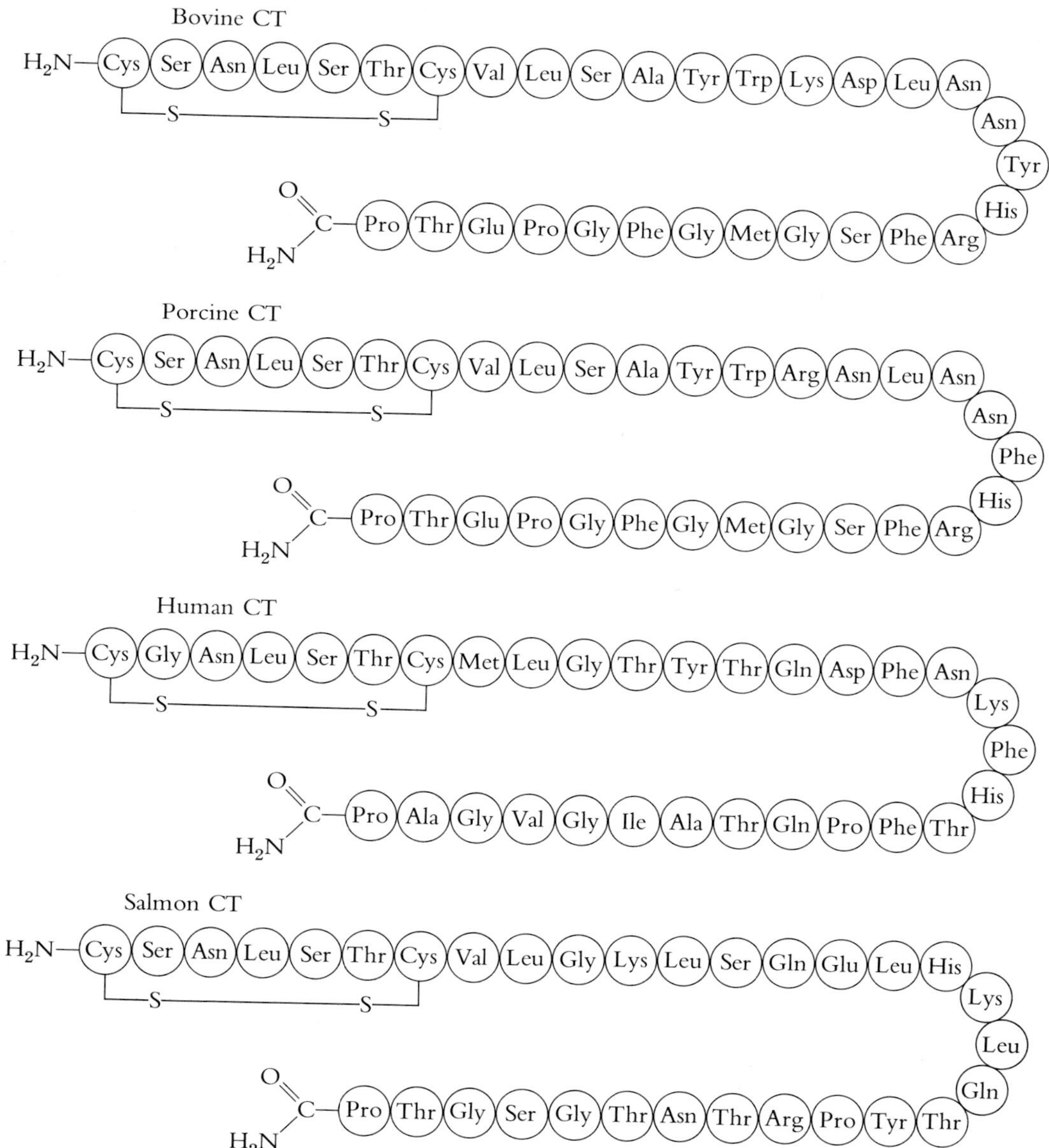

FIG. 12-5. Comparison of amino acid sequences of bovine, porcine, human and salmon calcitonin.

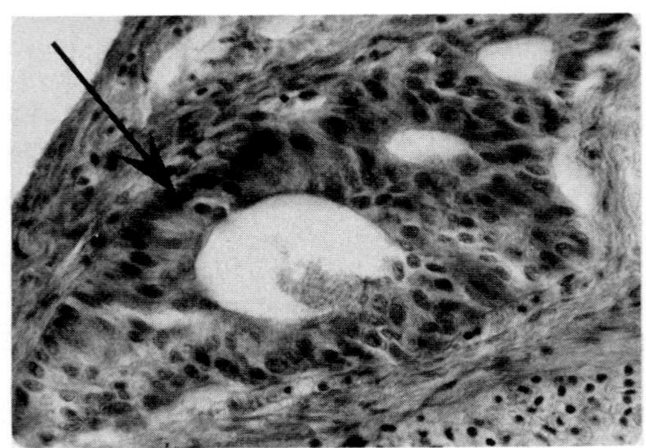

Fig. 12-6. Ultimobranchial tissue *(arrow)* from rainbow trout *Salmo gairdneri,* juvenile, 63 mm body length.

chicken and quail tissues have confirmed the origin of the CT-secreting cells of the ultimobranchial body from neural crest cells.[41] Parafollicular cells also contain somatostatin and ultrastructurally resemble the D-cells found in the intestinal lining[4] (see Table 14-1).

Calcitonin. Production of a potent mammalian hypocalcemic factor by cells of the parathyroid gland was first reported by Copp and associates; it was named calcitonin.[19] Other investigators provided evidence that the source of this hypocalcemic factor was, in fact, the thyroid gland and suggested the alternative name of thyrocalcitonin to reflect its origin. It was soon discovered that ultimobranchial glands of sharks and chickens contained a powerful hypocalcemic factor.[20,68] These observations were soon reconciled with the ultimobranchial origin of the parafollicular cells of the thyroid that had been shown to be responsible for synthesizing CT.

Mammalian CT is a small, single-chain polypeptide consisting of 32 amino acids with a disulfide link between residues 1 and 7. There are no active fragments of CT, and the entire molecule is necessary for biological activity. The amino acid sequence for CT is provided in Figure 12-5. It is synthesized as a larger peptide (136 amino acids). The CT sequence actually is cleaved from the middle of the prohormone.[34]

Skin, Liver, Kidney

The actions of PTH on bone and possibly kidney require the presence of a certain derivative of vitamin D. The D vitamins are all steroid molecules (see Chap. 9) that may be obtained through the diet or synthesized by the skin from cholesterol in the presence of adequate sunlight. Generally either vitamin D or vitamin D_3 (cholecalciferol) is converted sequentially by the liver to 25-hydroxycholecalciferol and then by the kidney to *1,25-dihydroxycholecalciferol* (1,25-DHC) (Fig. 12-7). This last compound is the necessary cofactor that facilitates the actions of PTH on bone and is itself responsible for intestinal absorption of Ca^{++}. The synthesis of 1,25-DHC by the kidney may be influenced positively by PTH, thus indirectly affecting intestinal absorption of calcium.

Some investigators have proposed that 1,25-DHC should be given the status of a true hormone,[40] a suggestion that, if it were adopted, might require some additional modification of our present concept of "hormone" since at least three tissues (skin, liver and kidney) participate actively in its synthesis (Fig. 12-7).

Interactions of Parathyroid Hormone, Calcitonin and 1,25-Dihydroxycholecalciferol

The major disturbance to calcium homeostasis is the influx of Ca^{++} following ingestion of a meal.[62] In addition, pregnancy and lactation may provide a relatively short-term stress on calcium homeostasis in females (see p. 325). The small intestine, kidney and bone are the primary sites where regulatory hormones (PTH, CT, 1,25-DHC) produce their actions during times of calcium excess or deficiency to maintain calcium homeostasis.

Actions of Parathyroid Hormone and Calcitonin on Bone. Two hypotheses have been advanced to explain the actions of PTH on bone. Which of these mechanisms might be the more important has not been determined, and both may be involved in the normal regulatory process. The first hypotheses deals with the proposed action on the osteoclasts, whereas the second deals with osteoblasts. Osteocytes embedded in the bone matrix may be influenced by both mechanisms and are considered by some researchers to be important targets of PTH.

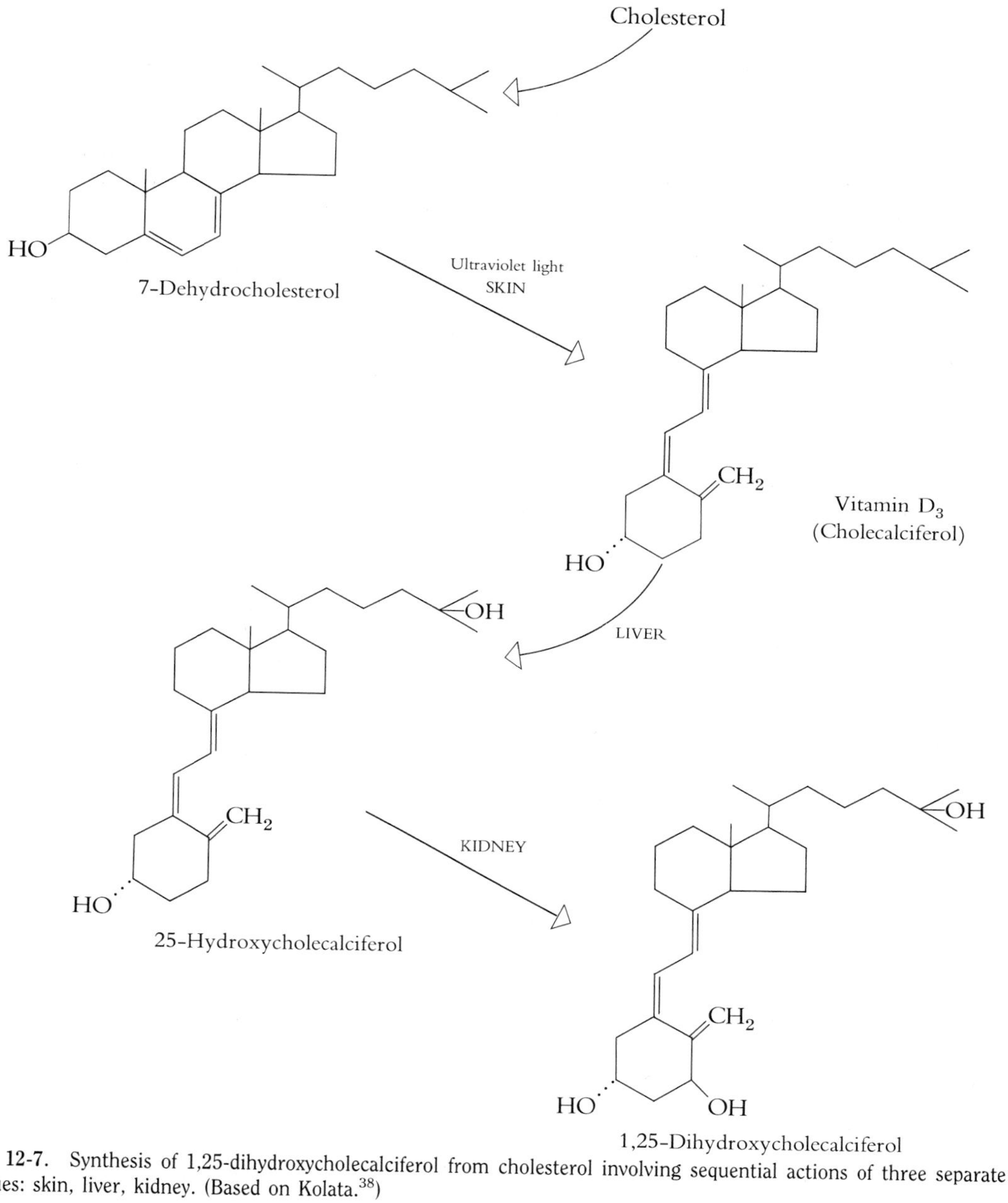

Cholesterol

HO

7-Dehydrocholesterol

Ultraviolet light
SKIN

Vitamin D_3
(Cholecalciferol)

CH_2

HO

LIVER

OH

CH_2

HO

25-Hydroxycholecalciferol

KIDNEY

OH

CH_2

HO

OH

1,25-Dihydroxycholecalciferol

FIG. 12-7. Synthesis of 1,25-dihydroxycholecalciferol from cholesterol involving sequential actions of three separate tissues: skin, liver, kidney. (Based on Kolata.[38])

Osteoclasts. Parathyroid hormone stimulates osteoclast activity and may cause an increase in the number of osteoclasts in bone. Only the mechanism of the former action has been investigated. The action of PTH on the osteoclast first involves intracellular synthesis of small lipid molecules known as prostaglandins[57] (see Chap. 15). These prostaglandins in turn activate the enzyme adenyl cyclase, resulting in an increase in cAMP within the osteoclast. Apparently an increase in cAMP is related to the release of lysosomal enzymes from cytoplasmic lysosomes. It is the action of these hydrolytic lysosomal enzymes that is responsible for bone resorption and release of Ca^{++} and HPO_4^{-2} to the plasma. Calcitonin apparently interferes with this sequence of events, presumably by interfering with the activation of adenyl cyclase by the prostaglandins.[36]

Osteoblasts. Several investigators have contributed to the following hypothesis suggesting that the osteoblasts of the endosteal membrane are influenced by PTH.[23,67] According to this hypothesis the osteoblasts contain a pumping mechanism analogous to the one described for intestinal uptake of Ca^{++}. In this case, however, PTH, through activation of adenyl cyclase and cAMP formation, increases the flux of Ca^{++} into the osteoblast from the bone surface and out of the osteoblast on the blood side of the endosteal membrane. A reverse mechanism has been used to explain the inhibition of bone deposition when PTH stimulates osteoclast activity.

There is evidence to suggest that at normal physiological levels PTH stimulates bone formation rather than bone resorption through an increase in osteoblast activity.[21,55] The observed effects of PTH on osteoclast activity requires considerable elevation of PTH levels and may occur only under conditions of calcium deprivation. Calcitonin may influence osteoblast functions to a limited extent and alter efflux of Ca^{++} and HPO_4^{-2} from bone. The major site for action of CT, however, appears to be the osteoclast.[44]

Actions of PTH and CT on Kidney. Calcium reabsorption by the kidney may be an important physiological action of PTH,[55] although some investigators believe the increased excretion of phosphate is more important. Parathyroid hormone increases the enzymatic formation of 1,25–DHC in kidney and may enhance intestinal calcium absorption indirectly. Estrogens and prolactin also enhance formation of 1,25-DHC, and these actions may be essential in pregnant and lactating mammals, respectively.

Calcitonin antagonizes the action of PTH on bone resorption but does not influence either renal or intestinal processes in normal animals. It has not been possible to demonstrate renal actions of CT except in parathyroidectomized mammals in which CT may cause dramatic changes in phosphate excretion.[35] It will be assumed that the physiological site of action for CT is bone.

Actions of 1,25–Dihydroxycholecalciferol on Intestinal Uptake of Ca^{++}. According to one scheme, Ca^{++} uptake by the intestinal mucosal cell is dependent upon a calcium-binding protein within these cells that is linked to a calcium-activated ATPase.[22] Calcium is actively absorbed by this protein-ATPase complex at the mucosal surface that is in contact with the lumen of the gut. Once in the cell these Ca^{++} ions enter the mitochondria

Table 12-2. *Hormones That Influence Calcium Metabolism in Mammals*[28]

HORMONE	CHEMICAL NATURE	SOURCE	ACTION
1,25-Dihydroxycholecalciferol	Steroid	Skin, liver, then kidney	Facilitates calcium absorption in small intestine
Parathyroid hormone	Polypeptide	Parathyroids	Stimulates bone resorption and renal calcium reabsorption
Calcitonin	Polypeptide	Thyroid C cells	Antagonizes action of PTH on bone
Growth hormone	Large polypeptide	Pituitary	Stimulates bone growth and calcium utilization
Thyroid hormones	Iodothyronines	Thyroid follicular cells	Permissive effect for GH
Estradiol	Steroid	Ovary	Causes closure of epiphysial plate and blocks further bone growth

and are somehow transported to the opposite serosal border of the cell where Ca^{++} ions diffuse into the interstitial fluid and then into the blood capillaries. Phosphate ions passively follow the movements of Ca^{++}. Synthesis of a calcium-transport protein (the calcium-binding protein or the calcium-activated ATPase or both) is stimulated by 1,25–DHC.

Actions of Calcitonin on Intestinal Uptake of Ca^{++}. No role has been hypothesized for CT in this intestinal mechanism for calcium uptake. Following the influx of Ca^{++} ions, however, calcitonin is released partly in response to the increase in plasma Ca^{++} but may also be released by *gastrin,* a gastrointestinal hormone released from the gastric mucosa during the early phase of digestion of a meal (see Chap. 14). This increased level of CT inhibits the action of PTH on bone osteoclasts and favors addition of the absorbed dietary Ca^{++} to the bone matrix.

Calcitonin becomes indispensable during pregnancy and lactation with respect to Ca^{++} mobilization.[69] Its role is apparently to protect the maternal skeleton from excessive destruction in meeting the calcium requirements of fetus or neonate and allow dietary Ca^{++} to be diverted to it. The relative importance of CT in different species varies markedly according to the precise demands for maternal calcium (Table 12–3).

A Proposed Role for Parathyroid Hormone in Acid-base Balance. It has been suggested that the parathyroid glands and PTH evolved in terrestrial vertebrates to deal with the problems of acid-base balance when water was in short supply.[74] A change in acid-base regulation was supposedly necessitated by the loss of gills and the ready availability of water in which to dispose of excess hydrogen ions. This hypothesis proposes that calcium regulation was a secondary acquisition and that carbonate and phosphate regulation related to acid-base regulation was primitive. The absence of parathyroid glands and cellular bone among the fishes is believed to support this hypothesis. Although this may seem to be an interesting hypothesis at first, it has been strongly criticized on theoretical grounds.[2] Nevertheless, it would seem that the "sudden" appearance of parathyroids in tetrapods may be related to more than the problem of calcium homeostasis.

Major Clinical Disorders Associated with Calcium Metabolism

Hypercalcemia

Excessive plasma calcium levels (greater than 10 mg/dl) can result from a variety of causes. Primary hypercalcemia is characterized by chronically elevated levels of PTH. The most common cause is a single parathyroid adenoma (90% of cases). Carcinomas of the parathyroids are very rare and may account for less than 1% of primary hypercalcemic cases. Approximately one-third of these cases are without overt symptoms, and the remainder exhibit rather generalized and nonspecific symptoms such as weakness, nausea and anorexia. Serum calcium levels are 10.2 to 11.0 mg/dl and are usually accompanied by lowered phosphate levels. Often, elevated serum levels of calcium are not seen because the kidney compensates with increased calcium excretion (hypercalcuria).

Among the many causative factors that can induce secondary hypercalcemia are lung squamous cell carcinoma and renal cell carcinoma that spontaneously secrete PTH. Breast

Table 12-3. *Calcium Content of Maternal Milk and Rate of Growth of Suckling Young Mammals*[33]

Species	Days to Double Birth Weight	% Calcium in Maternal Milk
Human	180	0.02
Bovine	47	0.12
Canine	7	0.32

carcinomas may produce vitamin D-like sterols that increase calcium absorption. Chronic immobilization can bring about extensive bone resorption and elevate blood calcium levels.

Hypocalcemia

There are many different conditions that can lead to hypocalcemia. In most cases there is a reduction in PTH secretion. This may be caused by abnormal development of the parathyroid glands, accidental damage or removal by surgery. Hypomagnesemia impairs PTH secretion and indirectly can cause hypocalcemia. In some cases (e.g., psuedo-hypoparathyroidism) the target organs do not respond to PTH and in others an abnormal PTH is secreted that will not activate tissue receptors. Reductions in 1,25-DHC due to failure to convert 25-HC or to synthesize vitamin D also lead to hypocalcemia. Most cases are without serious overt symptoms. Tetany may be inducible under calcium stress but otherwise is absent.

Osteoporosis

This disease is characterized by decalcification of the skeleton resulting in shrinkage, distortion and increased brittleness of the bones. Osteroporosis accompanies aging and is most common among postmenopausal women. Osteoporosis is eight times times more common in women than men largely as a consequence of women having smaller bone calcium reserves. Maximum adult bone mass is achieved in women at about age 35 after which calcium losses exceed calcium gain. During menopause (see Chap. 11) there is a gradual reduction in estrogen levels causing a disproportionate decrease in bone mass by allowing increased bone resorption to take place. Estrogen therapy is sometimes employed to arrest this condition. Increased calcium intake by pre- and postmenopausal women may lessen the impact of calcium losses in later life and retard development of osteoporosis.

Paget's Disease

This disorder is caused by increased osteoclast activity resulting in accelerated bone resorption. It occurs in 3% of the population over age 40, and occurs with greatest frequency in people of Western European or Mediterranean descent. About one-third of the people afflicted with Paget's disease do not exhibit any overt symptoms, but the bones become brittle as the disease progresses. Serum levels of calcium and phosphate are usually normal because the excess ions are excreted in the urine. Salmon CT has been used with some success to treat Paget' disease, because it has a much longer biological half-life in mammals than does mammalian CT.

Aspects of Calcium and Phosphate Homeostasis in Nonmammalian Vertebrates

An attempt to discuss the evolutionary aspects of this problem is complicated by major differences, indeed a distinct dichotomy, between the fishes and the tetrapods. Many fishes lack true bone (class Agnatha, class Chondrichthyes), and many of the bony fishes possess acellular bone rather than cellular bone. Scales may provide a source of calcium to bony fishes, and the surrounding waters have been hypothesized to be a more important source of calcium than even the skeleton.[51] Furthermore, parathyroid glands are lacking in fishes as is PTH, and no homologous structures are known. Calcium metabolism appears to be regulated by the pituitary and the corpuscles of Stannius located in the kidneys.[11] The parathyroids and PTH appear suddenly, fully differentiated in the amphibians. Even though most fishes have ultimobrachial glands that contain potent hypocalcemic factors when assayed in tetrapods, these structures do not seem to be important for calcium regulation in fishes. Finally, the comparative approach is hampered by the lack of detailed information concerning calcium and phosphate regulation in fishes. In fact, virtually nothing is known about calcium-phosphate metabolism in cyclostomes.

Estrogenic hormones elevate circulating calcium levels indirectly in females of most nonmammalian species during the process of vitellogenesis associated with oocyte growth.[21]

Synthesis of vitellogenic proteins by the liver is stimulated by estrogens. These proteins are released into the blood, through which they travel to the ovaries where they are incorporated into growing oocytes as yolk protein. Vitellogenic proteins readily bind Ca^{++}, indirectly decrease free plasma Ca^{++} levels and consequently stimulate release of more Ca^{++} from reservoirs such as bone. The presence of vitellogenic proteins elevates total plasma levels of Ca^{++}, although free Ca^{++} remains about the same. The relationship between reproductive hormones and vitellogenesis is discussed in more detail in Chapter 11.

Class Agnatha

Cyclostomes do not appear to have any hormonal regulatory mechanisms for calcium and phosphate metabolism.[21] Whatever regulatory mechanisms are employed, they are not as efficient as those found in other vertebrates as evidenced by circulating levels of calcium. Marine species exhibit an intermediate level of plasma Ca^{++} between that of sea water and plasma of tetrapods, whereas the plasma Ca^{++} level in freshwater lampreys is intermediate between that found in plasma of freshwater teleosts and fresh water.[21]

Class Chondrichthyes

These fishes occur in sea water, for the most part, where calcium availability is not a serious problem. Although these fishes lack true bone tissue, calcium salts are added to their cartilaginous skeletons for additional strength, especially in the larger species. The elasmobrach ultimobranchial glands contain a potent hypocalcemic factor when assayed in mammals.[20] Extracts of shark ultimobranchial glands, salmon CT and porcine CT, however, are all ineffective in altering plasma calcium in sharks.[50] Estrogens do not produce any appreciable alteration in plasma calcium as they do in bony fishes and tetrapods.[21] No experimental evidence has been reported for an adenohypophysial factor that would directly affect plasma calcium. Studies of the Nicaraguan freshwater shark might provide some interesting insight since these fishes live in very low calcium environments.

Class Osteichthyes: Actinopterygii

Calcium regulation appears to be under the control of a hypercalcemic adenohypophysial factor and a hypocalcemic factor associated with the corpuscles of Stannius (CS).[50] Hypophysectomy of either *Anguilla* (which has cellular bone) or *Fundulus* (acellular bone) results in a decrease in serum calcium and induction of tetany.[50] Recent studies suggest that the pituitary factor is PRL and that it is the primary hormone controlling calcium levels in low-calcium environments, that is, fresh water. There is also evidence for a parathyroid hormone-like peptide in pituitaries of codfish and eels that has been given the name of *hypercalcin.*[55] This hypercalcemic peptide may prove to be a more potent factor in teleosts than is prolactin, but more studies are needed for confirmation.

The CS are discrete bodies found embedded within the kidney of most actinopterygians. The number of CS varies greatly among the species that have been examined. It has been suggested that the CS are steroidogenic structures, but there is little evidence to support such a claim.[27] Little experimental work has been performed with species other than teleosts, and only a few of these fishes in fact have been examined. Removal of CS (stanniectomy) from the eel *A. anguilla* results in an increase in serum calcium, and administration of CS extracts reduces calcium to normal levels.[26] Surgical stanniectomy of freshwater *A. japonica* is followed by decreased urinary Ca^{++} levels and increased urinary HPO_4^{-2} levels.[6] It is possible that the CS are mainly active in reducing Ca^{++} levels in fish adapted to high calcium environments such as sea water.[50] The active hypocalcemic agent in the CS may be a peptide called *hypocalcin.*[53]

Calcitonin treatment generally has been ineffective in teleosts with respect to lowering calcium,[11,50,53] although some positive responses have been reported.[24,43,73] The gill may be a major site where CT regulates Ca^{++} transport.[45] Removal of the ultimobranchial glands from *A. japonica* caused effects just opposite to stanniectomy: an increase in Ca^{++} excretion accompanied by a decrease in HPO_4^{-2}, at least suggesting the possible existence of a PTH-like factor.[6]

Table 12-4. *Comparison of Relative Activity of Purified Human, Salmon and Porcine Calcitonin Determined by a Standard Bioassay*

SOURCE	ACTIVITY IN MRC[a] UNITS/MG HORMONE
Porcine	200
Human	120
Salmon	5000

[a]Medical Research Council of England

Salmon CT has been found to be a powerful hypocalcemic agent when tested in avian or mammalian systems[17] (Table 12-4), and it is now employed clinically to reduce pathological hypercalcemia (Paget's disease). This potency of salmon CT is related, at least in part, to its persistence in the circulation, that is, its long biological half-life as compared to mammalian CT (Table 12-5). It would seem almost that CT evolved prior to the evolution of its function in calcium homeostasis. The correct explanation for this apparent anomaly is more likely related to ignorance of the possible role for CT in fishes and the endocrine regulation of calcium homeostasis.

Some teleost kidneys possess sufficient enzyme necessary for the second hydroxylation of cholecalciferol to form 1,25-DHC.[21] This hormone is apparently not necessary for Ca^{++} uptake by the intestine, but large doses of 1,25-DHC enhances Ca^{++} uptake.[66]

Thyroid State and Calcium Homeostasis. Serum calcium may be influenced by thyroid state, but the physiological importance of these observations has not been established.

Table 12-5. *Biological Half-Life for Purified Vertebrate Calcitonins When Incubated in Either Mammalian or Avian Blood Plasma*

SOURCE	HALF-LIFE (MIN.)
Porcine	2
Salmon	20
Chicken	90

Serum calcium levels are decreased in juvenile steelhead trout *(Salmo gairdneri)* that were radiothyroidectomized prior to complete resorption of the yolk sac (Table 12-6). It is not possible to distinguish between general effects of radiation that may have damaged some calcium-regulating mechanism and effects due to the absence of thyroid hormones, however. Growth of the skeleton is also abnormal following radiothyroidectomy,[39] supporting an involvement of thyroid hormones at least indirectly. Abnormal skeletal growth could be related to ineffective action of growth hormone in the absence of thyroid hormones (see Chap. 8).

Table 12-6. *Serum Calcium Levels in Radiothyroidectomized Steelhead Trout,* Salmo gairdneri

	TOTAL SERUM CALCIUM ± SEM OR RANGE ( ) (MG/100 ML)	REFERENCE
Radiothyroidectomized as fingerlings	10 (4–12)	38
Intact controls	11 (9–15)	38
Radiothyroidectomized prior to yolk-sac resorption	11.8 ± 1.01	47
Intact controls	14.9 ± 0.51	47

Class Osteichthyes: Sarcopterygii

The lungfishes lack parathyroid glands and are relatively insensitive to tetrapod calcium-regulating hormones. It is both surprising and somewhat disappointing that in this one case they do not exhibit some tetrapod-like feature. Parathyroid extracts, PTH and salmon CT are all ineffective in altering Ca^{++} levels in the South American lungfish *Lepidosiren paradoxa.*[54] Surprisingly, however, CT and PTH are diuretic and antidiuretic respectively in these fishes. The physiological importance of these observations is not altogether clear, but these substances are certainly not involved in calcium homeostasis. Perhaps CT has some diuretic action in actinopterygian fishes as well.

Class Amphibia

Studies of amphibians have not shed any light on the origin of the parathyroid glands and the evolution of calcium regulation in tetrapods. Ultimobranchial and parathyroid glands are present in the Apoda, Anura and Caudata, and calcium regulation is similar to that observed in other tetrapods. It may well be that the explanation lies within the fossil record of fishes ancestral to the Amphibia or in fossil Amphibia themselves.

Pituitary. A hypercalcemic factor is present in pituitaries of urodele amphibians, and it is of greater importance in the more aquatic species.[52] Parathyroid glands are not present in some urodeles until after metamorphosis, and parathyroids never develop in some permanently neotenic aquatic species such as *Necturus*.[11] These glands are more important in calcium balance of early terrestrial urodeles and especially of anurans.

Ultimobranchial Glands. The amphibian ultimobranchial glands develop from the fifth pharyngeal arches. Most urodeles have only one ultimobranchial gland (usually on the left side). In apodans, anurans and some urodeles (for example, *Necturus* and *Amphiuma*) the ultimobranchial glands are paired. Calcitonin has been demonstrated immunologically in the ultimobranchial glands of *Rana temporaria* and *R. pipiens.*[71] Cytologically the ultimobranchial gland consists of one or more simple follicles containing only one epithelial cellular type. This cell has been termed a C cell and is one of the APUD cellular types (see Chap. 1). The C cell may appear in either a "dark" form (relatively electron dense) or in a less electron-dense "light" form, at least in anurans.[15]

In addition to the C cells, the ultimobranchial gland of *Chthonerpeton indistinctum,* an apodan, contains two types of neuronal endings, presumably cholinergic and purinergic.[72] Although the presence of sympathetic neurons has been demonstrated in the frog *R. pipiens,*[58] most anurans investigated do not exhibit innervation of the ultimobranchial glands. The condition of the urodele ultimobranchial gland with respect to innervation has not been described.

Parathyroid Glands. The parathyroid glands appear to develop from the third and fourth pharyngeal pouches as they do in mammals. Careful histological studies conducted on developing *R. temporaria* indicate that the parathyroid cells actually arise from neuroectodermal pharyngeal components rather than from endoderm.[54] In apodan parathyroids, only chief cells are present.[72] Two cellular types have been described for anurans, but they appear to be two forms of chief cells that occur in light and dark phases.[14] In contrast to the condition of apodans and anurans, two distinct cellular types have been reported for parathyroids in the urodele *Cynops pyrrhogaster.*[64] One of these cells is considered to be only a "supportive" cell, however.

Endolymphatic Sacs. In addition to cellular bone, the endolymphatic sacs located at the base of the skull appear to be major targets for factors regulating calcium homeostasis. These sacs contain large amounts of calcium carbonate and may be important reservoirs of these ions, particularly during metamorphosis and subsequent ossification of bones.[59,60] These structures may also provide bicarbonate ions for buffering the blood following the dissociation of calcium carbonate.

Calcium and Phosphate Homeostasis. The parathyroids, pituitary gland and ultimobranchial glands have been implicated in calcium and phosphate metabolism.[11,59,60] The vitamin D complex seems to be related to at least some actions of PTH in amphibians.[60] Removal of the ultimobranchial glands in frogs generally causes an increase in osteoclast activity and a consequent increase in blood calcium levels.[61] The ultimobranchial glands also prevent removal of calcium from the endolymphatic sacs and block uptake of calcium through the gut.[59]

Parathyroidectomy causes a decrease in plasma Ca^{++} in anurans[60] and in the newt *C. pyrrhogaster.*[48,60] No changes in serum Ca^{++} occur following parathyroidectomy of immature giant salamanders, *Megalobatrachus davidianus*[49] and additional studies are needed in urodeles to clarify this apparent dichotomy. Administration of bovine PTH to frogs increases plasma Ca^{++} and decreases plasma HPO_4^{-2}, implying that the kidney may also be a target for PTH. There appears to be a seasonal variation in the activity of parathyroid glands in frogs that also influences the activity of the ultimobranchial bodies.[61] In general the amphibians regulate plasma Ca^{++} and HPO_4^{-2} similarly to mammals.

Class Reptilia

The regulation of calcium and phosphate in lizards has been well studied, and in recent years these investigations have been extended to include snakes and turtles.[9,10] Both ultimobranchial glands and parathyroids have been described, and regulation of calcium is essentially like that in other tetrapods. The major sites for endocrine regulation of calcium metabolism are the kidney, cellular bone and the endolymphatic sacs, which in lizards, as in amphibians, are important reserves of calcium and carbonate ions.

Ultimobranchial Glands. The ultimobranchial glands of reptiles are located near the thyroid and parathyroid glands. They are small glands consisting primarily of follicles. All the reptilian ultimobranchials are innervated, although the nature of these neuronal endings has not been examined extensively. In crocodilians, chelonians and in some snakes the ultimobranchial glands are paired. In lizards only the left gland persists. Seasonal changes in the cytology of ultimobranchial glands have been reported for a few species, but the relationship between these changes and physiological and environmental parameters has not been ascertained.

Parathyroid Glands. Four reptilian parathyroids develop from the third and fourth pharyngeal pouches as described for the amphibians, and they resemble the mammalian parathyroids cytologically. Adult lizards and crocodilians have only one pair of parathyroid glands, whereas snakes and turtles retain all four glands. In addition to cellular cords, the presence of follicles containing PAS (+) material is a common feature of reptilian parathyroids.[8] The functional significance of these parathyroid follicles is not known. Figure 12-8 shows the parathyroid gland of *Graptemys pseudogeographica,* the false map turtle.

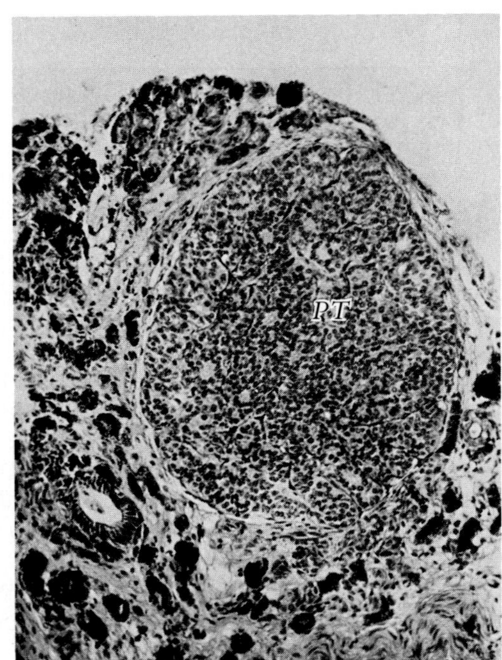

Fig. 12-8. Parathyroid gland of the false map turtle *Graptemys pseudogeographica,* surrounded by ultimobranchial tissue. *PT,* parathyroid. (Photomicrograph courtesy of Dr. Nancy B. Clark.)

Calcium and Phosphate Homeostasis. Parathyroidectomy of lizards and snakes causes a marked decrease in plasma Ca^{++} accompanied by tetany. However, there is little or no change in circulating Ca^{++} in turtles following a similar operation, and tetany does not occur in turtles. This insensitivity of turtles to parathyroidectomy is apparently a consequence of the immense calcium reservoir represented by the shell. Treatment with mammalian PTH causes increased plasma Ca^{++} and urinary HPO_4^{-2} as well as decreased urinary Ca^{++} and plasma HPO_4^{-2} in both lizards and turtles.

The renal action of mammalian parathyroid extracts on HPO_4^{-2} excretion is marked in parathyroidectomized snakes (four species of *Natrix*) although calcium excretion is probably not affected significantly.[13] Thus it appears that reptiles possess basically the same regulatory control of calcium homeostasis as exhibited by mammalian parathyroids.

The role of CT in reptiles is uncertain.[9,10] Extracts of reptilian ultimobranchial glands produce hypocalcemia when injected into rats, and salmon CT has been shown to lower Ca^{++} in the green iguana.[37] As with fishes and amphibians, when reptilian ultimobranchial factors are tested in mammals the presence of hypocalcemic factors is noted, but their endogenous physiological roles are not known.

Class Aves

There are typically four parathyroid glands in birds, and ultimobranchial glands are present. Cytologically the parathyroid glands resemble those of mammals, and the ultimobranchial cells are like the mammalian C cell. The regulation of calcium and phosphate homeostasis is typically mammalian with only minor differences.[1,3,12] It should be noted, however, that few avian species have been investigated thoroughly, and most of the studies have been conducted with domestic birds.

Parathyroid Glands. Avian parathyroid glands are separate and usually distinct, except for a few species, such as the domestic chicken, in which some fusion of the separate parathyroids may occur. Cytologically the parathyroid glands contain only chief cells; no oxyphils have been reported.

Ultimobranchial Glands. The ultimobranchial glands are usually separate structures although some fusion with the thyroid gland occurs in the pigeon. There are both light and dark cells in chicken ultimobranchials. The light cell is more abundant and resembles the mammalian C cell cytologically. A rich vagal innervation (parasympathetic) has been described for the chicken,[2] but its importance has not been elucidated.

Calcium and Phosphate Homeostasis. Parathyroidectomy in birds usually causes marked hypocalcemia accompanied by tetanic seizures and death within 24 hours. This degree of sensitivity to parathyroidectomy is not manifest on this time scale in amphibians or reptiles and may be related to the much higher body temperature of birds. Treatment with mammalian parathyroid extracts produces marked increases in plasma Ca^{++}. Dietary deprivation of Ca^{++} or vitamin D causes marked hypertrophy and hyperplasia of the parathyroid glands, whereas high Ca^{++} diets result in regression of the parathyroids.[1] As in mammals, estrogens and parathyroid extracts both increase levels of 1,25-DHC in Japanese quail.[63]

Mammalian parathyroid extract stimulates renal excretion of phosphate in normal starlings but does not seem to alter renal treatment of calcium.[12] The effect of mammalian parathyroid extract or PTH on avian bone is similar to that described for mammals.

Calcitonins that are structurally similar to mammalian CT have been isolated from chickens and turkeys and are potent hypocalcemic agents in both birds and mammals[1] (Table 12-7). Dietary levels of calcium are directly related to ultimobranchial activities, and high levels of Ca^{++} cause marked stimulatory changes.[7,46]

Summary

Precise regulation of calcium and phosphate homeostasis is necessary for many processes in vertebrates. In birds and mammals this regula-

Table 12-7. *Calcitonin Activity in Tissue Extracts from Domestic Chicken and Pig as Bioassayed in Sprague-Dawley Rats*[68]

TISSUE	EXTRACTION PROCEDURE	BIOLOGICAL ACTIVITY UNITS/mg
Chicken ultimobranchial	Urea-HCl-Cysteine	553
Chicken thyroid	Urea-HCl-Cysteine	1.6
Pig thyroid[a]	Urea-HCl-Cysteine	261
Chicken ultimobranchial	Hot-HCl	238
Chicken thyroid	Hot-HCl	0
Pig thyroid[a]	Hot-HCl	115

[a]Includes parafollicular or C cells of ultimobranchial origin.

tion is accomplished through secretion of hypercalcemic PTH from the parathyroid glands and hypocalcemic CT produced by the C-cells embedded between the follicles of the thyroid gland (mammals) or by the ultimobranchial glands (birds). Parathyroid hormone increases plasma calcium levels through direct and indirect action on bone, kidney and intestine. Parathyroidectomy invariably brings about tetany and usually death as a consequence of the decrease in circulating Ca^{++} following this operation. This condition can be alleviated through administration of PTH or calcium. The actions of PTH on bone may be anabolic (bone formation mediated through the osteoblasts) or catabolic (bone reabsorption via the osteoclasts). In addition to the effect of PTH on calcium, PTH stimulates renal excretion of phosphate ions. Both the resorption of bone and the kidney action of PTH may be dependent on a derivative of vitamin D, 1,25-DHC. The uptake of calcium through the intestinal wall requires 1,25-DHC. Synthesis of 1,25-DHC involves sequential intermediates produced in the skin, altered in the liver and finally converted to 1,25-DHC in the cortical portion of the kidney. This enzymatic conversion in the kidney may be influenced by PTH as well as by estrogens and prolactin.

Calcitonin has been isolated from mammalian parafollicular thyroid tissue and from bird ultimobranchial glands. The major site of action for CT is bone, where it antagonizes the action of PTH on osteoclasts.

The comparative aspects of calcium and phosphate regulation are complicated by the absence of parathyroid glands in fishes. Cyclostomes and elasmobranchs have not been studied sufficiently to provide any insight into the endocrine regulation of these ions. Among bony fishes, calcium regulation appears to be accomplished by a hypercalcemic pituitary factor (prolactin or hypercalcin) and a hypercalcemic factor (hypocalcin) from the CS embedded in the kidneys of some bony fishes. The pituitary factors appears to be the more important regulator in fresh water and the CS appears to regulate calcium in sea water. Calcitonin can decrease blood calcium, and the major target appears to be the gills. Salmon CT is a more potent vertebrate hypocalcemic factor than mammalian CT, and this greater potency may be a result of its relative resistance to clearance from the circulation and degradation. It is currently used for clinical treatment in situations of CT insufficiency.

Parathyroid glands are distinct in amphibians and reptiles, and the effects of PTH and parathyroidectomy are similar to those observed in birds and mammals but occur with lessened intensity. The pituitary may have a hypercalcemic role in aquatic amphibians. Amphibians and some reptiles possess endolymphatic sacs, which may be important sites for calcium carbonate storage. These endolymphatic sacs may be involved in acid-base balance through the actions of PTH. No role for CT has been demonstrated in these groups, although extracts of their ultimobranchial glands have hypocalcemic activity when tested in birds or mammals.

One feature which appears to be dominant throughout the tetrapods examined is the strong tendency for innervation of the ultimobranchial glands, although the nature of this innervation (e.g., cholinergic, adrenergic) and biological significance are not clear. Mammalian parafollicular cells contain both CT and somatostatin implying a paracrine role for these cells.

A second consistent relationship appears in all oviparous species except the cyclostomes and possibly the elasmobranchs. Estrogens increase the production of vitellogenic proteins by the liver which bind Ca^{++} when they are secreted into the blood. Consequently, there is an elevation in total plasma calcium associated with vitellogenesis in females which appears to be a mechanism whereby increased Ca^{++} ions become available for production of egg shells (birds and reptiles) and/or for incorporation into the eggs. Egg stores of Ca^{++} ions are used for early developmental processes prior to hatching and feeding by the offspring. A similar mechanism operates in mammals whereby maternal dietary calcium is directed during development or during lactation to the offspring with minimal damage to the maternal skeleton. Estrogens also stimulate production of 1,25-DHC in both birds and mammals.

References

1. Assenmacher, I. (1973). The peripheral endocrine glands. In D.S. Farner and J.R. King, eds., Avian Biology. Academic Press, New York, Vol. 3, pp. 183–286.
2. Barzel, U.S. (1970). Role of parathyroid hormone in acid-base homeostasis. Lancet 2:1363.
3. Belanger, L.F. (1971). The ultimobranchial gland of birds and the effects of nutritional variations. J. Exp. Zool. 178:125–138.
4. Buffa, R., J.P. Chayvaille, P. Fontana, L. Usellini, C. Capella and E. Solcia (1979). Parafollicular cells of rabbit thyroid store both calcitonin and somatostatin and resemble gut D cells ultrastructurally. Histochemistry 62:281–288.
5. Canalis, E. (1983). The hormonal and local regulation of bone formation. Endocrine Revs. 4:62–77.
6. Chan, D.K.O. (1972). Hormonal regulation of calcium balance in teleost fish. Gen. Comp. Endocrinol. Suppl. 3:411–420.
7. Chan, D.K.O., J.C. Rankin and I. Chester Jones (1969). Influence of the adrenal cortex and the corpuscles of Stannius on osmoregulation in the European eel (*Anguilla anguilla L.*) adapted to fresh water. Gen. Comp. Endocrinol. Suppl. 2:342–353.
8. Clark, N.B. (1967). Parathyroid glands in reptiles. Am. Zool. 7:869–881.
9. Clark, N.B. (1971). The ultimobranchial body of reptiles. J. Exp. Zool. 178:115–124.
10. Clark, N.B. (1972). Calcium regulation in reptiles. Gen. Comp. Endocrinol. Suppl. 3:430–440.
11. Clark, N.B. (1983). Evolution of calcium regulation in lower vertebrates. Am. Zool. 23:719–727.
12. Clark, N.B., E.J. Braun and R.F. Wideman, Jr. (1976). Parathyroid hormone and renal excretion of phosphate and calcium in normal starlings. Am. J. Physiol. 231:1152–1158.
13. Clark, N.B. and W.H. Dantzler (1972). Renal tubular transport of calcium and phosphate in snakes: Role of parathyroid hormone. Am. J. Physiol. 223:1455–1464.
14. Coleman, R. (1969). Ultrastructural observations on the parathyroid glands of *Xenopus laevis* Daudin. Z. Zellforsch. 100:201–214.
15. Coleman, R. (1975). The development and fine structure of ultimobranchial glands in larval anurans. Cell Tissue Res. 164:215–232.
16. Cooper, C.W., W.H. Schwesinger, A.M. Mahgoub and D.A. Ontjes (1971). Thyrocalcitonin: Stimulation of secretion by pentagastrin. Science 172:1238–1240.
17. Copp, C.W., (1969). Review. Endocrine control of calcium homeostasis. J. Endocrinol. 43:137–161.
18. Copp, D.H. (1972). Calcium regulation in birds. Gen. Comp. Endocrinol. Suppl. 3:441–447.
19. Copp, D.H., E.C. Cameron, B. Cheney, A.G.F. Davidson and K.G. Henze (1962). Evidence for calcitonin—a new hormone from the parathyroid that lowers blood calcium. Endocrinology 70:638–649.
20. Copp, D.H., D.W. Cockroft and Y. Kueh (1967). Calcitonin from ultimobranchial glands of dogfish and chickens. Science 158:924–925.
21. Dacke, C.G. (1979). Calcium Regulation in Submammalian Vertebrates. Academic Press, New York.
22. DeLuca, H.F. (1971). The role of vitamin D and its relationship to parathyroid hormone and calcitonin. Recent Prog. Horm. Res. 27:479–510.
23. DeLuca, H.F., H. Moril and M.J. Melancon (1968). The interaction of Vitamin D, parathyroid hormone and calcitonin. In R.V. Talmage and F.F. Belander, eds., Parathyroid Hormone and Thyrocalcitonin (Calcitonin). Excerpta Medica, Amsterdam, pp. 448–454.
24. Fleming, W.R., J. Brehe and R. Hanson (1973). Some complicating factors in the study of the calcium metabolism of teleosts. Am. Zool. 13:793–798.
25. Fontaine, J. (1979). Multistep migration of calcitonin cell precursors during ontogeny of the mouse pharynx. Gen. Comp. Endocrinol. 37:81–92.
26. Fontaine, M. (1964). Corpuscles de Stannius et regulation ionique (Ca, K, Na) du millieu interieur de l'anguille *(Anguilla anguilla* L.). C.R. Acad. Sci. 259:875–878.
27. Ford, P. (1959). Some observations on the corpuscles of Stannius. In A. Gorbman, ed., Comparative Endocrinology. John Wiley and Sons, New York, pp. 728–734.
28. Frieden, E. and H. Lipner (1971). Biochemical Endocrinology of the Vertebrates. Prentice-Hall, Englewood Cliffs, N.J.
29. Godwin, M.C. (1937). Complex IV in the dog with special emphasis on the relation of the ultimobranchial body to interfollicular cells in the post-natal thyroid gland. Am. J. Anat. 60:299–340.
30. Greep, R.O. (1948). The physiology and chemistry of the parathyroid hormone. In G. Pincus and K.V. Thimann, eds., The Hormones. Academic Press, New York, Vol. 1, pp. 255–300.
31. Habener, J., B.W. Kemper, A. Rich, and J.T. Potts, Jr. (1977). Biosynthesis of parathyroid hormone. Recent Prog. Horm. Res. 33:249–398.
32. Hodges, R.D. and R.P. Gould (1969). Partial nervous control of the avian ultimobranchial body. Experientia 25:1317–1319.
33. Irving, J.T. (1973). Calcium and Phosphorus Metabolism. Academic Press, New York.
34. Jacobs, J.W., R.H. Goodman, W.W. Chin, P.C. Dee, J.F. Habener, N.H. Bell and J.T. Potts, Jr. (1981). Calci-

tonin messenger RNA encodes multiple polypeptides in a single precursor. Science 313:457–459.

35. Katz, A.I. and M.D. Lindheimer (1977). Actions of hormones on the kidney. Annu. Rev. Physiol. 39:97–134.

36. Klein, D.C. and L.G. Raisz (1970). Prostaglandins: Stimulation of bone resorption in tissue culture. Endocrinology 86:1436–1440.

37. Kline, L.W. (1981). A hypocalcemic response to synthetic salmon calcitonin in the green iguana, *Iguana iguana*. Gen. Comp. Endocrinol. 44:476–479.

38. Kolata, G. (1975). Vitamin D: Investigations of a new steroid hormone. Science 187:635–636.

39. LaRoche, G., A.N. Woodall, C.L. Johnson and J.E. Halver (1966). Thyroid function in the rainbow trout (*Salmo gaidnerii* Rich). II. Effects of thyroidectomy on the development of young fish. Gen. Comp. Endocrinol. 6:249–266.

40. Lawson, D.E.M., D.R. Fraser, E. Kodicek, H.R. Morris and D.H. Williams (1971). Identification of 1,25-dihydrocholecalciferol, a new kidney hormone controlling calcium metabolism. Nature 230:228–230.

41. LeDouarin, N. and C. LeLièvre (1970). Demonstratiion de l'origine neurale des allules á calcitonine du corps ultimobranchial chez l'embryon de poulet. C.R. Acad. Sci. 270:2857–2860.

42. Lofts, B. and H.A. Bern (1972). The functional morphology of steroidogenic tissues. In D.R. Idler, ed., Steroids in Non-mammalian Vertebrates. Academic Press, New York, pp. 37–125.

43. Louw, G.N., W.S. Suton, and A.D. Kenny (1967). Action of thyrocalcitonin in the teleost fish *Ictalurus melas*. Nature 215:888–889.

44. Luben, R.A., G.L. Wong and D.V. Cohn (1976). Biochemical characterization with parathormone and calcitonin of isolated bone cells: Provisional identification of osteoblasts and osteoblasts. Endocrinology 99:526–534.

45. Milhaud, G., L. Bolis and A.A. Benson (1980). Calcitonin, A major gill hormone. Proc. Natl. Acad. Sci. (U.S.) 77:6935–6936.

46. Mueller, G.L., C.S. Anast and R.P. Breitenbach (1970). Dietary calcium and ultimobranchial body and parathyroid gland in the chicken. Am. J. Physiol. 218:1718–1722.

47. Norris, D.O. Unpublished observations.

48. Oguro, C. (1969). Are the parathyroid glands necessary to the life of the newt, *Cynops pyrrhogaster?* Endocrinol. Jap. 16:555–556.

49. Oguro, C. (1973). Parathyroid gland and serum calcium concentration in the giant salamander, *Megalobatrachus davidianus*. Gen. Comp. Endocrinol. 21:565–568.

50. Pang, P.K.T. (1973). Endocrine control of calcium metabolism in teleosts. Am. Zool. 13:775–792.

51. Pang, P.K.T., R.W. Griffith, J. Maetz and P. Pic (1980). Branchial calcium uptake in fishes. In B. Lahlou, ed., Epithelial Transport in the Lower Vertebrates. Cambridge University Press, Cambridge, pp. 121–132.

52. Pang, P.K.T., A.D. Kenny and C. Oguro (1980). Evolution of endocrine control of calcium regulation. In P.K.T. Pang and A. Epple, eds., Evolution of Vertebrate Endocrine Systems. Texas Tech Press, Lubbock, Texas, pp. 323–356.

53. Pang, P.K.T., R.K. Pang and W.H. Sawyer (1974). Environmental calcium and the sensitivity of killfish *(Fundulus heteroclitus)* in bioassays for the hypocalcemic response to Stannius corpuscles from killfish and cod (*Gadus morhua*). Endocrinology 94:548–555.

54. Pang., P.K.T. and W.H. Sawyer (1975). Parathyroid hormone preparations, salmon calcitonin and urine flow in the South American lungfish, *Lepidosiren paradoxa*. J. Exp. Zool. 193:407–412.

55. Parsons, J.A. (1979). Physiology of parathyroid hormone. In L.J. DeGroot et al., eds., Endocrinology. Grune and Stratton, New York, pp. 621–629.

56. Pearse, A.G.E. and T. Takor Takor (1976). Neuroendocrine embryology and the APUD concept. Clin. Endocrinol. 5, Suppl. 229s–244s.

57. Powles, T.J. (1973). Aspirin inhibition of *in vitro* osteolysis stimulated by parathyroid hormone and PGE. Nature 255:83–84.

58. Robertson, D.R. (1967). The ultimobranchial body in *Rana pipiens*. III. Sympathetic innervation of the secretory parenchyma. Z. Zellforsch. 78:328–340.

59. Robertson, D.R. (1971). Endocrinology of amphibian ultimobranchial glands. J. Exp. Zool. 178:101–114.

60. Robertson, D.R. (1972). Influence of the parathyroids and ultimobranchial glands in the frog *(Rana pipiens)* during respiratory acidosis. Gen. Comp. Endocrinol. Suppl. 3:421–429.

61. Robertson, D.R. (1977). The annual pattern of plasma calcium in the frog and the seasonal effect of ultimobranchialectomy and parathyroidectomy. Gen. Comp. Endocrinol. 33:336–343.

62. Sammon, P.J., R.E. Stacey and F. Bronner (1970). Role of parathyroid hormone in calcium homeostasis and metabolism. Am. J. Physiol. 218:479–485.

63. Sedran, S.H., T.G. Taylor and M. Akhtar (1981). The regulation of 25-hydroxycholecaliferol metabolism in the kidney of Japanese quail *(Coturnix coturnix japonica)* by sex steroids and by parathyroid extract. Gen. Comp. Endocrinol. 44:514–523.

64. Setogouchi, T., H. Isono and S. Sakurai (1970). Electron microscopic study on the parathyroid gland of the newt *Triturus pyrrhogaster* (Boie) in natural hibernation. J. Ultrastruct. Res. 31:46–60.

65. Sherwood, L.M., G.P. Mayer, C.F. Ramberg, Jr., D.S. Kronfield, G.D. Aurbach and J.T. Potts, Jr. (1968). Regulation of parathyroid hormone secretion: Proportional control by calcium, lack of effect of phosphate. Endocrinology 83:1043–1051.

66. Swarup, K. and S.P. Srivastava (1982). Vitamin D_3-induced hypercalcemia in male catfish, *Clarias batrachus*. Gen. Comp. Endocrinol. 46:271–274.

67. Talmage, R.F., C.W. Cooper and H.Z. Park (1970). Regulation of calcium transport in bone by parathyroid hormone. Vitam. Horm. 38:103–140.

68. Tauber, S.D. (1967). The ultimobranchial origin of thyrocalcitonin. Proc. Natl. Acad. Sci. 58:1684–1687.

69. Taylor, T.G., P.E. Lewis and O. Balderstone (1975). Role of calcitonin in protecting the skeleton during pregnancy and lactation. J. Endocrinol. 66:297–298.

70. Urist, M.R., R.J. DeLange and G.A.M. Finerman (1983). Bone cell differentiation and growth factors. Science 220:680–686.

71. Van Noorden, S., and A.G.E. Pearse (1971). Immunofluorescent localisation of calcitonin in the ultimobranchial gland of *Rana temporaria* and *Rana pipiens*. Histochemie 26:95–97.

72. Welsch, U. and C. Schubert (1975). Observations on the fine structure, enzyme histochemistry and innervation of parathyroid gland and ultimobranchial body of *Chthonerpton indistinctum* (Gymnophiona, Amphibia). Cell Tissue Res. 164:105–119.

73. Wendelaar Bonga, S.E. (1981). Effect of synthetic salmon calcitonin on protein-bound and free plasma calcium in the teleost *Gasterosteus aculeatus*. Gen. Comp. Endocrinol. 43:123–126.

74. Wills, M.R. (1970). Fundamental physiological role of parathyroid hormone in acid-base homeostasis. Lancet 2:802–804.

75. Zarrow, M.X., J.M. Yochin and J.L. McCarthy (1964). Experimental Endocrinology: A Source-book of Basic Techniques. Academic Press, New York.

13·The Endocrine Pancreas

The Mammalian Pancreas

The mammalian pancreas plays essential roles in digestion and metabolism. The digestive role is accomplished by the exocrine glandular portion of the pancreas which produces digestive enzymes. The endocrine portion of the pancreas influences metabolism by secreting hormones that regulate carbohydrate, lipid and protein metabolism.

The exocrine or acinar pancreas secretes digestive juices into the pancreatic duct whereby they reach the lumen of the small intestine. (An acinus is similar in structure to a follicle except that the lumen of the acinus makes contact with a duct through which the secretion products of the epithelium [acinar cells] are transported.) This pancreatic juice contains digestive enzymes and bicarbonate ions that buffer the acidic material entering the small intestine from the stomach.

The endocrine pancreas consists of small masses or islands or islets of endocrine cells scattered among the acinar tissue (Figs. 13-1–13-3). The pancreatic islets secrete *insulin, glucagon, somatostatin* (growth hormone release-inhibiting hormone) and an additional peptide known as *pancreatic polypeptide.* Insulin is primarily a hypoglycemic agent that lowers blood glucose, whereas glucagon is hyperglycemic. Both of these hormones produce effects on lipid and protein metabolism as well. The roles for pancreatic somatostatin and pancreatic polypeptide are not established.

Recognition for the role of the endocrine pancreas in blood glucose regulation originated from observations of the clinical syndrome *diabetes mellitus.* This disease was first described by the Greek physician Aretaeus in about 1500 B.C. as a condition where "flesh and bones run together" and are siphoned into the urine. The term diabetes, a siphon, comes from the Greek word diabainein: *dia* through + *bainein* to go. Indian physicians reported the sweet taste of the diabetic's urine in the 6th century. The term mellitus referring to the presence of glucose in the urine was added in the 18th century. This condition was always fatal. There is more than one form of diabetes mellitus, but here we refer to the type related to insufficient production of insulin.

Diabetes mellitus is characterized by the production of large quantities of glucose-containing urine. Normally little or no glucose should appear in the urine. It was the presence of glucose in the urine of pancreatectomized dogs that first linked diabetes mellitus to a possible disorder of the pancreas.[57]

The occurrence of glucose in the urine results from excessively high circulating levels of glucose as a result of the failure by the endocrine pancreas to secrete adequate amounts of insulin. Blood levels of glucose become elevated, resulting in more glucose in the glomerular filtrate produced in the kidney. The proximal convoluted portion of each nephron transports all glucose that appears in the glomerular filtrate back into the blood under normal conditions. However, should blood sugar levels be sufficiently high, so much glucose enters the glomerular filtrate that the recovery transport mechanism is saturated, and all of the glucose cannot be returned to the blood. Some glucose remains in the nephron, and its presence in the urine upsets the osmotic balance between urine and blood. Consequently

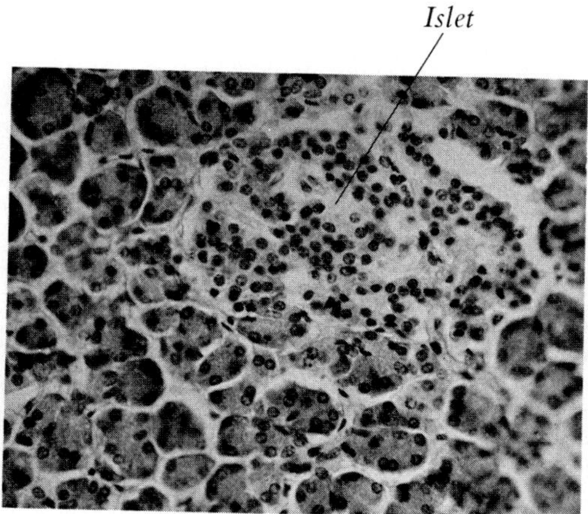

FIG. 13-1. Mammalian pancreatic islet embedded within acinar cells.

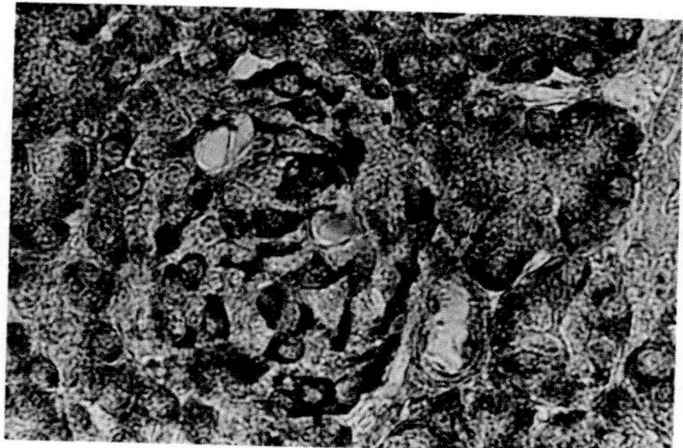

FIG. 13-3. Pancreatic islet of owl monkey (*Aotes* sp.). This islet exhibits mixture of cellular types characteristic of adult primate islets. The number of D cells *(black)* is somewhat higher than normal. (Courtesy of Dr. August Epple.)

less water can be reabsorbed and a greater volume of urine is produced. Because of the increased water loss associated with the loss of glucose in the urine this syndrome achieved the descriptive title of the pissing evil during the Middle Ages.

Other consequences of the inadequacy of insulin production contribute to water losses as well. Reduction in glucose availability causes increased utilization of fats and proteins for energy (see Chap. 19). Proteins are hydrolyzed to amino acids that are in turn deaminated to produce carbohydrates plus ammonia. Most of the highly toxic ammonia is converted to urea and excreted through the urine. Urea excretion places an additional demand on water required for removal, contributing to increased urine production. Lipid stores are mobilized to help compensate for carbohydrate shortages in the diabetic. Fats are hydrolyzed to glycerol and fatty acids, which in turn are oxidized directly for energy. In the process of fatty acid oxidation a number of by-products accumulate, including β-hydroxybutyrate, acetone and acetoacetic acid. These substances are known as *ketone bodies,* and their generation is referred to as *ketogenesis.* Ketone bodies increase in the blood (ketonemia) and consequently appear in the urine (ketonuria) and contribute to additional water losses through increased urine production.

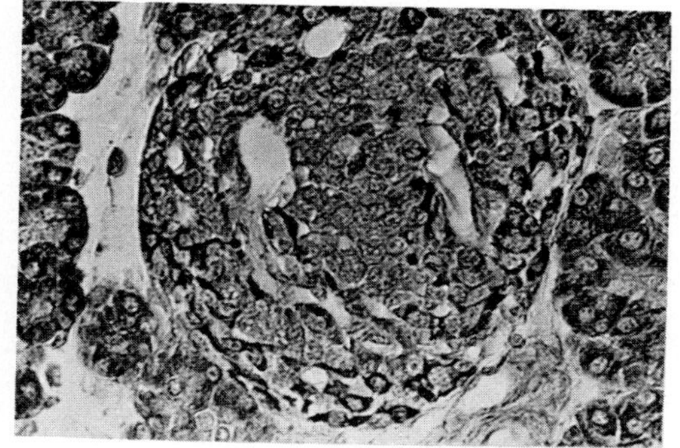

FIG. 13-2. Pancreatic islet of young chimpanzee (*Pan* sp.). Islet exhibits peripheral arrangement of D cells *(black)* as seen in human fetal islets. A cells *(unstained)* are scattered among D cells. The central portion of the islet is occupied by B cells. (Courtesy of Dr. August Epple.)

The diabetic individual suffers from an important nutrient loss, and metabolic alterations occur in an attempt to compensate for these losses. The loss of glucose into the urine and increased production of nitrogenous wastes and ketone bodies all contribute to a process of desiccation.

Development of the Mammalian Pancreas

The vertebrate pancreas develops from the endodermal lining of the primitive or embryonic gut (endoderm). A dorsal bud from the embryonic intestine fuses with one or two ventral buds to form the definitive pancreas. Usually only the dorsal connection to the intestine is retained as the exocrine pancreatic duct. The exocrine tissue in the developing pancreas can be identified by the formation of small ductules. These ductules coalesce into larger ducts until they form one or more large pancreatic ducts connecting the exocrine pancreas with the lumen of the small intestine. Small buds develop from the ductules and can be identified as solid clumps or islands of cells dispersed among the exocrine tissue. The clumps are referred to as the *islets of Langerhans*. In addition, some of the endocrine cells may be scattered singly or in groups of only a few cells throughout various regions of the pancreas.

Although the islets originate as outgrowths from the pancreatic ductules the actual origin for these cells is not clear. It has been suggested that they arise from mesoderm, from neural crest cells of neuroectodermal origin and from endoderm of the gastrointestinal tract.[1,17,48,51] The islet cells are not derived from neural crest, at least in birds,[2] and it is probable that mammalian islet cells are not derived from either neural crest or other neuroectoderm.[50] Transplantation of quail neural crest cells containing a unique cytological marker into chick embryos confirms their incorporation into the avian pancreas, but they do not give rise to the pancreatic endocrine cells.[21] Instead they differentiate into parasympathetic ganglia. Until this matter is clarified, it might be legitimate to refer to the endocrine pancreas as being of endodermal origin.

Several functional schemes have been proposed for the origins of the endocrine pancreatic cells that are divorced from their possible germ layer origins.[16] It is possible that these endocrine cells represent modified gastrointestinal mucosal cells that initially synthesized "inducers." Exocrine cells in teleosts that are homologous to avian and mammalian islet cells often possess a zymogen mantle, presumably induced by secretions of the adjacent pancreatic endocrine cells. Another suggestion is that these cells originally secreted hydrolytic enzymes related to digestion but that these "enzymes" have lost their catalytic properties and become hormones.[55] In either event these modified mucosal cells presumably lost their contact with the gut mucosa and specialized as centers for internal secretion. The similarity of peptides produced in the islet cells and those of the gastrointestinal tract (see Chap. 14) supports a common origin for these pancreatic and intestinal cells.

Cellular Types in Vertebrate Pancreatic Islets

At least five different cellular types have been identified in the endocrine pancreas: B, A, D, PP and an unnamed type. The so-called clear cell appears to be a fixation artifact since clear cells are most prevalent in Bouin-fixed material but "disappear" with other fixation procedures.[8] (Bouin's fixative is a standard solution used for preparing tissues for histological and cytological observation.) There are four general vertebrate patterns with respect to the dominant cellular types present in the endocrine pancreas (Tables 13-1, 13-2, 13-3). However, careful analyses indicate that it is misleading to characterize classes of vertebrates as exhibiting a particular pattern (Table 13-4).

B Cells. B cells (β-cells) stain with aldehyde fuchsin (AF+) and pseudoisocyanin (PIC+) following oxidation. The latter staining procedure has been claimed to be specific for insulin granules, but it stains other intracellular structures as well (for example, neurosecretory granules). Immunofluorescent techniques have verified that insulin is produced and stored in the B cell. Several drugs, such as alloxan and streptozotocin, selectively destroy

Table 13-1. *General Patterns of Islet Cellular Type Distributions in Vertebrates with Respect to A and B Cells*

CATEGORY	DOMINANT CYTOLOGY	REPRESENTATIVES
I	B cells mostly	Cyclostomes
II	More than 50% B cells	Teleosts, amphibians, mammals
III	Approx. 50% X cells	Chimaeras
IV	More than 50% A cells	Most lizards, birds

Modified from Epple et al.[14] and Epple A. and T.L. Lewis[16].

TABLE 13-2. *Comparative Cytology of the Endocrine Pancreas with Respect to Relative Predominance of A, B, D and PP cells*

CLASS	A CELLS	B CELLS	D CELLS	PP CELLS
Agnatha				
Hagfish	○	++++	+	?
Chondrichthyes				
Elasmobranchs	+++	++++	+	+
Osteichthyes				
Teleosts	+++	++++	+	+
Amphibia				
Anura and Urodela	+++	++++	+	+
Reptilia				
Sauria	++++	+	+	+
Crocodilia	+++	+++	+	?
Aves	+++++	+++	+	+
Mammalia	++	+++++	+	+

Compiled from many sources.
NOTE: The number of + marks in each column represents only an attempt to show relative abundance and should not be construed as precise ratios.

the B cells and impair the ability of the pancreas to secrete insulin. The affected B cells undergo a process of *hydropic degeneration* that is characterized by clumping of nuclear chromosomal material (formation of pyknotic nuclei) and eventual cell death. This technique of chemically induced degeneration is often used in experimental animals to selectively remove the insulin-secreting cells without altering the ability of the islets to secrete other pancreatic peptides.

A CELLS. The A cells (α_2-cells) of the pancreatic islets are generally acidophilic and argyrophilic (affinity for silver-staining techniques). They do not stain with AF or PIC procedures. The A cell is considered to be the source of the second major pancreatic hormone, glucagon. In some species A cells may contain other peptide hormones in addition to glucagon.[26,54] The round secretory granules in the cytoplasm of the A cells are morphologically distinct from the angular insulin granules of the B cells, making these cells easy to distinguish with the electron microscope (Fig. 13-5). This difference in granule shape is not found in all mammals, however. Treatment with cobalt selectively impairs the ability of A cells to secrete glucagon, but such treatment does not lead to the destructive degeneration such as alloxan produces in the B cells.

TABLE 13-3. *Size of Cytological Granules Representing Stored Hormones in Human Pancreatic Cells*

CELLULAR TYPE	HORMONE PRESENT	GRANULE SIZE (nm)
B cell	Insulin	300
A cell	Glucagon	235
D cell	Somatostatin	230
PP cell	Pancreatic polypeptide	125

Modified from Floyd, J.C., Jr. et al.[19]
NOTE: See text for explanation of cellular types.

D CELLS. D cells (α_1-cells or δ-cells) can be cytochemically distinguished from A cells by applying the toluidine blue staining procedure. They can be further distinguished from A cells and B cells by their staining with PIC following methylation but not following oxidation. Immunoreactive somatostatin has been localized in the D cells, although the physiological significance of somatostatin in the pancreas is not clear. The release of both insulin and glucagon is inhibited in paracrine fashion by somatostatin, and the D cell may influence the secretory activities of the A and B cells.[27] An early suggestion for the role of the D cell

TABLE 13-4. *Percentages of B Cells in the Pancreatic Islets of Selected Adult Mammals*

ORDER	SPECIES	% B CELLS
Rodentia	Rat	60–80
	Guinea pig	60–85
	Golden hamster	80.9
Lagomorpha	Rabbit	
Chiroptera	Bat *(Myotis myotis)*	78.9
Cetacea	Beluga whale	25–97
Carnivora	Dog	75
	Cat	83.2
Perissodactyla	Horse	45–67
Artiodactyla	Cattle	80
	Sheep	30–50
Primates	Monkey *(Maçaca cynomolgus)*	60–74
	Human	60–90
Marsupialia	Red kangaroo	8.1
	Grey kangaroo	15.9
	Brush-tailed possum	52.7

Modified from White and Harrop.[58]

was the production of pancreatic polypeptide. This substance has been localized in a separate cellular type, however, and is apparently not produced by the D cell.

THE PANCREATIC POLYPEPTIDE-SECRETING CELLS. Pancreatic polypeptide (PP) has been localized by immunofluorescence techniques in cells found at the periphery of the endocrine islets as well as in cells scattered throughout the exocrine pancreas.[19] These cells are distinct cytologically and immunologically from B, A and D cells. The distribution of these PP-secreting cells on the periphery of the islets varies greatly among different species, and it is difficult to generalize for all mammals.

AMPHOPHILS. Amphophilic cells have been demonstrated in many mammalian species as well as in sharks, teleosts, amphibians and reptiles, but no conclusions have been generated regarding their functional roles. They may represent either differentiating or degenerating forms, or both, of the other four cellular types that have been implicated in hormonal secretion.

Hormones of the Endocrine Pancreas

The two major pancreatic hormones are the hypoglycemic hormone, insulin, and the hyperglycemic hormone, glucagon. In addition, the pancreatic endocrine cells produce somatostatin and PP. The physiological significance of PP is unknown, but its increase in the circulation following ingestion of a meal suggests a role in postabsorptive metabolism. Somatostatin appears to regulate insulin and glucagon release and may influence release of PP as well.

INSULIN: THE HYPOGLYCEMIC HORMONE. Von Mering and Minkowski in 1889 observed the first correlation between the pancreas and blood sugar regulation when they induced diabetes mellitus in dogs following pancreatectomy.[57] The suspected hypoglycemic factor of the pancreas was later named "insuline" to emphasize its origin from the islets of Langerhans. Purified insulin, however, was not isolated until a physician, Frederick Banting, and a graduate student in physiology and biochemistry, Charles Best, teamed up at the University of Toronto in the summer of 1921. Much of their success was due to the collaborative efforts of J.B. Collip and the project's director, J.J.R. Macleod. Banting and Best traveled the poorer sections of Toronto in their Model-T Ford, nicknamed The Pancreas, purchasing dogs at $1.00 each for their experiments.

The presence of proteolytic enzymes in the exocrine pancreas had thwarted earlier attempts to extract insulin from a whole pancreas. Since it had been shown that tying off the pancreatic duct caused degeneration of the acinar pancreatic tissue but did not affect the islet tissue, Banting suggested they employ this technique to avoid contamination of their extracts with digestive enzymes. The hypoglycemic factor they isolated was first named isletin, but they later changed its name to conform to the earlier proposed name. The importance of the successful isolation of insulin and its use to alleviate the fatal symptoms of diabetes mellitus led to the awarding of the Nobel Prize in Physiology and Medicine for 1923 to Banting and Macleod. Best and Collip were not officially recognized in the award, although the recipients acknowledged them for their contributions.

Techniques for Measurement of Insulin. The standard challenge for the ability of the pancreas to secrete insulin is the *glucose tolerance test.* Following a period of fasting, a glucose load (excessive amount of glucose) is administered orally or intravenously, and its rate of disappearance (clearance) from the blood is measured. The clearance rate for a given glucose load is directly proportional to the secretion of insulin and hence reflects the ability of the pancreas to respond to hyperglycemia with insulin secretion (Table 13-5).

Insulin may also be bioassayed in vitro for its abilities to stimulate uptake of glucose from the medium into cells. Muscle cells from the rat diaphragm are often employed in this bioassay. Radioimmunoassay (RIA), however, is routinely employed to measure circulating insulin levels, and many commercial RIA kits are available for performing these analyses. Insulin RIAs are highly specific, and some can detect the difference between porcine and human insulins that vary in only one amino acid substitution.

Chemistry and Synthesis of Mammalian Insulins. The insulin molecule is a small protein composed of two different polypeptide chains linked together by disulfide bridges. The A chain consists usually of 21 amino acids, and the B chain has 30 amino acid residues. Although insulin was the first protein whose primary structure was elucidated,[52] attempts to synthesize the molecule in cell-free systems were unsuccessful because of the inability to induce proper formation of the disulfide bridges between the two polypeptide chains. Later it was discovered that the B cell synthesizes insulin by first forming a much larger single polypeptide chain that is folded by formation of disulfide bonds (Fig. 13-4). This preproinsulin is synthesized at the rough endoplasmic reticulum and cleaved to a smaller proinsulin molecule. Proinsulin is so constructed that A and B chains of insulin are connected by a chain of amino acids called the C peptide. Hydrolysis of proinsulin occurs at the Golgi apparatus as the result of actions of two proteolytic enzymes. One of these enzymes is trypsin-like in its action, and the other behaves like carboxypeptidase B. The resulting secretion granules contain crystals of insulin and C peptide fragments. The insulin fragment forms a complex with available zinc ions to produce a crystalline hexamer within the se-

Table 13-5. *Comparison of Human Responses to a Standard Glucose Tolerance Test.*

	VENOUS GLUCOSE LEVELS(mg/dl)			
	FASTING	30-MIN.	60-MIN.	120-MIN.
Normal Person	<100	<160	<160	<100
Probable Diabetic	<100 or 100–120	130–159	160–180	110–120
Diabetic	<100 or >110	>150	>160	>120

An abnormal glucose tolerance test can also occur from factors other than diabetes mellitus including improper feeding prior to test, malnutrition, obesity, infection, fever, hyperthyroidism or hypothyroidism, acromegaly, kidney disease and islet cell tumors.

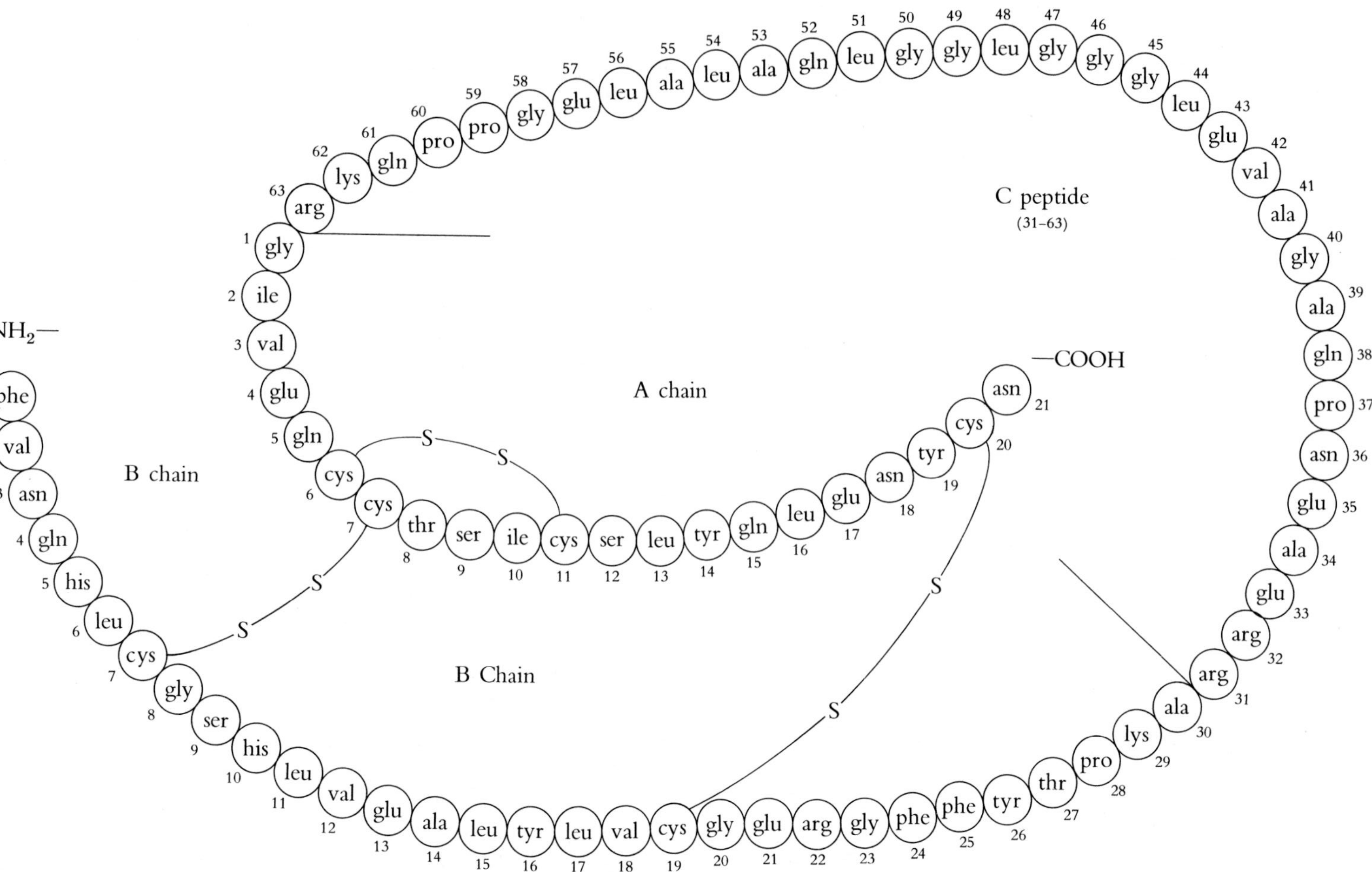

FIG. 13-4. Amino acid sequence of a mammalian proinsulin molecule. Note how the insulin molecule can be formed by cleaving this polypeptide chain at two locations to liberate the C peptide.

cretory granule. It is this crystalline structure that imparts the unique structure to insulin secretion granules in the B cell (Fig. 13-5).

When the contents of the secretory granules are released from the B cells by exocytosis, both insulin and the C peptide enter the blood as does a small amount of unhydrolyzed proinsulin. No function is known for either proinsulin or the C peptide once they have entered the general circulation. The events of synthesis and release of insulin are summarized in Figure 13-6.

Regulation of Insulin Release. Hyperglycemia can directly stimulate release of insulin through a direct action of glucose on the B cell. It is apparently not the presence of glucose but events associated with its metabolism by the B cell that stimulate insulin secretion.[40] Decreases in circulating glucose cause reduction in the secretion of insulin, and it appears that the basic regulatory control mechanism is directed through changes in blood levels of glucose. Any agent capable of elevating circulating glucose levels will also evoke insulin release.

In recent years the importance of nervous regulation of insulin secretion has been demonstrated. Nonmyelinated axonal fibers are present in the islets, and vagal (parasympathetic) stimulation induces insulin release. Similarly, acetylcholine stimulates insulin release, whereas the anticholinergic drug atropine blocks insulin release. Epinephrine, which is a hyperglycemic agent affecting liver, muscle and adipose tissue, also directly blocks the release of insulin. Thus, circulating epinephrine can potentiate its own hyperglycemic action by blocking the normal response of the B cell to increased blood glucose. This action of epinephrine is mediated via β-receptors on the surface of the B cell (see Appendix II).

Somatostatin has been shown to directly inhibit release of insulin from the B cell,[27] and it may play a paracrine role in regulating insu-

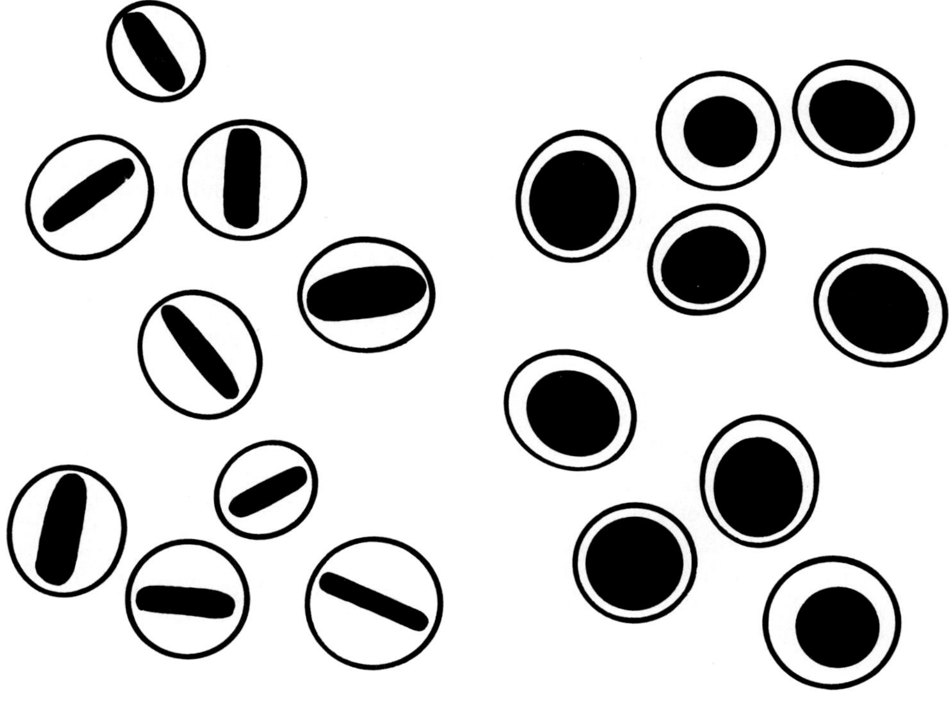

FIG. 13-5. Insulin and glucagon crystals in pancreatic cells. (Drawn from an electron photomicrograph in Fawcett, D.W. (1966). The Cell. W.B. Saunders Co.)

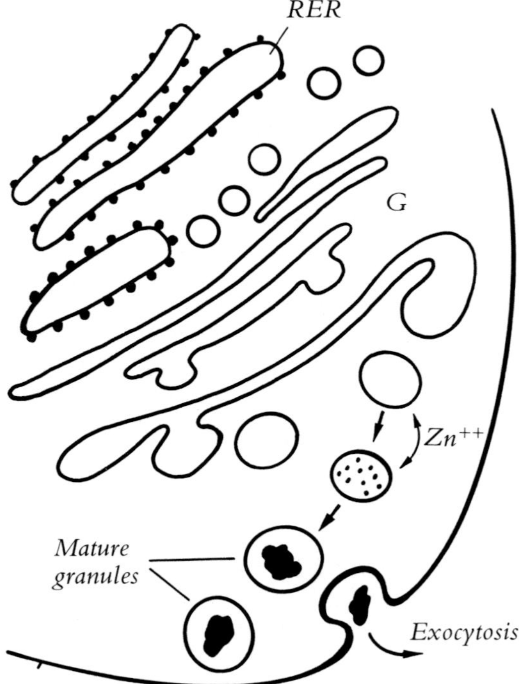

FIG. 13-6. Cellular events associated with the synthesis and release of insulin. Preproinsulin is synthesized at the ribosomes of the rough endoplasmic reticulum *(RER)*. It is cleaved to proinsulin that travels via the cisternae to the Golgi apparatus *(G)* where it is packaged into secretion granules. The proinsulin is hydrolyzed to free insulin within the secretion granule where it forms a complex with zinc ions *(Zn^{++})* to produce the crystals seen in the mature granules. The insulin and the C peptide derived from proinsulin exit from the cell via exocytosis.

lin release locally in the pancreas. It is not known what regulates somatostatin release from the pancreatic D cells.

Actions of Insulin on Target Tissues. Insulin promotes anabolic metabolism and growth through three types of action.[39] After binding to membrane receptors there is an immediate increase in the transport of glucose, amino acids, fatty acids, nucleotides and various ions into the target cell. Within a few minutes enhancement of anabolic pathways and a decrease in catabolic pathways occur (see Chap. 19 for more detail). Finally some hours later, cellular growth is stimulated. This growth-promoting action is due to an interaction between insulin and certain *insulinlike growth factors.*[33] There are a number of these factors including insulinlike growth factors I and II (IGF I, IGF II), somatomedins and multiplication-stimulating factor (MSA). Most of these factors occur in the blood. MSA is a substance isolated only from calf serum and from cultures of liver cells. These factors are all moderately sized polypeptides (7000–9000 daltons) with about 50% amino acid sequence homology to insulin. Nevertheless, these growth factors all have separate membrane receptors from those for insulin (Fig. 13-7). Once insulin binds to its receptor, a proteolytic step is initiated causing formation of glycopeptides which are rapidly internalized.[37] It is the glycopeptides which are believed to regulate the metabolic actions of insulin and to interact with the insulinlike growth factors.

Insulin appears to bring about hypoglycemia through stimulating increased uptake of nutrients from the blood (glucose and amino acids). These nutrients in turn alter metabolic pathways within the responsive cells. Some of these actions are summarized in Table 13-6. Insulin facilitates transport of glucose into muscle and fat cells as well as transport of amino acids into muscle cells. As a consequence, insulin stimulates glucose oxidation and lipogenesis (adipose tissue) and protein synthesis (muscle). Insulin also prevents glycogen breakdown (glycogenolysis) and enhances glycogen synthesis following uptake of glucose in muscle and liver.

Glucose oxidation increases the intracellular pools of precursors for fat synthesis, that is, glycerol, acetylcoenzyme A and fatty acids. In addition to indirectly enhancing lipogenesis, insulin inhibits lipolysis and hence reduces

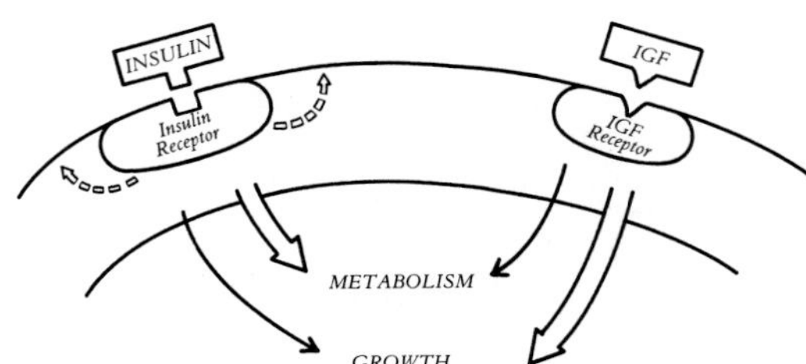

FIG. 13-7. Interaction of insulin and insulinlike growth factors (IGFs) on metabolism and growth. Glycopeptides released after insulin binding to its receptor may mediate insulin's effects on membrane permeability (dotted arrows).

TABLE 13-6. *Actions of Insulin on Various Mammalian Cellular Types*

CELL OR TISSUE	GLUCOSE UPTAKE	RESPONSE		
		GLYCOGENESIS	LIPID UPTAKE	NET TRIGLYCERIDE SYNTHESIS
Skeletal muscle	+	+	0	
Cardiac muscle	+	+		
Adipocytes	+	+	+	+
Cartilage	+	+		
Bone	+	+		
Fibroblasts	+	+		
Leukocytes	+	+		
Mammary gland (during lactation)	+	+		
Erythrocytes, kidney, testis, intestine, lymphoid tissue, brain	0	0		

fatty acid oxidation and formation of ketone bodies (ketogenesis), the by-products of fatty acid oxidation. These actions of insulin on adipose tissue and lipid metabolism are marked in carnivores, but there is little effect of insulin on either glucose metabolism or lipogenesis in herbivorous mammals. Consequently carnivorous mammals are more sensitive to pancreatectomy than are herbivores.

The increase in intracellular glucose and amino acids in both liver and muscle cells promotes protein synthesis. These are important actions of insulin in the postabsorptive state, that is, immediately following ingestion of a meal and the entry of large quantities of digestive products such as glucose and amino acids into the blood.

The details of the mechanism of action for insulin in these cells is not clear even after several decades of intensive research. Many of insulin's effects on muscle and adipose tissues can be explained simply on the basis of changes in permeability of the plasmalemma following the binding of insulin.[22] An extension of this hypothesis is the idea that insulin interacts with structural molecules associated with the plasmalemma and initiates a series of molecular rearrangements that are propagated along the membrane and into the interior of the cell.[37] This event could account for all other observed effects of insulin. Changes in enzyme concentrations reported by many investigators may be a secondary result of altered metabolism stemming from permeability changes associated with binding of insulin to the plasmalemma, and these enzymatic changes may not be the primary cause of the altered metabolism observed.

Insulin may enter the target cell itself, and its mechanism of action may relate to its binding to some intracellular site. On the other hand, internalization of insulin may be only a step in its metabolic degradation. It is very clear that insulin does not operate via activation of adenyl cyclase and formation of a second messenger in the form of cyclic adenosine 3′,5′-monophosphate (cAMP). Insulin may influence the intracellular levels of cyclic guanosine 3′,5′-monophosphate, however, and thus secondarily influence cAMP levels (see Chap. 1).

"Oral Insulins". "Oral insulin" refers to the synthetic hypoglycemic drugs known as *sulfonylureas* and related compounds (Fig. 13-8). Because they are not proteins and thereby not subject to enzymatic degradation in the gut, the sulfonylureas may be taken orally and can relieve the symptoms of diabetes mellitus. Oral insulins thus have considerable therapeutic value in certain types of insulin-deficiency dis-

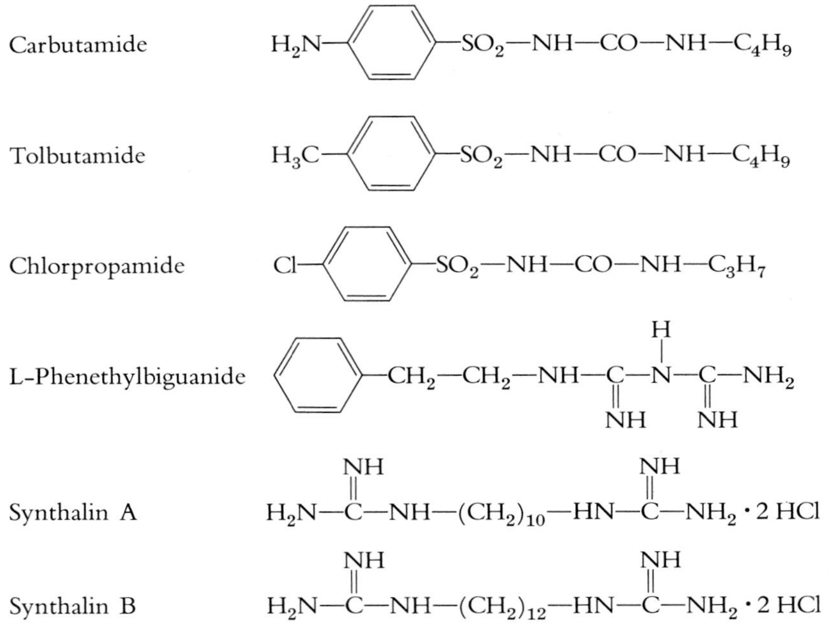

Carbutamide $H_2N-C_6H_4-SO_2-NH-CO-NH-C_4H_9$

Tolbutamide $H_3C-C_6H_4-SO_2-NH-CO-NH-C_4H_9$

Chlorpropamide $Cl-C_6H_4-SO_2-NH-CO-NH-C_3H_7$

L-Phenethylbiguanide $C_6H_5-CH_2-CH_2-NH-C(=NH)-N(H)-C(=NH)-NH_2$

Synthalin A $H_2N-C(=NH)-NH-(CH_2)_{10}-HN-C(=NH)-NH_2 \cdot 2\ HCl$

Synthalin B $H_2N-C(=NH)-NH-(CH_2)_{12}-HN-C(=NH)-NH_2 \cdot 2\ HCl$

Fig. 13-8. Structures of some "oral insulins."

orders. The effectiveness of these drugs may be related to their abilities in displacing insulin from nonspecific binding and noneffective linkages in serum, connective tissues and islet cells to provide marginally effective quantities of insulin for binding to effective (target) sites.[36] If too high a dose is employed, the oral insulins may also block the effective sites as well, and no hypoglycemic effect is observed. The oral insulins are useful only in disorders related to insulin insufficiency and would not be useful in totally pancreatectomized animals or in humans who can not produce insulin. Furthermore, oral insulins are effective only if diet is controlled.[53]

Glucagon: A Hyperglycemic Hormone. The discovery of glucagon was not marked by great publicity or special prizes as was that of insulin, and this second pancreatic hormone has always been overshadowed by the clinical importance of insulin. Glucagon is only one of several hyperglycemic factors, and more attention has been given to growth hormone and epinephrine as hyperglycemic hormones. Glucagon becomes more important in fasting carnivores and in herbivores than it appears to be in fed humans or carnivores.

Bioassay of Glucagon. Related to its role in fasting mammals, glucagon is often bioassayed in the fasting cat in which it induces hyperglycemia. As in the case of insulin, however, rapid RIAs have been developed for measuring blood glucagon levels, and these are employed routinely.

Chemistry of Glucagon. Glucagon is a straight-chain polypeptide hormone consisting of 29 amino acid residues and with a molecular weight of 3485 daltons (Fig. 13-9). The circulating form of glucagon is derived from a prohormone by hydrolysis prior to release. Structurally, glucagon is similar to the family of gastrointestinal hormones that includes secretin and pancreozymin-cholecystokinin (see Chap. 14).

Actions of Glucagon on Target Tissues. Glucagon promotes glycogenolysis in liver

his—ser—Gln—gly—thr—phe—thr—ser—asp—tyr—ser—lys—tyr—leu—asp—ser—arg—arg—ala—Gln—asp—phe—val—Gln—try—leu—met—Asn—thr
1 2 3 4 5 6 7 8 9 10 11 12 13 14 15 16 17 18 19 20 21 22 23 24 25 26 27 28 29

Fig. 13-9. Amino acid sequence of mammalian pancreatic glucagon.

cells, its primary target with respect to raising circulating glucose levels. This effect appears to be mediated through stimulation of adenyl cyclase and production of intracellular cAMP. Increased glycogenolysis accompanied by decreased intracellular oxidation of glucose directs the movement of glucose into the blood.

Lipolysis is stimulated by glucagon in both liver and adipose tissue of fasting animals. This increase in fatty acids following lipolysis results in fatty acid oxidation accompanied by ketogenesis. Glucagon-induced lipolysis depresses glucose metabolism and adds to the hyperglycemic effect.

Extrapancreatic Glucagon. There is one cellular type in the duodenal region of the intestine that stains very much like the pancreatic A cell and is ultrastructurally identical to the A cell (see Chap. 14). This cell produces an immunologically reactive polypeptide that is very similar but slightly larger than pancreatic glucagon (mol wt about 6000–10,000 daltons). After a meal this *enteroglucagon* (*enteron* gut) increases in the blood and may even exceed levels of pancreatic glucagon. Apparently calcium ions in the lumen of the gut stimulate release of enteroglucagon, which in turn elicits release of calcitonin from the parafollicular cells (C cells) of the thyroid.[20] A role for enteroglucagon in carbohydrate or lipid metabolism, however, has not been demonstrated.

Another extrapancreatic glucagon-like hyperglycemic factor has been characterized in extracts of submaxillary salivary glands obtained from rats, mice, rabbits and humans.[38] Release of this *salivary glucagon* is influenced in vitro in the same manner as pancreatic glucagon. Somatostatin, however, does not block release of salivary glucagon.

The biological importance of these extrapancreatic glucagons is not clear, although they might explain the presence of immunoreactive glucagon in the circulation of pancreatectomized and even pancreatectomized-eviscerated rats. To avoid confusion, the term glucagon will henceforth be used to indicate glucagon of pancreatic source. Extrapancreatic glucagons will always be designated according to their source as enteroglucagon or salivary glucagon.

Somatostatin: Regulator of Pancreatic Hormone Release? The D cell is believed to be the source of pancreatic somatostatin that is chemically identical with hypothalamic somatostatin. Levels of pancreatic somatostatin in rats have been reported to be equivalent to hypothalamic levels.[3] Somatostatin is believed to inhibit the release of insulin, glucagon and pancreatic polypeptide in a paracrine fashion.[19,27]

Pancreatic Polypeptide: A Third Metabolic Hormone? Pancreatic polypeptide has been purified from ovine, bovine, porcine and human pancreatic tissue. The average molecular weight for PP is 4200, and all peptides isolated consist of 36 amino acid residues (Fig. 13-10). The physiological role of PP is unknown, although there are several reasons for giving PP hormonal status.[16] In man, ingestion of a protein meal such as ground beef causes an increase in plasma levels of PP from preingestion levels of 57 pg/ml plasma to 229 pg/ml, 400 pg/ml and 580 pg/ml respectively in 5, 10 and 240 minutes. Infusion or ingestion of glucose does not evoke this sort of increase in hPP, and it appears that the rapid increase in plasma hPP following ingestion of protein is at least in part a neural response mediated via the vagus nerve. This release of hPP can be blocked by somatostatin, although it is not known whether this latter additional pancreatic agent is involved in the normal regulation of PP release.

Bovine PP is reported to be a potent inhibitor of pancreatic exocrine secretion, but it does not seem to influence carbohydrate (glucose) metabolism.[19] Avian PP has been reported to be a potent stimulator of gastric acid and pepsin secretion,[29] but this effect has not been reported in mammals. It is too early to decide whether these reports are related to the physiological roles of PP or not.

Clinical Aspects of Pancreatic Function

Diabetes Mellitus

Diabetes mellitus is a complex, heterogeneous assemblage of disorders having the common feature of the appearance of glucose in the urine. Diabetes mellitus is always fatal if not treated, and even if treated, serious com-

Source	1	2	3	4	5	6	7	8	9	10	11	12	13	14	15	16	17	18
bPP	Ala	Pro	Leu	Glu	Pro	Gln	Tyr	Pro	Gly	Asp	Asp	Ala	Thr	Pro	Glu	Gln	Met	Ala
oPP	Ala	Ser	Leu	Glu	Pro	Gln	Tyr	Pro	Gly	Asp	Asp	Ala	Thr	Pro	Glu	Gln	Met	Ala
pPP	Ala	Pro	Leu	Glu	Pro	Val	Tyr	Pro	Gly	Asp	Asp	Ala	Thr	Pro	Glu	Gln	Met	Ala
hPP	Ala	Pro	Leu	Glu	Pro	Val	Tyr	Pro	Gly	Asn*	Asp*	Ala	Thr	Pro	Glu	Gln	Met	Ala
aPP	Gly	Pro	Ser	Glu	Pro	Thr	Tyr	Pro	Gly	Asp	Asp	Ala	Thr	Pro	Glu	Asp	Leu	Ile

Source	19	20	21	22	23	24	25	26	27	28	29	30	31	32	33	34	35	36
bPP	Gln	Tyr	Ala	Ala	Glu	Leu	Arg	Arg	Tyr	Ile	Asn	Met	Leu	Thr	Arg	Pro	Arg	$Tyr-NH_2$
oPP	Gln	Tyr	Ala	Ala	Glu	Leu	Arg	Arg	Tyr	Ile	Asn	Met	Leu	Thr	Arg	Pro	Arg	$Tyr-NH_2$
pPP	Gln	Tyr	Ala	Ala	Glu	Leu	Arg	Arg	Tyr	Ile	Asn	Met	Leu	Thr	Arg	Pro	Arg	$Tyr-NH_2$
hPP	Gln	Tyr	Ala	Ala	Asp	Leu	Arg	Arg	Tyr	Ile	Asn	Met	Leu	Thr	Arg	Pro	Arg	$Tyr-NH_2$
aPP	Arg	Phe	Tyr	Asp	Asn	Leu	Gln	Gln	Tyr	Leu	Asn	Val	Val	Thr	Arg	His	Arg	$Tyr-NH_2$

*Asn may occur in either position 10 or 11.

FIG. 13-10. Amino acid sequences of vertebrate pancreatic polypeptides. Boxes indicate identical amino acid residues in all five molecules. Note that there are few substitutions in the four mammalian molecules, but the avian pancreatic polypeptide (aPP) is considerably different. PP, pancreatic polypeptides: bPP, bovine; oPP, ovine; pPP, porcine; hPP, human.

plications may develop including blindness, kidney disease, and circulatory problems. Approximately 5% of the U.S. population is afflicted with diabetes mellitus, and the incidence of the disease is increasing at the rate of 6% a year. Since the availability of insulin, relatively few deaths in diabetics are directly related to ketoacidosis of the blood and coma. Prior to this, ketoacidosis was the most common cause of death. Nevertheless, diabetes mellitus is responsible directly for about 38,000 deaths annually. Cardio-renal-vascular complications resulting from diabetes mellitus are responsible for an additional 300,000 deaths annually, making diabetes a leading cause of death in the United States.

Most cases of diabetes mellitus can be characterized as either *maturity onset diabetes* (ketosis-resistant; insulin-independent) or as *juvenile onset diabetes* (ketosis-prone; insulin-dependent). "Maturity" and "juvenile" are not entirely appropriate terms since the former can occur occasionally in children and adolescents, whereas the latter can occur with low frequency in middle-aged or older adults. These two types of diabetes are compared in Table 13-7. There are some additional forms of diabetes now recognized, but these are rare and are not discussed here.

Maturity onset diabetes (MOD), accounting for approximately 90 to 95% of the reported cases, typically occurs in overweight people (80% of cases) who are over 40 years of age. It has a slow onset with no obvious pancreatic disease, and can usually be controlled by manipulating the diet. Insulin levels in MOD are usually normal or in excess of normal. Apparently, the target cells become insensitive to insulin, possibly due to a decrease in receptor populations or to a deficiency in the mechanism of action of insulin after it is bound to the cell. Another possible cause might be an increase in non-specific binding of insulin to non-target cells. Whatever the defect, dietary regulation and the removal of excess weight will bring these patients back into normal carbohydrate balance, and the regulation of carbohydrate metabolism will return to normal. Oral hypoglycemic agents (e.g., sulfonylureas) generally are effective at reducing blood glucose levels in these patients, provided dietary intake is controlled rigidly.

There is evidence to support a familial or genetic component in MOD. A series of studies

TABLE 13-7. *Comparison of Juvenile and Maturity Onset Diabetes Mellitus.*

	JUVENILE ONSET	MATURITY ONSET
Age of onset	Usually during childhood or puberty	Frequently over 45
Type of onset	Abrupt	Usually gradual
Genetic Basis	Frequently positive relationship	Commonly positive relationship
Nutritional Status	Usually undernourished	Usually obesity present to some degree (about 80% of cases)
Symptoms	(a) Polydipsia, polyphagia, polyuria	(a) May be none
	(b) Ketosis frequently present	(b) Ketosis uncommon except under stress
	(c) Hepatomegaly rather common	(c) Hematomegaly uncommon
	(d) Blood glucose fluctuates widely in response to small changes in insulin dose, exercise and infection.	(d) Blood sugar fluctuations less marked than for juvenile onset
Fasting Blood Sugar Levels	Elevated	Often normal
Requirement for Insulin	Necessary for all patients	Necessary for 20–30% of patients
Effectiveness Oral Agents	Rarely effective	Effective when diet is controlled

Compiled from several sources

on twins indicates that if one twin develops MOD after age 50, the other twin develops MOD in almost every case.

Juvenile onset diabetes (JOD) usually develops in persons under 20 years of age and is characterized by an abrupt onset of symptoms. A small percentage of people over 40 who contract diabetes mellitus exhibit this form of the disease. Typically, the pancreatic B-cells are reduced markedly (usually to less than 10% of normal), and insulin levels are very low or absent. Glycogen stores are depleted readily and fatty acid metabolism is accelerated, resulting in accumulation of ketone bodies in the blood (e.g., acetone, β-hydroxybutyrate). This accumulation of ketone bodies produces ketoacidosis in about 48 hours and eventually leads to coma and death unless insulin is administered. Patients with JOD have an absolute requirement for insulin for the rest of their lives. Because of this reliance on exogenous insulin and difficulties in administering the appropriate dose when needed, the diabetic must always be prepared for the onset of hypoglycemia following excessive insulin. This usually can be counteracted by consuming a high glucose source.

No strong evidence for a genetic link has been offered for JOD; however, there is some evidence to suggest a role of infection. The symptoms of JOD appear abruptly, and there is a higher incidence of onset during the fall and winter months when infectious diseases also increase. In certain genetic strains of mice, JOD has been linked to a specific virus. There also appears to be a correlation between the occurrence of certain viral diseases (e.g., mumps, rubella *in utero*) and the later appearance of JOD.

Dietary restrictions are similar for both MOD and JOD patients although a reduction in total caloric intake is necessary for overweight MOD patients. Specific diets must be determined individually for every patient. Carbohydrates are still essential to the diabetic diet but need to be in the form of polysaccharides (e.g., starch). Mono- and disaccharides are usually avoided because of rapid uptake and resultant hyperglycemia soon after ingestion. The ingestion of simple sugars is less a problem for the MOD patient as the pancreas can respond with some insulin release.

Comparative Aspects of the Endocrine Pancreas

Five anatomical arrangements for pancreatic islet systems can be distinguished readily by examination of the major vertebrate groupings.[13]

1. *Cyclostome type.* The cyclostome type is composed of aggregations of islet cellular types with no obvious relationship to the homologous intraintestinal equivalent of mammalian acinar cells. In hagfishes islets surround the base of the common bile duct, and in lampreys they are located on the surfaces of the intestine (epi-intestinal), within the intestinal mucosa (intraintestinal) and even within the liver (intrahepatic). The lamprey pattern of islet distribution is considered to be the most primitive pattern in vertebrates. Exocrine pancreatic elements are embedded in the intestinal lining.

2. *Primitive gnathostome type.* Islet tissue of elasmobranchs, holocephalans and the sarcopterygian coelacanth *(Latimeria)* occurs as layers surrounding the smaller ducts of a compact, extraintestinal pancreas as well as some scattered cells throughout the exocrine pancreas.

3. *Actinopterygian type.* Usually the exocrine pancreatic cells are scattered (diffused) along the bile ducts, abdominal blood vessels and on the outer surfaces of the gastrointestinal tract, gallbladder and liver. An intrahepatic pancreas has been observed in several species. The islet tissue often accumulates as clumps near the common bile duct but is not usually separated from the acinar tissues.

4. *Lungfish type.* The pancreas of lungfishes is a compact, intraintestinal structure with a number of encapsulated islets.

5. *Tetrapod type.* Tetrapods typically exhibit a compact, extraintestinal pancreas containing scattered islets and occasionally some scattered individual endocrine cells. In some tetrapods (for example, birds and the toad *Bufo*), islets may be concentrated in particular lobes of the pancreas and not evenly distributed.

There are some generalizations concerning the origin of the various components of the pancreas and their relationship to the distribution of islets.[7] The dorsal pancreatic bud gives rise to the tail and body of the pancreas (also known as the splenic portion) and the ventral buds give rise to the head or duodenal portion. Islets associated with the splenic lobe typically are larger and consist mainly of B, A and D cells. The islets of the duodenal pancreas are smaller and may contain many PP cells.

Comparative Structure of Insulin

Insulin is a conservative protein in that few amino acid substitutions have occurred at the critical sites related to its structure and biological activity.[17,55] The amino acid sequences for a number of vertebrate insulins are provided in Figures 13-11 and 13-12. The C peptide of proinsulin "tolerates" a greater number of substitutions, yet portions of this peptide also remain rather conservative, for example, the glycine-rich central core of the C peptide. Single amino acid substitutions may have profound effects on the resultant molecule. One substitution in hagfish insulin is believed responsible for the observation that hagfish insulin does not bind Zn^{++} and therefore does not form the typical hexamer crystals characteristic of most vertebrate insulins. The number of amino acids in the B chain varies when insulins from different vertebrate classes (especially reptiles) are compared.

Comparative Structure of Glucagon

Mammalian glucagons that have been characterized chemically exhibit no amino acid substitutions.[20] Turkey glucagon differs from mammalian glucagons only at position 28 where serine is substituted for asparagine.[41] Chicken glucagon is identical to turkey glucagon, whereas duck glucagon has threonine at position 16 instead of serine.[25] Glucagon has been isolated from the spiny dogfish shark *Squalus acanthias,* but the primary structure of this glucagon has not been reported.[17]

A CHAIN

	1	2	3	4	5	6	7	8	9	10	11	12	13	14	15	16	17	18	19	20	21
Human	Gly	Ile	Val	Glu	Gln	Cys	Cys	Thr	Ser	Ile	Cys	Ser	Leu	Tyr	Gln	Leu	Glu	Asn	Tyr	Cys	Asn
Guinea pig				Asp				Ala	Gly	Thr		Thr	Arg	His			Gln				
Avian								His	Asn	Thr											
Teleost			Leu					His	His	Pro		Asn	Lys	Phe	Asp		Gln	Ser			
Hagfish								His	Lys	Arg			Ile		Asx	. . .	. . .	. . .	. . .	. . .	. . .

B CHAIN

	1	2	3	4	5	6	7	8	9	10	11	12	13	14	15	16	17	18	19	20
Human	Phe	Val	Asn	Gln	His	Leu	Cys	Gly	Ser	His	Leu	Val	Glu	Ala	Leu	Tyr	Leu	Val	Cys	Gly
Guinea pig			Ser	Arg						Asn			Thr				Ser			Gln
Avian	Ala	Ala																		
Teleost	Ala	Ala	Ala										Asp							
Hagfish	Arg	Thr	X	Gly					Lys	Asp			Asn	Ala	. . .	. . .	. . .	. . .	. . .	. . .

B CHAIN (Cont.)

	21	22	23	24	25	26	27	28	29	30
Human	Glu	Arg	Gly	Phe	Phe	Tyr	Thr	Pro	Lys	Thr
Guinea pig	Asp	Asp					Ile			Asp
Avian							Asn	Ser		
Teleost	Asp						Asn	Ser		—
Hagfish	. . .	. . .	. . .	. . .	. . .	. . .	. . .	. . .	. . .	. . .

FIG. 13-11. Comparison of amino acid sequences in some vertebrate insulins. A chains and B chains are compared. Blanks indicate that residues at that position are identical to human insulin. Dots indicate no data.

	1	2	3	4	5	6	7	8	9	10	11	12	13	14	15	
NH_3^+ -	Glu -	Ala -	*Glu* -	Asp -	Leu -	Gln -	Val -	Gly -	Gln -	Val -	Glu -	*Leu* -	Gly -	*Gly* -	Gly -	MAN
NH_3^+ -	Glu -	Ala -	*Glu* -	Asp -	Pro -	Gln -	Val -	Gly -	Gln -	Val -	Glu -	*Leu* -	Gly -	*Gly* -	Gly -	MONKEY
NH_3^+ -	Glu -	Ala -	*Glu* -	Asp -	Pro -	Gln -	Val -	Gly -	Glu -	Val -	Glu -	*Leu* -	Gly -	*Gly* -	Gly -	HORSE
NH_3^+ -	Glu -	Val -	*Glu* -	Asp -	Pro -	Gln -	Val -	Pro -	Gln -	Leu -	Glu -	*Leu* -	Gly -	*Gly* -	Gly -	RAT I
NH_3^+ -	Glu -	Val -	*Glu* -	Asp -	Pro -	Gln -	Val -	Ala -	Gln -	Leu -	Glu -	*Leu* -	Gly -	*Gly* -	Gly -	RAT II
NH_3^+ -	Glu -	Ala -	*Glu* -	Asn -	Pro -	Gln -	Ala -	Gly -	Ala -	Val -	Glu -	*Leu* -	Gly -	*Gly* -	Gly -	PIG
NH_3^+ -	Glu -	Val -	*Glu* -	Gly -	Pro -	Gln -	Val -	Gly -	Ala -	Leu -	Glu -	*Leu* -	Ala -	*Gly* -	Gly -	COW, LAMB
NH_3^+ -	Asp -	Val -	*Glu* -									- *Leu* -	Ala -	*Gly* -	Ala -	DOG

16	17	18	19	20	21	22	23	24	25	26	27	28	29	30	31		
- Pro -	Gly -	Ala -	Gly -	Ser -	*Leu* -	Gln -	Pro -	Leu -	Ala -	Leu -	Glu -	Gly -	Ser -	Leu -	*Gln* -	CO_2^-	MAN
- Pro -	Gly -	Ala -	Gly -	Ser -	*Leu* -	Gln -	Pro -	Leu -	Ala -	Leu -	Glu -	Gly -	Ser -	Leu -	*Gln* -	CO_2^-	MONKEY
- Pro -	Gly -	Leu -	Gly -	Gly -	*Leu* -	Gln -	Pro -	Leu -	Ala -	Leu -	Ala -	Gly -	Pro -	Gln -	*Gln* -	CO_2^-	HORSE
- Pro -	Glu -	Ala -	Gly -	Asp -	*Leu* -	Gln -	Thr -	Leu -	Ala -	Leu -	Glu -	Val -	Ala -	Arg -	*Gln* -	CO_2^-	RAT I
- Pro -	Gly -	Ala -	Gly -	Asp -	*Leu* -	Gln -	Thr -	Leu -	Ala -	Leu -	Glu -	Val -	Ala -	Arg -	*Gln* -	CO_2^-	RAT II
- Leu -	Gly -			- Gly -	*Leu* -	Gln -	Ala -	Leu -	Ala -	Leu -	Glu -	Gly -	Pro -	Pro -	*Gln* -	CO_2^-	PIG
- Pro -	Gly -	Ala -	Gly -	Gly -	*Leu* -						- Glu -	Gly -	Pro -	Pro -	*Gln* -	CO_2^-	COW, LAMB
- Pro -	Gly -	Glu -	Gly -	Gly -	*Leu* -	Gln -	Pro -	Leu -	Ala -	Leu -	Glu -	Gly -	Ala -	Leu -	*Gln* -	CO_2^-	DOG

FIG. 13-12. Comparison of C peptides of mammalian insulins. The basic residues that link the C peptide to the active insulin molecule are omitted at either end. Identical residues for all species are italicized. Steiner, D.F. et al.[55]

Occurrence of Vertebrate Pancreatic Hormones in Invertebrates

B cells and insulin activity have been identified in the guts or digestive organs of a number of nonchordate invertebrate animals (Table 13-8). Mammalian insulin reduces blood sugar levels and promotes glycogen synthesis in a gastropod mollusc, *Strophocheilus oblongus.*[17] Insulinlike molecules have even been found in protozoans, bacteria and fungi. Insulin is therefore a widely distributed factor that is capable of regulating carbohydrate metabolism in a great variety of organisms and possibly does so. The evolution of insulin must involve a long and interesting history, most of which remains to be discovered.

Immunoreactive glucagon has been localized in the digestive glands of a crab, *Cancer pagurus,* and two gastropod molluscs, *Patella caerulae* and *Helix pomatia.* A glucagon-like molecule is present in extracts of invertebrate chordates, including tunicates and cephalochordates.[5]

Class Agnatha: Cyclostomata

Hagfish "islet" tissue (Fig. 13-13) consists almost exclusively of B cells plus some "light" cells that could represent precursor or "spent" secretory cells. Some B cells occur in the gut mucosa as do immunologically reactive A cells.[43] Lamprey islets (Fig. 13-14) exhibit insulin-secreting B cells as well as four acidophilic cellular types for which functions have not been identified.[10,13] Cyclostomes do not have A cells and do not respond to injections of glucagon.[14]

Insulin has been purified following the extraction of islet tissue obtained from several

TABLE 13-8. *Blood Sugar Levels in Selachians (Elasmobranchs) and Holocephalans (Ratfish)*

SPECIES	PLASMA GLUCOSE (mg/dl ± S.E.M.)
Squalus acanthias	90 ± 49
	6.6 ± 0.55
	9.12 ± 25.1
	49.2 ± 2.1
	50.3 ± 4.9
	40.1 ± 2.9
Raja erinacea	53.5 ± 17.6
	44.2 ± 14.9
Hydrolagus colliei	62.2 ± 1.6

Data from numerous studies summarized from Patent.[46]

NOTE: Methods of capture and blood sampling differed markedly, but glucose was determined in each instance by the glucose oxidase method.

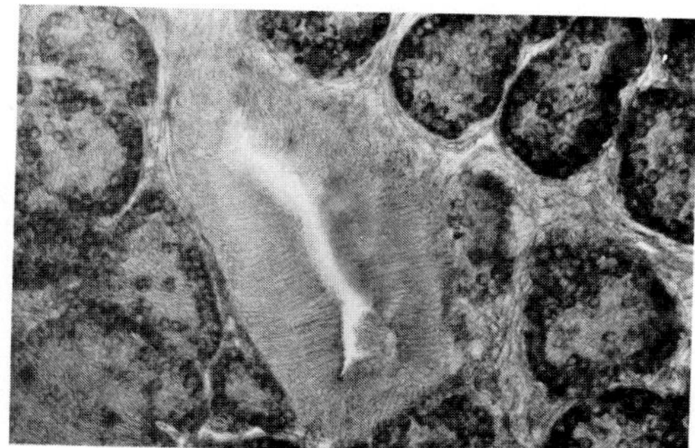

Fig. 13-13. Islet tissue of the hagfish *(Eptatretus burgeri)*. Follicles of islet tissue surround the lower bile duct *(center)*. Stained with pseudoisocyanin. (Courtesy of Dr. August Epple.)

thousand hagfishes, and its partial structure is indicated in Figure 13-11. Hagfish B cells synthesize insulin through processes that appear to be identical to those described for mammals.[55] Insulin has also been extracted from islet tissue of the river lamprey *Lampetra fluviatilis.*[17]

Hagfish insulin behaves similarly to other insulins in mammalian assays. The biological activity of purified hagfish insulin in mammals, however, is only about 4- to 7% of that reported for mammalian insulins,[17] indicating the evolution of greater specificity in target cells as well as some changes in the insulin molecule itself. Both mammalian and hagfish insulins cause hypoglycemia when injected into hagfish. Hagfish insulin stimulates both glycogen and protein synthesis in hagfish skeletal muscle but only stimulates protein synthesis in liver.[12] Amino acids are known to stimulate insulin release in lampreys providing additional support for insulin's role as a regulator of protein metabolism.[14] Known insulin antagonists, such as epinephrine, glucagon, T_4, corticotropin and prolactin (containing growth hormone as a contaminant) were all ineffective in altering blood sugar levels.[18] Curiously, isletectomy of *Myxine* does not cause hyperglycemia, and the response to a glucose load in isletectomized hagfish is normal.[17] Hypophysectomy has no effect on islet cytology or blood sugar levels.[18] There must be an explanation for the presence of insulin and the demonstration of its hypoglycemic action in the hagfish with the number of negative observations just mentioned, but it will require more research to reconcile these contradictory data.

Class Chondrichthyes

The endocrine pancreas of a number of species of selachians and holocephalans has been examined (Fig. 13-15, Table 13-8).[3] Normal blood sugar levels for three of those species (a skate, a shark and the ratfish) are provided in Table 13-9. The selachian pancreatic islets contain B, A, D, and PP cells.[7,13] Both insulin and glucagon have been extracted from the

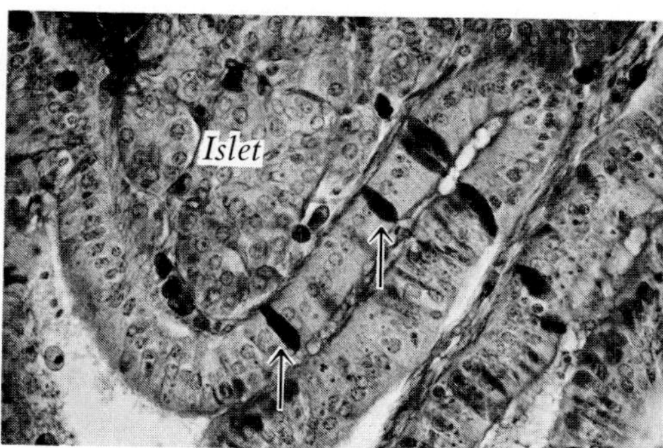

Fig. 13-14. Cephalic islet tissue of lamprey *(Petromyzon marinus)*. Note that the *islet* tissue is located in the submucosa of the intestine and is totally separate from the black presumptive exocrine pancreas equivalents *(arrows)*. (Courtesy of Dr. August Epple.)

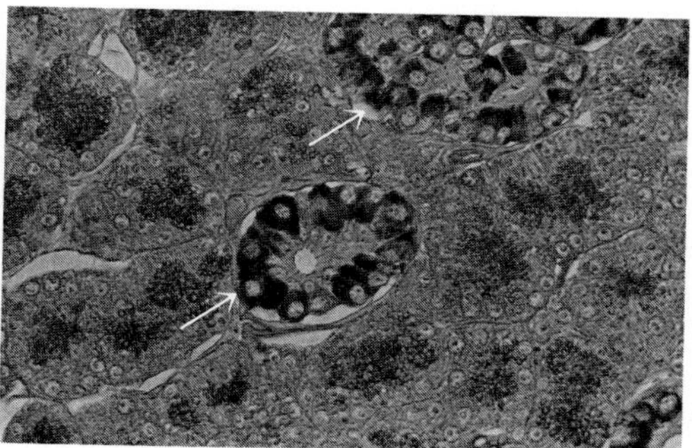

Fig. 13-15. Pancreas with islet tissue of dogfish *(Scyliorhinus canicula)*. The most primitive islet organization known for vertebrates is seen in the center with the endocrine cells surrounding a small unstained ductule (resembles early embryonic stages of human islets). Several small ductules congregate to form a primitive islet *(upper right)*. (Courtesy of Dr. August Epple.)

TABLE 13-9. *Blood Sugar Levels in Some Representative Vertebrates (Values May Include Both Starved and Fed Animals)*

CLASS	SPECIES	NO. INVESTIGATIONS	AVERAGE BLOOD SUGAR LEVEL (mg/dl)	RANGES REPORTED (mg/dl)
Agnatha	*Myxine glutinosa*	1	17	12–23
Chondrichthyes	*Raja erinacea* (skate)	2	49	20–89
	Squalus acanthias (shark)	1	49	8–193
	Hydrolagus colliei (ratfish)	1	62	15–112
Osteichthyes				
Teleosts				
	Scomber scombous	1	63	
	Opsanus tau	1	15	
	Pneumatophorus colus	1	91	
Amphibia	*Bufo* (2 spp)	7	27	20–36
	Rana (4 spp)	19	36	14–58
	Amphiuma means (urodele)	1	–	4–88
	Taricha torosa (urodele)	1	25	
	Ambystoma annulatum (urodele)	1	52	30–90
	Necturus maculosus (urodele)	1	64	35–110
	Eurycea lucifuga (urodele)	1	167	77–600
Reptilia	Chelonia (6 spp)	15	78	49–112
	Sauria (13 spp)	23	136	54–224
	Serpentes (18 spp)	26	46	19–90
	Crocodilia (1 sp)	16	76	45–138
Aves	Duck	1	208	
Mammals	Rabbit	1	136	
	Ferret	1	95	
	Mouse	1	138	

Data from summaries provided by Assenmacher,[4] Falkmer and Matty,[18] Gorbman and Bern,[24] McMillan and Wilkinson,[42] Patent,[46] Penhos and Ramey.[49]

pancreas of the spiny dogfish *Squalus acanthias.*[17] In the ratfish *Hydrolagus colliei,* approximately 50% of the islet cells are of a type referred to as *X cells.* These cells resemble both A and D cells but also possess some unique cytological features of their own.[16] It is not clear whether these X cells represent a transient stage between known cellular types or perform some unique function yet unknown.

It appears that blood sugar regulation is not very precise in these fishes, and blood sugar may vary considerably even within a species. Administration of mammalian insulin evokes hypoglycemia in these fishes, and glucagon has been shown to induce hyperglycemia in some species. Epinephrine also elevates the blood glucose level, and the effect of injected epinephrine occurs very rapidly. On a superficial basis it appears that regulation of carbohydrate metabolism is similar to the mammalian pattern.

There are many unusual features of metabolism in these fishes that require further study. Although liver glycogen levels in dogfish sharks conform with predicted responses to fasting and force feeding, the liver of holocephalans is apparently incapable of storing glycogen.[46] Injection of a glucose load does not alter tissue glycogen even though circulating glucose is increased. These observations may explain the inability of glucagon to increase blood glucose in the ratfish. Protein and lipid metabolism with respect to the actions of pancreatic hormones have not been studied. Lipid metabolism in these fishes should be of special interest since hepatic fat content may be as high as 70% in the dogfish and 80% in the ratfish.[45]

Class Osteichthyes

Most species possess isolated masses of pancreatic islet tissue called *Brockmann bodies.* A given species may have a number of Brockmann bodies, or the islet tissue may be concentrated largely in one "principal islet" as in the Atlantic eel *Anguilla anguilla* or the bullhead *Ictalurus* spp. Brockmann bodies of actinopterygian fishes contain A, B, and D cells, but PP cells occur only in Brockmann bodies located in the pyloric region.[7]

Insulin and glucagon are produced by the B and A cells respectively.[9] Somatostatin is apparently synthesized by the D cells of the pancreas of the angler fish,[43] implying that the role of somatostatin in pancreatic function is not unique to mammals. A fourth cellular type of undefined function has been reported in catfishes,[9] and definite PP cells have been reported in *Xiphophorus helleri.*[36]

The lungfish *(Protopterus annectens)* pancreas is located intraintestinally and contains a number of scattered encapsulated islets.[10] The islet tissue of the lungfish possesses A, B, and D cells.[8] There are probably PP cells present, but they have not been identified.

Insulins prepared from several teleosts appear to be similar to mammalian insulins. Glucagon has been isolated from the anglerfish.[56] It consists of 29 amino acid residues that differ somewhat from those of mammalian glucagons. It is produced from a larger proglucagon peptide. Generally insulin is hypoglycemic and glucagon is hyperglycemic in bony fishes. Injections of glucose or the amino acid leucine stimulate insulin secretion in the toadfish *Opsanus tau* and in the European silver eel *A. anguilla.*[32,47] Purified codfish insulin is a potent hypoglycemic agent in Northern pike, *Esox lucius.* Furthermore, insulin increases uptake and incorporation of labeled glucose and glycine into muscle lipids and protein.[31] Administration of mammalian glucagon increases blood glucose in channel catfish (Table 13-10). Glycogenolysis in isolated hepatocytes (liver cells) of goldfish is stimulated by glucagon and epinephrine.[6] Some representative blood glucose levels for teleosts can be found in Tables 13-9 and 13-10.

Class Amphibia

The anatomy of the pancreas of anurans and urodeles is similar to that of the other tetrapods. Data are lacking for apodans. The islets are distributed in the acinar tissue, although in at least one anuran, *Bufo arenarum,*

TABLE 13-10. *Effect of Glucagon on Blood Glucose Level of the Indian Catfish* Channa punctatus ± *SE (n)*

TIME (HR)	BLOOD GLUCOSE (mg/dl)	BLOOD GLUCOSE (mg/dl)
	Control	Glucagon (2.0 mg/kg[a])
½	51 ± 2.00 (2)	82.6 ± 13.39 (3)
1	54 ± 6.01 (2)	107.5 ± 5.18 (4)
3	54.5 ± 2.555 (2)	74 ± 2.00 (4)
13	47 ± 3.00 (2)	72 ± 16.18 (3)
24	47 ± 2.00 (2)	78 ± 0.70 (4)
48	53.5 ± 6.53 (2)	75 ± 3.00 (4)
72	50 ± 10.03 (2)	69.3 ± 12.71 (3)
96	50 ± 2.00 (2)	56.5 ± 13.61 (4)
120	52 ± 7.01 (2)	53 ± 3.87 (4)

Modified from Gill, T.S. and S.S. Khanna.[23]
[a]0.5 mg glucagon/kg also elevated blood glucose level, but the effect was significant only at 1 hr postinjection.

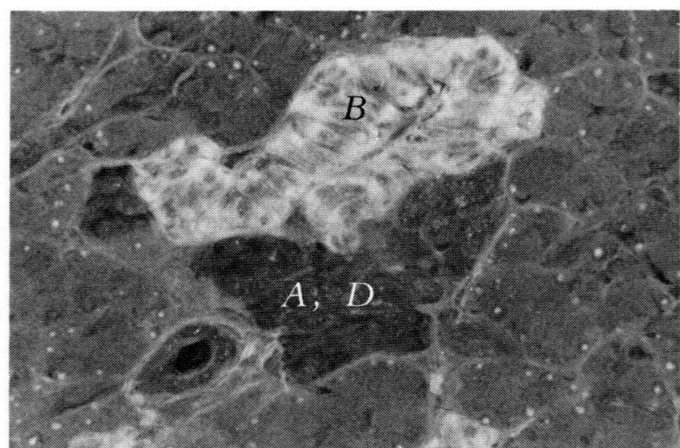

Fig. 13-16. Endocrine pancreas of the toad *(Bufo bufo)*. The light area consists of B cells with fluorescent granules. The dark area is occupied mainly by A cells, but some D cells are present. (Courtesy of Dr. August Epple.)

many of the islets are concentrated in one lobe of the pancreas. The islets of anuran amphibians resemble those of mammals cytologically with A, B, D, PP and a fifth unidentified cellular type present.[7,14] Although B cells predominate in amphibians, there are almost equal proportions of A and B cells (Fig. 13-16), whereas A cells comprise only about 10%–20% of the islets of most mammalian species. D cells are also present. The "islets" of *Necturus maculosus* are not encapsulated and occur as groups of cells.[10] Most urodeles, however, exhibit the typical tetrapod type of islet arrangement (Fig. 13-17).

Mammalian insulin and glucagon produce effects in amphibians similar to those observed in mammals.[49] Insulin induces hypoglycemia in anurans and in urodeles (Table 13-11), stimulates incorporation of amino acids into proteins and lowers fatty acid levels.[11,14,42,59] The response to a glucose load in anurans and the effects of pancreatectomy do indicate an endogenous role for insulin. Mammalian glucagon causes hyperglycemia in anurans (Table 13-12) and in the salamander *Ambystoma annulatum*.[42] Although mammalian glucagon has been found to be ineffective in some amphibians,[15,59] glucagon treatment is effective in raising blood glucose levels at certain times of year.[14]

Epinephrine is also hyperglycemic in tadpoles and adults of *Xenopus laevis*.[58] Administration of epinephrine or norepinephrine causes reduction in liver and muscle glycogen as well.

Research on the amphibian pancreas has led to a widely employed procedure for research into mammalian diabetes mellitus. It was in the toad *B. arenarum* that the antagonism of pituitary hormones and blood glucose of pancreatectomized or insulin-deficient animals was discovered by Bernardo A. Houssay almost 50 years ago. This discovery led to the widespread use of hypophysectomy to alleviate extreme diabetic conditions in experimental animals, and such doubly operated-on dogs and cats and other laboratory beasts became known commonly as Houssay animals. This action of hypophysectomy in the pancreatic-deficient animal is termed the Houssay effect.

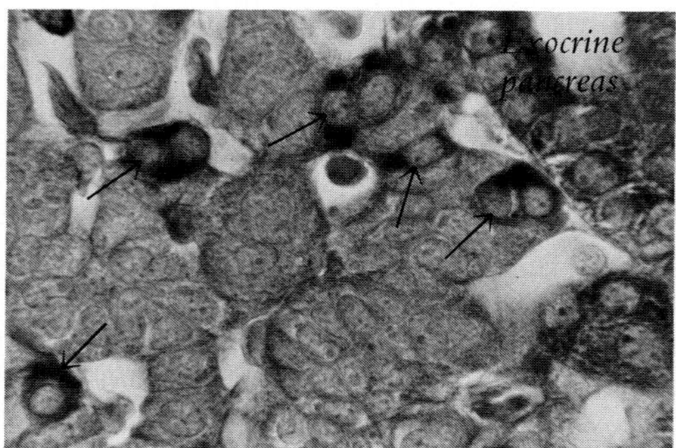

Fig. 13-17. Endocrine pancreas of the Mexican axolotl *(Ambystoma mexicanum)*. The large islets consist mainly of B cells (unstained) with other cellular types at the periphery. *Arrows* designate D cells stained with toluidine blue. (Courtesy of Dr. August Epple.)

Class Reptilia

Reptiles have a distinct pancreas containing both acinar and islet tissues.[13] There is a predominance of A cells in lizard islets (ratio of 4:1 over B cells), and there is some tendency for the islets to concentrate in the caudal (splenic) lobe of the pancreas. In contrast, the B cells represent about 50% of the islet cellular types in the alligator. D cells are present also in the reptilian pancreas but are not a dominant type. PP cells have not been described.

Reptiles exhibit mammalian-like responses to injected insulin (Table 13-13) and glucagon (Table 13-14) and to glucose loading (Table 13-15). Lizards, however, are particularly in-

TABLE 13-11. *Reponse to Injections of Crystalline Insulin during the Spring by Fasted (7 Days) Male Toads* Bufo marinus *and Frog* Rana catesbeiana

DOSE OF INSULIN (U/kg)	MEAN BLOOD SUGAR (mg/dl) AT INTERVALS (HR) 0	1	5	9	24	48	72	96	120
				Bufo marinus					
1.0	30	31	18	15	21	26	31	29	
10.0	33	28	15	8	11	15	26	36	
				Rana catesbeiana					
1.0	39	41	26	12	8	17	35	36	
10.0	45	41	13	4	12	10	19	36	43

Modified from Penhos, J.C. and E. Ramey.[49]

TABLE 13-12. *Response of Fasting (7 Days) Male Anurans to Mammalian Glucagon during the Spring*

GLUCAGON DOSE (MG/KG)	BLOOD GLUCOSE (mg/dl) AT INTERVALS (HR) 0	1	2	3	4	6	24
			Bufo marinus				
10.0	27	31	29	30	27	31	28
100.0	31	73	61	57	48	36	27
			Rana catesbeiana				
10.0	32	34	28	33	26	23	31
100.0	28	96	118	79	63	53	31

Modified from Penhos, J.C. and E. Ramey.[49]

TABLE 13-13. *Response of Male Reptiles to Injections of Crystalline Insulin during the Spring in Fasted (10 Days) Animals*

INSULIN DOSE (U/KG)	MEAN BLOOD SUGAR (mg/dl) AT INTERVALS (DAYS) 0	1	2	3	4	5	6	8	10	12	14
				Tupinambis tequixin (lizard)							
10.0	97	57	69	91	101						
100.0	92	50	23	6	22		69				
				Xenodon merremii (snake)							
10.0	46	13	28	44	48						
50.0	48	9	6	19	29	42					
				Alligator mississippiensis							
1.0	77	18	13	21	28	37	46	58	71	81	
1.0	81	16	10	12	10	19	26	37	51	70	79

Modified from Penhos, J.C and E. Ramey.[49]

TABLE 13-14. *Response of Fasting (10 Days) Male Reptiles to Mammalian Glucagon during the Spring*

GLUCAGON DOSE (mg/kg)	BLOOD GLUCOSE (mg/dl) AT INTERVALS (HR) 0	2	4	8	24	48	96	240	432
			Tupinambis tequixin (lizard)						
10.0	108	173	202	196	115	98	103		
100.0	97	209	297	342	269	217	193	104	
			Xenodon merremii (snake)						
10.0	42	79	117	131	89	53	45		
100.0	39	132	196	279	266	221	170	87	46
			Alligator mississipiensis						
10.0	86	98	97	98	99	89	80		
100.0	80	119	142	195	270	203	167	83	

Modified from Penhos, J.C. and E. Ramey.[49]

sensitive to insulin, and large quantities of mammalian insulin are required to invoke hypoglycemic responses. It is virtually impossible to induce insulin shock with massive doses (Table 13-16). Pancreatectomy does induce a hyperglycemic state in lizards as it does in snakes and alligators. These observations suggest that in spite of the predominance of A cells in lizard islets, insulin may plan an important endogenous role in carbohydrate regulation in lizards as well as in other reptiles.

Glucagon has not been isolated from reptiles, and its role in carbohydrate metabolism has been inferred from observations of the actions of mammalian glucagon administered to reptiles. Mammalian glucagon is ineffective in hypophysectomized snakes,[16] suggesting that pituitary hormones may be more important hyperglycemic agents. Perhaps the effects of injected mammalian glucagons are somehow dependent on pituitary hormones.

Insulin has been purified from rattlesnakes, *Crotalis atrox,* and partially characterized chemically.[35] The amino acid composition of rattlesnake insulin is considerably different from bovine insulin with some uncommon substitutions occurring in the B chain. Comparative analyses of reptilian insulins may shed some light on pancreatic regulation of carbohydrate metabolism in reptiles, especially the apparent insensitivity of many species to mammalian insulins. Cyclostome insulin is more like mammalian insulins than is rattlesnake insulin, which points out the difficulties of inferring evolutionary events from molecular structures.

Of particular interest is the absence of studies in which lipid and protein metabolism of reptiles were examined. Insulin and other "metabolic" hormones have not been examined for their roles in lipid or protein metabolism. Until all aspects of the hormonal regula-

TABLE 13-15. *Effects of a Glucose Load on Blood Sugar Levels of Fasting Anurans (7 Days) and Reptiles (10 days)*

	BLOOD GLUCOSE (mg/dl) AT INTERVALS (HR) 0	1	2	4	8	24	48
Bufo arenarum (toad)	30	135	195	258	54	34	
Rana catesbeiana (bullfrog)	34	136	220	324	136	32	
Tupinambis tequixin (lizard)	99	306	453	539	333	186	88
Xenodon merremii (snake)	52	253	319	402	271	117	56

Data from Penhos and Ramey.[49]

TABLE 13-16. *Fatal Doses of Insulin for Various Vertebrates*

ANIMAL	IU INSULIN/kg BODY WEIGHT
	Nonmammals
Salamander	50
Lizard	>10,000[a]
Canary	1000–4000
Pigeon	400–1200
Duck	50–500
	Mammals
Rabbit	4–8
Mouse	7–50
Rat	29–36
Dog	16–300

Modified from Gorbman, A. and H.A. Bern.[24]
NOTE: High doses of insulin cause intense hypoglycemia, followed by coma and death.
Animals with fewer B-cells are less sensitive.
[a]10,000 IU insulin had no effect on survival of lizards.

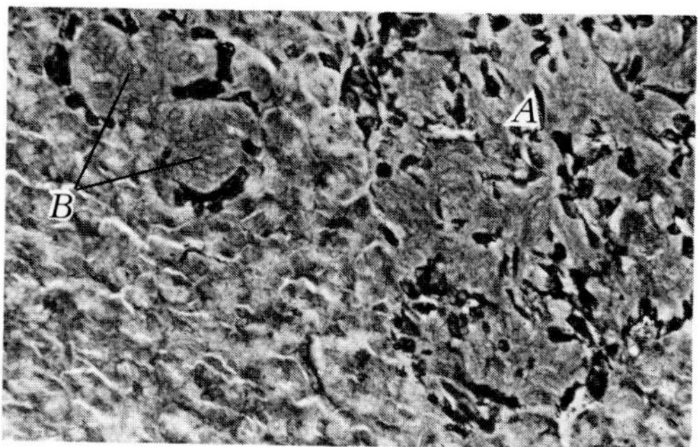

FIG. 13-18. Endocrine pancreas of domestic chicken. The A cells generally are located in separate islets from the B cells. The 8-shaped B islet *(B)* is surrounded by black D cells (and probably some pancreatic polypeptide-secreting cells). Some D cells are scattered through the large A islet *(A)*. (Courtesy of Dr. August Epple.)

tion of metabolism in reptiles are integrated with the observations of effects of insulin and glucagon, a complete picture for the roles of reptilian pancreatic hormones will not emerge.

Class Aves

The avian pancreas consists of dorsal, ventral and splenic lobes. In some species a fourth lobe occurs (inappropriately called the "third" lobe). The dorsal embryonic pancreatic bud gives rise to the splenic lobe (and "third" lobe when present), whereas the ventral buds produce the dorsal and ventral lobes.[7] Unlike the condition for other vertebrates, there appear to be two cytologically distinct types of islets in the avian pancreas (Fig. 13-18). The first type consists of A and D cells. These islets are called A islets. The B islets are composed primarily of B and D cells. Both types of islets are distributed throughout the pancreas although the splenic lobe contains predominantly A islets. Hyperglycemia initially observed following pancreatectomy is now believed to have been a result of overlooking the splenic lobe during pancreatectomy.[16] Total pancreatectomy results in hypoglycemia rather than hyperglycemia and suggests that glucagon plays a major role in avian blood sugar regulation. This suggestion is further supported by observations that a high glucose load is required to induce insulin release in the duck and by the relative insensitivity of avian tissues to insulin (Tables 13-16, 13-17). Elevated glucose levels depress glucagon release, whereas high circulating levels of free fatty acids induce glucagon release.[4] PP cells are uncommon in islets of the splenic lobe but occur in islets of ventral and dorsal lobes.

Avian tissues respond with hyperglycemia, glycogenolysis and lipolysis following administration of mammalian glucagon.[28] The avian pancreas contains about five to ten times the extractable glucagon per gram of pancreas as compared to mammals, emphasizing its importance to metabolic regulation in birds. In one of the few studies performed in wild birds, mammalian glucagon stimulates both plasma levels of free fatty acids and glucose in penguins, whereas insulin causes a reduction in blood glucose.[25] Additional studies with wild avian species representing diverse taxonomic groupings would be welcome in order to confirm or alter generalizations based upon observations of domestic species.

Insulin has been extracted from the avian pancreas, and its structure has been examined (Fig. 13-11). Chicken insulin is more effective in inducing hypoglycemia in birds than it is in mammals, and it is more potent in birds than is mammalian insulin. Glucagon has been extracted and its primary structure determined

Table 13-17. *Effect of Experimental Manipulations on Plasma Glucose, Insulin and Glucagon Levels in Domestic Ducks*

EXPERIMENTAL TREATMENT	MEAN PLASMA GLUCOSE (mg/dl)	MEAN PLASMA INSULIN (mM/ml)	MEAN PLASMA GLUCAGON (ng/ml)
Starvation	208	18	1.15
Pancreatectomy (3–22 hr)	96	6	0.20
Glucose load (1.75 mg/kg)	596	47	0.75

Data from Assenmacher.[4]

for duck, turkey and chicken hormones.[28] These hormones are almost identical structurally to mammalian glucagon.

In the process of extraction and purification of insulin from chickens, a third biologically active peptide was isolated and named avian PP. Like mammalian PP, aPP consists of 36 amino acid residues and has a molecular weight of approximately 4200 daltons. Its primary structure is provided in Figure 13-10. Avian PP, unlike its mammalian counterpart, appears to have a strong stimulatory influence on gastric acid secretion in chickens. The physiological role for aPP, however, is uncertain at this time.

Summary

The predominant cellular types in the vertebrate endocrine pancreas are the A cell, B cell and D cell. The A cell and B cell have been identified as the sources for glucagon and insulin respectively. The D cell produces somatostatin. A fourth cellular type located at the periphery of the mammalian pancreatic islet produces PP. These four cellular types plus a fifth type of unknown function are found in most vertebrate groups. It is not certain as to the germ layer origins for the endocrine cells. They do not come from the neural crest in spite of the amine precursor uptake and decarboxylation characteristics, and it is not clear whether they are of endodermal or ectodermal origin.

Five patterns of islet morphology can be distinguished: (1) cyclostome type, (2) primitive gnathostome type, (3) actinopterygian type, (4) lungfish type and (5) tetrapod type. It is assumed that the most primitive anatomical arrangement for the endocrine pancreatic tissue occurs in lampreys as the follicles of Langerhans embedded in the gut lining. The equally if not more primitive hagfishes, however, have a definite endocrine pancreas. Bony fishes tend to have discrete islets but lack an acinar (exocrine) pancreas. Elasmobranchs, holocephalans and *Latimeria* all exhibit the primitive gnathostome type. Tetrapods have distinct pancreatic organs containing both acinar and islet tissues.

Glucagon is one of several hyperglycemic factors in vertebrates, and it stimulates glycogenolysis and lipolysis in liver and adipose cells while inhibiting glucose oxidation. These actions of glucagon appear to be mediated through activation of adenyl cyclase and formation of cAMP. Low blood sugar levels stimulate glucagon release, and somatostatin blocks glucagon release. High levels of circulating free fatty acids stimulate glucagon release in birds and herbivorous mammals. Glucagon may be the primary regulator of carbohydrate metabolism in birds and reptiles with insulin playing only a minor role. Glucagon seems to be hyperglycemic in amphibians and fishes. Immunoreactive glucagon is present in several invertebrate phyla including Arthropoda, Mollusca and the invertebrate Chordata.

Insulin is the only naturally occurring hypoglycemic factor in vertebrates. It has been extracted from all of the major vertebrate classes except Amphibia, in which extraction has not been attempted. Insulin is present in many invertebrate species as well and may even function there as a hypoglycemic factor. The actions of insulin include permeability effects on the plasmalemma, resulting in the increased uptake of glucose and amino acids into muscle cells and uptake of glucose by adipose cells. Lipogenesis increases following the binding of insulin to the plasmalemma of adipose cells because of the increased availability of substrates following glucose uptake and oxidation and active inhibition of lipolysis. Although the mechanisms of insulin action are not certain, it does not seem to operate via the activation of adenyl cyclase. It has been proposed that the primary action of insulin is a change in permeability of the plasmalemma and release of glycopeptides that determines all subsequent effects observed. Growth effects occur in cooperation with insulinlike growth factors.

High circulating glucose levels stimulate release of insulin from the B cells of the pancreatic islets. It is the uptake and metabolism of this glucose that actually is responsible for causing insulin release. Neural factors (parasympathetic) and other hormones (for example, secretin) may also stimulate insulin release. Low blood glucose levels, somatostatin, epinephrine and gastrin all inhibit release.

It has been proposed that the most primitive function for insulin is the effect on amino acid incorporation into protein.[14] Glucose administration does not evoke insulin release in lampreys, lizards or birds, and insulin stimulates only protein synthesis in hagfish liver. These observations suggest limited involvement of insulin in carbohydrate metabolism of nonmammals. The effects of insulin on lipid metabolism may be largely a mammalian occurrence.

References

1. Adelson, J.W. (1971). Enterosecretory proteins. Nature 229:321–325.
2. Andrew, A. (1976). An experimental investigation into the possible neural crest origin of pancreatic APUD (islet) cells. J. Embryol. Exp. Morphol. 35:577–593.
3. Arimura, A., H. Sata, A. Dupont, N. Nishi and A.W. Schally (1975). Somatostatin: Abundance of immunoreactive hormone in rat stomach and pancreas. Science 189:1007–1009.
4. Assenmacher, I. (1973). The peripheral endocrine glands. In D.S. Farner and J.R. King, eds., Avian Biology. Academic Press, New York, Vol. 3, pp. 183–286.
5. Barrington, E.J.W. (1975). An Introduction to General and Comparative Endocrinology. Clarendon Press, Oxford.
6. Birnbaum, M.J., J. Schultz and J.N. Fain (1976). Hormone-stimulated glycogenolysis in isolated goldfish hepatocytes. Am. J. Physiol. 231:191–197.
7. Bonner-Weir, S. and G.C. Weir (1979). The organization of the endocrine pancreas: a hypothetical unifying view of the phylogenetic differences. Gen. Comp. Endocrinol. 38:28–37.
8. Brinn, J.E. (1973). The pancreatic islets of bony fishes. Am. Zool. 13:653–666.
9. Brinn, J.E. (1975). Pancreatic islet cytology of Ictaluridae (Teleostei). Cell Tissue Res. 162:357–365.
10. Brinn, J.E. and A. Epple (1976). New types of islet cells in a cyclostome, *Petromyzon marinus* L. Cell Tissue Res. 171:317–329.
11. Copeland, P.L. and R. DeRoos (1971). Effect of mammalian insulin on plasma glucose in the mudpuppy. *(Necturus maculosus)*. J. Exp. Zool. 178:35–43.
12. Emdin, S.O. (1982). Effects of hagfish insulin in the Atlantic hagfish, *Myxine glutinosa*. The *in vivo* metabolism of (^{14}C) glucose and (^{14}C) leucine and studies on starvation and glucose-loading. Gen. Comp. Endocrinol. 47:414–425.
13. Epple, A. and J.E. Brinn, Jr. (1975). Islet histophysiology: Evolutionary correlations. Gen. Comp. Endocrinol. 27:320–349.
14. Epple, A., J.E. Brinn and J.B. Young (1980). Evolution of pancreatic islet functions. In P.K.T. Pang and A. Epple, eds., Evolution of Vertebrate Endocrine Systems. Texas Tech Press, Lubbock, Texas, pp. 269–321.
15. Epple, A., C.B. Jorgensen and P. Rosenkilde (1966). Effect of hypophysectomy on blood sugar, fat, glycogen, and pancreatic islets in starving toads (*Bufo bufo* (L.)). Gen. Comp. Endocrinol. 7:197–202.
16. Epple, A. and T.L. Lewis (1973). Comparative histophysiology of the pancreatic islets. Am. Zool. 13:567–590.
17. Falkmer, S., J.F. Cutfield, S.M. Cutfield, G.G. Dodson, J. Gliemann, S. Gammeltoft, M. Marques, J.D. Peterson, D.F. Steiner, F. Sundby, S.O. Emdin, N. Havu, Y. Östberg, and L. Winbladh (1975). Comparative endocrinology of insulin and glucagon production. Am. Zool. 15, Suppl. 1:255–270.
18. Falkmer, S. and A.J. Matty (1966). Blood sugar regulation in the hagfish, *Myxine glutinosa*. Gen. Comp. Endocrinol. 6:334–346.

19. Floyd, J.C., Jr., S.S. Fajans, S. Pek and R.E. Chance (1977). A newly recognized pancreatic polypeptide: Plasma levels in health and disease. Recent Prog. Horm. Res. 33:519–570.

20. Foa, P.P. (1973). Glucagon: An incomplete and biased review with selected references. Am. Zool. 13:613–624.

21. Fontaine, J., C. LeLievre and N.M. LeDouarin (1977). What is the developmental fate of the neural crest cells which migrate into the pancreas in the avian embryo? Gen. Comp. Endocrinol. 33:394–404.

22. Fritz, I.B. (1972). Insulin actions on carbohydrate and lipid metabolism. In G. Litwack, ed., Biochemical Actions of Hormones Vol. 2. Academic Press, New York, pp. 165–214.

23. Gill, T.S. and S.S. Khanna (1975). Effect of glucagon upon blood glucose level of the fresh water fish *Channa punctatus* (Bloch). Indian J. Exp. Biol. 13:298–300.

24. Gorbman, A. and H.A. Bern (1962). A Textbook of Comparative Endocrinology. John Wiley and Sons, New York.

25. Groscolas, R. and J. Bezard (1977). Effect of glucagon and insulin on plasma free fatty acids and glucose in the emperor penguin, *Aptenodytes forsteri.* Gen. Comp. Endocrinol. 32:230–235.

26. Grube, D., V. Maier, S. Raptis and W. Schlegel (1978). Immunoreactivity of the endocrine pancreas. Evidence for the presence of cholecystokinin-pancreozymin within the A-cell. Histochemistry 56:13–35.

27. Guilleman, R. and J.E. Gerich (1976). Somatostatin: Physiological and clinical significance. Annu. Rev. Med. 27:379–388.

28. Hazelwood, R.L. (1973). The avian endocrine pancreas. Am. Zool. 13:699–709.

29. Hazelwood, R.L., S.D. Turner, J.R. Kimmel and H.G. Pollock (1973). Spectrum effects of a new polypeptide (third hormone?) isolated from the chicken pancreas. Gen. Comp. Endocrinol. 21:485–497.

30. Hodgkin, D.C. (1974). Insulin, its chemistry and biochemistry. Proc. Roy. Soc. Lond. 186:191–215.

31. Ince, B.W. and A. Thorpe (1976). The *in vivo* metabolism of ^{14}C-glucose and ^{14}C-glycine in insulin-treated northern pike (*Esox lucius* L.). Gen. Comp. Endocrinol. 28:481–486.

32. Ince, B.W. and A. Thorpe (1977). Glucose and amino acid-stimulated insulin release *in vivo* in the European silver eel (*Anguilla anguilla* L.) Gen. Comp. Endocrinol. 31:249–256.

33. Kahn, R.C., K.L. Baird, J.S. Flier, C. Grunfeld, J.T. Harmon, L.C. Harrison, F.A. Karlson, M. Kasuga, G.L. King, U.C. Lang, J.M. Podskalny and E. Obberghen (1981). Insulin receptors, receptor antibodies, and the mechanism of insulin action. Rec. Prog. Horm. Res. 37:477–538.

34. Kaneto, A., E. Miki and K. Kosaka (1974). Effects of vagal stimulation on glucagon and insulin secretion. Endocrinology 95:1005–1010.

35. Kimmel, J.R., M.J. Maher, H.G. Pollock and W.H. Vensel (1976). Isolation and characterization of reptilian insulin: Partial amino acid sequence of rattlesnake *(Crotalus atrox)* insulin. Gen. Comp. Endocrinol. 28:320–333.

36. Klein, C. and S. van Noorden (1980). Pancreatic polypeptide (PP) and glucagon cells in the pancreatic islet of *Xiphophorus helleri* H. (Teleostei). Correlative immunohistochemistry and electron microscopy. Cell Tiss. Res. 205:187–198.

37. Larner, J., K. Cheng, C. Schwartz, K. Kunimi, S. Tamura, S. Creacy, R. Dubler, G. Galasko, C. Pullin and M. Katz (1982). Insulin mediators and the control of metabolism through protein phosphorylation. Rec. Prog. Horm. Res. 38:511–556.

38. Lawrence, A.M., S. Tan, S. Hojvat and L. Kirsteins (1977). Salivary gland hyperglycemic factor: An extrapancreatic source of glucagon-like material. Science 195:70–72.

39. Levine, R. (1982). Insulin: the effects and mode of action of the hormone. Vit. Horm. 39:145–173.

40. Malaisse, W.J., D.G. Pipeleers, E. VanObberghen, G. Somers, G. Devis, M. Marichal and F. Malaisse-Lagae (1973). The glucoreceptor mechanism in the pancreatic beta-cell. Am. Zool. 13:605–612.

41. Markussen, J., E. Frandsen, L.G. Heding, and F. Sundby (1972). Turkey glucagon: Crystallization, amino acid composition and immunology. Horm. Metab. Res. 4:360–363.

42. McMillan, J.E. and R.F. Wilkinson, Jr. (1972). The effect of pancreatic hormones on blood sugar in *Ambystoma annulatum.* Copeia 1972:664–668.

43. Noe, B.D., D.J. Fletcher, G.E. Bauer, G.C. Weir and Y. Patel (1978). Somatostatin biosynthesis occurs in pancreatic islets. Endocrinology 102:1675–1685.

44. Östberg, Y., S. VanNoorden and A.G.E. Pearse (1975). Cytochemical, immunofluorescence, and ultrastructural investigations on polypeptide hormone localization in the islet parenchyma and bile duct mucosa of a cyclostome, *Myxine glutinosa.* Gen. Comp. Endocrinol. 25:274–291.

45. Patent, G. (1970). Comparison of some hormonal effects on carbohydrate metabolism in an elasmobranch *(Squalus acanthias)* and a holocephalan *(Hydrolagus colliei).* Gen. Comp. Endocrinol. 14:215–242.

46. Patent, G.J. (1973). The chondrichthean endocrine pancreas: What are its functions? Am. Zool. 13:639–652.

47. Patent, G.J. and P.P. Foa (1971). Radioimmunoassay of insulin in fishes, experiments *in vivo* and *in vitro.* Gen. Comp. Endocrinol. 16:41–46.

48. Pearse, A.G.E. and J.M. Polak (1971). Neural crest origin of the endocrine polypeptide (APUD) cells of the gastrointestinal tract and pancreas. Gut 12:783–788.

49. Penhos, J.C. and E. Ramey (1973). Studies on the endocrine pancreas of amphibians and reptiles. Am. Zool. 13:667–698.

50. Pictet, R.L., L.B. Rall, P. Phelps and W.J. Rutter (1976). The neural crest and the origin of the insulin-producing and other gastrointestinal hormone-producing cells. Science 191:191–192.

51. Pictet, R. and W.J. Rutter (1972). Development of the embryonic endocrine pancreas. Handbook of Physiology, Sec. 7, Endocrinology. Williams & Wilkins, Baltimore, Vol. I, pp. 25–66.

52. Sanger, F. (1959). Chemistry of insulin. Science 129–1340–1344.

53. Seltzer, H.H. (1980). Efficacy and safety of oral hypoglycemic agents. Ann. Rev. Med. 31:261–272.

54. Smith, P.H., F.W. Merchant, D.G. Johnson, W.T. Fujimoto and R.H. Williams (1977). Immunocytochemical localization of a gastric inhibitory polypeptide-like material within A-cells of the endocrine pancreas. Amer. J. Anat. 149:585–590.

55. Steiner, D.F., J.D. Peterson, H. Tager, S. Emdin, Y. Östberg and S. Falkmer (1973). Comparative aspects of proinsulin and insulin structure and biosynthesis. Am. Zool. 13:591–604.

56. Trakatellis, A.C., K. Tada, K. Yamaji, and P. Gordiki-Kouidou (1975). Isolation and partial characterization of anglerfish proglucagon. Biochemistry 14:1508–1512.

57. Von Mering, J. and O. Minkowski (1889). Diabetes mellitus nach Pankreasextirpation. Arch. Exp. Pathol. Pharmakol. 26:371. Cited by Gorbman and Bern.[24]

58. White, A.W. and C.J.F. Harrop (1975). The islets of Langerhans of the pancreas of macropodid marsupials: A comparison with eutherian species. Aust. J. Zool. 23:309–319.

59. Wong, K.L. and W. Hanke (1977). The effects of biogenic amines on carbohydrate metabolism in *Xenopus laevis* Daudin. Gen. Comp. Endocrinol. 31:80–90.

60. Wurster, D.H. and M.R. Miller (1960). Studies on the blood glucose and pancreatic islets of the salamander, *Taricha torosa*. Comp. Biochem. Physiol. 1:101–109.

14·The Gastrointestinal Peptides

With the identification by Bayliss and Starling of the first blood-borne chemical messenger, *secretin,* produced by the duodenal mucosa, and the proposal for *gastrin,* from the antral stomach a few years later by Edkins, the existence of endocrine regulation of the mammalian digestive system was established and the discipline of endocrinology was born.[5,19] Ironically the gastrointestinal (GI) hormones have been among the last to be chemically characterized, and it was only after isolation of the purified hormones in the 1960s that it became possible to confirm the diffusely distributed cellular types responsible for their secretion. Because of the lack of precision in observations, the complications of sorting out neutral and proposed endocrine factors, effects of known pharmacological agents and rapid proliferation of unsubstantiated factors, the entire area of GI endocrine research was easily overshadowed when the nature of certain medically important hormones was discovered. Research with corticosteroids, reproductive hormones, thyroid hormones, insulin and epinephrine occupied the mainstream of endocrine research, whereas advances associated with GI factors were uncommon.

In recent years, there has been rapid expansion in GI peptide research, and there are now many peptides that have been isolated and chemically characterized. Yet we do not understand the physiological roles for many of these peptides. For others, the assignment of their physiological roles changes so frequently that it is bewildering. Even their names seem to be in a state of flux. Some GI peptides appear to function as classic hormones, others are paracrine secretions and still others may be neurotransmitters. Many GI peptides have been identified within the central nervous system and in certain endocrine glands. For simplicity, all of these regulatory substances are referred to here as GI peptides.

Endocrine regulation of digestion must be considered an integral portion of the entire digestive process. Consequently it is necessary to review the entire digestive process to illustrate the regulatory actions of GI peptides. The following discussion emphasizes the human digestive system, including the mouth, pharynx, esophagus, stomach and small intestine (Fig. 14-1). In addition to the roles played by these portions of the alimentary canal, digestion is aided by three essential exocrine glands: (1) the several pairs of salivary glands that secrete into the mouth, (2) the liver and (3) the exocrine pancreas; the last two secrete materials into the small intestine (Fig. 14-1). The reader should keep in mind the many anatomical and functional differences that exist between the human digestive system and those of mammalian carnivores and herbivores with respect to the specific details of the following account. The metabolic fate of absorbed products of digestion and their endocrinological implications are discussed in Chapter 19.

The Human Digestive System

The first detailed and systematic knowledge of human digestive processes came from the observations of William Beaumont on his patient Alexis St. Martin, a French Canadian who, while visiting Fort Mackinac, Michigan, was accidentally shot in the chest from close range by a shotgun; two ribs were fractured, the lungs lacerated and the stomach perforated. Although Beaumont assumed that St. Martin would not live the night, he miraculously survived. The wound in St. Martin's stomach, however, never healed completely, resulting in a permanent opening to the outside (a *gastric fistula*) through which Beaumont was able to observe the progression of gastric digestion under varying conditions over a period of years.[7] It was these pioneering observations by Beaumont that stimulated much of the later interest in gastric physiology.

The accidental production of a gastric fistula in St. Martin provided the inspiration for a variety of surgical techniques, including production of gastric fistulas and gastric or intestinal pouches (isolated pouches no longer connected with the lumen of the gut). Transplantation of denervated pouches or pieces of digestive tract or pancreas to sites under the skin where revascularization can occur has enabled investigators to separate endocrine and nervous regulatory mechanisms. Finally the development of crossed circulatory systems between experimental animals was used to confirm the transfer of chemical factors (hormones) through the blood to target tissues. *In-vitro* studies of pancreatic slices or mucosal tissues from various regions of the gut have been employed profitably to ascertain details of the actions of the various GI peptides and factors regulating their release.

Table 14-1 summarizes the action the some GI peptides in mammals.

Oral Events

When food is ingested it is first torn and ground by the teeth and is mixed with *saliva* secreted from the exocrine salivary glands. Salivation is under direct neural control and can be stimulated by sight, smell or simply the thought of food or by the presence of food in the mouth. Saliva is a basic fluid containing the hydrolytic enzyme *salivary amylase,* which hydrolyses starches to disaccharides. The saliva and partially digested chewed food are mixed thoroughly to form a bolus that is pushed back into the pharynx by the tongue. After entry into the pharynx the bolus is swallowed by a reflexive series of events that propel it down the esophagus and into the stomach.

Gastric Events

Upon entering the stomach the bolus of food is in an acidic environment due to secretion of *hydrochloric acid* by glands located in the *mucosa* (epithelial lining) of the *fundus* or main body of the stomach (Fig. 14-1). The specific source of HCl is the *parietal cell* of the mucosa. These cells can be distinguished by staining fixed tissue sections with modification of the Zimmermann technique, following which the parietal cells appear yellow.[40] Hydrochloric acid reduces the pH of the stomach contents, thereby activating the proteolytic enzyme *pepsin,* which is secreted in an inactive form, *pepsinogen,* by the *chief cells* of the gastric glands. Chief cells are stained blue by the modified Zimmermann technique. The acidity of the gastric contents softens fibrous material, kills some bacteria ingested with the food and extracts calcium salts from bone and cartilage. In addition, HCl brings about slow inactivation of salivary amylase as the acid penetrates the bolus and blocks further starch digestion.

It is not known how the parietal cell is able to secrete concentrated hydrogen ions (HCl) without damage to itself. The presence of tight junctions between the mucosal cells and the high mitotic rate observed for gastric mucosal cells in part explain how the stomach contains such a caustic solution without causing irreparable destruction. These tight junctions prevent the penetration of acid and proteolytic enzyme (pepsin) into the mucosa. This outer layer is continuously replaced by mitotic activity to maintain the integrity of the mucosal barrier.

The Gastrin Theory and Acid Secretion. Edkins in 1905 showed that extracts prepared from the most posterior portion of the stomach, the *antrum,* stimulated acid secretion by the fundic glands, and he suggested the name of *gastrin* for the active substance in these extracts.[19] He found no gastrin activity in extracts prepared from the fundic portion of the stomach. Edkin's gastrin hypothesis temporarily lost credibility with the discovery of *histamine,* a potent stimulator of gastric acid secre-

TABLE 14-1. *Actions of Some Gastrointestinal Peptides in Mammals*

PEPTIDE	CELLULAR SOURCE[a]	MAJOR ESTABLISHED PHYSIOLOGICAL ACTIONS	CONSEQUENCES OF ACTIONS
Gastrin	G cell	Stimulates HCl secretion by parietal cell in fundic mucosa	Activates pepsinogen and accelerates protein digestion
Secretin	S cell	Stimulates release of basic pancreatic juice into duodenum via pancreatic duct	Converts acidic chyme entering duodenum to basic medium facilitating further digestion; helps protect duodenum from harmful effects of acid
Pancreozymin-cholecystokinin (PZCCK)	I cell	Stimulates release of pancreatic enzymes into pancreatic juice	Completes digestion of proteins to peptides begun in stomach; completes digestion of carbohydrates to disaccharides begun in mouth; hydrolyzes fats to fatty acids and glycerol
		Stimulates contraction of gallbladder smooth muscle and relaxation of Sphinchter of Oddi controlling the exit from the gallbladder	Flow of bile into duodenum to aid fat digestion through emulsification of fat droplets
Glucose-dependent insulinotropic peptide,[b] (GIP)	K cell	Released by elevated glucose and stimulates release of insulin	Slows gastric events when more time is required for processing materials already in duodenum
Motilin	EC cell	Stimulates pepsinogen secretion; stimulates gastric motility	Accelerates gastric digestion; antagonizes action of GIP and reinitiates higher rate of gastric processing
Vasoactive intestinal peptide (VIP)	H cell	Increases blood flow to viscera	Presumably aids in digestion and absorption by increasing vascular supply
Enteroglucagon	EG_1 cells	Unclear; may have glucagon-like effects on pancreas; possibly augments secretion of calcitonin	
Somatostatin	D cell	Paracrine inhibition of release of other peptides	Stops digestive process

[a]Designations for these cells used by Jaffe.[29]
[b]Formerly gastric inhibitory peptide.

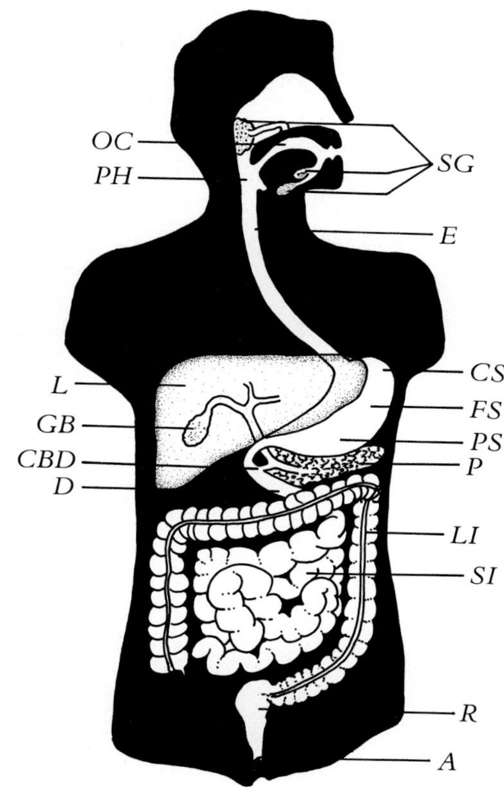

Fig. 14-1. The human digestive system. *OC,* oral cavity; *SG,* salivary glands; *PH,* pharynx; *E,* esophagus; *L,* liver; *CS,* cardiac stomach; *FS,* fundic stomach; *PS,* pyloric stomach; *GB,* gallbladder; *CBD,* common bile duct; *P,* pancreas; *D,* duodenum; *LI,* colon or large intestine; *SI,* jejunem and ileum of small intestine; *R,* rectum; *A,* anus.

tion, and the demonstration of histamine in extracts of the gastric mucosa. It was almost 30 years before it was shown that histamine-free extracts from the mucosa of the antral portion of the stomach possessed the ability to stimulate acid secretion by the parietal cells. Nevertheless it was not until gastrin was finally isolated and characterized chemically that the term gastrin theory was discarded.

At least two similar peptides with gastrin activity have been isolated (gastrin I and gastrin II) from the antral stomach. Both of the molecules are composed of 17 amino acids; their only difference is that the C-terminal tyrosine of gastrin II is sulfated. A molecule of 34 amino acids has also been found in the circulation; it consists of gastrin I or II together with a third 17 amino acid peptide component. This big gastrin constitutes only about 5% of the circulating gastrin. The preprohormone for gastrin is composed of 104 amino acids. This molecule is cleaved enzymatically several times to release big and little gastrins.[23] Most of the biological activity of these gastrins resides in the four carboxy-terminal amino acids consisting of *Trp-Met-Asp-Phe-*NH_2. Several peptides that possess this terminal sequence have been shown to stimulate acid secretion (see Fig. 14-2). A synthetic pentapeptide *(pentagastrin)* that incorporates the terminal tetrapeptide sequence is frequently used for experimental studies.

The gastrin theory for control of acid secretion combines the observations that parasympathetic stimulation, acetylcholine (ACh), histamine and gastrin all cause acid secretion, whereas atropine (an anticholinergic drug), procaine (an anesthetic), sympathetic stimulation or certain antihistamines tend to reduce acid secretion under some experimental conditions.[31] Presumably parasympathetic stimulation through release of ACh causes release of gastrin from the *G cell* in the antral mucosa. Gastrin travels via the blood to the fundus of the stomach where it stimulates the release of histamine from cells situated in the mucosa. Gastrin activates the synthesis of histidine decarboxylase, the enzyme responsible for histamine synthesis. Histamine in turn stimulates release of HCl from the parietal cell, probably via an adenyl cyclase-cyclic adenosine 3′,5′-monophosphate (cAMP) mechanism, resulting in decreased pH of the stomach contents. Gastrin may stimulate parietal cells directly without employing histamine as an intermediate, and some investigators conclude that histamine is not involved in endogenous acid secretion.[31] Vagal stimulation or application of ACh may stimulate the parietal cells directly to secrete HCl.

During active digestion the pH of the stomach may be between 1 and 2. Low pH in the antral portion of the stomach (especially near the pyloric sphincter) reduces gastrin release.

Secretion of Pepsinogen. The major gastric enzyme is the protease pepsin that is secreted by the chief cells in an inactive form, pepsinogen. Conversion of inactive pepsinogen to pepsin is accomplished by the presence of an excess of hydrogen ions supplied by HCl

	Secretin	Glucagon	GIP	PZCCK	Caerulein	Human Gastrin II
1	His	His	Tyr			
2	Ser	Ser	Ala			
3	Asp	Gln	Glu			
4	Gly	Gly	Gly			
5	Thr	Thr	Thr			
6	Phe	Phe	Phe			
7	Thr	Thr	Ile			
8	Ser	Ser	Ser			
9	Glu	Asp	Asp			
10	Leu	Tyr	Trp			
11	Ser	Ser	Ser			
12	Arg	Lys	Ile			
13	Leu	Trp	Ala			
14	Arg	Leu	Met			
15	Asp	Asp	Asp			
16	Ser	Ser	Lys			
17	Ala	Arg	Ile			(1) Glu
18	Arg	Arg	Arg			(2) Glu
19	Leu	Ala	Gln			(3) Pro
20	Gln	Gln	Gln			(4) Try
21	Arg	Asp	Asp			(5) Leu
22	Leu	Phe	Phe			(6) Glu
23	Leu	Val	Val			(7) Glu
24	Gln	Gln	Asn		(1) Gln	(8) Glu
25	Gly	Trp	Trp		(2) Gln	(9) Glu
26	Leu	Leu	Leu	Asp	(3) Asp	(10) Glu
27	$ValNH_2$	Met	Leu	Tyr (SO_3H)	(4) Tyr ((SO_3H)	(11) Ala
28		Asn	Ala	Met	(5) Thr	(12) Tyr (SO_3H)
29		Thr	Gln	Gly	(6) Gly	(13) Gly
30			Lys	Trp	(7) Trp	(14) Trp
31			Gly	Met	(8) Met	(15) Met
32			Lys	Asp	(9) Asp	(16) Asp
33			Lys	Phe-NH_2	(10) Phe-NH_2	(17) Phe-NH_2
34			Ser			
35			Asp			
36			Trp			
37			Lys			
38			His			
39			Asn			
40			Ile			
41			Thr			
42			Gln			

Fig. 14-2. Comparison of amino acid sequences of polypeptide hormones from the digestive system. Overlapping sequences are enclosed in boxes. Numbers in parentheses indicate actual sequence numbers in which small peptides have been aligned with the carboxyl terminal octapeptide sequence of pancreozymin-cholecystokinin *(PZCCK)*. *GIP*, glucose-dependent insulinotropic peptide. Caerulein is a molecule first isolated from frog skin that has gastrin-like activity.

secreted from parietal cells. The optimum pH for vertebrate pepsins lies between 1 and 2, the normal pH range observed in the stomach following stimulation of acid secretion. The presence of acid on the surface of the gastic mucosa may activate a cholinergic reflex that evokes pepsinogen release.[30] Parasympathetic stimulation via the vagus nerve causes release of pepsinogen, but hormonal control of pepsinogen secretion has not been established. A duodenal peptide motilin (see p. 371), has been implicated in regulating pepsinogen secretion. Gastrin causes release of pepsinogen only when applied in doses great enough to *inhibit* acid secretion by the parietal cells, implying that gastrin is not the normal factor causing pepsinogen release from the chief cells. Several other GI peptides can invoke pepsinogen release but do so only when applied in pharmacological doses.

Phases of Gastric Regulation. Gastric secretion is controlled via two levels. The *cephalic phase* involves stimulation of secretion via parasympathetic discharges elicited by the same stimuli that cause salivation; that is, sight, smell, taste, thought or presence of food. In the *gastric phase* of secretory control the presence of food in the stomach elicits secretion through vagovagal reflexes and/or through the gastrin mechanism. It has not been possible to determine which of these mechanisms is more important in controlling gastric secretion; probably all of these mechanisms operate in the normal digestive process.

Intestinal Events

While in the stomach, the bolus of food become saturated with the acidic gastric juices. These substances are thoroughly mixed by peristaltic contractions of the stomach to form an acidic, viscous fluid called *chyme.* Motility of the stomach, which is stimulated by the parasympathetic system, is responsible for churning the food mass and mixing it with gastric juices to form chyme. If the pH of the chyme in the antrum is sufficiently low (that is, less than 4.5) and of proper viscosity, the pyloric sphincter opens, and acidic chyme is squirted into the first segment of the small intestine, the *duodenum.* The exact mechanism controlling ejection of chyme from the stomach is not understood. Secretions also enter the duodenum from the exocrine pancreas and liver, through the *common bile duct,* in response to events taking place in the duodenum.

The duodenal mucosa contains many secretory cells, including cells responsible for digestive enzyme secretion as well as a variety of hormone-secreting cells and mucus-secreting cells. The intestinal mucosa is organized into thousands of tiny finger-like projections called *villi.* The presence of villi greatly increases the total surface area of the small intestine for both secretion and absorption of digestive products. The duodenum possesses more villi and secretory cells than do the more posterior sections of the small intestine (*jejunum* and *ileum.*) The degree of specialization in the mucosa decreases progressively from anterior to posterior.

Secretin and Pancreozymin. The presence of acidic chyme (pH less than 4.5) in the duodenum directly stimulates the *S-type cell* in the duodenal mucosa to release the peptide *secretin* into the blood. Bayliss and Starling discovered the existence of this factor that stimulates the pancreas to secrete basic juice and helps to neutralize the acidity of the chyme that has entered the small intestine.[5] Although secretin levels in the blood do not increase following ingestion of a meal, the action of secretin on the exocrine pancreas is potentiated by another intestinal peptide hormone, *cholecystokinin,* that increases the blood following ingestion.[31]

Originally it was believed that secretin was also responsible for stimulating secretion of the digestive enzymes normally present in the pancreatic juice, including the proteases chymotrypsin and trypsin, pancreatic lipase, pancreatic amylase and nucleases (DNase and RNase). After 40 years of controversy following the demonstration of secretin it was confirmed finally by Harper and Raper that purified secretin stimulates secretion of pancreatic fluid that is rich in sodium bicarbonate and poor in digestive enzymes.[25] A second duodenal peptide, named *pancreozymin,* was found to contaminate some secretin preparations but not others, depending on the methods of preparation. Since *zymogen granules* represent vesicles of stored enzyme within the acinar (exocrine) pancreatic cell, the peptide that causes extrusion of zymogen granules from pancreatic acinar cells is logically called pancreozymin (pancreas-zymogen). It was postulated that the release of pancreozymin into the blood in response to the presence of peptides and amino acids in the chyme is due to direct actions of these molecules on pancreozymin-producing cells, similar to the action of hydrogen ions on the S-type cell. Sometimes the term *secretagogue* is applied to substances present in food, products secreted from the mucosa into the gut lumen or products of digestion that induce gastric or intestinal secretions.

Cholecystokinin. It was proposed in 1928 by Ivy and Goldberg that the presence of fat in the chyme or some of the digestive products stimulated release of yet another intestinal peptide that they named *cholecystokinin* (*chole* bile + *kystis* bladder + *kinein* move). Cholecystokinin travels via the blood to the gallbladder where it stimulates contraction of the smooth muscles comprising the walls of the gallbladder. At the same time it causes relaxation of the sphincter muscle that controls exit of bile from the gallbladder (the sphincter of Oddi). As a result, bile is expelled from the gallbladder, enters the bile duct (bile-bladder-move) and is transported to the duodenum. Bile is a viscous, complex mixture consisting largely of bile salts and bile pigments. Bile salts are powerful emulsifiers of fats (detergents). Bile pigments are breakdown products of hemoglobins, and they provide to bile and feces their characteristic colorations. Many other substances produced by the liver are present in bile, including metabolites of steroid hormones (Chap. 9) and inorganic iodide from deiodination of thyroid hormones (Chap. 8). When bile enters the small intestine the bile salts emulsify globules of fat, causing them to be dispersed as small fat droplets within the aqueous digestive fluids. The emulsification of fats allows for marked reduction in the volume-to-surface ratio of the fat droplets, facilitating hydrolytic attack by pancreatic lipase to release glycerol and fatty acids for absorption.

Pancreozymin-Cholecystokinin. Isolation and purification of GI peptides was finally accomplished by Mutt and Jorpes in Sweden more than half a century after the discovery of secretin by Bayliss and Starling. Investigators have since succeeded in identifying many distinct GI peptides. Secretin was confirmed as a separate peptide consisting of 27 amino acids.[32] Purified secretin stimulated secretion of pancreatic juice that was low in enzyme content. However, the biological functions previously ascribed to PZ and CCK were found to reside in the same peptide consisting of 33 amino acids.[33] Consequently the rather cumbersome name *pancreozymin-cholecystokinin* (PZCCK or CCKPZ) has been proposed to designate the single peptide that has been described in the literature under separate names for these separate functions. The *I-type* cell in the intestinal mucosa has been identified as the synthetic source for PZCCK.[29,37]

The separate functional roles of secretin and PZCCK have been demonstrated elegantly in vitro with slices of exocrine pancreas. Physiological levels of PZCCK do not evoke release of basic pancreatic juice except in the presence of secretin,[31] implying a permissive role. The action of secretin is markedly enhanced by PZCCK. Addition of purified PZCCK causes extrusion of zymogen granules from the acinar cells. Acetylcholine also causes extrusion of zymagen granules, suggesting a role for parasympathetic control over enzyme release from the exocrine pancreas. Parasympathetic influence and PZCCK probably operate via separate mechanisms. Atropine blocks the action of ACh but not of PZCCK. Purified secretin does not induce zymogen granule extrusion in these preparations. These data support the hypothesis for direct vagal (parasympathetic) influence over pancreatic enzyme release as being part of the normal regulatory mechanism; however, PZCCK does not require neural factors for its action.

Glucose-dependent Insulinotropic Peptide. Another intestinal GI peptide *enterogastrone,* was proposed in 1930 by Kosaka and Lim to be released in response to arrival of fat from the stomach.[35] Enterogastrone was believed to inhibit gastric motility (peristalsis) as well as reduce acid secretion by the parietal cells. These actions would slow the entrance of fat into the small intestine and allow more time for proper processing of fat.

A peptide has been isolated from the intestine that inhibits gastric function. It was named *gastric-inhibitory peptide* (GIP) and is produced by the K cell in the duodenal mucosa. Chemically, GIP is similar to glucagon and secretin (Fig. 14-2) but is larger (42 amino acids). This peptide blocks gastric peristalsis and secretion of acid and enzyme. However, these effects occur only in the experimentally denervated stomach.[10] It also stimulates release of insulin from the endocrine pancreas. This insulin-releasing action is now believed to be the physiological role for GIP. Following glucose uptake,[10,31] GIP is secreted into the blood and causes release of insulin. Because of this action, GIP's name has been changed to *glucose-dependent insulinotropic peptide* while retaining the same acronym.

Neither bile secretion by the liver nor the secretion of *Brunner's glands* in the intestinal mucosa are influenced by GIP. Brunner's glands secrete viscid alkaline mucus that is believed to neutralize gastric juice entering through the pylorus. These glands are concentrated in the region of the pyloric sphincter and gradually decrease in frequency posteriorly, only occasionally being present in the most anterior portion of the jejunum. These cells also may secrete mucus in response to the presence of acidic chyme in the duodenum.

Motilin. A unique small peptide (22 amino acids) that stimulates both motility and secretion of pepsinogen by the stomach has been isolated from the duodenum (Fig. 14-3). This peptide, *motilin,* is structurally unlike the other GI peptides. Motilin is released from the *EC-type* cells when alkaline conditions are present in the duodenum, but the actual regulatory mechanism(s) governing its release is (are) uncertain. The physiological significance of this effect has been questioned since very alkaline conditions (pH 8.5–10) are required for releasing motilin.[29,31] Acidification may cause motilin release under certain conditions in humans.[29]

Vasoactive Intestinal Polypeptide. Another peptide isolated from the intestinal mucosa has been shown to relax smooth muscle,[51] thereby increasing the flow of blood to the viscera. This *vasoactive intestinal polypeptide* (VIP) consists of 28 amino acids and is structurally similar to both glucagon and secretin as well as to GIP. Vasoactive intestinal peptide is produced in neurons and by a pyramidal-shaped *H cell* found in the small intestine and in the colon of some species.[29] Sufficiently high doses of VIP have been shown to produce secretin-like effects on the pancreas as well as a hyperglycemic response. These actions of VIP on the exocrine pancreas and blood sugar levels may be pharmacologic.

A major role for VIP is that of an inhibitory neurotransmitter produced by intestinal nerves.[9] It inhibits vascular smooth muscle but stimulates glandular epithelia.[20] It is the inhibitory action on vascular smooth muscle that increases blood flow into intestinal tissues. The immunoactive VIP found in the brain is structurally identical to intestinal VIP.

Enterocrinin. In 1938 intestinal extracts were shown to stimulate intestinal secretion itself, and a hormone immediately was postulated in the usual manner to account for this activity. The purported hormone was named *enterocrinin.* However, both VIP and GIP have been shown to be capable of evoking secretion by the small intestine. Secretin and PZCCK are ineffective.[2] Enterocrinin is probably not a descrete peptide but it remains to be demonstrated that intestinal secretion during normal digestion is controlled by either VIP or GIP or both.

Enteroglucagon. In addition to those hormones isolated from the small intestine, the *EG_1-type cells* produce *enteroglucagon,* which is structurally and functionally like pancreatic glucagon. Enteroglucagon is extractable in a small and a large form. The latter has been named *glicentin* and consists of 69 amino acids.[43] This may be a prehormone form since it contains the glucagon sequence enclosed within peptide fragments of 8 and 30 amino acids. The physiological role for enteroglucagon and its relationship to pancreatic glucagon and glucose metabolism are open for speculation. A relationship to release of calcitonin (CT) and calcium regulation has been proposed (see Chap. 13).

Other Gastrointestinal Peptides. A peptide isolated from the duodenum of the pig

Phe-Val-Pro-Ile-Phe-Thr-Tyr-Gly-Glu-Leu-Gln-
Arg-Met-Gln-Glu-Lys-Glu-Arg-Asn-Lys-Gly-Gln

Fig. 14-3. Amino acid sequence for motilin. Molecular weight, 2700 daltons. (From Jaffe.[29])

specifically stimulates release of the inactive protease chymotrypsinogen.[1] When activated in the duodenum, chymotrypsin enzymatically converts trypsinogen into the active protease trypsin. This peptide has been named *chymodenin.* This finding may represent a specialized refinement in control of specific enzymes from the pancreas according to the particular composition of the food mass.

A *gastrin-releasing peptide* (GRP) has been isolated from the antral gastric mucosa of dogs. It is composed of 27 amino acids and is structurally similar to *bombesin,* a peptide that may function as an enteric neurotransmitter.[43,50]

Somatostatin is produced by neurons and paraneurons (D cells) located throughout the small intestine.[50] It seems to function in paracrine fashion by inhibiting release of all other GI peptides.[38] Somatostatin has been demonstrated in the arterial circulation of dogs following a meal and may act as a hormone to inhibit release of gastrin, insulin and pancreatic polypeptide.[53] Two forms of somatostatin have been isolated.[43] The first is identical to the hypothalamic tetradecapeptide neurohormone. The second consists of somatostatin plus an additional 14 amino acids. This may be a presomoatostatin form. *Dynorphin,* a heptadecapeptide from the central nervous system and pituitary gland is also present in the intestine.[43] *Neurotensin* (tridecapeptide) and *substance P* (onadecapeptide) are neurotransmitters of the central nervous system that are also found in the intestine. Substance P was the first peptide to be identified in both the intestine and brain (in 1931). It is not clear whether substance P and neurotensin are neurotransmitters only or if they have paracrine functions in the intestine.

The new biochemical methodologies for isolating and sequencing of peptides are allowing the isolation of new GI peptides faster than physiological studies can be performed to find a function for them! Porcine histidine isoleucine heptacosapeptide (PHI) is such a peptide.[43] It consists of 27 amino acids, is structurally similar to the secretin family of peptides and is in need of a good, stable function.

Some Proposed GI Peptides. Numerous different peptides have been postulated to influence intestinal and gastric physiology, including *coherin* from neurohypophysial extracts,[22] *villikinin, duocrinin, bulbogastrone, urogastrone, oxyntomodulin, sorbin* and several others from the gut.[31,43] However, none of these proposed regulators has been shown to be an important, integral part of the digestive control mechanisms.

Phases of Intestinal Regulation. Three stages or phases of intestinal regulation can be identified involving neural and endocrine mechanisms. There appears to be a distinct *cephalic phase* mediated via vagal stimulation that influences pancreatic secretion. The *gastric phase* involves vagal and vagovagal stimulation of gastrin release that appears to influence pancreatic secretion. Finally, and certainly the most important regulatory mechanism, the *intestinal phase* relies primarily on release of peptides stimulated by the composition of the intestinal contents.

Chemistry of Mammalian Gastrointestinal Peptides

A number of specific peptides have been isolated from the GI tract of man and several domestic mammals. As described previously, these peptides exhibit the biological activities classically associated with secretin, gastrin and PZCCK and more recently with GIP, VIP, motilin and others. The sequences of amino acids that have been worked out for some of these peptides suggest that three chemical classes of GI peptides have evolved. The first group includes the gastrins, PZCCK and some related peptides (Fig. 14-2). Secretin, enteroglucagon, VIP, GIP and PHI form the second group. The third group is composed of bombesin, GRP, substance P and a number of related peptides that have been isolated from amphibian skin (physalaemin, phyllomedusin, etc.) and molluscs (eledoisin). This last group are known also as tachykinins.[27] Motilin and somatostatin are each unique peptides and are not similar to the peptides in any of these groups.

Embryonic Origin of Gastrointestinal Endocrine Cells

Although the use of immunological and fluorescent techniques has enabled investigators to identify the actual cellular sources for many of the GI peptides, there is still considerable disagreement with respect to the embryonic origin or origins of these cells in mammals. Pearse proposed that all of these GI cellular types as well as calcitonin-secreting C cells of the thyroid gland, parathyroid chief cells, α- and β-cells of the pancreatic islets, melanin-containing cells, adenohypophysial cells and the chromaffin cells of the adrenal medulla belong to the so-called APUD cellular series (amine content and amine precursor uptake and decarboxylation) (see Chap. 1). These APUD cells are derivatives of neural crest or other neural ectoderm cells, suggesting that GI endocrine cells are of ectodermal rather than endodermal origin and that they have migrated into the intestinal mucosa early during development. An alternative view might be that at least some of these different cellular types have independently acquired APUD characteristics subsequent to or coincident with their differentiation from endodermal cells. The occurrence of certain GI peptides such as VIP in neural tissue argues strongly for a neural origin for these peptide hormone-secreting cells.[52] A single origin for GI endocrine cells is supported further by observations that immunoreactive gastrin, CCK and glucagon appear to be localized in a single cellular type in the invertebrate chordate amphioxus and in the cyclostomes.[17]

Complex Interactions of Gastrointestinal Peptides

Many studies have been published in the past few years that involve observation of the effects of administering combinations of GI peptides as well as the influences of one peptide on the release of another. Studies of this type indicate considerable overlap in the functional roles of the various peptides (for example, glucagon-like activity in secretin) although pharmacological doses usually were employed. At the present time it is difficult to sort out interactions due to structural similarities, pharmacological doses or both from those interactions that might represent true synergisms, functional overlaps or inhibitions. Consequently there is considerable literature concerning such interactions that will not be discussed here. The reader is encouraged to study literature and to find order in the chaos.

Influence of Gastrointestinal Peptides on Other Endocrine Systems

The influence of GIP on insulin release has already been mentioned, and it is possible that enteroglucagon release would also stimulate insulin secretion. Consequently GI peptides might influence the metabolism of carbohydrates, amino acids and fats after absorption (see Chap. 19).

Pentagastrin administered in small doses stimulates release of calcitonin from the C cells of the mammalian thyroid.[10] Since experimental hypercalcemia produced by systemic infusion of calcium results in elevated levels of circulating gastrin, it has been proposed that uptake of calcium from the gut acting through the release of gastrin as a mediator effects release of CT. This increase in CT levels would enhance deposition of calcium in bones and offset any effects of parathyroid hormone

TABLE 14-2. *Distribution of Some Peptides in Layers of the Intestine*

PEPTIDE	MUCOSA (pmol/g)	SUBMUCOSA (pmol/g)	MUSCLE AND NERVE (pmol/g)
Bombesin	<1.5	16–30	32
CCK8	2–5	6–11	7–14
Met-enkephalin	100	1000	400–1300
Leu-enkephalin	6	100	140
Neurotensin	8	<0.02	<0.02
Somatostatin	132	239	172
Substance P	33	135	240–360
VIP	83	119	135

From Costa and Furness.[12]

(PTH) on this target tissue. The early release of gastrin during the processing of a meal may represent an "anticipation" of the consequent uptake of calcium that will occur so that CT released by gastrin lowers plasma Ca^{++}, thereby stimulating PTH release, which in turn would influence Ca^{++}/HPO_4^{-2} management by the kidney and indirectly enhance uptake of calcium from the gut (see Chap. 12). The action of PTH on bone would be blocked by CT. Enteroglucagon has also been suggested to evoke CT release in a similar manner.[21]

Comparative Aspects of Gastrointestinal Peptides

There have been few studies concerning endocrine regulation of GI physiology in submammalian vertebrates, and most of these studies have been performed since the advent of purified mammalian peptides. Obviously the investigation into comparative regulation was hampered by the lack of understanding and interest in the general physiology of digestion in submammalian species. For example, although extensive research in teleosean fishes of commerical importance has been accomplished with respect to diets, growth and feeding ecology, few experiments have been concerned with physiological control mechanisms. The following brief account should serve to further emphasize the neophyte status of this area of comparative endocrinology and, it is hoped, encourage some developments in the study of comparative aspects of GI peptides.

Invertebrates

Immunoreactive gastrin has been extracted from the GI tract of two molluscan species.[57] The levels of extractable gastrin are comparable to those of mammals. Gastrin has also been demonstrated in the neuroendocrine cells of an insect, *Manduca septa,* supporting possible neural origins for this peptide.[36] These data suggest a broad phylogenetic distribution of these peptides associated with digestive functions. Peptides characteristic of invertebrate systems are turning up in vertebrate guts and nervous systems. For example, the head inducing substance of *Hydra* has been found in human brain and intestine.[43] The implications of these isolated observations may become more meaningful through studies of other invertebrate groups.

Class Agnatha: Cyclostomata

Cytological studies by Ostberg and coworkers on the intestine of the Atlantic hagfish *Myxine glutinosa* have revealed the presence of primitive open-type endocrine cells.[49] These cells extend from the basal portion of the intestinal epithelium to border on the lumen of the gut. Hagfish intestinal endocrine cells do not possess APUD characteristics, although APUD-type cells have been reported in the pancreatic islets that differentiate into insulin-producing B-cells.[49] Antibody to human gastrin, pentagastrin and porcine glucagon binds to endocrine cells in the *Mxyine* gut. These intestinal endocrine cells in the Atlantic hagfish do not resemble zymogen cells either, suggesting a separate origin for the endocrine and enzyme-secreting cells. In contrast, the intestinal epithelium of larval and adult lampreys (*Lampetra* spp.) contains APUD-type cells that react to antibodies prepared against mammalian glucagon and gastrin.[59,60]

Secretin-like and PZCCK-like activities have been demonstrated in intestinal extracts prepared from river lampreys, *Lampetra fluviatilis,* and sea lampreys, *Petromyzon marinus.*[3] Both secretin and PZCCK activities were assayed by monitoring pancreatic secretions in the anesthetized cat. Similar observations have been reported for *M. glutinosa.*[46] Gallbladder strips prepared from a Pacific hagfish, however, did not respond in vitro with contractions to porcine PZCCK although ACh caused contractions.[61] Secretion of intestinal lipase in this same species is stimulated by porcine PZCCK.[63] These observations suggest that the evolution of gallbladder receptors for PZCCK occurred after the appearance of molecules in the intestine that possess PZCCK-like activities.

Somatostatin is not present in the intestines of hagfishes.[55] It does occur in the pancreas.

Class Chondrichthyes

In their classical studies Bayliss and Starling reported the presence of secretin-like activity in extracts prepared from dogfish shark and skate intestines when these preparations were assayed in mammals. The activity they measured may have been due to secretin-like or PZCCK-like factors (or to both) present in these extracts.[6] Intestinal extracts prepared from the holocephalan *Chimaera monstrosa* also possess PZCCK activity.[45] Porcine PZCCK stimulates contractions in strips of gallbladder prepared from dogfish sharks, and the intensity of the response is proportional to the dose of PZCCK.[61]

Class Osteichthyes: Teleostei

Only a few species of teleosts have been investigated within the entire class of bony fishes. The first published observations are those of Bayliss and Starling who reported that intestinal extracts prepared from salmon *(Salmo salar?)* possessed secretin-like activity (possibly also PZCCK activity as well).[6] Similar activities were reported for pike, *Esox lucius,* and cod, *Gadus morhua,* when intestinal extracts were assayed in either birds or mammals. The magnitude of these responses was similar to those induced by purified mammalian VIP.[16] PZCCK activity has been reported in the intestine of the Atlantic eel, *Anguilla anguilla* and the pike.[4,15] Isolated strips of gallbladder from Pacific salmon *(Oncorhynchus)* contract in the presence of porcine PZCCK, indicating sensitivity of the salmon gallbladder to the mammalian peptide.[62]

A gastrin-histamine type of mechanism is present in the teleost stomach. Extracts from the gastric mucosa of sunfish *(Lepomis macrochirus)* stimulate acid secretion in bullfrogs,[47] and large doses of histamine (10–15 mg/kg weight) induced acid secretion in the European catfish *Silurus glanis*.[24] Histamine-induced acid secretion in cod (15 mg/kg) is blocked by certain antihistamines,[26] supporting the existence of a mammalian-like regulatory system.

Somatostatin and motilin were not demonstrable in the intestine of *Gillichthyes mirabilis.*[55,56]

Class Amphibia

Regulation of gastric mechanisms has been studied more extensively in frogs than in any other nonmammalian species. It appears that amphibians possess mechanisms very much like those of mammals, involving both neural and endocrine mechanisms. Stomachs of intact frogs or isolated gastric mucosa prepared from frogs (including *Rana pipiens, R. catesbeiana, R. temporaria* and *R. esculenta*) respond with acid secretion when subjected to ACh, histamine, pentagastrin or crude gastrin preparations from nonmammals or mammals.[14,34,41,47,54] Similarly gastric mucosa isolated from a urodele, *Necturus,* secretes acid in response to pentagastrin.[44] Treatment with atropine or surgical vagotomy reduces acid secretion in frogs as it does in mammals.[34,42] Supposedly the release of pepsinogen in *R. esculenta* can be effected by increasing parasympathetic activity.[57] Caerulein, a peptide previously thought to be present only in anuran skin and which is known to stimulate acid secretion from stomach mucosa in a variety of vertebrates, appears to be the endogenous "gastrin" in *R. temporaria.*[39]

Bayliss and Starling reported that extracts from frog intestines would evoke pancreatic secretion in dogs,[6] providing evidence for the presence of secretin-like or PZCCK-like factors or both. Frog gallbladders will contract in the presence of porcine PZCCK in vitro,[61] which supports the possible existence of a PZCCK-like factor in amphibians as well as a role for PZCCK in regulation of gastric processes.

Class Reptilia

The only observation with respect to GI regulation in reptiles dates back to the observation by Bayliss and Starling that a factor or factors capable of causing pancreatic secretion in mammals is present in the intestine of a tortoise.[6] Immunoreactive somatostatin is present in the intestine of the lizard *Anolis carolinensis,* but motilin is not.[55,56] It is remarkable that additional studies have not been reported or if reported have escaped recognition. Certainly the field is open for some careful comparative studies.

Class Aves

Mammalian gastrin can stimulate acid secretion in birds, and large amounts of PZCCK cause release of enzymes from the avian exocrine pancreas.[64] However, no good evidence has been presented for a physiological role for these hormones in birds. Glucagon and GIP have no effects on pancreatic secretion. Extracts prepared from chicken intestines are strong stimulants of pancreatic secretion when assayed in turkeys, but these extracts are only weak stimulants in mammals (cat, rat). Purified porcine secretin only weakly stimulates exocrine pancreatic secretion in turkeys, but purified mammalian VIP is a potent stimulator.[16] These data suggest that secretin-like activity in birds may reside in a molecule that is more like mammalian VIP than it is like secretin. However, chicken VIP has been isolated and differs structurally from porcine VIP at only four positions.[20] Somatostatin and motilin have been demonstrated in the intestines of Japanese quail,[55,56] but nothing is known about their functions.

Summary

The existence of three major GI hormones postulated at the beginning of this century has been established, and their primary chemical structures have been elucidated. Gastrin is produced by the G cell of the antral gastric mucosa in response to the presence of food. The parietal cell of the fundic portion of the stomach secretes HCl in response to gastrin or direct neural (vagal) stimulation. Histamine may play a role as an intermediate in the action of gastrin on the parietal cell. Parasympathetic stimulation (vagal, ACh) also evokes secretion of pepsinogen from the chief cell in the fundic mucosa. Secretin is produced by the S cell of the intestinal mucosa in response to the presence of acidic chyme entering from the stomach. The major action of secretin is to cause release of basic juices from the exocrine pancreas. The presence of peptides, amino acids or fats in the chyme causes release of PZCCK from the I cell of the intestinal mucosa, which in turn stimulates secretion of pancreatic enzymes and release of bile from the gallbladder. Neural stimulation may be involved to a limited degree in the intestinal phases, but the endocrine factors predominate.

Four additional peptides that may deserve hormone status have been isolated from the mucosa of the small intestine. GIP from the K cell stimulates release of insulin from the pancreas. Motilin from the EC cell stimulates gastric motility and secretion of pepsinogen but does not influence acid secretion. The factors controlling release of motilin have not been identified. VIP is a neurotransmitter that stimulates blood flow to the viscera. Enteroglucagon produced by the EG_1 cells has been identified in the intestinal mucosa, but its physiological role is uncertain.

Secretin, enteroglucagon (like pancreatic glucagon), GIP and VIP are very similar peptides with many common amino acids. VIP apparently has some secretin-like properties when assayed in birds. Gastrin and PZCCK have similar C-terminal portions and are chemically distinct from the secretin grouping. Bombesin, substance P and GRP form a third chemical grouping. The first two may be neurotransmitters. Motilin, somatostatin and some others appear to be unique peptides chemically unlike any of the other GI factors.

Comparative studies of GI hormones are limited, and only a few generalizations may be ventured here. It appears that intestinal peptides with GI hormone activities occurred early in vertebrate evolution (class Agnatha), although endogenous roles for these substances in agnathans have not been confirmed. Studies of hagfishes suggest that GI endocrine cells are probably not derived from neural crest cells and have acquired APUD characteristics independently. Furthermore, these endocrine cells do not seem to represent modified zymogen cells. Gastrin-like, PZCCK-like and secretin-like factors seem to be present in bony fishes, with the latter two factors also shown for cartilaginous fishes (selachians). Among the Amphibia there is good evidence for a mammalian-type control of gastric secretion (both neural and endocrine control), although little is known concerning the intestinal events. No generalizations concerning reptiles are possible; however, it would not be surprising to learn that the generalized mammalian pattern of regulation is operating. Avian systems appear to be basically like mammals. Unfortunately knowledge of avian digestive regulation is based upon a few highly domesticated species, and little is known about wild species.

References

1. Adelson, J.W. and S.S. Rothman (1974). Selective pancreatic enzyme secretion due to a new peptide called chymodenin. Science 183:1087–1089.

2. Barbezat, G.O. and M.I. Grossman (1971). Intestinal secretion: Stimulation by peptides. Science 174:422–424.

3. Barrington, E.J.W. and G.J. Dockray (1970). The effect of intestinal extracts of lampreys (*Lampetra fluviatilis* and *Petromyzon marinus*) on pancreatic secretion in the rat. Gen. Comp. Endocrinol. 14:170–177.

4. Barrington, E.J.W. and G.J. Dockray (1972). Cholecystokinin-pancreozymin-like activity in the eel *(Anguilla anguilla)*. Gen. Comp. Endocrinol. 19:80–87.

5. Bayliss, W.M. and E.J. Starling (1902). Mechanism of pancreatic secretion. J. Physiol. 28:352–353.

6. Bayliss, W.M. and E.J. Starling (1903). On the uniformity of the pancreatic mechanism in Vertebrata. J. Physiol. 29:174–180.

7. Beaumont, W. (1833). Experiments and observations on the Gastric juice and the Physiology of Digestion. F.P. Allen, Plattsburgh.

8. Bersimbaev, R.I., S.V. Argutinskaya and R.I. Salganik (1971). The stimulating action of gastrin pentapeptide and histamine on adenylcyclase activity in rat stomach. Experientia 27:1389–1390.

9. Bitar, K.N. and G.M. Makhlouf (1982). Relaxation of isolated gastric smooth muscle cells by vasoactive intestinal peptide. Science 216:531–533.

10. Bloom, S.R. and J.M. Polak (1980). Establishing the physiology of gastrointestinal hormones. In R.F. Beers, Jr. and E.G. Bassett, eds., Polypeptide Hormones. Raven Press, New York, pp. 421–438.

11. Brown, J.C., J.R. Dryburgh, S.A. Ross and J. Dupré (1975). Identification and actions of gastric inhibitory polypeptide. Recent. Prog. Horm. Res. 31:487–532.

12. Costa, M. and J.B. Furness (1982). Neuronal peptides in the intestine. Br. Med. Bull. 38:247–252.

13. Cooper, C.W., W.H. Schwesinger, A.M. Mahgoub and D.A. Ontjes (1971). Thyrocalcitonin: Stimulation of secretion by pentagastrin. Science 172:1238–1240.

14. Davidson, W.D., O. Urushibara and J.C. Thompson (1969). Comparison of the effects of human and porcine gastrin on isolated gastric mucosa of the bullfrog. Proc. Soc. Exp. Biol. Med. 130:204–206.

15. Dockray, G.J. (1974). Extraction of a secretin-like factor from intestines of pike *(Esox lucius)*. Gen. Comp. Endocrinol. 23:340–347.

16. Dockray, G.J. (1975). Comparative studies on secretin. Gen. Comp. Endocrinol. 25:203–210.

17. Dockray, G.J. (1979). Comparative biochemistry and physiology of gut hormones. Annu. Rev. Physiol. 41:83–95.

18. Dockray, G.J. (1980). Gastrointestinal hormones: nature and heterogeneity. In R.F. Beers, Jr. and E.G. Bassett, eds., Polypeptide Hormones. Raven Press, New York, pp. 357–370.

19. Edkins, J.S. (1905). On the chemical mechanism of gastric secretion. Proc. Roy. Soc. Ser. B 76:376.

20. Fahrenkrug, J. and P.C. Emson, (1982). Vasoactive intestinal peptide: functional aspects. Br. Med. Bull. 38:265–270.

21. Foa, P.P. (1973). Glucagon: An incomplete and biased review with selected references. Am. Zool. 13:613–624.

22. Goodman, I. and R.B. Hiatt (1972). Coherin: A new peptide of the bovine neurohypophysis with activity on gastrointestinal motility. Science 178:419–421.

23. Gregory, R.A. (1982). Heterogeneity of gut and brain regulatory peptides. Br. Med. Bull. 38:271–276.

24. Gzgzyan, D.M., M.G. Zaks and O.F. Tanisiychuk (1968). Effect of histamine and pituitrin "P" on the gastric secretion of the European catfish (*Silurus glanis* L.). Prob. Ichthyol. 8:97–100.

25. Harper, A.A. and H.S. Raper (1943). Pancreozymin, a stimulant of the secretion of pancreatic enzymes in extracts of the small intestine. J. Physiol. 102:115–125.

26. Holstein, B. (1977). Effect of atropine and SC-15396 on stimulated gastric acid secretion in the Atlantic cod, *Gadus morhua.* Acta Physiol. Scand. 101:185–193.

27. Iverson, L.L. (1982). Substance P. Br. Med. Bull. 38:277–282.

28. Ivy, A.C. and E. Goldberg (1928). A hormone mechanism for gallbladder contraction and evacuation. Am. J. Physiol. 86:599–613.

29. Jaffe, B.M. (1979). Hormones of the gastrointestinal tract. In L.J. DeGroot et al., eds., Endocrinology. Grune and Stratton, New York, pp. 1669–1698.

30. Johnson, L.R. (1972). Regulation of pepsin secretion by topical acid in the stomach. Am. J. Physiol. 223:847–850.

31. Johnson, L.R. (1977). Gastrointestinal hormones and their functions. Annu. Rev. Physiol. 39:135–158.

32. Jorpes, J.E. (1968). The isolation and chemistry of secretin and cholecystokinin. Gastroenterology 55:157–164.

33. Jorpes, J.E. and V. Mutt (1966). Cholecystokinin and pancreozymin, one single hormone? Acta Physiol. Scand. 66:196–202.

34. Kasbekar, D.K., H.A. Ridley and J.G. Forte (1969). Pentagastrin and acetylcholine relation to histamine in H^+ secretion by gastric mucosa. Am. J. Physiol. 216:961–967.

35. Kosaka, T. and R.K.S. Lim (1930). Demonstration of the humoral agent in fat inhibition of gastric secretion. Proc. Soc. Exp. Biol. Med. 27:890–891.

36. Kramer, K.J., R.D. Soeirs and C.N. Childs (1977). Immunochemical evidence for a gastrin-like peptide in insect neuroendocrine system. Gen. Comp. Endocrinol. 32:423–426.

37. Kubes, L. and K. Jirasek (1974). Possible cellular localization of cholecystokinin-pancreozymin. Experientia 30:961–963.

38. Larsson, L.-I., N. Goltermann, L. De Magistris, J.F. Rehfeld, and T.W. Schwartz (1979). Somatostatin cell processes as pathways for paracrine secretion. Science 205:1393–1395.

39. Larsson, L.-I. and J.F. Rehfeld (1977). Evidence for a common evolutionary origin of gastrin and cholecystokinin. Nature 269:335–338.

40. Marks, I.N. and K.M. Drysdale (1957). A modification of Zimmermann's method for differential staining of gastric mucosa. Stain Technol. 32:48.

41. Morrissey, S.M. and Y.C. So (1970). The effect of gastrin on gastric secretion in *Rana catesbeiana* (American bullfrog). Comp. Biochem. Physiol. 34:521–533.

42. Morrissey, S.M. and B.Y.C. Wan (1970). The influence of mammalian gastric stimulants on *in vivo* secretion of acid in frogs. Comp. Biochem. Physiol. 34:507–520.

43. Mutt, V. (1982). Chemistry of the gastrointestinal hormones and hormone-like peptide and a sketch of their physiology and pharmacology. Vit. Horm. 39:231–427.

44. Nakajima, S., R.L. Shoemaker, B.I. Hirschowitz and G. Sachs (1970). Comparison of actions of aminophylline and pentagastrin on *Necturus* gastric mucosa. Am. J. Physiol. 219:1259–1262.

45. Nilsson, A. (1970). Gastrointestinal hormones in the holocephalian fish *Chimaera monstrosa* (L.). Comp. Biochem. Physiol. 32:387–390.

46. Nilsson, A. and R. Fange (1970). Digestion proteases in the cyclostome *Myxine glutinosa* (L.). Comp. Biochem. Physiol. 32:237–250.

47. Norris, D.O. and J.S. Norris (1971). Evidence for a gastric factor from bluegill sunfish that stimulates gastric acid secretion in the frog, *Rana pipiens*. J. Colo.-Wyo. Acad. Sci. 7:109 (Abstract).

48. Ostberg, Y., L. Boquist, S. VanNoorden and A.G.E. Pearse (1976). On the origin of islet parenchymcal cells in a cyclostome, *Myxine glutinosa.* A fluorescence microscopical and ultrastructural study with particular reference to endocrine cells in the bile duct mucosa. Gen. Comp. Endocrinol. 28:228–246.

49. Ostberg, Y., S. VanNoorden, A.G.E. Pearse and N.W. Thomas (1976). Cytochemical, immunofluorescence, and ultrastructural investigations on polypeptide hormone containing cells in the intestinal mucosa of a cyclostome. *Myxine glutinosa.* Gen. Comp. Endocrinol. 28:213–227.

50. Polak, J.M. and S.R. Bloom (1980). Gastrointestinal hormones: distribution and tissue localization. In R.F. Beers, Jr. and E.G. Bassett, eds., Polypeptide Hormones. Raven Press, New York, pp. 371–394.

51. Said, S.I. and V. Mutt (1970). Polypeptide with broad biological activity: isolation from small intestine. Science 169:1217–1218.

52. Said, S.I. and R.N. Rosenberg (1976). Vasoactive intestinal polypeptide: Abundant immunoreactivity in neural cell lines and normal nervous tissue. Science 192:907–908.

53. Schusdziarra, V., E. Zyznar, D. Rouiller, G. Boden, J.C. Brown, A. Arimura, and R.H. Unger (1980). Splanchnic somatostatin; a hormonal regulator of nutrient homeostasis. Science 207:530–532.

54. Sedar, A.W. (1961). Electron microscopy of the oxyntic cell in the gastric glands of the bullfrog, *Rana catesbeiana.* II. The acid-secreting gastric mucosa. J. Biophys. Biochem. Cytol. 10:47–57.

55. Seino, Y., D. Porte, Jr. and P.H. Smith (1979). Immunohistochemical localization of somatostatin-containing cells in the intestinal tract: a comparative study. Gen. Comp. Endocrinol. 38:229–233.

56. Seino, Y., D. Porte, Jr., N. Yanaihara and P.H. Smith (1979). Immunocytochemical localization of motilin-containing cells in the intestines of several vertebrate species and a comparison of antisera against natural and synthetic motilin. Gen. Comp. Endocrinol. 38:234–237.

57. Smit, H. (1964). The regulation of pepsin secretion in the edible frog, *Rana esculenta* (L.). Comp. Biochem. Physiol. 13:129–141.

58. Straus, E., R.S. Yalow and H. Gainer (1975). Molluscan gastrin: Concentration and molecular forms. Science 190:687–689.

59. VanNoorden, S., J. Greenberg and A.G.E. Pearse (1972). Cytochemical and immunofluorescence investigations on polypeptide hormone localization in the pancreas and gut of the larval lamprey. Gen. Comp. Endocrinol. 19:192–199.

60. VanNoorden, S. and A.G.E. Pearse (1974). Immunoreactive polypeptide hormones in the pancreas and gut of the lamprey. Gen. Comp. Endocrinol. 23:311–324.

61. Vigna, S. (1979). Distinction between cholecystokinin-like and gastrin-like biological activities extracted

from gastrointestinal tissues of some lower vertebrates. Gen. Comp. Endocrinol. 39:512–520.

62. Vigna, S.R. and A. Gorbman (1977). Effects of cholecystokinin, gastrin and related peptides on coho salmon gallbladder contraction *in vitro*. Amer. J. Physiol. 232:E485–E491.

63. Vigna, S. and A. Gorbman (1979). Stimulation of intestinal lipase secretion by porcine cholecystokinin in the hagfish, *Eptatretus stouti*. Gen. Comp. Endocrinol. 38:356–359.

64. Ziswiler, V. and D. Farner (1972). Digestion and the digestion system. In D.S. Farner and J.R. King, eds., Avian Biology, Academic Press, New York, Vol. 2, pp. 343–430.

15·Miscellaneous Regulatory Substances

This chapter contains discussions of a number of vertebrate regulatory substances that do not fit easily into any of the previous chapters. They are either found only in mammals or are too general to classify with respect to their origins, actions or both. A kidney hormone, *erythropoietin,* several growth factors, the ubiquitous *prostaglandins* and related compounds, and the *thymus hormone* or hormones are discussed as they occur in mammals. *Kallikreins* and *kinins* are discussed, although they are often not included as hormones per se. Nevertheless their formation is similar to those events involved with the renin-angiotensin system, and they are included here. Chemical substances that function as chemical messages between organisms and influence physiology and behavior are known for most vertebrate groups. These chemical substances are known collectively as *semiochemicals.* Finally the *epiphysial complex,* including the pineal gland, is discussed. The *caudal neurosecretory system* of teleostean fishes and its neurohemal organ, the *urophysis,* are discussed in Chapter 16.

Erythropoietin

Erythropoietin is a glycoprotein hormone (mol wt 60,000–70,000) produced in mammals in response to hypoxia (reduced oxygen availability). The hormone was so named for its ability to stimulate erythropoiesis (erythrocyte or red blood cell formation) in bone marrow, and it is an essential factor in both fetal erythropoiesis and in adaptation to respiratory distress in adult mammals (Fig. 15-1). These adaptations include increases in hematocrit, in life span of red blood cells and in hemoglobin content of these red blood cells. All of these changes contribute to greater oxygen-carrying capacity of the blood.

Erythropoietin is produced from a plasma substrate under control of the kidney via a mechanism similar to the renin-angiotensin system described in Chapter 10. Erythropoietin acts on erythropoietin-responsive cells (ER cells) in the bone marrow, causing them to differentiate into erythroblasts (erythrocyte-forming cells), which differentiate into reticulocytes and erythrocytes. At the molecular level erythropoietin induces synthesis of hemoglobin in the ER-cell, which marks the conversion of the ER cell to an erythroblast.

The kidney produces an erythropoietic factor termed *erythrogenin* that contains erythropoietin in an inactive form. An unidentified factor in the serum causes erythropoietin to be released from erythrogenin.[139] The fixed macrophages (Kupffer cells) in the liver may also produce erythrogenin especially during liver regeneration.[127]

Regulation of erythropoietin production is determined by availability of oxygen to kidney or liver cells. Hypoxia increases production and hyperoxia reduces production of erythropoietin. Similarly agents that normally increase oxygen consumption, such as thyroxine and dinitrophenol, increase erythropoietin

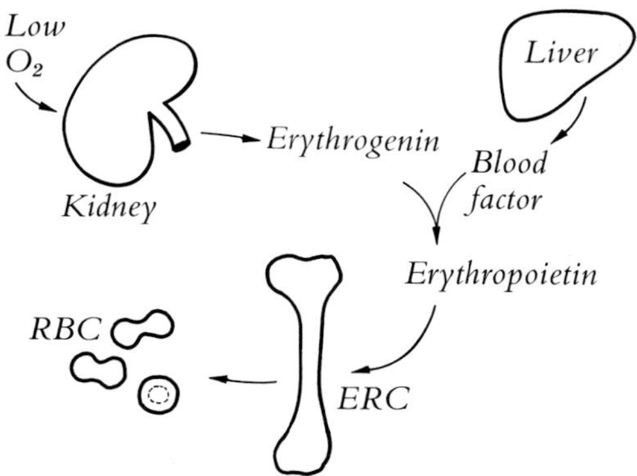

FIG. 15-1. Erythropoietin. Under conditions of hypoxia (low O_2) the kidney produces a polypeptide, erythrogenin, that interacts with a blood factor from the liver to release erythropoietin. Erythropoietin stimulates bone marrow cells *(ERC)* to produce more erythrocytes *(RBC)* which enhance O_2 transport.

production. Factors that bring about a reduction in oxygen consumption (hypophysectomy, goitrogens, starvation) decrease its production.

Growth Factors

Somatomedins

Early studies on the actions of growth hormone (GH) indicated that GH stimulated the liver to produce a blood-borne factor which mediated the action of GH on cartilage. This product was named *somatomedin,* but is known now to be several different peptides: somatomedin A, somatomedin C, insulinlike growth factors I and II (IGF I, IGF II), and multiplication stimulating activity (MSA).[173] All of these peptides (1) are dependent upon GH for their synthesis, (2) enhance incorporation of sulfate into cartilage and (3) exert insulinlike effects on extraskeletal tissues. (Another peptide, somatomedin B, has been dropped from this list since it does not stimulate sulfate incorporation.) The four peptides comprising the MSA complex are the most potent of these factors for stimulating cell division (mitogenic).

The insulinlike activity of these peptides is a consequence of their structural similarity to insulin. They are all small proteins (5000–9000 daltons) consisting of two peptide chains with as much as a 50% overlap in amino acid sequences with insulin. Somatomedin C and IGF I are similar and in fact may be identical peptides. In plasma the levels of IGF II far exceed those of IGF I. The activity of IGF II is more like insulin than IGF I and does not support cartilage growth as well as IGF I.

Insulin is not responsible for all of the insulinlike activity observed in the blood. After removing insulin by treating blood with antibodies prepared against insulin, most of the insulin's biological activity remains. The name for the proteinaceous preparation responsible for this residual activity is *nonsuppressible insulinlike activity soluble peptide* or NSILA-S. It is a heterogenous collection of peptides that has been difficult to characterize since it probably includes some or all of the other insulinlike peptides.

At least some of these "somatomedins" are essential intermediates in the actions of pituitary GH (see Chap. 5). They cooperate with insulin to produce mitogenic effects sometimes attributed to insulin action (see Chap. 13).

Other Growth Factors

Growth factors comprise a family of proteins that stimulate various aspects of embryonic development. They are also known to cause proliferation of cells or tumors in culture.[38,173] These growth factors include *nerve growth factor* (NGF) and *epidermal growth factor* (EGF) isolated from the mouse sub-maxillary gland. *Ovarian growth factor* (OGF), *fibroblast growth factor* (FGF) and *myoblast growth factor* (MGF) have been isolated from the bovine pituitary gland. A *platelet-derived growth factor* (PGF) is produced by platelets. All of these compounds are named for their source or for a major cellular type they stimulate. They vary in size from about 6,000 to 35,000 daltons. Nerve growth factor actually exhibits structural similarity to insulin but lacks the cartilage stimulation and relationship to GH that characterize the insulinlike growth factors. Roles for these growth factors in normal physiology have not been established and their endocrinological significance is questionable.

Urogastrone is a peptide isolated from the intestine that is capable of blocking acid secretion by the stomach. Once its chemical structure became known, it was found to be almost identical to EGF from the salivary glands. Both consist of 54 amino acid residues and differ at only 12 locations with respect to specific amino acids. During pregnancy of mice and humans these peptides increase and may play important roles in fetal development.[84] EGF activity also appears in human milk and may influence growth of the newborn as well.

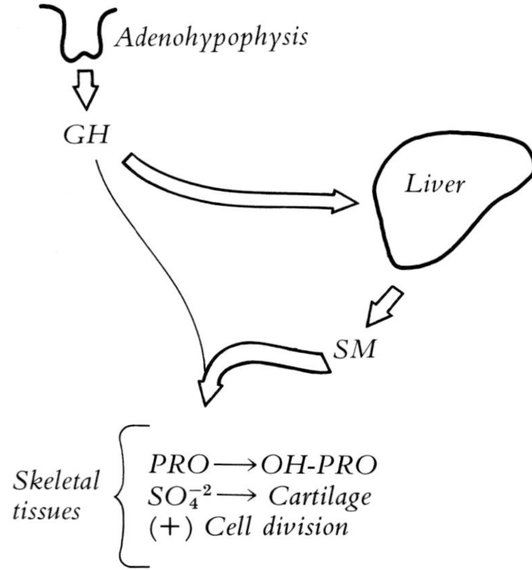

Fig. 15-2. Somatomedin. Growth hormone *(GH)* stimulates liver production of somatomedin *(SM)* and interacts with somatomedin to stimulate cartilage and bone formation, including conversion of proline *(PRO)* to hydroxyproline *(OH-PRO)* essential for collagen fiber synthesis, incorporation of sulfate *(SO_4^{-2})* into the cartilage matrix, and proliferation of cellular elements.

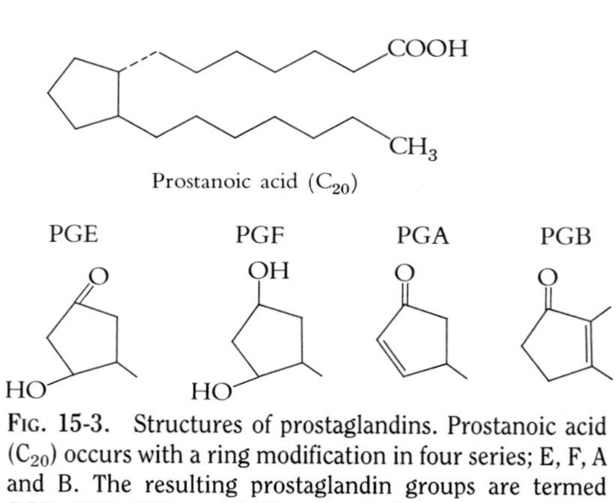

Eicosanoids

Eicosanoids are small lipids.[122] They are derived from a common precursor, *arachidonic acid,* which is synthesized from linolenic acid. Arachidonic acid liberated enzymatically from phospholipids can be converted to four groups of eicosanoids. Cyclooxygenase transforms arachidonic acid into endoperoxides. These endoperoxides are used to synthesize *prostaglandins, prostacyclin* or *thromboxanes.* Drugs such as aspirin and indomethacin inhibit cyclooxygenase and block their syntheses. A separate enzyme, 5-lipoxygenase, forms the *leucotrienes* from arachidonic acid. This enzyme is not inhibited by aspirin and indomethacin. Elucidation of these compounds and their synthetic pathways resulted in the awarding of the 1982 Nobel Prize in Physiology or Medicine to three principal researchers: Sune Bergstrom, Bengt Samuellson and John Vane.

Prostaglandins

In 1933 Maurice Goldblatt in England discovered some lipids in human seminal plasma with some peculiar properties. At about the same time, U.S. von Euler in Sweden found similar substances in extracts prepared from sheep vesicular glands, and he later named these compounds *prostaglandins* (PGs) based upon what he believed to be their source in man, the prostate gland. In 1956 Sune Bergstrom succeeded in elucidating the structures for 16 PGs. They are all related to the basic structure of prostanoic acid, and they can be separated into four classes (E, F, A, and B) on the basis of structural differences (Fig. 15-3). The most commonly occurring PGs are PGE_1, PGE_2 and $PGF_{2\alpha}$ (Fig. 15-4). Prostaglandins are not restricted to the male genital tract, and they have been found in most tissues of both males and females.

The PGs have pronounced effects on smooth-muscle contraction in the intestine, uterus and blood vessels. They produce vasodi-

COOH
CH_3
Prostanoic acid (C_{20})

PGE PGF PGA PGB

Fig. 15-3. Structures of prostaglandins. Prostanoic acid (C_{20}) occurs with a ring modification in four series; E, F, A and B. The resulting prostaglandin groups are termed *PGE, PGF, PGA,* and *PGB* respectively.

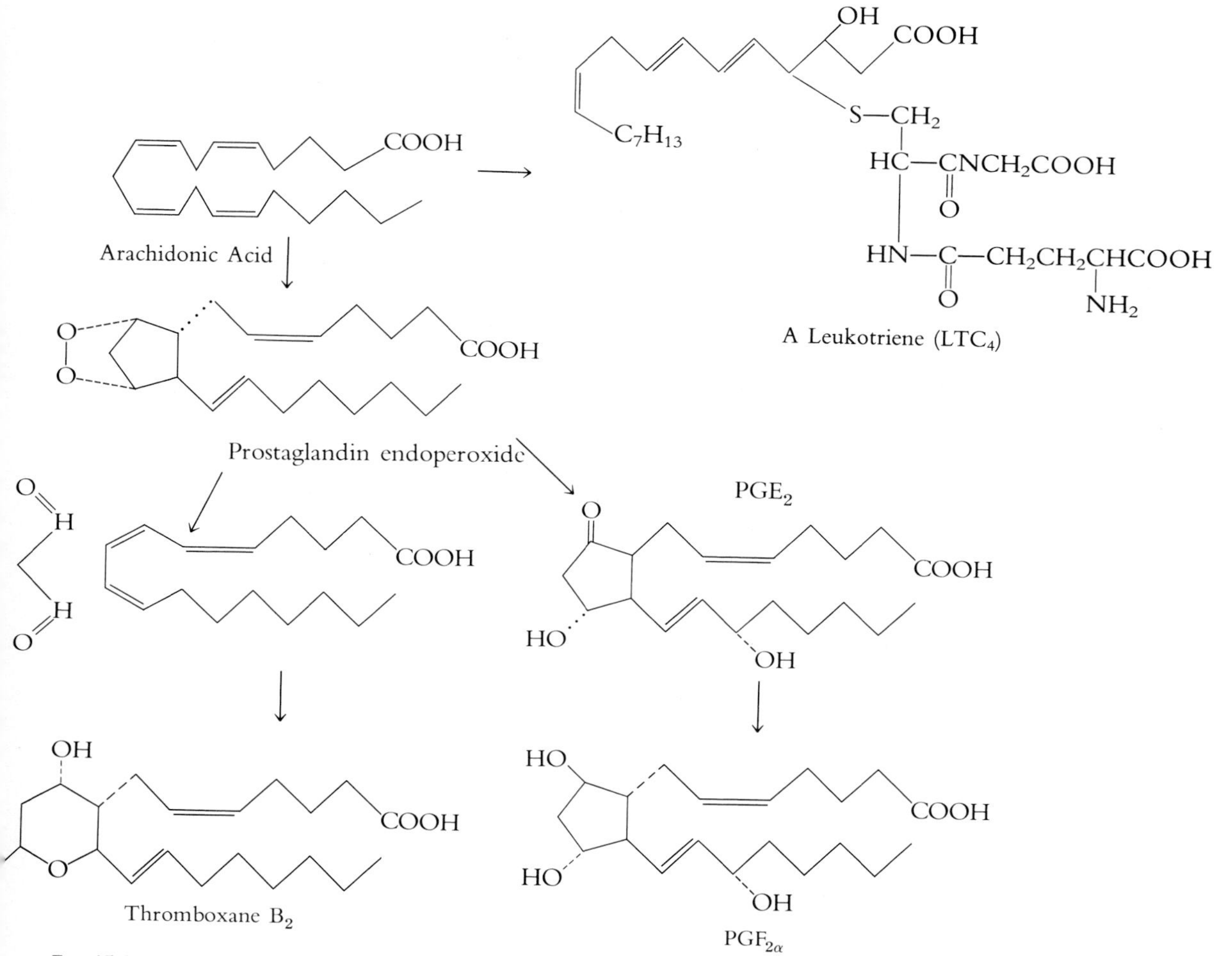

Fig. 15-4. Relationship of leukotrienes, prostaglandins and thromboxanes. Two of the most common prostaglandins are shown *(PGE_2, $PGF_{2\alpha}$)*. See text for explanation.

lation but may cause vasoconstriction in certain vessels such as those of the placenta. Prostaglandins stimulate contractions in uterine and intestinal smooth muscle. Bioassays for PGs capitalize on these smooth-muscle effects or on vasodepressor effects.

Prostaglandins at first seem to be involved in a wide variety of unrelated physiological processes in addition to effects on smooth muscles and blood vessels. For example, they may modulate central nervous system function or stimulate synthesis of specific enzymes, testosterone and corticosteroids.[64,77,82,169] One PG ($PGF_{2\alpha}$) is believed to be the uterine luteolytic substance in certain mammalian species (see Chap. 11). The presence of an intrauterine contraceptive device in rats causes increased synthesis and release of PGs from the uterus[100] and could explain the basis for how such devices inhibit pregnancy in some species. Prostaglandins also reduce progesterone synthesis by the corpus luteum, induce ovulation and lactation in rodents and may be involved in induction of labor. Because of their stimulatory actions on the smooth muscles of the pregnant uterus,[81] PGs are now being employed as arbortifacients.

Prostaglandins may be involved with the inflammatory response.[118] The anti-inflammatory action of aspirin and indomethacin is a consequence of inhibition of PG synthesis and blocking of early inflammatory events. The antipyretic (fever-decreasing) action of aspirin is also related to inhibition of PG synthesis. Consequently, these drugs have proved to be useful tools in studying the physiology of PGs.[34] Glucocorticoids are also anti-inflammatory, but they produce their effects by interfering with the participation of leukotrienes and kinins in the normal inflammatory response (see below). Because of the differences in mechanisms involved, aspirin and indomethacin are termed *nonsteroid anti-inflammatory drugs* (NSAID) to distinguish them from glucocorticoids.

A different role for PGs may be as mediators in the mechanism of action of peptide hormones that stimulate cAMP production in target cells such as for luteinizing hormone(LH), thyrotropin (TSH) and parathyroid hormone.[99,147,182] Prostaglandins may also mediate the effects of estrogens on release of pituitary LH.[164] One must not generalize too broadly on the role of PGs with respect to cAMP formation since the effects may be highly tissue specific.[85] For example, PGE_1 mimics corticotropin (ACTH) and TSH in the adrenal and thyroid gland respectively by stimulating cAMP formation. In adipose tissue where cAMP formation and lipolysis are stimulated by epinephrine and glucagon, PGE_1 inhibits cAMP formation and blocks lipolysis.

Prostacyclin

Prostacyclin (PGI_2), a compound closely related to the prostaglandins of the E, F, A and B series, is generated by the walls of many blood vessels.[123] This eicosanoid is a potent inhibitor of blood platelet aggregation and inhibits blood clotting. Prostacyclin is synthesized from the same precursors as the prostaglandins.

Thromboxanes

Researchers discovered the thromboxanes during studies on prostaglandin metabolism and action. Thromboxane A_2 causes translocation of free calcium ions to bring about changes associated with the shape of the platelet. It is this change in platelet shape that allows platelets to aggregate and facilitate clotting. Thromboxanes also may be released from the platelet and cause local constriction of vascular smooth muscle. This might enhance clotting by reducing the diameter of the arterioles and slowing blood flow through the capillary beds.

Leukotrienes

Leukotrienes (Fig. 15-4) are a novel group of at least 15 related compounds occurring in five structural classes (A, B, C, D, and E).[176] Their formation from arachidonic acid was discovered in 1979, and there is still much to be learned concerning their physiological roles. They are synthesized and released by white blood cells in response to injury or invasion of foreign antigens. Leukotrienes contribute to inflammatory or allergic response by causing contraction of vascular smooth muscle and increasing vascular permeability. Glucocorticoids may produce their anti-inflammatory effects by limiting the availability of free arachidonic acid and thereby blocking synthesis of the leukotrienes. Synthesis of leukotrienes is not influenced by NSAIDs.

The Thymus Gland

The function of the mammalian thymus (Fig. 15-5) was unknown until after the middle of the twentieth century when its role in the immune response system was recognized.[105] Prior to 1961 it was presumed to play some ill-defined role in juveniles but not in adults, since its rapid deterioration began at puberty. Jacques F.A.P. Miller discovered that thymectomy of newborn mice was followed by a short period of normal growth after which the animals suddenly became ill and soon died of a wasting disease. Autopsy revealed these mice were severely deficient in lymphocytes, which normally account for 70% of the mouse white blood cells. It was soon established that the thymus serves as the source or "seed bed" of lymphocytes normally found in other lymphoid tissues, including the spleen, lymph nodes and the small concentrations of lymphoid tissue in the wall of the intestine (Peyer's patches). Not only are thymectomized mice

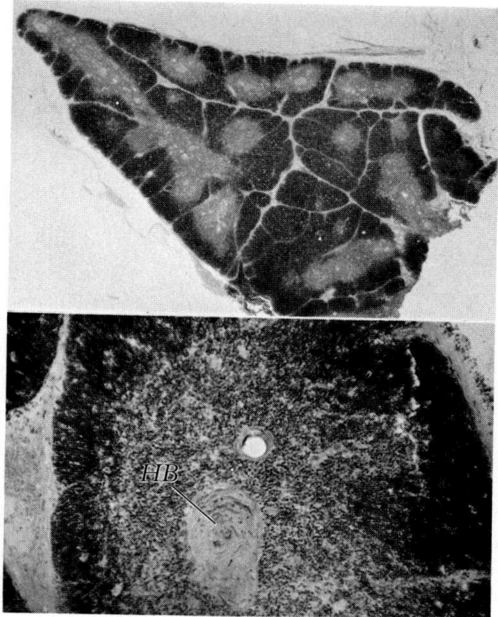

FIG. 15-5. The thymus gland. A mammalian thymus gland *(top)* consists of lobules of lymphatic tissue, each composed of cortical (dark) and medullary components (light). An enlargement of one lobule *(bottom)* reveals a large Hassal's body *(HB)*. The functional importance of Hassal's bodies is unknown.

deficient in lymphocytes, but their ability to produce circulating antibody is also impaired. Furthermore, thymectomized mice readily accept foreign tissue grafts. Inoculation of thymectomized mice with foreign lymphocytes may result in a "graft-versus-host" reaction in which the foreign cells immunologically "reject" the host. These observations led to the conclusion that lymphocytes participate in immunological responses. Such interactions are referred to as cell mediated.

Thymectomized mice that receive grafts of thymus from mice of the same inbred strain (to reduce occurrence of graft-versus-host reactions) do not develop the wasting disease, and their lymphoid tissues produce lymphocytes at normal rates. When the grafted thymus came from a mouse with a cytologically distinct abnormal chromosome (chromosome marker), it was discovered that the lymphocytes being produced were genetically like cells of the host and did not contain the marker chromosome of the graft donor. These results suggested that the thymus does more than just produce lymphocytes mitotically and laid the basis for suspecting existence of a thymus hormone that controlled differentiation and maturation of lymphocytes.

We know now that the thymus stimulates differentiation and maturation of *T-lymphocytes* in the thymus as well as in other lymphoid tissues. These T-lymphocytes are responsible for cell-mediated immunity including transplant rejection, graft-versus-host reactions, delayed hypersensitivity to foreign antigens, resistance to viruses and immune surveillance of tumor cells. Humoral immunity (circulating antibody) is also influenced by T-lymphocytes. Circulating antibody is produced by *plasma cells,* derived from another type of lymphocyte, the *B-lymphocyte,* which resides in the bone marrow. There are different populations of T-lymphocytes that can aid or suppress antibody formation. Failure of T-lymphocytes to differentiate in the absence of thymus hormone explains observations originally made for thymectomized mice.

The thymus actually produces a variety of stimulatory and inhibitory humoral agents that seem to be important in differentiation, immune response, endocrine functions, calcium regulation, cell growth and metabolism. Ten agents have been isolated from thymus tissue that might be considered candidates for thymic hormones[72,105], and at least eight more factors are suspected. Only five of these agents have been reasonably characterized chemically. All of these agents are present in thymus, and all disappear from the circulation following thymectomy.

The most promising preparation for hormone status is one termed *thymosin.*[72,73] There are actually at least two thymosin peptides. Thymosin-α_1 consists of 28 amino acids (M.W. = 3108) and stimulates mitosis in T-lymphocytes. The gene for thymosin-α_1, has been synthesized. Thymosin-β_4 is a slightly larger peptide (43 amino acids, 4982 daltons).

One of the other candidates isolated from thymus is *lymphocyte-stimulating hormone* (LSH), which occurs as a small heat-labile protein (molecular weight 8000) and as a conjugated form (mol wt about 15,000).[72] Both of these LSH substances increase the proportion of lymphocytes among the white blood cells and confer the ability to synthesize antibody to a foreign antigen. *Thymosterin* is a steroid derivative isolated from thymus that inhibits tumor growth and stimulates antibody synthesis and lymphocytopoiesis.[72] The *homeostatic thymic hormone*[36] is a relatively small molecule (mol wt about 2000) that contains amino acids, amino sugars and possibly a nucleotide. This substance appears to play a permissive role in the negative feedback effects of several hormones on the hypothalamo-hypophysial axis as well as being immunologically active itself. *Thymopoietin* has been characterized chemically as a peptide (49 amino acids, 5562 daltons) which stimulates bone marrow to produce thymic lymphocytes.[72]

Kinins

Kallikreins are serine proteases that bring about release of small peptides called *kinins*.[177] All kallikreins are glycoproteins with molecular weights between 25,000 and 40,000. They were first found in pancreas and blood, and were named from *kallikreas,* the Greek word for pancreas. The name is a misnomer because kallikreins have been characterized from pancreas, urine (kidney), blood and salivary glands and also reported in lung, intestine, brain and nerve. Kallikreins are structurally and functionally similar to the proteolytic enzymes of snake venom and to trypsin. All of these enzymes can cause release of kinin from the substrate *kininogen* (Fig. 15-6). There are different kininogens that correspond to specific kallikreins. These kininogens are large glycoproteins (about 120,000 daltons). Kinins are hypotensive agents. A specific kinin, the nonapeptide *bradykinin,* is produced by renal kallikreins and is thought to relax smooth muscle of arterioles in the renal vascular bed.

Pancreatic kallikrein is found in zymogen granules and is released into pancreatic juice rather than blood. Kallikreins may activate digestive enzymes (trypsin, chymotrypsin, etc.). They are also believed to convert many prohormones to active hormones (e.g., prorenin, proinsulin, proglucagon). In addition, kallikreins are implicated in fertilization (proteolytic penetration by spermatozoa), implantation, cell growth and possibly in embryonic development and differentiation. Kallikreins are found in secretory granules containing growth factors and may be responsible for release of peptides such as EGF and NGF.

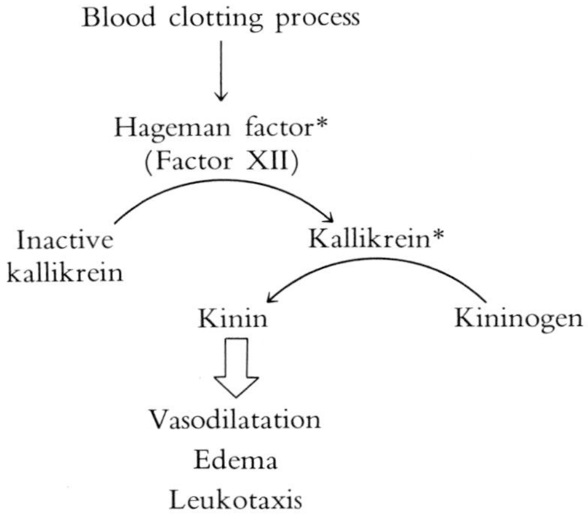

FIG. 15-6. Kinin production and action. Kininogen, an inactive precursor for kinin, is converted by active (*) kallikrein that is in turn activated by one of the normal agents in blood clotting, active (*) Hageman factor or Factor XII. Kinins produce effects related to combating infection that are frequently observed following physical trauma (vasodilation, edema and leukotaxis).

Kinins have been reported from mammals, birds and most reptiles but have not been demonstrated in snakes, amphibians, teleosts, holocephalans or elasmobranchs.[46,59,101,150,180] The absence of kinins in anamniote vertebrates has not been explained.

Chemical Communication

The phenomenon of chemical communication among animals includes a variety of compounds or semiochemicals that are secreted externally and affect the physiology or behavior or both of other individuals.[154] Such compounds may function as intraspecific signals, as interspecific signals or both. A classification of such compounds is provided in Table 15-1, but only two categories will be discussed here. The first category includes conspecific semiochemicals termed *pheromones,* and the second category consists of the interspecific (or transspecific) *allelomones.*

TABLE 15-1. *Classification of Vertebrate Semiochemicals*

PHEROMONES (Intraspecific)	
Primer pheromones	Reproductive maturation; growth inhibitors/stimulants
Signal pheromones	Courtship, mating; territorial and trail marking; recognition: sex, species, parent/young, dominant/subordinate; alarm; location of food; use of garlic by man to keep his house free of vampires
ALLELOMONES (Interspecific)	
Allomones (advantageous to emitter)	Repellents; venoms; growth inhibitors
Kairomones (advantageous to recipient)	Attractants from prey organisms; alarm

The intraspecific category of pheromones includes conspecific semiochemical signals that influence the physiology and/or behavior of the recipient. These chemical substances are involved with sexual attraction, group aggregation, avoidance or dispersal (alarm) responses, synchrony of gamete maturation, induction of mating behavior, trail or territory marking, individual recognition and food location. Pheromones may be subdivided into *primer* and *releaser* pheromones. Primer pheromones initiate a chain of physiological events in the recipient animal such as the hormonal events discussed in Chapter 11 that lead to ovulation in female mammals. Releaser pheromones elicit a more or less immediate behavioral response in the recipient such as the induction of copulatory behavior in male monkeys. A more appropriate term for these substances might be *signal pheromones* in that the recipient may be made aware of the sexual state of the emitter, for example, but may choose not to respond at that moment to the signal. In general, pheromones are highly species-specific molecules, and in some cases even two closely related species produce chemically distinct molecules for the same purpose that do not elicit responses by the other species.

There are two subcategories of allelochemic substances or allelomones. The first consists of *allomones,* which are substances that change the behavior of the recipient so that the emitter benefits. The "perfume" emitted by skunks is a good example of an allomone. Interspecific substances that benefit only the recipient and not the emitter are termed *kairomones.* The attraction of mosquitos by L-lactic acid, a component of human sweat, is an example.[1] These functional definitions cause some confusion, for one molecular species may be classified as more than one type of semiochemical.

All of these semiochemicals are compounds of small molecular weight that readily diffuse through water or air. These substances are extremely potent, and only a few hundred molecules arriving at an appropriate chemoreceptor are necessary to elicit a response. This sensitivity is not unexpected when one considers the problem of directing a chemical into the environment appropriately to reach the intended recipient in sufficient concentration to elicit a response.

Although the concept of semiochemicals has achieved scientific respectability only in recent years, their existence was suggested in early writings. Reproduction of the partridge *Perdix* was described in the 12th century Bestiary as follows: "Desire torments the females so much that even if a wind blows towards them from the males, they become pregnant from the smell."[79] Even earlier, a Roman, Pliny the Elder, reported a variety of substances that could function as abortifacients such as menstrual secretions of other women or castoreum secreted by the beaver. These agents reportedly were effective when a pregnant woman came near. They were also burned in lamps during orgies. It is difficult to see how such substances would naturally function in chemical communications as do currently recognized pheromones, allomones and kairomones.

Much of the research with semiochemicals has been performed with insects and vertebrates, but this phenomenon is widespread in the animal kingdom as well as in plants, protistans and monerans. The discussion here will be limited to vertebrates. The interested reader should consult the reading list (Appendix III) for references to chemical communication in other groups of organisms.

Mammalian Pheromones

For centuries scientists have known that mammals use glandular secretions or urine to mark territories.[151] Rabbits possess a chin gland that secretes a pheromone used for marking territory boundaries, and the behavior of male dogs in marking upright objects with their urine is known to scientist and layman alike. Musk-secreting glands are found in many sexually mature mammals and may be involved in a variety of behaviors, including territory marking, defense and mating. Pheromones have also been implicated in alarm signaling, individual or group recognition, including maternal-young interactions, and in promotion of aggression.

Sex Pheromones in Mammals. Many reports have appeared with respect to sexual pheromones in laboratory mammals, including mice, gerbils, guinea pigs and hamsters (Table 15-2). Crowded female mice enter anaestrus when no males are present (Lee-Boot effect). However, simply the odor from a male mouse can cause them to synchronously reenter estrus (Whitten effect). The endocrinological basis for these effects is suggested by observations that pheromones from female mice suppress pituitary release of follicle-stimulating hormone (FSH), whereas male pheromone stimulates FSH release that is followed in normal sequence by LH release and ovulation.[8] A newly mated female will abort if placed with a "strange" male (not the previous mate), and the incidence of abortion increases with genetic dissimilarity of the strange male to the male with whom she was mated. If offspring result, they are always from the second mating (Bruce effect). This effect has also been observed in voles and may not be peculiar to laboratory mice.[178,179,185]

The sexual pheromones involved in the Lee-Boot and Bruce effects are probably modified steroids (steroid metabolites) and are transmitted via the urine of the male to the olfactory apparatus of the female. Male mouse urine induces and accelerates estrous cycles of females (Whitten effect), and the effect is most pronounced on Lee-Boot groups of females. The time of vaginal closing in females is also influenced by male urine.[90] Anosmic females (animals whose nostrils have been blocked or whose olfactory bulbs have been removed surgically) do not respond to male urine.[125]

Pregnant and lactating rats produce pheromones that influence other females.[110] Odors from pregnant females shorten the estrous cycle of nonpregnant females so that more females will be pregnant at the same time. Presumedly it is advantageous to have many females give birth at the same time so that the females can cooperate in pup care. In contrast, odors from a lactating female with pups lengthens estrous cycles of nonpregnant females. Thus a socially dominant lactating female can suppress fertility of other females until she is again in estrus herself. A similar

Table 15-2. *Some Mammalian Responses to Primer Pheromones*

Bruce effect	A newly impregnated female will abort and return to estrus if exposed to odor from a strange male.
Whitten effect	An odor transmitted via male urine accelerates and synchronizes the estrous cycles in females.
Lee-Boot effect	Crowding of large numbers of females causes suppression of estrous cycles; smaller groups tend to exhibit pseudopregnancies.
Ropartz effect	Adrenal enlargement and increased production of corticosterone occurs when isolated mouse is exposed to the odor of other mice.
Vandenberg effect	Odor from a male accelerates sexual maturation in a female.

Note: These effects were originally observed in mice and could be related to the same primer pheromone.[27]

lactating pheromone may be produced by gerbils.

Males may also be influenced by female pheromones. Pairing of a previously paired male mouse with a strange female results in elevation of plasma testosterone, indicating that endocrine responses of both males and females may be influenced through bisexual encounters.[108] Proximity of ewes in estrus increases plasma testosterone levels in mature rams, implying that a female estrogen-dependent pheromone is responsible.[87] The display of estrous odor preference in male beagles is an androgen-dependent behavior induced by female pheromones.[4] Removal of the olfactory bulbs has no effect on sexual behavior of male hamsters, but removal of the vomeronasal organ as well as the olfactory bulbs abolishes copulatory behavior.[146] Removal of only the vomeronasal organ blocks copulatory behavior in only about one third of the hamsters, indicating an important interaction between this organ and olfactorily influenced sexual behavior.

The precise sources of many pheromones are not known. Those transmitted via the urine may originate in either the liver or kidney or both. Some steroids are converted by apocrine epidermal glands to pheromones in rabbits, and these pheromones readily diffuse into the air from the surface of the animal.[53] Musk is a steroid derivative (Fig. 15-7) that is produced by specialized epidermal glands. However, not all semiochemicals produced by mammals are derived from steroids. For example, the distinctive allomone of skunks consists of several mercaptans. Phenylacetic acid has been identified as the scent-marking pheromone secreted by the ventral scent-marking gland of male Mongolian gerbils,[190] and the

Musk odor of human urine

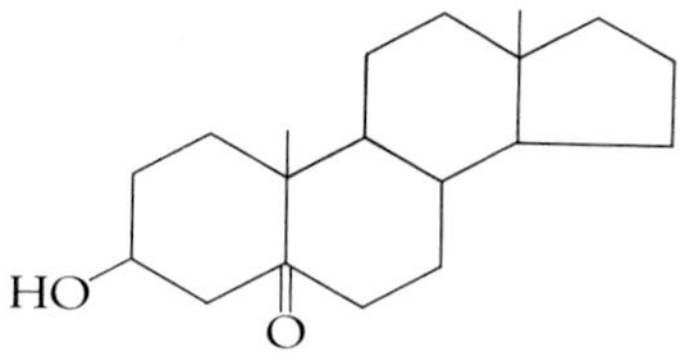

HO, O

Territory-marking pheromone from black-tailed deer

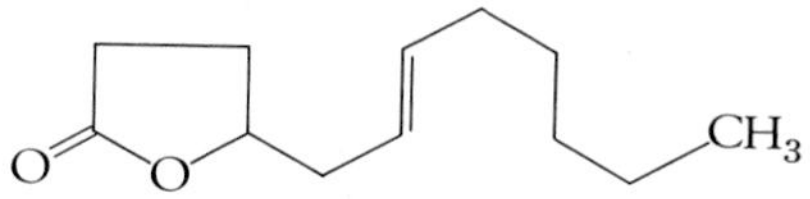

O, O, CH_3

Antelope scent-marking pheromone

$(CH_3)_2CHCH_2COOH$
Isovaleric acid

Gerbil scent-marking pheromone

O—CO—CH_3

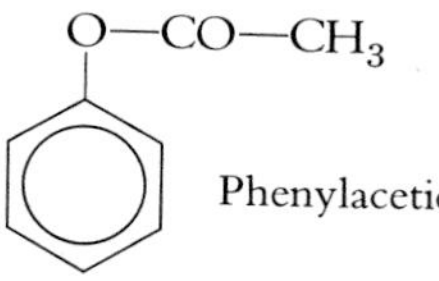

Phenylacetic acid

Sex attractant complex of volatile fatty acids from vaginal secretions of female rhesus monkey

CH_3COOH Acetic acid

CH_3CH_2COOH Propionic acid

$(CH_3)_2CHCOOH$ Isobutyric acid

$(CH_3(CH_2)_2COOH$ Butyric acid

$(CH_3)_2CHCH_2COOH$ Isovaleric acid

FIG. 15-7. Structures of some mammalian pheromones. See text for explanation.

active substance secreted by the male pronghorn antelope to mark territory is isovaleric acid, a small fatty acid.[124] The secretion of the tarsal gland of black-tailed deer is also a nonsteroidal lipid.[35] Dimethyl disulfide has been identified as the attractant pheromone of vaginal smears obtained from hamsters,[184] and its production may be estrogen dependent. Many of the pheromonal secretions of males described above appear to be influenced by androgens.[126] Although all sexual pheromones may not be steroids or steroid derivatives, it is clear that secretions of most male or female sexual pheromones or the responses to them are dependent upon androgens or estrogens.

Primates also produce semiochemicals utilized in territorial marking and reproduction.[121] Female rhesus monkeys produce a mixture of fatty acids of low molecular weight in vaginal secretions that stimulates sexual interest of males and may induce mounting behavior and ejaculation. The major volatile fatty acids produced are acetic acid, butanoic acid, propanoic acid, methylbutanoic acid and methylpropanoic acid. Synthetic mixtures of these fatty acids in appropriate ratios stimulate male interest in females. Males are not interested in females receiving steroidal contraceptives, suggesting that the releasers of overt male sexual behavior are hormone-dependent agents associated with the normal ovulatory cycle. Estrogens stimulate fatty acid secretions, and progesterone is inhibitory; observations that correlate well with levels of fatty acids observed in vaginal secretions throughout the menstrual cycle. Human vaginal discharges exhibit a similar variation in fatty acid composition (Fig. 15-8), although human females produce a much greater percentage of acetic acid than do rhesus monkeys. The use of oral contraceptives effectively obliterates the preovulatory increase in volatile fatty acids. The behavioral implications of these observations are not clear.

Although studies with humans are complicated by a number of psychological and social considerations, some evidence exists for production of pheromones and their roles in reproduction. A "dormitory effect" of menstrual synchrony has been described for all-female living groups.[109] Even though it is generally accepted that the olfactory sense in humans is

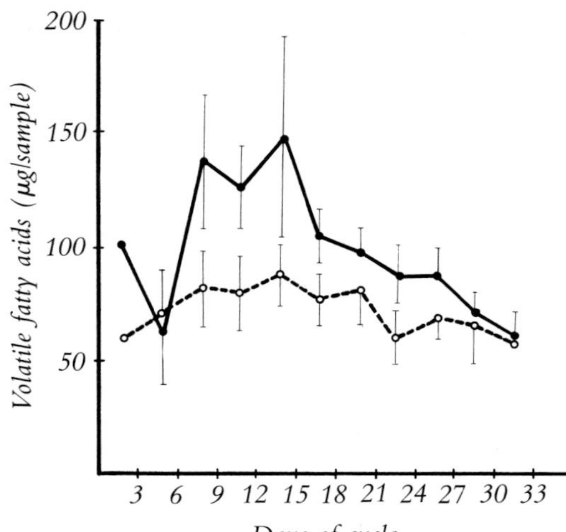

Fig. 15-8. Oral contraceptives and effects on composition of vaginal secretions collected over 3-day intervals. Volatile fatty acid content of vaginal secretions of 47 normal women *(black line)*. Midcycle rise in volatile fatty acid content does not occur in women taking oral contraceptives *(dashed line)*. Ovulation occurred around day 14 in 14 normal subjects. (After Michael, R.P., R.W. Bonsall and P. Warner.[120])

limited as compared to most mammals, several studies have shown definite sensitive olfactory discriminations, including sexually based differences in the abilities to perceive certain odors.[58] Trained perfumers can apparently distinguish olfactorily between different skin and hair types, and some psychiatrists claim to be able to smell schizophrenics because of abnormal production and elimination of trans-3-methylhexanoic acid.[184] The ability to detect some odors is sex dependent, such as the greater sensitivity of women to "boar taint" associated with spoiled pork. Whether these differences are related to possible pheromone production and behavior in humans remains to be shown.

Chemical Communication in Teleostean Fishes

Intraspecific chemical communication is employed by teleosts for sexual and individual recognition, sexual attraction, induction of courtship behavior, parent-young interactions, aggregation (schooling) and dispersal (alarm) behavior.[14] Homing in prespawning migratory teleosts involves perception of chemical cues and is discussed in Chapter 18. Purified semiochemicals have not been isolated and verified under natural conditions, and it must be recognized that the use of such terms as pheromone requires verification.

Individual chemical recognition has been shown in the minnow *Phoxinus,* the blind goby *Typhlogobius californiensis* and the yellow bullhead *Ictalurus natalis.*[12,14] Studies of the last species demonstrated that a dominant bullhead could recognize subordinates and distinguish them from intruders. When threatened, subordinate fish sought out shelter controlled by the dominant bullhead, who would tolerate their presence until the danger was past. Intruders were not tolerated even under these conditions. Anosmic fish (olfaction blocked experimentally) could not make these distinctions.

Evidence for sexual attracting substances and substances that elicit courtship behavior have been suggested for sticklebacks, shad, salmon, brown bullhead, several blennies and a goby.[12,14] Experimental studies with *Bathygobius soporator* have confirmed production by the female of a pheromone that elicits courtship behavior in males.[188] The pheromone appears to come from the ovary. Segregated anosmic males show no courtship response to introduction of ovarian pheromone to their aquarium. A similar response occurs in the goldfish *Carassius auratus.*[137] The early claim for production of a pheromone (copulin) by male guppies, *Poecilia reticulata,* which stimulated copulatory responses in female guppies has not been confirmed.[12]

Several species including *I. nebulosus, T. californiensis, Heterochromis bimaculatus, Nannacara anomala* and *Cichlasoma nigrofasciatum* can distinguish their own broods of young fish from other young of the same species on the basis of olfactory cues.[12,14] In the jewel fish *H. bimaculatus,* the young presumably produce a pheromone that stimulates certain aspects of parental behavior that is recognized by only the parents.[98] Fry of *Cichlasoma citrinellum* also exhibit chemical recognition of parental odors.[13]

Although schooling behavior includes a very strong visual component, experimental evidence supports a role for an aggregating pheromone in at least one species.[12,14] This *aggregating pheromone* reduces swimming activity and causes individuals to remain near one another. Evidence for dispersing or *alarm pheromones* has been found.[14,141] There is some lack of specificity among closely related species in responses to these alarm pheromones, and they might be more appropriately termed kairomones. However, interfamilial responses are slight, as are responses of species that are closely related phylogenetically but are geographically isolated. Certain species do exhibit a flight reaction when presented with the scent of a common predator. Brown bullheads have been observed to guard their nests in response to scent from a potential predator of their young.[12]

Chemical Communication in Amphibians

Evidence for chemical communication in amphibians comes primarily from studies performed with urodeles. Salamanders and newts utilize semiochemical as well as tactile information, especially in courtship. Urodeles possess *hedonic glands* or *cloacal glands* or both that appear to be sources for pheromones. Anurans on the other hand lack hedonic and cloacal glands, and there are no convincing data to support the use of pheromones or allelomones in anuran reproductive behavior.[116]

Plethodontid and desmognathid salamanders rely largely on tubular *mental* (chin) hedonic glands for stimulation of courtship behavior. Most of these salamanders are nonmigratory, largely terrestrial species. Migratory or nonmigratory semiaquatic salamanders (for example, Ambystomidae, Salamandridae) rely more on cloacal glands, particularly the abdominal gland of males that supposedly produces hedonic-type secretions.[39,128] The other cloacal glands are responsible for production of spermatophores.[97,181] Many behavioral observations on salamanders (*Ambystoma*) and several newts (*Taricha, Triturus, Notophthalmus, Cynops*) have implicated involvement of cloacal secretions in courtship.[116,175]

Attractant pheromones have been reported for *Taricha granulosa.* Males are attracted upstream to a sponge soaked in female odor.[197]

Laboratory experiments employing a simple olfactometer device demonstrate that male *T. granulosa* exhibit directed movements toward air passing over either males or females, but females exhibit random movements with respect to "newt air" versus "non-newt air" (Table 15-3).

Evidence for territorial marking has been reported for *Plethodon cinereus* and *P. jordani* involving chin-touching and nosetouching behaviors.[115,192] Scent production may be related to either the epidermal hedonic mental glands or to unsaturated lipids secreted by *nasolabial glands.* Only plethodontid salamanders possess nasolabial glands, and the use of nosetouching to transfer chemicals is probably unique to these salamanders.

Many amphibians have granular integumentary *poison glands* distributed over various areas of the body that probably discourage would-be predators. These glands secrete alkaloid toxins that readily meet the definition of allomones. Some of these toxins are extremely potent, and the simple act of handling the animal may produce irritation to the skin. Attempted consumption of a western newt (*Taricha*) may be a terminal event in a dog, although other organisms, such as garter snakes, do not appear to be affected by this toxin. Ingestion of these newts is fatal to humans, too. Certain South American frogs (for example, dendrobatids) secrete powerful neurotoxins used by Indians to tip their poison arrows. The interested reader is referred to G. Kingsley Noble's classical treatise on *The Biology of the Amphibia* (1931) for a discussion of amphibian poison glands.

A curious relationship has been documented for a possible growth-inhibiting pheromone in anurans. Crowding of tadpoles causes reduced growth rates, presumably due to secretions from the largest tadpoles.[3,104,167,168,204] This growth retardation was first attributed to the presence of an algal cell in the feces.[162,163] However, it is not clear whether the algal cell produces the growth-inhibitor pheromone or whether the tadpole does, since the phenomenon has been observed in the absence of any algal cells.[204] Conditioned medium (that is, water that has contained crowded tadpoles) prepared from cultures of *Rana pipiens* tadpoles inhibits growth of tadpoles of ten other anuran species,[104] indicating this pheromone could function as an allomone as well. Other studies have suggested that these effects are only consequences of crowding, and resultant behavioral interactions.[74,91] Additional research may resolve these conflicting interpretations.

Anuran larvae may produce recognition pheromones. The ability of tadpoles to distinguish siblings from nonsiblings is thought to involve detection of chemical cues.[24]

Chemical Communication in Reptiles

The use of semiochemicals (at least pheromones and allomones) for communication can

TABLE 15-3. *Sex-dependent Conspecific Odor Preferences in* Taricha granulosa: *Directed Locomotor Response of Newts to Newt and Non-Newt Odors, Examined in a Simple Olfactometer*

NO. OF TESTS	SEX OF TEST NEWT	SEX OF STIMULUS NEWT	RATIO OF S[a]/NS[b]	PROBABILITY THAT CHOICES WERE RANDOM
10	Male	Male	7/3	0.0570
10	Male	Female	10/0	0.0003
20	Male	Male/Female	17/3	0.0004
10	Female	Male	4/6	0.625
10	Female	Female	6/4	0.625
20	Female	Male/Female	10/10	0.987

Unpublished data of M. Schwartz, D. Duvall and D.O. Norris.
[a] Subject chose air from stimulus animal.
[b] Subject chose air from nonstimulus source (no newt).

be inferred from experimental data gathered for all major reptilian groups. However, visual information appears to be the primary mode for communication as it is in their feathered descendants, the birds. This is especially true in certain families of lizards (for example, Iguanidae, Agamidae) in which visual signals are primary determiners of both courtship and territorial interactions.[37] Nevertheless, pheromones may be important chemical signals for eliciting male to male aggression[48] and other behaviors.

Lizards of several families (Scincidae, Lacertidae, Teidae, Gekkonidae) possess holocrine *femoral glands* on the midventral surface of each thigh and apocrine glands associated with the proctodeum (cloaca). These glands are prominent in males and show an androgen-dependent increase in secretory activity during the breeding season.[29,33] Many behavioral observations suggest that olfaction plays an important role in courtship and territorial behavior in lizards possessing femoral glands,[60,61] and the femoral glands or the proctodeal apocrine glands or both may be sources of pheromones. Considerable research must be done before a pheromonal function of these glands can be confirmed, however.

Snakes, unlike their legged relatives, are well known for the role olfaction plays in their life histories and generally have well-developed glandular structures associated with the cloaca. Emission of a somewhat disagreeable material (allomone?) under the stresses of handling are known to even small children who have attempted to collect garter snakes (genus *Thamnophis*). Numerous studies have demonstrated involvement of odors in snake behavior, including trail-following behavior, sex recognition and preference for (aggregation) or avoidance of conspecifics.[45,65,129,130,145,202] Distinct chemical differences for the lipid portion of cloacal emissions have been found for 25 species of snakes representing three families.[133] These observations provide a chemical basis for species-specificities in cloacal emissions and a potential for species-recognition mechanisms.

When rattlesnakes are given a choice of a freshly envenomed mouse or a mouse killed by cervical dislocation, the snakes prefer the envenomed mouse.[49] These observations suggest that either the venom itself or some substance released by the envenomed mouse attracts the snake and acts as a releaser of swallowing behavior.

Holocrine mental glands of terrestrial and semiterrestrial chelonians produce saturated and unsaturated fatty acids that appear to have communicative significance. Models coated with mental gland secretions from male *Gopherus belandieri* attracted both males and females.[166] Moreover, the model elicited aggressive behavior from the males. Apparently sex recognition can be accomplished through mental gland secretions. The size of these glands and the quantity of secretion may be an expressin of dominance in male tortoises. Inguinal and axillary glands (collectively termed Rathke's glands) in chelonians secrete musk and appear to be involved in defensive behavior.[56] Furthermore, Rathke's glands are involved with sexual behavior in mud turtles and musk turtles.[117] Chelonians also have cloacal glands that have been implicated in trail marking and other behaviors.[7,88,89]

Crocodilians have been suspected of employing pheromones dispersed via secretion of musk glands. Both male and female alligators, *Alligator mississippiensis,* release musk scents during excitement and courtship. Semiochemicals may also be involved in territorial displays.[30,44,113] Similar behavioral observations have been reported for the Nile crocodile *Crocodylus niloticus,*[144] although no pheromones have been identified experimentally.

Chemical Communication in Birds

Birds are known to be highly oriented toward visual displays as well as vocalizations. Much of their physiology and resultant behaviors are influenced by photoperiod and temperature. Although a few studies have established the role of olfaction in location of prey,[203] there is little evidence for either pheromones or allomones in birds. A possible sexual attractant has been reported for the duck, *Anas platyrhynchos.*[11] Considering the importance of olfaction in nonavian vertebrates with respect to intraspecific and interspecific chemical communication, it is unexpected to find an entire vertebrate class without even suggestive evidence for these substances. But then, birds are certainly unique in many other respects, so maybe it is not so surprising after all. Obviously the apparent absence of pheromones and allomones has not hindered their evolutionary success.

The Epiphysial Complex

Almost all vertebrates exhibit one or two epithalamic structures that constitute the epiphysial complex (Fig. 15-9). The components of this complex are the *pineal organ* and a more anterior projection, the *parapineal organ.* In fishes, amphibians and some reptiles (lizards), these organs are basically sac-like diverticula that are more or less open to the third ventricle of the brain. They consist of a basal portion composed of sensory and ependymal (supportive) cells and may have an attached stalk with a distal end vesicle that contacts the dorsal brain case. These structures probably arose in primitive fishes as a pair of diverticula that later changed positions relative to one another.[83] A well-developed parapineal organ has been retained only in cyclostomes and lizards, whereas the pineal organ is found in all vertebrate groups with the exception of crocodilians. In anamniotes as well as in lizards the pineal organ has retained its sensory functions, but in other reptiles, birds and mammals the pineal appears to be only an endocrine structure and is often termed the *pineal gland.*

Two additional prominent dorsal evaginations of the brain occur in this same region:

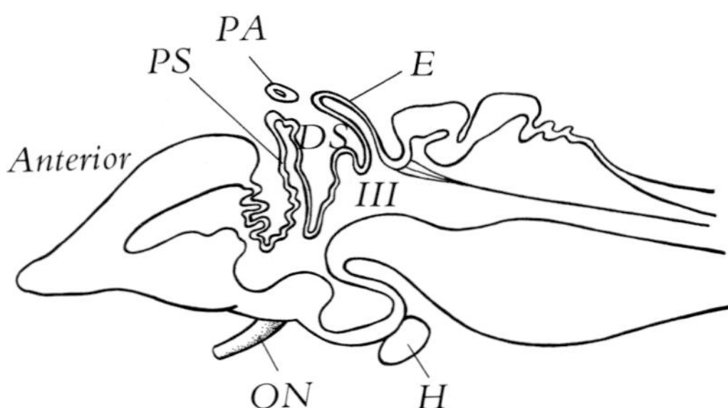

FIG. 15-9. The generalized epiphysial complex. *E,* Epiphysis cerebri or pineal organ; *PA,* parietal or parapineal organ; *PS,* paraphysis; *DS,* dorsal sac; *III,* third ventricle; *ON,* optic nerve; *H,* hypophysis.

the paraphysis and the dorsal sac. The anteriormost evagination that actually develops from the telencephalon is known as the *paraphysis.* The paraphysis is best seen in amphibians as a highly vascularized, sac-like diverticulum (Fig. 15-10); it may function similarly to the choroid plexus in producing cerebrospinal fluid. The *dorsal sac* arises in most vertebrates as a diencephalic (epithalamic) evagination just posterior to the paraphysis but anterior to the epiphysial complex. It is especially prominent in the ganoid fishes (Chondrostei, Holostei) and becomes less conspicuous in teleosts. In most vertebrates the dorsal sac contributes to formation of the choroid plexus.

The pineal complex is connected to an adjacent ependymal structure, the *subcommissural organ* of Dendy (SCO).[5,135] The ependymal cells of the SCO produce an aldehyde-fuchsin positive secretion rich in disulfide bonds and cysteine similar to that observed in the pineal ependyma. The major secretory product of the SCO is a noncellular fiber that in some species extends into the central canal of the spinal cord for its entire length. This structure is known as *Reissner's fiber.* Its significance is not clear. The SCO and its Reissner's fiber have been described in vertebrates from cyclostomes to mammals. Originally it was supposed that Reissner's fiber was involved in regulating posture through tension produced in it by flexion of the body. This tension presumably operated through influences of Reissner's fiber on pressure-sensitive neurons. A more plausible suggestion is the possibility that Reissner's fiber contributes to formation of cerebrospinal fluid. Formation and dissolution of the fiber into the cerebrospinal fluid has been documented as a temperature-dependent process in the frog *Rana esculenta.*[42] Reissner's fiber also binds biogenic amines (epinephrine, norepinephrine) present in the fluid in both *R. esculenta* and in mammals (cow, cat),[80] suggesting still another role. Studies with mammals and reptiles imply a relationship among the pineal complex, the SCO and the adrenal cortex,[6,135,199] but the nature of that relationship remains somewhat obscure. Cytological activation of the SCO in the lizard *Lacerta s. sicula* has been correlated positively with seasonal activities of adrenal cortical cells and of testicular Leydig

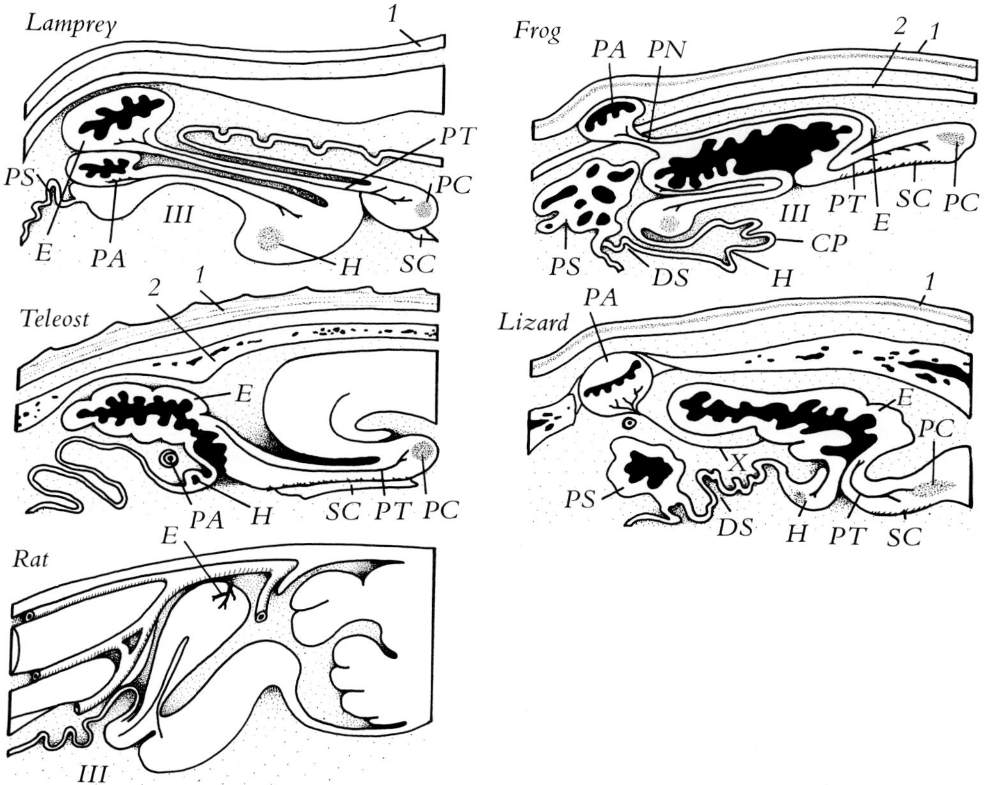

FIG. 15-10. Selected epiphysial complexes. *1*, skin, *2*, skull; *III*, third ventricle; *CP*, choroid plexus; *DS*, dorsal sac; *E*, epiphysis cerebri or pineal organ; *H*, habenular commissure; *PA*, parietal or parapineal organ; *PC*, posterior commissure; *PN*, pineal nerve; *PS*, paraphysis; *PT*, pineal tract; *SC*, subcommissural organ; *X*, parietal nerve. (Redrawn from Bentley.[17])

cells.[47,199] The actual role or roles for the SCO and its secretory products must await further research, but preliminary data would suggest it is somehow related to activity of the pineal complex.

The human pineal gland was described by Galen during the second century as a structural (supportive) element within the brain. Much later, in 1646, Rene Descartes discussed it as a small gland in the brain in which "the soul exerted its function more particularly than in any other part."[158] It was, however, three centuries later that scientists determined what it was that the soul was doing through the pineal gland. McCord and Allen observed that pineal extracts caused blanching (lightening of the skin) of amphibian larvae by causing a concentration of melanin within the melanophores (see Chap. 6).[111] Many years later Lerner and his co-workers succeeded in isolating and characterizing the active skin-lightening agent, 5-methoxyl-N-acetyltryptamine or *melatonin*[102] (Fig. 15-11). Since that time a number of biologically active agents and related compounds have been isolated from pineal tissue including *serotonin* (5-HT), *N-acetylserotonin, 5-methoxytryptophol* (5-MTP) and *5-hydroxytryptophol* (5-HTP).[114] The initial substrate for their synthesis is the amino acid tryptophan (Fig. 15-11). Two enzymes have been studied extensively with respect to their role in regulating melatonin synthesis: *N-acetyltransferase* (NAT) and *hydroxyindole-O-methyltransferase* (HIOMT). N-acetyltransferase converts 5-HT to N-acetylserotonin, which in turn is converted to melatonin by HIOMT. The conversion of 5-HTP to 5-MTP is also catalyzed by HIOMT. Another enzyme complex, *monoamine oxidase* (MAO), acts upon 5-HT, converting it to *5-hydroxy-*

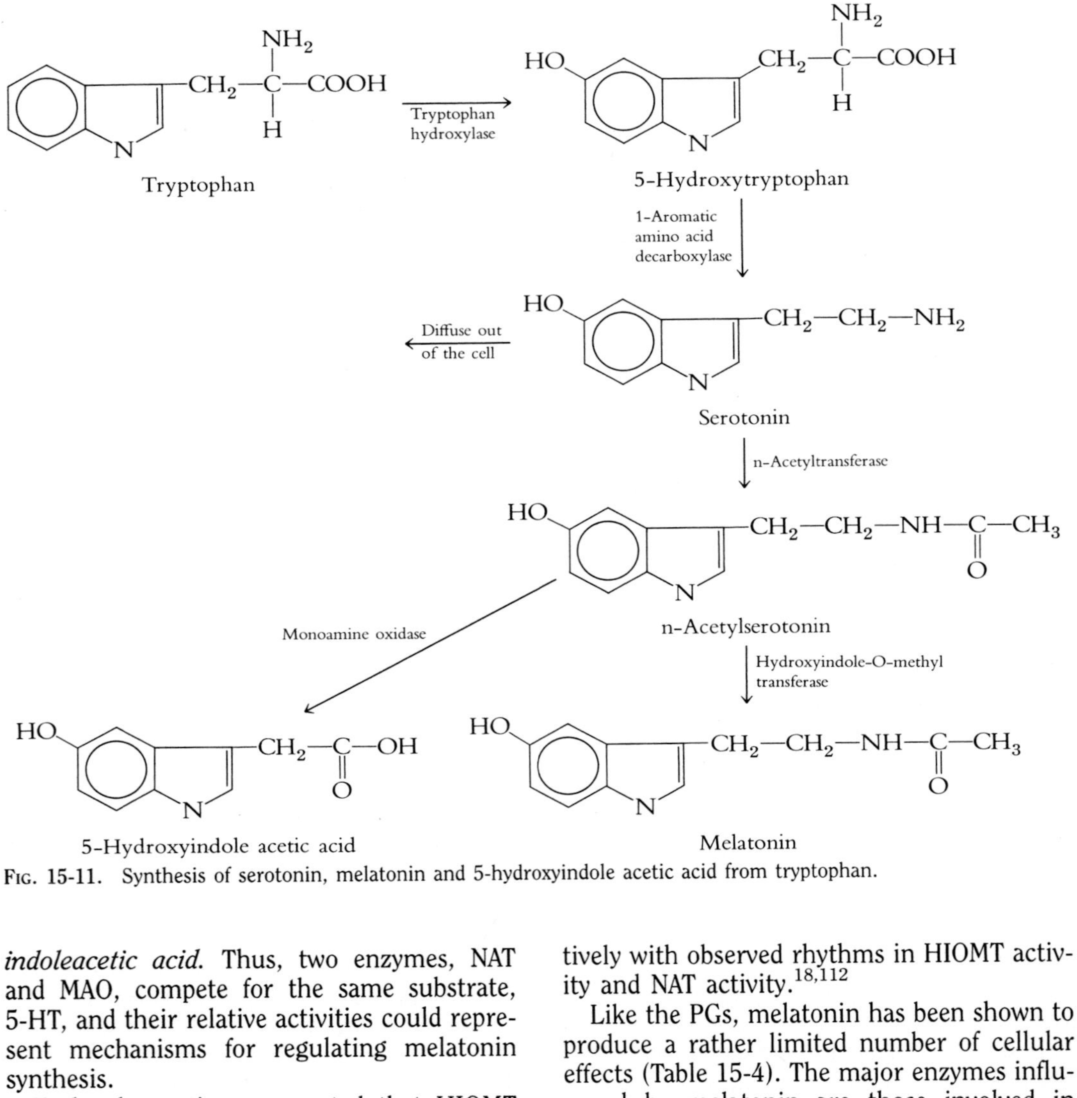

Tryptophan

5-Hydroxytryptophan

Serotonin

n-Acetylserotonin

5-Hydroxyindole acetic acid

Melatonin

FIG. 15-11. Synthesis of serotonin, melatonin and 5-hydroxyindole acetic acid from tryptophan.

indoleacetic acid. Thus, two enzymes, NAT and MAO, compete for the same substrate, 5-HT, and their relative activities could represent mechanisms for regulating melatonin synthesis.

Early observations suggested that HIOMT was the rate-limiting enzyme for melatonin synthesis, and several studies describe correlations between HIOMT activity and melatonin synthesis. More recent studies, however, have established NAT as the rate-limiting enzyme in melatonin synthesis.[18,19]

The mammalian and avian pineals are innervated by sympathetic fibers, and variations in norepinephrine synthesis are correlated with pineal functions. Circadian rhythms in tyrosine hydroxylase activity, the rate-limiting enzyme for norepinephrine synthesis, have been reported in rats. Moreover, the rhythm associated with this enzyme correlates positively with observed rhythms in HIOMT activity and NAT activity.[18,112]

Like the PGs, melatonin has been shown to produce a rather limited number of cellular effects (Table 15-4). The major enzymes influenced by melatonin are those involved in steroid transformations, for example, 5α-reductase and MAO. The actions of melatonin on MAO activity and consequent effects on tissue 5-HT levels may explain effects observed on pancreas, pituitary, testes and the pineal itself following administration of melatonin.[57]

Pineal and Rhythms

Melatonin levels in the blood exhibit a distinct diurnal rhythm being greater at night than during the day. This circadian rhythm persists under constant dark conditions.

TABLE 15-4. *Summary of Nonreproductive Actions of Melatonin and the Pineal in Mammals*[149]

TARGET	DESCRIPTION
Melanophores (melanocytes)	Melatonin implants in weasels, *Mustela erminea,* causes them to grow white coats (typical of winter) in the spring instead of brown coats.
Hair	Melatonin inhibits hair growth of intact or pinealectomized mice.
Connective tissue	Pinealectomy reduces permeability of subcutaneous connective tissue.
Adrenal cortex	Pineal substance, adrenoglomerulotropin, claimed to stimulate aldosterone release.
	Pineal may alter release of ACTH from adenohypophysis.
Parathyroid	Pinealectomy of rat caused hypertrophy of parathyroids, which was reduced by administration of pineal extract or melatonin.
Cardiovascular system	Vasopressor activity reported for pineal extracts, probably due to presence of AVT.
Immune response	Chronic administration of pineal extracts caused leukocytosis, lymph node hypertrophy and an increase in mitotic activity in the spleen. Probably it was a simple immunological response to antigens in the extract.
Thyroid	Melatonin or pineal extracts inhibit thyroid function, possibly through regulation of TSH release from the adenohypophysis.

Plasma melatonin rhythm is a consequence of a circadian rhythm in NAT activity.[19] This enzymatic rhythm is controlled by neural signals from the suprachiasmatic nucleus of the hypothalamus.[187] Information on photoperiod detected by the retina is responsible for entraining the suprachiasmatic nucleus to light dark cycles. The suprachiasmatic nucleus probably controls a number of circadian rhythms in mammals.

Pineal Secretion and Reproduction

So many potential physiological roles of the pineal gland have been reported that it is second only to prolactin (PRL) and the PGs in the number of possible roles.[67] The major effects of the pineal gland in mammals probably relate to reproduction. In 1941 Fiske reported that keeping rats under conditions of constant light increased the frequency of estrus. Several years later Wurtman discovered that pinealectomy also increased the frequency of estrus in rats maintained under normal photoperiods, and a surge of investigation was launched into possible roles of photoperiod, the pineal gland and melatonin in controlling sexual maturity and reproductive cycles in mammals. A mass of data appeared that suggested melatonin released from the pineal gland acted through either the blood or cerebrospinal fluid or through both on the hypothalamus or directly on the pituitary to lower circulating LH levels. The early morning increase of circulating PRL in male rats has also been correlated with the release of some agent from the pineal.[165] Presumably light inhibits sympathetic input to the pineal, resulting in decreased melatonin synthesis and increased levels of LH. Increased LH was considered the basis for increased estrus. The mechanism governing PRL has not been elucidated.

Recent studies have provided a different explanation for the effects of light on estrus. Pinealectomy or injection of massive doses of melatonin never produces marked effects on rat reproduction, and some workers have not found any effect of melatonin on rat reproduction.[15] One study, in fact, reported stimulation of rat gonads by melatonin treatments.[189] The golden hamster *Mesocricetus auratus* exhibits marked gonadal collapse when subjected to short photoperiods (less than 12 hours of light per day). Pinealectomized hamsters do not exhibit gonadal collapse when subjected to short photoperiods, and subdermal melatonin implants (in Silastic capsules) cause testicular atrophy in hamsters maintained on long photoperiods.[160,193–195] If rats are made anosmic (olfaction blocked either mechanically or surgically) and are blinded, more marked gonadal atrophy occurs than was seen following pinealectomy. Furthermore, pinealectomy or melatonin treatment negates the effects of blinding and anosmia in rats as it does in hamsters. Additional support for a stimulatory gonadal role for melatonin has been reported for the ferret, in which melatonin may be responsible for bringing the animal out of photorefractoriness. Melatonin treatment restores the gonadal growth response to long photoperiod in postbreeding ferrets maintained on long photoperiods.[191]

If melatonin is not an antigonadal agent as previously thought, how are the data which indicate an antigonadal role for the pineal explained? Early observations on the nature of pineal extracts showed that, in addition to melatonin and related compounds, peptide fractions could be prepared that exhibited a variety of biological activities. It is known that ependymal cells of fetal human and rat pineals synthesize arginine vasotocin (AVT)[138] which has also been found in adult mammalian pineals. Arginine vasotocin may not be present in all mammalian pineals.[23] Furthermore, the AVT sequence identified immunologically in the pineal could be a fragment of a larger peptide. If AVT is administered to neonatal mice during the period when the brain is undergoing sexual differentiation, increased growth of reproductive organs upon entering adulthood is observed. In contrast, if AVT is administered after the brain has undergone sexual differentiation the growth of accessory organs and in some cases the gonads themselves is inhibited.[200]

The compensatory hypertrophy of the remaining ovary after unilateral ovariectomy is a response to increased gonadotropin levels caused by an effective reduction in circulating estrogens. Arginine vasotocin administered intraperitoneally or directly into the third ventricle of the brain prevents compensatory ovarian hypertrophy (COH). Much less AVT is required if it is administered through the third ventricle than if it is given intraperitoneally. Several related octapeptides including arginine vasopressin, lysine vasopressin and 4-Leu-AVT also inhibit COH, although oxytocin does not. All of the active compounds have an identical ring structure and a basic amino acid at position 8. Treatment of these active molecules with mercaptoethanol disrupts the disulfide bridges necessary for maintenance of the ring structure. Such reduced octapeptides no longer prevent COH; in fact, they enhance it. Melatonin is not as effective as melatonin-free preparations in preventing COH.[57]

Arginine vasotocin exhibits effects on 5α-reductase and MAO activities similar to those reported for melatonin. In fact, AVT or a similar peptide may prove to be the physiological regulator. An antigonadotropic peptide has been isolated from bovine pineals that prevents LH release from the pituitary.[16] This peptide is not AVT since it possesses no oxytocin-like activity in biological assays and has no arginine residues. Release of LH or FSH from rat adenohypophysial cells in culture, however, is not influenced by AVT over a concentration range of 10^{-18} to 10^{-7} moles/liter culture medium.[40] These data would support a role for AVT at the level of the hypothalamus. The presence of other hypothalamic peptides including oxytocin, arginine vasopressin, thyrotropin-releasing hormone and somatostatin has been demonstrated in human pineals.[23] Any of these might be candidates for the illusive pineal inhibitory peptide.

Reiter et al.[42] proposed a scheme that relates the actions of melatonin and pineal antigonadotropic peptides (PAGs) with respect to the observations discussed above as well as to the presence of calcium deposits *(corpora arenacea)* characteristic of some mammalian pineal glands (Fig. 15-12). Since the pineal peptides appear to be structurally similar to the neurohypophysial octapeptides they suggest that PAGs are also stored bound to a carrier protein. Neurophysin-like molecules have been obtained from bovine and human pineals.[98,156,157] These peptides may be related to the neurohypophysial octapeptides present in the pineal or to other pineal peptides synthesized in a similar manner. Consequently the mechanism for secretion of PAGs may also be similar. They suggest that PAGs are released into the interstitial fluids by exocytosis, which also deposits the walls of the secretory vesicles as "exocytotic debris." The PAG-carrier complex presumably interacts with calcium ions, producing a Ca^{++}-carrier protein complex that results in release of free PAGs that can

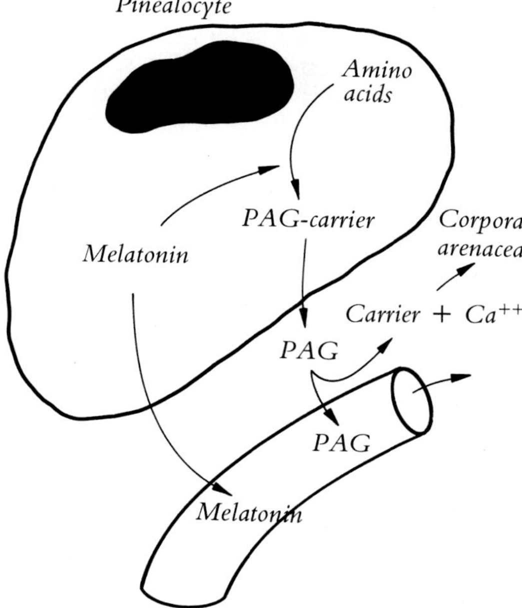

Fig. 15-12. Role proposed for pineal melatonin and pineal antigonadotropic peptides (PAGs) on reproduction. See text for explanation. (Based on Reiter et al.[159])

diffuse into the blood. The Ca^{++}-carrier protein complex interacts with exocytotic debris to produce corpora arenacea. Melatonin would act by inhibiting synthesis or release or both of PAGs in the pineal cell.

Other Factors Affecting the Pineal

In addition to the well-known actions of light on the pineal gland, hypophysectomy, stress and gonadal steroids all influence pineal function.[22,106] Androgens (testosterone, dihydrotestosterone) inhibit MAO activity in the pineal, which in turn causes increased melatonin synthesis. Estrogens have a reverse effect on MAO and pineal activity. Hypophysectomy or administration of histamine reduces melatonin synthesis by reducing activity of HIOMT.

Acute stress stimulates pineal activity, presumably through sympathetic stimulation. Chronic stress (for example, starvation) also increases melatonin synthesis but through a different mechanism. Elevated corticosteroids reduce pineal MAO activity and allow for increased melatonin production. All of these data are consonant with an antigonadal hypothesis for pineal function.

Extrapineal Sources of Melatonin

The harderian gland was described by Harder in 1694 in the red deer. It is located directly behind and around the eye in all vertebrates that possess nictitating membranes, with the possible exception of higher primates.[205] Reddish porphyrin pigments present in the harderian gland undergo fluctuations correlated with lighting conditions. Prior to 12 days of age the harderian gland contains little porphyrin pigment.[206] Blinded 12-day-old rats exhibit an increase in pineal serotonin as well as HIOMT activity during the scotophase (dark portion of photoperiod cycle), but this rhythm is abolished if the harderian glands are also removed.[205,207]

Melatonin has been demonstrated in the rat harderian gland,[28] and continuous illumination causes enlargement of the rat harderian gland and an increase in HIOMT. Harderian HIOMT differs from the HIOMT found in the pineal gland and from that found in the retina of the eye. In contrast, continuous illumination decreases pineal weight and pineal HIOMT activity.[201] The importance of these observations to overall involvement of pineal indoles or harderian indoles to observations on reproduction or other pineal-influenced processes remains to be determined.

The retina of the eye may be another viable source for melatonin,[70] but the nocturnal increase in circulating melatonin is of pineal origin. Melatonin has also been found in the colon of rats, but the significance of this observation is unknown.

Comparative Aspects of the Epiphysial Complex

Class Agnatha: Cyclostomata. The epiphysial complex of cyclostomes consists of a pineal organ and a parapineal organ, although the latter may be lacking in some species.[83] Both organs possess variably shaped end vesicles that project dorsally against the roof of the brain case. The end vesicles contain sensory and ependymal cells structurally organized to suggest that they are photoreceptors.[51] Efferent neural fibers from the pineal organ end at the posterior commissure, whereas those from the parapineal terminate at the habenular commissure. These organs probably relay photoperiodic information to other regions of the brain.

Nocturnal blanching has been observed in ammocetes larvae, and epiphysial levels of HIOMT are correlated with this nocturnal lightening in *Geotria australis.*[92] Removal of the epiphysial complex causes persistent expansion of melanophores in *Lampetra planeri* and *G. australis* but not in *Mordax mordacia* which lacks a parapineal organ. This melanophore response may be mediated via the parapineal.[55] Hypophysectomy of cyclostomes results in blanching due to melanophore contraction, and the action of the parapineal principle may be to inhibit release of melanotropin.

There is evidence for a possible antithyroid effect of the pineal organ. Pinealectomy may inhibit metamorphosis of the ammocetes in all of the above-mentioned lampreys,[54] but confirmatory data are needed.

Class Chondrichthyes. The shark pineal organ contains photosensory and supportive cells.[174] No experimental data, however, have been reported, and the functional importance of the pineal is not known for these fishes. A parapineal organ has not been described for any species in this group.

Class Osteichthyes: Teleostei. The epiphysial complex of teleosts consists of a pineal organ that is extremely variable in both size and degree of development.[83] There is usually a prominent lumen, which in some cases is open to the third ventricle. Photosensory cells and ependymal cells are present in the pineals of several species. A reduced parapineal has been described in some teleosts.

Pigmentation, responses to light and thyroid changes are influenced by the pineal organ. Melanophore changes have been reported in several species of teleost, including rainbow trout, following injection of pharmacological amounts of melatonin.[75,155] Some of these species also respond in a similar manner to epinephrine treatment. Other species respond only to epinephrine with no reaction to melatonin. Circulatory melatonin levels exhibit no correlations to adaptation by rainbow trout to different backgrounds, indicating that melatonin may not be a factor influencing normal pigmentary responses in this species.[134] Furthermore, levels of HIOMT in rainbow trout pineals are not altered by either continuous light or darkness.[76]

The white sucker *Catostomus commersoni,* is responsive to light intensity and/or thermal gradients. This sensitivity is mediated through the pineal.[94] Shielding the sucker's pineal from light causes the fish to choose the warmer portion of horizontal temperature gradients or the better illuminated portions of chambers maintained at a constant temperature. When the shield is removed, the fish returns to its original preference. The pineal may provide information on light intensity for use in mediating thermal behavior. When there is no temperature gradient, retinal receptors alone determine the location of the fish.

Structural correlations have been described between the pineal organ and phototactic responses by fishes.[25] Species with a translucent covering over the pineal organ (a definitive pineal spot) exhibit predominantly positive phototaxis, whereas species with a pigmented, opaque skeletal covering do not show phototaxis. Species that have pigment cells located so that dispersal and concentration of pigment granules could regulate the intensity of light reaching the pineal organ exhibit responses varying from positive phototaxis to no response. The pineal organ might be involved in some other functions for the species showing no phototaxis. The presence of a pineal spot is more common in deep-sea fishes than in freshwater or shallow-water marine species and may relate to the influence of light on vertical migrations performed by deep-sea fishes.[83]

Pinealectomy of *Poecilia reticulata* (guppy) causes pituitary enlargement and hyperplasia of the thyroid.[142] This effect also occurs in *Fundulus heteroclitus* if pinealectomy is performed during the winter months (December through March). Pinealectomy between February and June produces no effect on the thyroid, however.[136] Pituitary and thyroid of the characin, *Astyanax mexicanus,* are not affected by pinealectomy,[153] but both stimulation and inhibition of the goldfish thyroid have been described.[62,140] A possible influence of the pineal on gonadal development has been reported for *F. heteroclitus* and *F. similis*,[41,136] but no relationship was found in goldfish or in *A. mexicanus*.[140,153] Additional studies performed on a seasonal basis involving a large number of species are needed before any definitive statements can be made with respect to the pineal and reproductive or thyroid functions. Differences in photoperiod regimens could explain these differences.[41]

Melatonin has been measured in the retina of rainbow trout, and HIOMT is present in the retinas of several teleostean species.[67] Levels of melatonin in trout retina exceed levels reported in the pineal.

Class Amphibia. The epiphysial complex of amphibians, like that of most vertebrates, consists only of a pineal organ (Fig. 15-13). The frontal organ has not been investigated for its capacity to synthesize melatonin. The proximal or basal portion of the amphibian epiphysial complex as well as the retina of the eye contain HIOMT activity and melatonin.[67] Pinealectomy reduces circulating melatonin to daytime levels,[68] suggesting that the retina may be responsible for basal levels of melatonin in the blood.

As mentioned earlier, the role of melatonin on melanophores in larval Amphibia was first suggested by the observations of McCord and Allen.[111] Since that time it has been shown that melatonin is the pineal agent responsible for the blanching of tadpoles or larval salamanders when held in the dark.[9,26,96,102] As little as 0.0001 μg/ml medium causes aggregation of melanin granules in melanophores of *Xenopus laevis* tadpoles.[10]

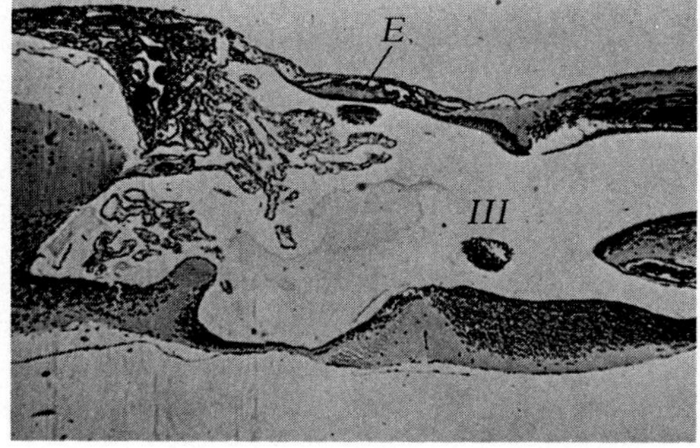

Fig. 15-13. Epiphysial complex of sexually mature tiger salamander larva (neotene). Sagittal section through the brain of a 100-g larva to show the rather minimally developed pineal body *(E)*. *III*, third ventricle. (Courtesy of Dr. William A. Gern.)

Attempts to relate pineal function or melatonin with thyroid function have been equivocal. Pinealectomy of tadpoles of the midwife toad *Alytes obstetricans* accelerates metamorphosis,[161] but a similar operation in larvae of the newt *Taricha torosa* was without effect.[95] Earlier observations in *Bufo americanus*, however, indicated that feeding mammalian pineal to tadpoles accelerated metamorphosis.[2] Pinealectomized larval tiger salamanders, *Ambystoma tigrinum*, exhibit decreased thyroidal uptake of injected radioiodide (^{131}I),[66,143] but neither purified melatonin nor commercial bovine pineal powder influences iodide uptake of intact larvae.[131] Certainly additional studies of the relationship of pineal factors to thyroid function would help to resolve some of these apparent contradictions.

Reproduction may be under inhibitory influence of the pineal organ, at least in anurans. Accelerated gonadal development follows pinealectomy of *A. obstetricans* and *Hyla cinerea*.[41,43,128] Gonadotropin-induced ovulation from *Rana pipiens* ovaries in vitro is inhibited by addition of melatonin to the culture medium.[132] Bovine pineal extract similarly inhibited human chorionic gonadotropin-induced spermiation in male *R. esculenta*, but purified melatonin had no effect.[93] This dichotomy of melatonin's influence in male and female anurans warrants further investigation. The possible influence of pineal principles on reproduction in urodeles has not been studied.

Unlike the other gnathostomous vertebrates some anurans have retained a well-developed end vesicle known as the *frontal organ* or *stirnorgan*[208] (Fig. 15-10). Because of the presence of photosensory cells the frontal organ is often referred to as the parietal eye.[50]

Class Reptilia. Reptiles can be separated into several groups on the basis of the anatomy of the epiphysial complex. Melatonin has been localized in the blood, pineal gland and retinas of snakes, lizards and turtles.[67] Although a pineal is absent in alligators, melatonin is present in the blood.[170] Presumably this melatonin is of retinal origin. Lizards possess an elaborate sac-like, pigmented pineal organ containing both sensory and ependymal cells.

The lumen of the lizard pineal lies close to the third ventricle but does not join with it. A parapineal organ penetrates the skull, forming a parietal spot on the surface. The parapineal is often termed the *parietal eye.* Turtles and snakes have retained only the basal portion of the pineal organ and have lost the end vesicle and stalk of the pineal organ as well as the complete parapineal organ. Nevertheless the turtle pineal organ is the best-developed epiphysial structure in vertebrates (Fig. 15-14). The crocodilians apparently "have seen fit to discard" the entire epiphysial complex.[83]

The parietal eye of lizards has been examined with respect to a number of events, including thyroid function, thermoregulation and reproduction. The lizard parietal contains HIOMT activity suggesting that it synthesizes melatonin.[148] Removal of the parietal eye stimulates thyroid hyperplasia and oxygen consumption.[32,86] These data suggest that melatonin or some other pineal principle influences pituitary function, as reported for teleosts, although direct effects are not ruled out entirely. It has been proposed that the reptilian parietal eye is a photothermal radiation dosimeter that monitors solar radiation and, in turn, regulates activity patterns of lizards.[71] Indeed, excision of the pineal or parietal eye alters thermal responses of lizards.[63] This suggestion has been expanded and supported with extensive documentation,[52,171,172] and it may well be the major functional role for the epiphysial complex in lizards.

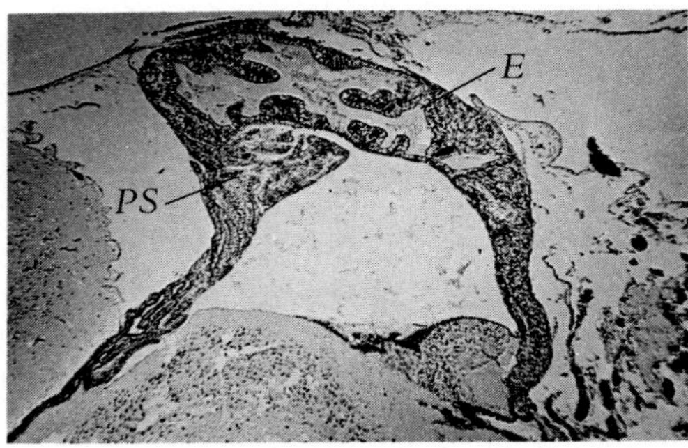

Fig. 15-14. Pineal *(E)* and paraphysis *(PS)* of the green sea turtle *Chelonia mydas.* This section is from a 1-month old specimen, courtesy of Dr. David A. Owens. Compare this not-yet fully developed gland to that exhibited by the sexually mature salamander (Fig. 15-13).

A definite effect of the epiphysial complex on reproduction has been reported.[103] Excision of the parietal eye of the lizard *Anolis carolinensis* stimulates ovarian development in reproductively quiescent animals. This effect is blocked by administration of melatonin. The onset of gonadal recrudescence in this lizard is induced by long photoperiod and warm temperatures. The parietal eye appears to be the transducer through which photoperiod influences reproduction.

Class Aves. The pineal organ of birds has been reduced to the glandular basal portion, the pineal gland. No parapineal or remnant thereof is present. Structurally the avian pineal exhibits considerable diversity, and it is composed of several cellular types. The avian pineal is innervated by sympathetic fibers as reported for mammals.

Avian pineals are biochemically like their mammalian counterpart. Variations have been reported in HIOMT and NAT activities with respect to lighting conditions, but the most dramatic effects involve NAT. Activity of this enzyme exhibits a marked increase with onset of the scotophase, a peak about the middle of the scotophase and a decrease rapidly following the onset of the photophase.[18,21,22] Brief exposure to light at the peak of NAT activity causes a rapid reduction to photophase levels. Melatonin rhythms that correlate with rhythms in pineal NAT activity have been reported for brain, pineal, retina and serum of birds.[67,152] The brain and especially the hypothalamus in birds may be the primary site of action for melatonin and may explain effects of melatonin on gonadal function, thermoregulation and locomotor activity.

The role of the pineal in the reproductive biology of birds may be progonadal.[31] Pinealectomy inhibits androgen synthesis, whereas administration of melatonin stimulates androgen synthesis, presumably by altering gonadotropin release from the adenohypophysis. Pinealectomy of quail delays ovarian development, an observation that also supports a progonadal role. Melatonin injections cause a decrease in gonadal weight suggesting that the progonadal agent might be a peptide. Marked species differences may occur, as evidenced by depression of testicular function in the duck following pinealectomy. However, no effects of melatonin treatment on parameters of gonadal development and their relationship to photoperiod could be demonstrated in either white-throated sparrows or border canaries.[186,196]

Pinealectomy abolishes endogenous body temperature rhythms as well as free-running locomotor activity rhythms in house sparrows, *Passer domesticus*.[20,119] Effects on locomotor activity appear to involve two pathways, one of which can bypass the pineal organ. Pinealectomized birds that have lost free-running locomotor activity in the dark still exhibit entrainment to light-dark cycles, supporting the presence of a bypass system. Both systems can be entrained by light, but the pineal has control over the bypass system (Fig. 15-15).

Evolution of Melatonin's Functions

An intriguing hypothesis for the original function of melatonin and the evolution of other functions is based on the presence of melatonin synthesizing systems in retinas, parietal eyes and pineals and the observations that pineals of more primitive vertebrate groups are photoreceptors.[67] Evidence suggests that both retinal and pineal melatonin exhibit night-time (scotophasic) peaks of synthesis. This hypothesis proposes that melatonin was initially a local hormone for regulating the distribution of melanosomes in the retina. During the day, melanosomes are dispersed in retinal pigment cells which protect the photoreceptors from intense light. At night, elevated melatonin causes concentration of melanosomes and allows dim light to maximally stimulate the photoreceptors. Similar mechanisms presumedly operate in the photoreceptive outer portion of the pineal, in the parietal eye and in the amphibian frontal organ. The increase in melatonin synthesis during the scotophase causes a greater proportion of melatonin to appear in the blood. Consequently, the scotophasic elevation in melatonin is a reliable internal cue for obtaining information about seasonal photoperiods. Information concerning length of the scotophase is reflected in circulating melatonin levels. Thus, according to this hypothesis, the diurnal rhythm in melatonin has been co-opted as the blood borne signal entraining a number of other internal events during the evolution of vertebrates.

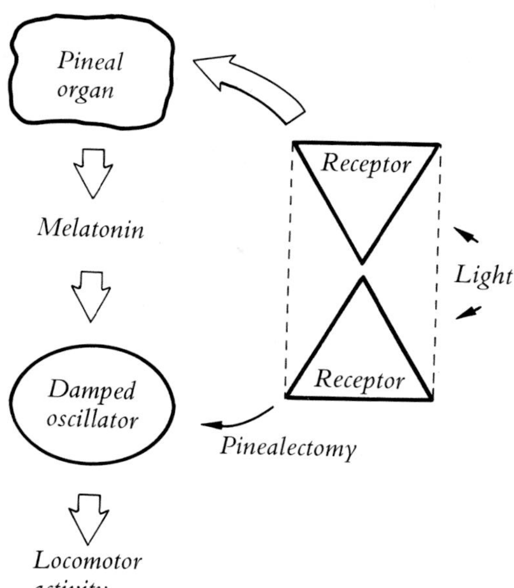

Fig. 15-15. Role of pineal in controlling circadian locomotor rhythm in birds. Circadian fluctuations in pineal activity entrains a damped oscillator that drives the locomotor activity. In the absence of pineal activity (that is, following pinealectomy) a separate endogenous pathway also entrained by photoperiod controls the rhythm. The action of the second pathway is normally overridden by the pineal influence. (Based on Menaker and Zimmerman.[119])

Summary

A cohesive summation of the individual endocrine phenomena discussed here is not possible, and so a simple listing of the systems covered and some generalizations of each will follow. It is recognized that this chapter has not been all inclusive, and other chemical messengers might have been included.

Erythropoietin is a polypeptide hormone produced from a kidney precursor, erythrogenin. It stimulates production of red blood cells from precursor cells in the bone marrow. Release of erythropoietin is stimulated by hypoxic conditions.

Somatomedins are produced by the liver and secreted into the blood under the influence of growth hormone. They mediate the effects of growth hormone on skeletal tissue, and mimic the action of insulin which they resemble chemically. Several other growth-promoting proteins are known including nerve growth factor and epidermal growth factor.

Eicosanoids are lipoidal substances that include prostaglandins, prostacyclin, thromboxanes and leukotrienes. Prostaglandins are small lipids synthesized by most tissues. They may be important mediators in the mechanisms of hormone action as well as in other physiological processes. The stimulatory effect of PGs on smooth muscle has led to their use as abortifacients. Prostacyclin inhibits platelet aggregation, whereas thromboxanes enhance aggregation. Leukotrienes contribute to inflammatory reactions. Synthesis of prostaglandins, prostacyclin and thromboxanes is blocked by NSAIDs. Glucocorticoids interfere with leukotriene synthesis.

The thymus gland produces several factors that promote lymphocyte differentiation in other lymphoid tissues.

Kinins are produced from blood borne factors through the action of kallikreins. They are hypotensive agents. Other actions of kinins include participation in activation of a number of pancreatic digestive enzymes, conversion of prohormones to their active forms, fertilization, implantation and development.

Semiochemicals are substances secreted into the environment that control the physiology and behavior of other organisms. Pheromones are intraspecific substances and allelomones are interspecific substances employed in chemical communications. Primer pheromones operate through neuroendocrine mechanisms, whereas signal pheromones produce immediate responses through the nervous system. Allelomones are subdivided into allomones and kairomones; allomones benefit the emitter and kairomones benefit the recipient. The importance of these semiochemicals in animal communication is now being recognized, and many behaviors have been shown to depend upon or be modified by these substances.

The epithalamic subcommissural organ (SCO) secretes Reissner's fiber that extends the length of the spinal cord in all vertebrate groups. The significance of this system is not understood.

The glandular portion of the vertebrate epiphysial complex produces melatonin, AVT and some other small peptides that are released into the blood, cerebrospinal fluid or both. In many vertebrates the output of these substances is influenced by photoperiodic stimuli operating via the eyes or extraretinal photoreceptors such as the "third eye" of amphibians and reptiles. Melatonin may have evolved as a local regulator of pigment distri-

TABLE 15-5. *Effects of Melatonin Treatment in Vertebrates.*

	(+/−)	AGNATHA	OSTEICHTHYES	AMPHIBIA	REPTILIA	AVES	MAMMALIA
Concentration of melanosomes or inhibition of melanin synthesis	yes/no	+	+	+	+		+
Preferred temperature	Increase/decrease		+	−	−		
Thermogenic effect on body temperature	Increase/decrease				−	−	+
Gonad function: adults	stimulate/inhibit		±	−	−	−	±
Gonad function: juvenile	stimulate/inhibit					+	
Thyroid function	stimulate/inhibit			−			−

From Gern and Karn,[67] Heldmaier et al.,[78] and Kavaliers.[94]

bution in vertebrate photoreceptors. Pineal principles probably influence release of adenohypophysial hormones (primarily thryotropin and gonadotropins) through effects at the level of the hypothalamus. Reproduction, thyroid function, pigment patterns, thermoregulation and locomotor activity may be influenced by pineal principles. The mammalian antigonadotropic pineal factor appears to be a peptide whose release may be influenced by melatonin. The scotophasic pulse of melatonin in blood has become an important internal cue for timing of physiological and behavioral events.

References

1. Acree, F., R.B. Turner, H.K.Gouck, M. Beroza and N. Smith (1968). L-lactic acid: A mosquito attractant isolated from humans. Science 161:1346–1347.
2. Addair, J. and F.E. Chidester (1928). Pineal and metamorphosis: The influence of pineal feeding upon the rate of metamorphosis in frogs. Endocrinology 12:791–796.
3. Akin, G.W. (1966). Self-inhibition of growth in *Rana pipiens* tadpoles. Physiol. Zool. 39:341–356.
4. Anisko, J.J. (1977). Hormonal substrate of estrous odor preference in beagles. Physiol. Behav. 18:13–17.
5. Ariens Kappers, C.U., G.C. Huber and E.C. Crosby (1936). The Comparative Anatomy of the Nervous System of Vertebrates Including Man. Hafner Publishing Co., New York.
6. Attila, U. and S. Talanti (1973). Incorporation of ^{35}S-labelled cysteine in the subcommissural organ of the rat after adrenalectomy and after treatment with hydrocortisone. Acta Physiol. Scand. 87:422–424.
7. Auffenberg, W. (1965). Sex and species discrimination in two sympatric South American tortoises. Copeia 1965:335–342.
8. Avery, T.L. (1969). Pheromone-induced changes in the acidophil concentration of mouse pituitary glands. Science 164:423–424.
9. Bagnara, J.T. (1960). Pineal regulation of the body lightening reaction in amphibian larvae. Science 132:1481–1483.
10. Bagnara, J.T. (1963). The pineal and the body lightening reaction of larval amphibians. Gen. Comp. Endocrinol. 3:86–100.
11. Balthazart J. and E. Schoffeniels (1979). Pheromones are involved in the control of sexual behavior in birds. Naturwissenschaften 66:55–56.
12. Bardach, J.E. and J.H. Todd (1970). Chemical communication in fish. In J.W. Johnston, Jr., D.G. Moulton and A. Turk, eds., Advances in Chemoreception, Vol. 1, Communication by Chemical Signals. Appleton-Century-Crofts, New York, pp. 205–240.
13. Barnett, C. (1977). Chemical recognition of the mother by the young of the cichlid fish *Cichlasoma citrinellum.* J. Chem. Ecol. 3:463–468.
14. Barnett, C. (1977). Aspects of chemical communication with special reference to fish. Biosci. Commun. 3:331–392.
15. Benson, B., B.R. Larsen, P.R. Findell and K.M. Orstead (1983). Participation of pineal peptides in reproduction. In S.M. McCann and D.S. Dhindsa, eds., Role of Peptides and Proteins in Control of Reproduction. Elsevier Science, New York, pp. 111–130.
16. Benson, B., M.J. Matthews and V.J. Hruby (1976). Characterization and effects of a bovine pineal antigonadotropic peptide. Am. Zool. 16:17–24.
17. Bentley, P.J. (1976). Comparative Vertebrate Endocrinology. Cambridge University Press.
18. Binkley, S. (1976). Comparative biochemistry of the pineal glands of birds and mammals. Am. Zool. 16:57–65.
19. Binkley, S.A. (1983). Circadian rhythms of pineal function in rats. Endo. Revs. 4:255–270.
20. Binkley, S., E. Kluth and M. Menaker (1971). Pineal function in sparrows: Circadian rhythms and body temperature. Science 174:311–314.
21. Binkley, S., S. MacBride, D.C. Klein and C.L. Ralph (1973). Pineal enzymes: Regulation of avian melatonin synthesis. Science 181:273–275.
22. Binkley, S., S. MacBride, D.C. Klein and C.L. Ralph (1975). Regulation of pineal rhythms in chickens: Refractory period and nonvisual light perception. Endocrinology 96:848–853.
23. Blask, D.E., M.K. Vaughan and R.J. Reiter (1983). Pineal peptides and reproduction. In R. Relkin, ed., The Pineal Gland. Elsevier Biomedical, New York, pp. 201–224.
24. Blaustein, A.R. and R.K. O'Hara (1982). Kin recognition cues in *Rana cascadae* tadpoles. Behav. Neural Biol. 36:77–87.
25. Breder, C.M. and P. Rasquin (1950). A preliminary report on the role of the pineal organ in the control of pigment cells and light reactions in recent teleost fishes. Science 111:10–12.
26. Brick, I. (1962). Relationship of the pineal to the pituitary-melanophore effector system in *Amblystoma opacum.* Anat. Rec. 142:229.

27. Bronson, F.H. (1974). Pheromonal influences on reproductive activities in rodents. In M.C. Birch, ed., Pheromones. North Holland Res. Monogr. 32:344–365.

28. Bubenik, G.A., G.M. Brown and L.J. Grota (1976). Immunochemical localization of melatonin in the rat Harderian gland. J. Histochem. Cytochem. 24:1173–1177.

29. Burkholder, G.L. and W.T. Tanner (1974). A new gland in *Sceloporus graciosus* males (Sauria: Iguanidae). Herpetolgica 30:368–371.

30. Burrage, B.R. (1965). Copulation in a pair of *Alligator mississippiensis.* Br. J. Herpetol. 3:207–208.

31. Cardinalli, D.P. and J.M. Rosner (1971). Effects of melatonin, serotonin and N-acetyl serotonin on the production of steroids by duck testicular homogenates. Steroids 18:25–37.

32. Clausen, H.J. and B. Mofshin (1939). The pineal eye of the lizard (*Anolis carolinensis*), a photoreceptor as revealed by oxygen consumption studies. J. Cell Comp. Physiol. 14:29–41.

33. Cole, C.J. (1966). Femoral glands in lizards: A review. Herpetologica 22:199–206.

34. Collier, H.O.J. (1971). Prostaglandins and aspirin. Nature 232:17–19.

35. Comfort, A. (1971). Communication may be odorous. New Scientist. See Science 166:398.

36. Comsa, J. (1973). Thymus replacement and HTH, the homeostatic thymic hormone. In T.D. Luckey, ed., Thymic Hormones. University Park Press, Baltimore, pp. 39–58.

37. Crews, D. (1975). Psychobiology of reptilian reproduction. Science 189:1059–1065.

38. Das, M. (1982). Epidermal growth factor: mechanisms of action. Int. Rev. Cytol. 78:233–256.

39. Dawson, A.B. (1922). The cloaca and cloacal glands of the male. *Necturus.* J. Morphol. 36:447–465.

40. DeMoulin, A., B. Hudson, P. Franchimont and J.J. Legros (1977). Arginine vasotocin does not affect gonadotropin secretion *in vitro.* J. Endocrinol. 72:105–106.

41. DeVlaming, V.L., M. Sage and C.B. Charlton (1974). The effects of melatonin treatment on gonadosomatic index in the teleost, *Fundulus similis,* and the tree frog, *Hyla cinerea.* Gen. Comp. Endocrinol. 22:433–438.

42. Diederen, J.H.B. (1975). Influence of ambient temperature on growth rate of Reissner's fibre in *Rana esculenta.* Cell Tissue Res. 156:267–271.

43. Disclos, P. (1964). Epiphysectomie chez le tetard d'Alytes. C.R. Acad. Sci. 258:3101–3103.

44. Ditmars, R.L. (1910). Reptiles of the World. Sturgis and Walton Co., New York.

45. Dundee, H.A. and M.C. Miller (1968). Aggregative behavior and habitat conditioning by the prairie ringneck snake *Diadophis punctatus arnyi.* Tulane Stud. Zool. Bot. 15:41–58.

46. Dunn, R.S. and A.M. Perks (1975). Comparative studies of plasma kinins: The kallikrein-kinin system in poikilotherm and other vertebrates. Gen. Comp. Endocrinol. 26:165–178.

47. D'uva, V., G. Ciarcia, A. Ciarletta and F. Angelini (1978) The subcommissural organ of *Lacerta s. sicula* Raf.: Effects of experimental treatment on castrated animals during winter. J. Exp. Zool. 205:285–292.

48. Duvall, D. (1979). Fence lizard chemical signals: Conspecific discriminations and release of social behavior. J. Exp. Zool. 210:321–326.

49. Duvall, D., D. Chiszar, J. Trupiano and C.W. Radcliffe (1978). Preference for envenomated rodent prey by rattlesnakes. Bull. Psychonom. Soc. 11:7–8.

50. Eakin, R.M. (1961). Photoreceptors in the amphibian frontal organ. Proc. Natl. Acad. Sci. 47:1084–1088.

51. Eakin, R.M. (1963). Lines of evolution of photoreceptors. In D. Mazia and A. Tyler, eds., General Physiology of Cell Specialization. McGraw-Hill, New York, pp. 393–425.

52. Eakin, R.M. (1973). The Third Eye. University of California Press, Berkeley.

53. Ebling, F.J. (1972). The response of the cutaneous glands to steroids. Gen. Comp. Endocrinol. Suppl. 3:228–237.

54. Eddy, J.M.P. (1969). Metamorphosis and the pineal complex in the brook lamprey, *Lampetra planeri.* J. Endocrinol. 44:451–452.

55. Eddy, J.M.P. and R. Strahan (1968). The role of the pineal complex in the pigmentary effector system of the lampreys, *Mordacia mordax* (Richardson) and *Geotria australis* Gray. Gen. Comp. Endocrinol. 11:528–534.

56. Ehrenfeld, J.G. and D.W. Ehrenfeld (1973). Externally secreting glands of freshwater and sea turtles. Copeia 1973:305–314.

57. Ellis, L.C. (1976). Periperal and CNS effects of the pineal gland: Target enzymes common to tissues and species. Am. Zool. 16:67–78.

58. Engen, T. (1970). Man's ability to perceive odors. In Johnston, J.W., Jr., D.G. Moulton and A. Turk, eds., Advances in Chemoreception, Vol. 1, Communication by Chemical Signals. Appleton-Century-Crofts, New York, pp. 361–384.

59. Erdös, E.G., I. Miwa and W.J. Graham (1967). Studies on the evolution of plasma kinins: Reptilian and avian blood. Life Sci. 6:2433–2439.

60. Evans, L.T. (1961). Structure as related to behavior in the organization of populations in reptiles. In W.F. Blair, ed., Vertebrate Speciation. University of Texas Press, Austin, pp. 148–178.

61. Evans, L.T. (1965). Introduction. In W.M. Milstead, ed., Lizard Ecology: A Symposium. University of Missouri Press, Columbia, pp. 83–86.

62. Fenwick, J.C. (1970). Demonstration of melatonin in a fish. Gen. Comp. Endocrinol. 14:86–97.

63. Firth, B. and H. Heatwole (1976). Panting threshold of lizards: The role of the pineal complex in panting responses in an agamid, *Amphibolurus muricatus.* Gen. Comp. Endocrinol. 29:388–401.

64. Flack, J.D., R. Jessup and P.W. Ramwell (1969). Prostaglandin stimulation of rat corticosteroidogenesis. Science 163:691–692.

65. Gelbach, F.R., J. Watkins and J. Kroll (1971). Pheromone trail-following studies of Typhlopid, Leplotyphlopid and Colubrid snakes. Behaviour 40:282–294.

66. Gern, W.A. and K.F. DeBoer (1973). Pineal thyroid relationships in neoteny. J. Colo.-Wyo. Acad. Sci. 7(4):32–33.

67. Gern, W.A. and C.M. Karn (1983). Evolution of melatonin's functions and effects. Pineal Res. Revs. 1:49–90.

68. Gern, W.A. and D.O. Norris (1979). Plasma melatonin in the neotenic tiger salamander (*Ambystoma tigrinim*): Effects of photoperiod and pinealectomy. Gen. Comp. Endocrinol. 38:393–398.

69. Gern, W.A., D.W. Owens and C.L. Ralph (1978). Plasma melatonin in the trout: Day-night change demonstrated by radioimmunoassay. Gen. Comp. Endocrinol. 34:453–458.

70. Gern, W.A. and C.L. Ralph (1979). Melatonin synthesis by the retina. Science 204:183–184.

71. Glaser, R. (1958). Increase in locomotor activity following shielding of the parietal eye in night lizards. Science 128:1577–1578.

72. Goldstein, A.L., T.L.K. Low, G.B. Thurman, M.M. Zatz, N. Hall, J. Chen, S.-K. Hu, P.B. Nalor and J.E. McClure (1981). Current status of thymosin and other hormones of the thymus gland. Rec. Prog. Horm. Res. 37:369–415.

73. Goldstein, A.L., F.D. Slater and A. White (1966). Preparation, assay and partial purification of a thymus-lymphocytopoietic factor. Proc. Natl. Acad. Sci. 56:1010–1017.

74. Gromko, M.H., F.S. Mason and S.J. Smith-Gill (1973). Analysis of the crowding effect in *Rana pipiens* tadpoles. J. Exp. Zool. 186:63–72.

75. Hafeez, M.A. (1970). Effect of melatonin on body coloration and spontaneous swimming activity in rainbow trout, *Salmo gairdneri.* Comp. Biochem. Physiol. 36:639–656.

76. Hafeez, M.A. and W.B. Quay (1970). Pineal acetylserotonin methyltransferase activity in the teleost fishes. *Hesperoleucus symmetricus* and *Salmo gairdneri,* with evidence for lack of effect of constant light and darkness. Comp. Gen. Pharmacol. 1:257–262.

77. Haynes, N.B., H.D. Hafs, R.J. Waters, J.G. Mannus and A. Riley (1975). Stimulatory effect of prostaglandin $F_{2\alpha}$ on the plasma concentration of testosterone in bulls. J. Endocrinol. 66:329–338.

78. Heldmaier, G., S. Steinlechner, J. Rafael and P. Vsiansky (1981). Photoperiodic control and effects of melatonin on nonshivering thermogenesis and brown adipose tissue. Science 212:917–919.

79. Hertzler, E.C. (1968). Airbourne pheromones. Science 162:813.

80. Hess, J. and G. Sterba (1973). Studies concerning the function of the complex subcommissural organ-liquor fibre: The binding ability of liquor fibre to pyrocatechin derivatives and its functional aspects. Brain Res. 58:303–312.

81. Hinman, J.W. (1970). Prostaglandins: A report on early clinical studies. Postgrad. Med. J. 46:562–575.

82. Hoffer, B.J., G.R. Siggins and F.E. Bloom (1969). Prostaglandins E_1 and E_2 antagonize norepinephrine effects on cerebellar Purkinje cells: Microelectrophoretic study. Science 166:1418–1420.

83. Hoffman, R.A. (1970). The epiphyseal complex in fish and reptiles. Am. Zool. 10:191–199.

84. Hollenberg, M.D. (1979). Epidermal growth factor-urogastrone, a polypeptide acquiring hormonal status. Vit. Horm. 37:69–110.

85. Horton, E.W. (1972). The prostaglandins. Proc. R. Soc. Lond. 182:411–426.

86. Hutton, K.E. and R. Ortman (1957). Blood chemistry and parietal eye of *Anolis carolinensis.* Proc. Soc. Exp. Biol. Med. 96:842–844.

87. Illius, A.W., N.B. Haynes and G.E. Lamming (1976). Effects of ewe proximity on peripheral plasma testosterone levels and behavior in the ram. J. Reprod. Fertil. 48:25–32.

88. Jackson, G., Jr. and J.D. Davis (1972). A quantitative study of the courtship display of the red-eared turtle, *Chrysemys scripta elegans.* Herpetologica 28:58–64.

89. Jackson, G., Jr. and J.D. Davis (1972). Courtship display behavior of *Chrysemys concinna suwanmiensis.* Copeia 1972:385–387.

90. Jesel, L. and C.L. Aron (1976). The role of pheromones in the regulation of estrous cycle duration in the guinea pig. Neuroendocrinology 20:97–109.

91. John, K.R. and D. Fenster (1975). The effects of partitions on the growth rates of crowded *Rana pipiens* tadpoles. Am. Midl. Nat. 93:123–130.

92. Joss, J.M.P. (1977). Hydroxyindole-O-methyl-transferase (HIOMT) activity and the uptake of ^{3}H-melatonin in the lamprey, *Geotria australis* Gray. Gen. Comp. Endocrinol. 31:270–275.

93. Juszkiewicz, T. and Z. Rakalska (1965). Lack of the

effect of melatonin on the frog spermatogenic reaction. J. Pharm. Pharmacol. 17:189–190.

94. Kavaliers, M. (1982). Effects of pineal shielding on the thermoregulatory behavior of the white sucker, *Catostomus commersoni.* Physiol. Zool. 55:155–161.

95. Kelly, D.E. (1958). Embryonic and larval epiphysectomy in the salamander, *Taricha torosa,* and observations on scoliosis. J. Morphol. 103:503–538.

96. Kelly, D.E. (1962). Pineal organs: Photoreception, secretion, and development. Am. Sci. 50:597–625.

97. Kingsbury, B.F. (1895). The spermatheca and methods of fertilization in some American newts and salamanders. Proc. Am. Microsc. Soc. 27:261–305.

98. Krass, M.E., F.S. LaBella, S.H. Shin and J. Minnich (1971). Biochemical features of the pineal compared with other endocrine and nervous structures. In H. Keller and K. Lederis, eds., Subcellular Organization and Function in Endocrine Tissues, Mem. Soc. Endocrinol. 19:49–76.

99. Kuehl, F.A., Jr., J.L. Humes, J. Tarnoff, V.J. Cirillo and E.A. Ham (1970). Prostaglandin receptor site: Evidence for an essential role in the action of luteinizing hormone. Science 169:883–885.

100. Lau, I.F., S.K. Saksena and M.C. Chang (1974). Prostaglandin F in the uterine horns of mice with intrauterine devices. J. Reprod. Fertil. 37:429–432.

101. Lavras, A.A., M. Fichman, E. Hiraichi, P. Schmuziger and P.Z. Picarelli (1969). Action of different kininogenases on snake plasma. Pharmacol. Res. Commun. 1:171.

102. Lerner, A.B., J.D. Case, Y. Takahashi, T.H. Lee and W. Mori (1958). Isolation of melatonin, the pineal gland factor that lightens melanocytes. J. Am. Chem. Soc. 80:2587.

103. Levey, I.L. (1973). Effects of pinealectomy and melatonin injections at different seasons on ovarian activity in the lizard. *Anolis carolinensis.* J. Exp. Zool. 185:169–174.

104. Licht, P. (1967). Environmental control of annual testicular cycles in the lizard, *Anolis carolinensis.* I. Interaction of light and temperature in the initiation of testicular recrudescene. J. Exp. Zool. 165:505–516.

105. Luckey, T.D. (1973). Thymic Hormones. University Park Press, Baltimore.

106. Lynch, H.J., M. Ho and R.J. Wurtman (1977). The adrenal medulla may mediate the increase in pineal melatonin synthesis induced by stress, but not that caused by exposure to darkness. J. Neural Transm. 40:87–97.

107. MacGinitie, G.E. (1939). The natural history of the blind goby, *Typhlogobius californiensis.* (Steindachner). Am. Midl. Nat. 21:489–505.

108. Macrides, F., A. Bartke and S. Dalterio (1975). Strange females increase plasma testosterone levels in male mice. Science 189:1104–1106.

109. McClintock, M.K. (1971). Menstrual synchrony and suppression. Nature 229:224–246.

110. McClintock, M.K. (1983). Modulation of the estrous cycle by pheromones from pregnant and lactating rats. Biol. Reprod. 28:823–829.

111. McCord, C.P. and F.P. Allen (1917). Evidences associating pineal gland function with alteration in pigmentation. J. Exp. Zool. 23:207–224.

112. McGreer, E.G. and P.L. McGreer (1966). Circadian rhythm in pineal tyrosine hydroxylase. Science 153:73–74.

113. McIlhenny, E.A. (1934). The Alligator's Life History. Christopher Publ. House, Boston.

114. McIsaac, W.M., G. Farrell, R.G. Taborsky and A.N. Taylor (1965). Indole compounds: Isolation from pineal tissue. Science 148:102–103.

115. Madison, D.M. (1975). Intraspecific odor preferences between salamanders of the same sex: Dependence on season and proximity of residence. Can. J. Zool. 53:1356–1361.

116. Madison, D.M. (1977). Chemical communication in amphibians and reptiles. In D. Muller-Schwartze and M.M. Mozell, eds., Chemical Signals in Vertebrates. Plenum Publishing Co., pp. 135–168.

117. Mahmoud, I.Y. (1967). Courtship behavior and sexual maturity in four species of kinosternid turtles. Copeia 1967:314–319.

118. Marx, J.L. (1972). Prostaglandins: Mediators of inflammation? Science 177:780–781.

119. Menaker, M. and N. Zimmerman (1976). Role of the pineal in the circadian system of birds. Am. Zool. 16:45–55.

120. Michael, R.P., R.W. Bonsall and P. Warner (1974). Human vaginal secretion: Volatile fatty acid content. Science 186:1217–1219.

121. Michael, R.P., R.W. Bonsall and D. Zumpe (1976). Evidence for chemical communication in primates. Vitam. Horm. 34:137–186.

122. Moncada, S. ed. (1983). Prostacyclin, thromboxane and leukotrienes. Br. Med. Bull. 39:209–295.

123. Moncada, S., R. Korbut, S. Bunting and J.R. Vane (1978). Prostacyclin is a circulating hormone. Nature 273:767–768.

124. Müller-Schwarze, D., C. Müller-Schwarze, A.G. Singer and R.M. Silverstein (1974). Mammalian pheromone: Identification of active component in the subauricular scent of the male pronghorn. Science 183:860–862.

125. Murphy, M.R. and G.E. Schneider (1970). Olfactory bulb removal eliminates mating behavior in the male golden hamster. Science 167:302–304.

126. Mykytowycz, R. (1972). The behavioral role of the mammalian skin glands. Naturwissenschaften 59:133–139.

127. Naughton, B.A., S.M. Kaplan, M. Roy, A.J. Burdowski, A.S. Gordon and S.J. Piliero (1977). Hepatic regeneration and erythropoietin production in the rat. Science 196:301–302.

128. Noble, G.K. (1931). The hedonic glands of the plethodontid salamanders and their relation to sex hormones. Anat. Rec. Suppl. 48:57–58.

129. Noble, G.K. (1937). The sense organs involved in the courtship of *Storeria, Thamnophis* and other snakes. Bull. Am. Mus. Nat. Hist. 73:673–726.

130. Noble, G.K. and H.J. Clausen (1936). The aggregation behavior of *Storeria deKayi* and other snakes with special reference to the sense organs involved. Ecol. Monogr. 6:269–316.

131. Norris, D.O. and J.E. Platt (1973). Effects of pituitary hormones, melatonin, and thyroidal inhibitors on radioiodide uptake by the thyroid glands of larval and adult tiger salamanders, *Ambystoma tigrinum* (Amphibia: Caudata). Gen. Comp. Endocrinol. 21:368–376.

132. O'Connor, J.M. (1969). Effect of melatonin on *in vitro* ovulation of frog oocytes. Am. Zool. 9:577.

133. Odlak, P. (1976). Comparison of the scent gland secretion lipids of 25 species of snakes. Implications for biochemical systematics. Copeia 1976:320–326.

134. Owens, D.W., W.A. Gern, C.L. Ralph and T.J. Boardman (1978). Nonrelationship between plasma melatonin and background adaptation in the rainbow trout (*Salmo gairdneri*). Gen. Comp. Endocrinol. 34:459–467.

135. Palkovits, M. (1965). Participation of the epithalmo-epiphyseal system in the regulation of water and electrolytes. In J.A. Kappers and J.P. Schade, eds., Structure and Function of the Epiphysis Cerebri. Elsevier Publishing Co., Amsterdam, p. 627–634.

136. Pang, P.K.T. (1967). The effect of pinealectomy on adult male killifish, *Fundulus heteroclitus.* Am. Zool. 7:715.

137. Partridge, B.L., N.R. Liley and N.E. Stacey (1976). The role of pheromones in the sexual behavior of the goldfish. Anim. Behav. 24:291–299.

138. Pavel, S., R. Goldstein, E. Ghinea and M. Calb (1977). Chromatographic evidence for vasotocin biosynthesis by cultured pineal ependymal cells from rat fetuses. Endocrinology 100:205–208.

139. Peschle, C. and M. Condorelli (1975). Biogenesis of erythropoietin: Evidence for pro-erythropoietin in a subcellular fraction of kidney. Science 190:910–912.

140. Peter, R.E. (1968). Failure to detect an effect of pinealectomy in goldfish. Gen. Comp. Endocrinol. 10:443–449.

141. Pfeiffer, W. (1977). The distribution of fright reaction and alarm substance cells in fishes. Copeia 1977:653–665.

142. Pflugfelder, O. (1956). Wirkungen von Epiphysan und Thyroxin auf die Schildrüse epiphysektomierter *Lebistes reticulatus.* Roux Arch. Entwickungsmech. Org. 148:463–473.

143. Platt, J.E. and D.O. Norris (1973). The effects of melatonin, bovine pineal extract and pinealectomy on spontaneous and induced metamorphosis and thyroidal uptake of ^{131}I in larval *Ambystoma tigrinum.* J. Colo.-Wyo. Acad. Sci. 7(4):40.

144. Pooley, A.C. and C. Gans (1976). The Nile crocodile. Sci. Am. 234:114–124.

145. Porter, R.H. and J.A. Czaplicki (1974). Responses of water snakes (*Natrix r. rhombifera*) and garter snakes (*Thamnophis sirtalis*) to chemical cues. Anim. Learn. Behav. 2:129–132.

146. Powers, J.B. and S.S. Winans (1975). Vomeronasal organ: Critical role in mediating sexual behavior of the male hamster. Science 187:961–963.

147. Powles, T.J., D.M. Easty, G.C. Easty, P.K. Bondy and A. Monro-Neville (1973). Aspirin inhibition of *in vitro* osteolysis stimulated by parathyroid hormone and PGE. Nature 245:83–84.

148. Quay, W.B. (1965). Retinal and pineal hydroxyindole-O-methyltransferase activity in vertebrates. Life Sci. 4:983–991.

149. Quay, W.B. (1970). Endocrine effects of the mammalian pineal. Am. Zool. 10:237–246.

150. Rabito, S.F., A. Binia and R. Segovia (1972). Plasma kininogen content of toads, fowl and reptiles. Comp. Biochem. Physiol. 41A:281–284.

151. Ralls, K. (1971). Mammalian scent marking. Science 171:443–449.

152. Ralph, C.L. (1976). Correlations of melatonin content in pineal gland, blood, and brain of some birds and mammals. Am. Zool. 16:35–44.

153. Rasquin, P. (1958). Studies in the control of pigment cells and light reactions in recent teleost fishes. Bull. Am. Mus. Nat. Hist. 115:1–68.

154. Regnier, F.E. (1971). Semiochemicals—structure and function. Biol. Reprod. 4:309–326.

155. Reed, B.L., B.C. Finnin and N.E. Ruffin (1969). The effects of melatonin and epinephrine to the melanophores of fresh water teleosts. Life Sci. 8:113–120.

156. Reinharz, A.C., P. Czernichow and M.B. Vallotton (1974). Neurophysin-like protein in bovine pineal gland. J. Endocrinol. 62:35–44.

157. Reinharz, A.C. and M.B. Vallotton (1977). Presence of two neurophysins in the human pineal gland. Endocrinology 100:994–1001.

158. Reiter, R.J. (1970). Introduction to the symposium: A précis of the pineal odyssey. Am. Zool. 10:189–190.

159. Reiter, R.J., A.J. Lukaszyk, M.K. Vaughn and D.E. Blask (1976). New horizons of pineal research. Am. Zool. 16:93–101.

160. Reiter, R.J., M.K. Vaughan, D.E. Blask and L.Y. Johnson (1975). Pineal methoxyindoles: New evidence concerning their function in the control of

pineal-mediated changes in the reproductive physiology of male golden hamsters. Endocrinology 96:206–213.

161. Remy, C. and P. Disclos (1970). Influence de l'epiphysectomie sur le developpement de la thyroide et des gonades chez les tetârds *d'Alytes obstetricans.* C.R. Soc. Biol. 164:1989–1993.

162. Richards, C.M. (1958). The inhibition of growth in crowded *Rana pipiens* tadpoles. Physiol. Zool. 31:138–151.

163. Richards, C.M. (1962). The control of tadpole growth by alga-like cells. Physiol. Zool. 35:285–296.

164. Roberts, J.S. and J.A. McCracken (1975). Prostaglandin $F_{2\alpha}$ production by the brain during estrogen-induced secretion of luteinizing hormone. Science 190:894–896.

165. Ronnekleiv, O.K., L. Krulich and S.M. McCann (1973). An early morning surge of prolactin in the male rat and its abolition by pinealectomy. Endocrinology 92:1339–1342.

166. Rose, F.L. (1970). Tortoise chin gland fatty acid composition: Behavioral significance. Comp. Biochem. Physiol. 32:577–580.

167. Rose, S.M. (1959). Failure of survival of slowly growing members of a population. Science 129:1026.

168. Rose, S.M. (1960). A feedback mechanism of growth control in tadpoles. Ecology 41:188–199.

169. Rosenfeld, M.G., I.B. Abrass and B. Chiang (1976). Hormonal stimulation of α-amylase synthesis in porcine pancreatic minces. Endocrinology 99:611–618.

170. Roth, J.J., W.A. Gern, E.C. Roth, C.L. Ralph and E. Jacobson (1980). Nonpineal melatonin in the alligator (*Alligator mississippiensis*). Science 210:548–550.

171. Roth, J.J. and C.L. Ralph (1976). Body temperature of the lizard (*Anolis carolinensis*). Effect of parietalectomy. J. Exp. Zool. 198:17–28.

172. Roth, J.J. and C.L. Ralph (1977). Thermal and photic preferences in intact and parietalectomized *Anolis carolinensis.* Behav. Biol. 19:341–348.

173. Rothstein, H. (1982). Regulation of the cell cycle by somatomedins. Int. Rev. Cytol. 78:127–232.

174. Rudeberg, C. (1969). Light and electron microscopic studies on the pineal organ of the dogfish, *Scyliorhinus canicula* L. Z. Zellforsch. 96:548–581.

175. Salthe, S.N. and J.S. Mecham (1974). Reproductive and courtship patterns. In B. Lofts, ed., Physiology of the Amphibia. Academic Press, New York, Vol. 2, pp. 310–522.

176. Samuellson, B. and S. Hammarstrom (1982). Leukotrienes: a novel group of biologically active compounds. Vit. Horm. 39:1–30.

177. Schachter, M. (1980). Kallikreins (kininogenases)—A group of serine proteases with bioregulatory actions. Pharmacol. Rev. 31:1–17.

178. Schadler, M.H. (1981). Postimplantation abortion in pine voles (*Microtus pinetorum*) induced by strange males and pheromones of strange males. Biol. Reprod. 25:295–297.

179. Schadler, M.H. (1983). Male siblings inhibit reproductive activity in female pine voles, *Microtus pinetorum.* Biol. Reprod. 28:1137–1139.

180. Seki, T., I. Miwa, T. Nakajima and E.G. Erdös (1973). Plasma kallikrein-kinin system in nonmammalian blood: Evolutionary aspects. Am. J. Physiol. 224:1425–1430.

181. Sever, D.M. (1978). Male cloacal glands of *Plethodon cinereus* and *Plethodon dorsalis* (Amphibia: Plethodontidae). Herpetologica 34:1–19.

182. Shenkman, L., Y. Imai, K. Kataoka, C.S. Hollander, L. Wan, S.C. Tang and T. Avruskin (1974). Prostaglandins stimulate thyroid function in pregnant women. Science 184:81–82.

183. Singer, A.G., W.C. Agosta, R.J. O'Connell, C. Pfaffman, D.V. Bowen and F.H. Field (1976). Dimethyldisulfide: An attractant pheromone in hamster vaginal secretion. Science 191:948–950.

184. Smith, K., G.F. Thompson and H.D. Koster (1969). Sweat in schizophrenic patients: Identification of the odorous substance. Science 166:398–399.

185. Stehn, R.A. and M.E. Richmond (1975). Male-induced pregnancy termination in the prairie vole, *Microtus ochrogaster.* Science 187:1211–1213.

186. Storey, C.R. and T.J. Nicholls (1978). Failure of exogenous melatonin to influence the maintenance or dissipation of photorefractoriness in the canary, *Serinus canarius.* Gen. Comp. Endocrinol. 34:468–470.

187. Takahashi, J.S. and M. Zatz (1982). Regulation of circadian rhythmicity. Science 217:1104–1111.

188. Tavolga, W.N. (1956). Visual, chemical and sound stimuli in the sex discrimatory behavior of the gobiid fish, *Bathygobius soporator.* Zoologica 41:49–64.

189. Thieblot, L., J. Berthelay and S. Blaise (1966). Effêts de la mélatonine chez le rat mâle et femelle. I. Action au niveau des gonades et des annexes. Ann. Endocrinol. 27:65–68.

190. Thiessen, D.D., F.E. Regnier, M. Rice, M. Goodwin, N. Isaacks and N. Lawson (1974). Identification of a ventral scent marking pheromone in the male Mongolian gerbil (*Meriones unquiculatus*). Science 184:83–85.

191. Thorpe, P.A. and J. Herbert (1976). Studies on the duration of the breeding season and photorefractoriness in female ferrets pinealectomized or treated with melatonin. J. Endocrinol. 70:255–262.

192. Tristram, D.A. (1977). Intraspecific olfactory communication in the terrestrial salamander, *Plethodon cinereus.* Copeia 1977:597–600.

193. Turek, F.W. (1977). Antigonadal effect of melatonin in pinealectomized and intact male hamsters. Proc. Soc. Exp. Biol. Med. 155:31–34.

194. Turek, F.W., C. Desjardins and M. Menaker (1975). Melatonin: Antigonadal and progonadal effects in male golden hamsters. Science 190:280–282.

195. Turek, F.W., C. Desjardins, and M. Menaker (1976). Melatonin-induced inhibition of testicular function in adult golden hamsters. Proc. Soc. Exp. Biol. Med. 151:502–506.

196. Turek, F.W. and A. Wolfson (1978). Lack of an effect of melatonin treatment via silastic capsules on photic-induced gonadal growth and the photorefractory condition in white-throated sparrows. Gen. Comp. Endocrinol. 34:471–474.

197. Twitty, V.C. (1955). Field experiments on the biology and genetic relationships of the California species of Triturus. J. Exp. Zool. 129:129–148.

198. Urry, R.L., K.A. Dougherty, J.L. Frehn and L.C. Ellis (1976). Factors other than light affecting the pineal gland: Hypophysectomy, testosterone, dihydrotestosterone, estradiol, cryptorchidism and stress. Am. Zool. 16:79–92.

199. Varano, L., V. LaForgia, V. D'uva, G. Ciarcia and A. Ciarletta (1978). Possible relationship between the activity of the adrenal gland and the subcommissural organ in the lizard *Lacerta s. sicula* Raf. Effects of ACTH administration during winter. Cell Tissue Res. 192:53–65.

200. Vaughan, M.K., G.M. Vaughan, D.E. Blask, M.P. Barnett and R.J. Reiter (1976). Arginine vasotocin: Structure-activity relationships and influence on gonadal growth and function. Am. Zool. 16:25–34.

201. Vlahakes, G.J. and R.J. Wurtman (1971). A new melatonin-forming enzyme in rat harderian gland. Abstract, Endocrine Society, 53rd Meeting, A-105.

202. Watkins, J.F., II, F.R. Gelbach and J.C. Kroll (1969). Attractant-repellent secretions of blind snakes (*Leptotyplops dulcis*) and their army ant prey (*Neivamyrmex nigrescens*). Ecology 50:1098–1102.

203. Wenzel, B.M. (1973). Chemoreception. In D.S. Farner and J.R. King, eds., Avian Biology, Academic Press, Vol. 3, pp. 389–416.

204. West, L.B. (1960). The nature of growth inhibitory material from crowded *Rana pipiens* tadpoles. Physiol. Zool. 33:232–239.

205. Wetterberg, L., E. Geller and A. Yuwiler (1970). Harderian gland: An extraretinal photoreceptor influencing the pineal gland in neonatal rats? Science 167:884–885.

206. Wetterberg, L., A. Yuwiler, E. Geller and S. Schapiro (1970). Harderian gland: Development and influence of early hormonal treatment on porphyrin content. Science 168:996–998.

207. Wetterberg, L., A. Yuwiler, R. Ulrich, E. Geller and R. Wallace (1970). Harderian gland: Influence on pineal hydroxyindole-O-methyltransferase activity in neonatal rats. Science 170:194–196.

208. Wurtman, R.J., J. Axelrod and D.E. Kelly (1968). The Pineal. Academic Press, New York.

PART IV

16·Endocrine Regulation of Iono-Osmotic Balance in Teleosts

Teleostean fishes have adapted to life in a variety of aquatic habitats from dilute fresh water to relatively high salinities. In this chapter, some of the endocrine factors are examined that facilitate survival under differing conditions of salinity. The purpose of this discussion is to emphasize how various endocrine factors are involved cooperatively in achieving balanced regulation of body fluids. For the most part, only generalizations are stressed, and the interested reader should consult the list of readings at the end of this chapter to obtain more detailed documentation. Considerable variations exist in how different species solve particular iono-osmotic problems, and the generalizations stressed in this chapter must be viewed with some reservations. The same processes may be involved, but the emphasis on particular processes varies. For example, in freshwater-adapted eels only about 1% of the total Na^+ influx occurs across the intestine,[52] whereas the same basic mechanism accounts for 25% of the Na^+ influx in goldfish.[40]

Most of the available data for this topic have been generated from studies employing *euryhaline* species; that is, fishes that can tolerate wide ranges of salinity. Some of these species in nature are strictly seawater fishes, some are strictly freshwater species and still others have capitalized on their wide range of osmoregulatory capabilities and may migrate between marine and freshwater habitats.

Fishes that cannot tolerate fluctuations in environmental salinity beyond a very narrow range are termed *stenohaline*. Unfortunately little research has been reported involving stenohaline species, although they too must have endocrine regulatory mechanisms similar to their euryhaline relatives. The following discussion focuses on euryhaline species. Similar mechanisms may be operating in stenohaline fishes. There is, however, little flexibility in altering these osmoregulatory mechanisms as compared to euryhaline fishes, which may account for the inability of stenohaline species to tolerate salinity fluctuations.

Teleosts evolved in freshwater (hypo-osmotic) environments, and their glomerular kidney is the major osmotic regulatory organ for removing excess water that has entered as a result of the large osmotic gradient between fresh water and body fluids. The blood of freshwater fishes is about one-fourth the osmotic concentration of sea water (about 300 mOsm/liter), and these fishes tend to gain a considerable volume of water via osmosis and lose salts through diffusion (Fig. 16-1). Freshwater fishes must actively accumulate salt and resist its diffusion and at the same time produce a large volume of dilute urine (Table 16-1).

Marine fishes have a blood osmotic concentration of approximately 400 mOsm/liter or about one-third the concentration normally found for sea water (1200 mOsm/liter). Most of

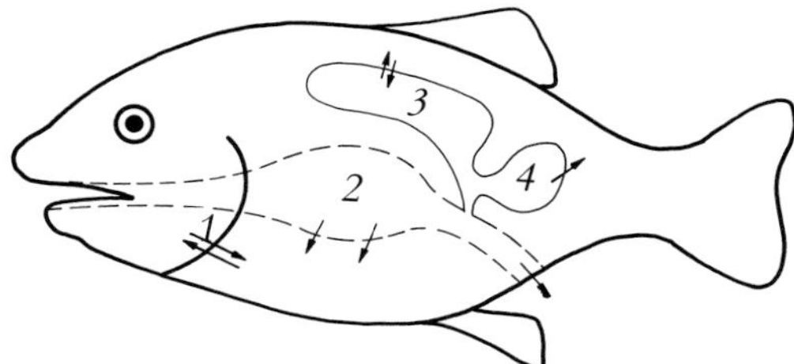

FIG. 16-1. Fish osmoregulatory organs. The gill *(1)* is a major site for ion exchange. The gut *(2)* is important for ion and water uptake. The kidney *(3)* functions primarily to remove water although some salt-balance activities are also performed. The urinary bladder *(4)* may be important for water and ion balance in some species.

this osmolarity is due to NaCl, and is part of the adaptations of teleosts to the marine environment. The blood of marine and seawater-adapted fishes is hypo-osmotic to sea water, and they have the opposite regulatory problems of freshwater fishes; that is, they tend to lose water and gain salt. Consequently marine and seawater-adapted fishes imbibe water and actively excrete excess salts, primarily through the gills and to a limited extent via the urine. The kidney of marine and seawater-adapted fishes is shut down to conserve water, and little urine is produced (Table 16-1). Some marine fishes have developed an aglomerular kidney and have thus reduced urine production. Other marine and many euryhaline fishes have vascular shunts whereby most of the blood will bypass the kidney, thus reducing the glomerular filtration rate (GFR) and urine output.

TABLE 16-1. *Chloride Composition of Blood and Plasma and Urine Production by Rainbow Trout* Salmo gairdneri *Adapted to Fresh Water or Sea Water*[68]

	SW-ADAPTED	FW-ADAPTED
ml urine/kg body weight/day	0.5–1	75–90
plasma chloride (mOsm/liter)	140	137.5
urine chloride (mOsm/liter)	200–220	5–12

The primitive teleostean kidney lacks an effective water reabsorption mechanism such as the one associated with the loop of Henle in birds and mammals. Consequently marine teleosts cannot produce urine that is hypertonic to the blood, and they are forced to utilize the gill and operular membrane for salt excretion. The only exception to this is a transitory production of urine hypertonic to the blood in euryhaline *Fundulus kansae* during osmoregulatory adjustments following transfer from fresh water to sea water.[75] The effective use of a blood-shunting mechanism is illustrated by rainbow trout, *Salmo gairdneri,* adapted to fresh water as compared to sea water (Table 16-1). In spite of drastic alterations in the volume of water excreted by regulating urine output, trout are able to maintain stable blood ionic composition following complete adaptation to the environmental salinity.

The urinary bladder and the kidney tubules may be involved with water or ion reabsorption in some species. For example, eels of the genus *Anguilla* exhibit a similar GFR whether adapted to sea water or fresh water, indicating that no shunting mechanism is employed to any significant extent. These fishes rely apparently upon "tubular" or bladder reabsorption of water or both to reduce urine flow when in sea water.

The major sites for salt and water exchange in fishes are the gills opercular membrane, kidney, bladder, gut and skin (Fig. 16-2). The importance of gills in ion and water exchange with the environment might be inferred simply from the immense surface area they exhibit. Branchial surface area may be from 10 to 60 times greater than that provided by the skin.[63] In the gills and opercular membrane are found specialized salt-transporting cells known as *Keys-Wilmer* or chloride cells. The ability to transport salt appears to be related directly to Na^+-K^+-activated adenosine triphosphatase (Na^+/K^+-ATPase) activity in the branchial salt-secreting cells. Keys-Wilmer cells are important for excretion of salt in marine and seawater-adapted fishes in which they account for about 90% of all the excreted salt. Stenohaline marine fishes exhibit four to five times the Na^+/K^+-ATPase activity in the gills, of stenohaline freshwater species,[34,41] emphasizing the greater role of the gill for salt excre-

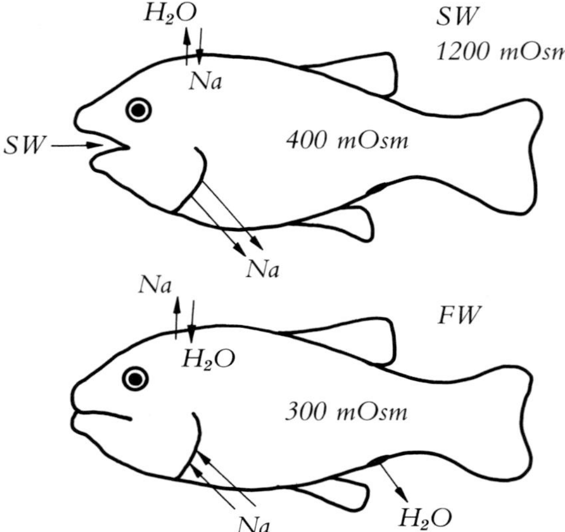

FIG. 16-2. Fish in sea water and fresh water. The seawater-adapted fish *(SW)* is hypo-osmotic to sea water and is in danger of desiccation. It drinks sea water, absorbs water and salt through the intestine and excretes excess salt through the gills. The kidney produces only a small quantity of glomerular filtrate, and urine production is very slight. In contrast, the freshwater-adapted fish *(FW)* readily takes up water osmotically and must excrete a large quantity of dilute urine. Salt tends to diffuse into the medium, and the gills must transport salt into the blood. Salts are also absorbed from the gut, but water is not. Osmotic concentration for blood of freshwater and seawater fishes and for sea water are indicated in mOsm.

tion in marine fishes than for salt accumulation under freshwater conditions. In freshwater or freshwater-adapted fishes the direction of branchial salt transport is reversed, but here it appears that salt uptake by cells in the gut may be more important than branchial transport.

As mentioned above, the kidney is not an effective agent for excreting salt because of its inability to produce urine hypertonic to the blood. Salt excretion via the urine would hence result in serious water losses for the marine and seawater-adapted fishes that are already losing water osmotically to the outside medium. Nevertheless the kidney does play a major role in freshwater and freshwater-adapted species as a vehicle for eliminating water and for selectively reabsorbing salts. The urinary bladder also may be a site for independently influencing urine composition in some species. In seawater-adapted or marine species, the kidney and urinary bladder become more involved with water conservation and selective ion excretion, especially the excretion of excess divalent ions such as magnesium.[56] Euryhaline species in general exhibit switching from using the kidney as a freshwater fish when adapted to fresh water and using it as would a marine fish when adapted to sea water.

The intestine is an important site for regulating salt and water balance as are the kidney and gill. In marine or seawater-adapted fishes the gut is a site for water reabsorption following active transportation of salts. This water and salt are ingested with food or by drinking. Sodium is actively absorbed from the intestinal lumen of freshwater or freshwater-adapted fish, but water uptake does not occur. The endocrine bases for these differences are described below.

The skin of teleosts does not appear to be a major site for regulating iono-osmotic events although water and a variety of ions diffuse across it. Water losses in marine and seawater-adapted fishes and water influx in freshwater and freshwater-adapted species can occur through the skin, but the emphasis for regulation is clearly upon the gills, gut, kidney and urinary bladder. Scales and the presence of mucus (especially prominent in freshwater or freshwater-adapted fishes) tend to reduce the permeability of the skin to both water and ions.

Endocrine Factors in Iono-Osmotic Regulation

The major hormones responsible for regulation of water and salt balance appear to be *prolactin* (PRL), *corticotropin* (ACTH), *cortisol* and *arginine vasotocin* (AVT). The *corpuscles of Stannius* located in the kidney and the *caudal neurosecretory system* with its neurohemal organ, the *urophysis,* located at the base of the tail may also play important roles. *Catecholamines, thyroid hormones* and others have been implicated as influencing ionic and osmotic regulation. Each of these factors will be discussed, first separately and then cooperatively, as they are involved in

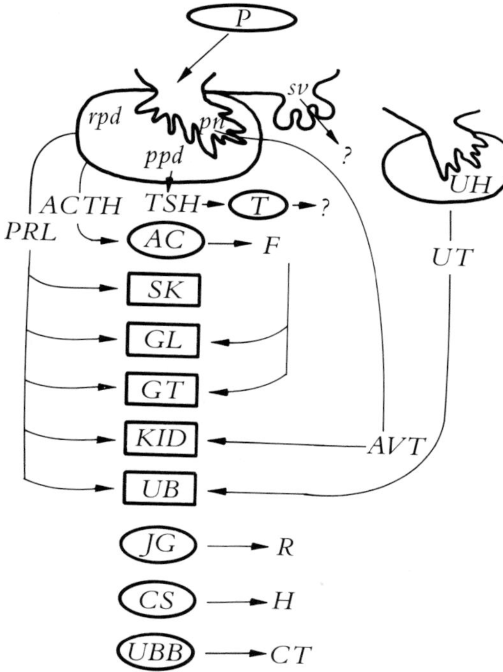

FIG. 16-3. Summary for endocrine regulation of iono-osmotic balance in teleosts. See text for explanation. (Modified from Johnson.[38]) ACTH, corticotropin; AVT, arginine vasotocin; CS, corpuscles of Stannius; CT, calcitonin; F, cortisol; GL, gill and opercular membranes; GT, gut; H, hypocalcin

AC, adrenocortical tissue; JG, juxtaglomerular cells; KID, kidney; P, pineal; pn, pars nervosa; ppd, proximal pars distalis; PRL, prolactin; R, renin; rpd, rostral pars distalis

SK, skin; sv, saccus vasculosus; T, thyroid; TSH, thyrotropin; UB, urinary bladder; UBB, ultimobranchial bodies; UH, urophysis; UT, urotensins. Effects of urotensins on gut, skin and opercular membrane are not shown.

adaptations to environments of high or low salinity. Figure 16-3 summarizes endocrine regulation of iono-osmotic balance in teleosts.

Prolactin

Hypophysectomized euryhaline killifish, *Fundulus heteroclitus,* soon die if retained in fresh water but live if placed in sea water.[66] This phenomenon has been observed in several other similar species.[70] Hypophysectomized freshwater *Poecilia latipinna* exhibit considerable sodium loss prior to death, and the loss in sodium is considered to be a major factor responsible for death following hypophysectomy. The greater sodium content of sea water allows such hypophysectomized animals to survive. This loss of sodium following hypophysectomy can be prevented by injection of mammalian PRL,[1,2,23,44,67] and PRL-treated hypophysectomized fishes survive in fresh water so long as PRL therapy continues. Treatment with pharmacological agents that block PRL release mimics hypophysectomy in these species.[50]

Not all species die in fresh water following hypophysectomy. Eels (*Anguilla* spp.), salmonids and goldfish *(Carassius auratus)* survive in fresh water but exhibit increased sodium loss.[10] Treatment of these species with PRL can prevent posthypophysectomy sodium loss.[17]

The above observations led to formulation of the hypothesis that pituitary PRL must be important for osmoregulation by fishes in fresh water but was not essential for all species of marine or seawater-adapted fishes.[7] Observations of pituitary cytology and PRL content in seawater-adapted euryhaline species (for example, *P. latipinna, Sarotherodon mossambicus*) as compared to freshwater-adapted individuals reveal more PRL-producing eta cells (Fig. 16-4) as well as more extractable PRL activity in the rostral pars distalis of freshwater-adapted individuals.[22,49] Injection of mammalian PRL into seawater-adapted fish elevates plasma sodium and can even lead to

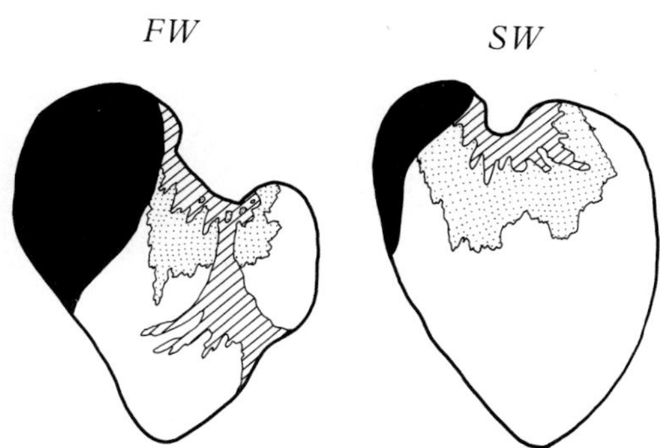

FIG. 16-4. Relative areas occupied by rostral pars distalis in the pituitary of freshwater-adapted *(FW)* and seawater-adapted *(SW)* tilapia, *Sarotherodon mossambica.* Black, rostral pars distalis containing prolactin-secreting cells; *stipple,* proximal pars distalis; *white,* pars intermedia; *diagonal lines,* nervous tissue. (Redrawn from Dharmamba and Nishioka.[16])

death.[15,76] Plasma levels of PRL are 6 to 10 times greater in freshwater-adapted tilapia than in seawater-adapted fish. Adaptation of seawater-adapted tilapia to fresh water is accompanied by increase in plasma PRL.[57] These observations support both the action of PRL on plasma sodium and its importance for freshwater fishes. This response of plasma sodium to PRL in teleosts has resulted in development of sensitive bioassays for fish PRL (see Chap. 5).

Another major effect of PRL in teleosts is its influence on water permeability. Hypophysectomy of freshwater-adapted brown trout, *Salmo trutta,* is followed by a decrease in water turnover that is returned to normal by PRL treatment.[58] Prolactin reduces permeability of the gills to water and reduces water transfer across the gut and urinary bladder.[38,60] The effect of PRL on urinary bladder permeability is not related to any change in sodium.[18]

A third important action of PRL in teleosts is the effect on water excretion via the kidney. Prolactin treatment causes an increase in GFR indirectly by altering the anatomical relationship between the vascular system and the kidney.[45,61] In seawater-adapted or hypophysectomized glomerular fishes a physical gap (the glomerular-renal capsular space) forms between the glomerulus and the kidney tubule (Fig. 16-5). This gap decreases the effectiveness of fluid transfer from the blood vascular system to the kidney and reduces urine formation. Freshwater-adapted fish of the same species exhibit close contact between the glomerulus and the renal capsule as do seawater-adapted or hypophysectomized fish treated with PRL. This anatomical arrangement presumably facilitates fluid transfer and is responsible for the effect of PRL on GFR. Prolactin has also been observed to decrease the permeability of kidney tubules in freshwater-adapted starry flounders and thereby facilitates water excretion.[28]

There is some evidence to suggest that PRL may have some influence on skin permeability in freshwater-adapted and freshwater fishes. Hypophysectomy of freshwater-adapted fishes causes reduction in mucus on the skin and gill surfaces. Prolactin stimulates mucus secretion and restores the mucus covering on hypophys-

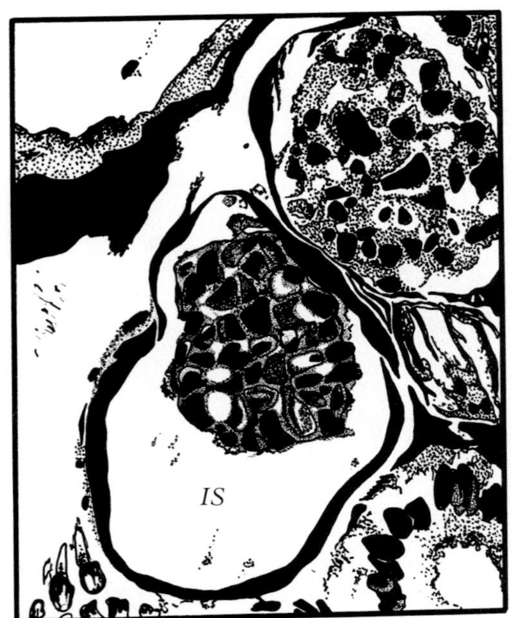

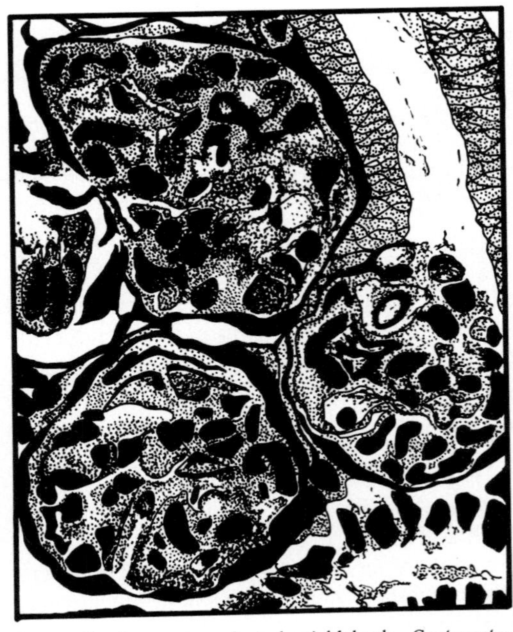

FIG. 16-5. Prolactin on glomerular structure in kidney. Glomeruli of seawater-adapted stickleback, *Gasterosteus aculeatus* form *trachurus (left).* Note prominent intracapsular space *(IS)* separating glomerulus from Bowman's capsule. Prolactin injections result in disappearance of this intracapsular space *(right)* and cause increased glomerular filtration. (Drawn from Lam and Leatherland.[45])

ectomized fishes. This mucus presumably reduces movement of ions and water across the skin.[54,59] The skin of seawater fishes does not appear to be permeable to water.[38]

Prolactin reduces water reabsorption from the bladder of seawater-adapted Platichthyes *stellatus* and in the long-jawed mudsucker *Gillichthyes mirabilis* and in vitro.[19,35,38] This effect is similar to placing seawater-adapted flounders in fresh water or other hypo-osmotic medium and supports the general role for PRL as being essential for adaptation to freshwater environments. This effect of PRL on the bladder would augment water diuresis in a hypo-osmotic medium.

Movement of fluid across the intestinal epithelium is influenced by PRL. Treatment of seawater-adapted eel and trout reduces absorption of sodium, chloride and water.[49] These observations correlate with the differences in pituitary PRL content noted for freshwater-adapted and seawater-adapted tilapia.[16]

In addition to effects described for it on water movements, PRL has been shown to influence salt transport directly. Prolactin stimulates reabsorption of Na^+ from the urinary bladder and causes an increase in Na^+/K^+-ATPase activity in both the urinary bladder and the kidney.[38] Conversely, efflux of Na^+ is decreased in gills of seawater-adapted flounder[39] and tilapia[15] following treatment with PRL and in several hypophysectomized species.[2,42,43] Prolactin may produce similar effects on the gills of freshwater fishes.

The hypercalcemic effect of PRL in freshwater fishes was discussed in Chapter 12. In the absence of parathyroid glands, PRL is believed to be the pituitary factor responsible for calcium homeostasis in these fishes. It has been suggested that blood calcium levels rather than blood sodium levels may be the factor correlating to pituitary PRL levels in some species.[31] A separate pituitary factor, *hypercalcin,* has also been claimed to be the pituitary hypercalcemic factor.[62] The role of the pituitary remains the same whether the agent is either PRL, hypercalcin, or both.

ACTH and Cortisol

Synthesis of cortisol, the principal mineralocorticoid of teleosts, by adrenocortical tissue is controlled by ACTH from the adenohypophysis (see Chap. 10). Most of the data on effects of cortisol on Na^+ movements have been gathered from European, North American and Asian eels (*Anguilla anguilla, A. rostrata* and *A. japonica* respectively), but similar actions have been observed in other species. Seawater-adapted eels exhibit a marked turnover of Na^+ (50%–60%/hour), but ion flux is very low in freshwater-adapted eels (less than 1%/hour). Cortisol increases Na^+/K^+-ATPase in Keys-Wilmer cells of the gills, in gut epithelial cells and in kidney cells.[24,65] Circulating cortisol levels are similar in freshwater-adapted and seawater-adapted eels.[30] Cortisol levels, however, are elevated for several days when seawater-adapted eels are transferred to fresh water, but they then return to those levels characteristic of seawater-adapted and freshwater-adapted eels.[34] Elevation of corticosteroids in freshwater salmonids prior to their seaward migration reflects changing osmoregulatory physiology.[72]

Adrenalectomy of seawater-adapted eels causes an increase in plasma Na^+, but the same operation performed in freshwater-adapted eels causes a decline. These effects of adrenalectomy in seawater-adapted or freshwater-adapted eels are overcome by cortisol injections.[11,12,32,55]

Hypophysectomy of freshwater-adapted eels lowers plasma Na^+ slowly,[10,26] and when the eels are placed in sea water they accumulate Na^+. Plasma cortisol is also reduced following hypophysectomy but can be restored to normal by treatment with ACTH.[34] Neither cortisol nor ACTH can restore completely normal ion balance in freshwater-adapted animals, which suggests that PRL is also necessary for normal ion balance. Mammalian ACTH can maintain interrenal structure in hypophysectomized fish, but PRL has no effect.[4]

These data support a role for cortisol in regulating sodium balance in both freshwater-adapted and seawater-adapted teleosts. In freshwater fishes, cortisol probably works in concert with PRL to regulate sodium balance. The major targets for cortisol appear to be the gill and the intestinal epithelium.

Arginine Vasotocin

Arginine vasotocin is an antidiuretic hormone acting primarily through effects on glomerular filtration in amphibians, reptiles and birds (see Chap. 7). In fishes AVT has been reported to be diuretic by causing an increase in GFR due to effects of vasoconstriction on kidney arterioles. This diuresis has been demonstrated in the goldfish *C. auratus* and the Atlantic eel *A. anguilla* as well as in lungfishes.[69] However, AVT has been shown to be antidiuretic in *A. anguilla* if only small doses are administered.[33] This effect of AVT is due to a decrease in GFR resulting from vasodilation of kidney arterioles and not to effects on tubular reabsorption. No data are available concerning circulating levels of AVT in teleost blood, and it is not possible to resolve whether AVT is diuretic or antidiuretic or if it has any physiological role in water balance. It is tempting to believe that the antidiuretic effects are "physiological" since lower doses were employed, but it is conceivable that both the diuretic and antidiuretic properties of AVT could be employed in physiological regulation of water balance, depending upon circumstances. Arginine vasotocin does not appear to be involved in the events following hypophysectomy of freshwater species,[4] but it may contribute to the failure to survive this experimental procedure.

Catecholamines

Epinephrine reduces excretion of sodium and chloride in seawater-adapted fishes by effects on the gills and opercular membrane.[27] At the same time it increases permeability of the gill to water. This latter effect is observed in freshwater-adapted fishes as well. The action of epinephrine on sodium extrusion is inhibited by administration of α-adrenergic blocking agents, whereas the effect on water permeability can be inhibited by β-adrenergic blocking agents. Because elevated epinephrine levels and attendant disturbances in ion and fluid balance can be induced readily by stress such as handling or forced swimming, it seems doubtful that catecholamines are directly involved in regulation of salt and water balance.[5]

Corpuscles of Stannius

The importance of the corpuscles of Stannius (CS) in calcium regulation by seawater-adapted fishes was discussed in Chapter 12. Stanniectomy of the seawater-adapted eel *A. anguilla* produces not only an increase in plasma calcium but also an increase in plasma potassium and a comparable decrease in sodium.[26] Bentley has suggested that effects observed on sodium and potassium may be a consequence of reduced cortisol production brought about by an effect of elevated calcium on the interrenal.[5] Corticosteroidogenesis may be inhibited by hypercalcemia in eels.[48]

Two cellular types have been described in the CS of certain migratory species, the euryhaline stickleback (*Gasterosteus aculeatus,* form *trachurus*) and the Atlantic eel (*A. anguilla*).[77] One type responds cytologically to calcium fluctuations in the external medium and could be the source of the proposed hypocalcemic factor, *hypocalcin*.[1,31] The second cellular type is unresponsive to calcium variations but cytologically appears to be more "active" in freshwater-adapted than in seawater-adapted forms, and this cell might be involved in iono-osmotic regulation. This second cellular type was not found in two marine species, the cod (*Gadus morrhua*) and the plaice (*Pleuronectes platessa*).

Small quantities of renin are present in CS but considerably less than found in kidneys of these same species. Higher renin levels in the kidney have been reported for freshwater-adapted than for seawater-adapted fish,[71] but the relationship of renin to either corticosteroidogenesis or sodium-potassium balance remains obscure.

The Caudal Neurosecretory System

Large neurosecretory (NS) cells in the posterior portion of the spinal cord of elasmobranchs and teleosts were reported by Dahlgren and by Speidel more than 60 years ago,[13,73,74] but the importance of this caudal NS system was not known until its "rediscovery" in teleosts by Enami in 1955.[20] The axonal endings of teleostean Dahlgren cells terminate in a unique posterior neurohemal structure, the *urophysis* (Figs. 16-6, 16-7). Originally this neurohemal structure was termed the urohypophysis because of its structural similarity to the more anterior pars nervosa. Cytologically it is not possible to distinguish elements of the caudal NS system from those of

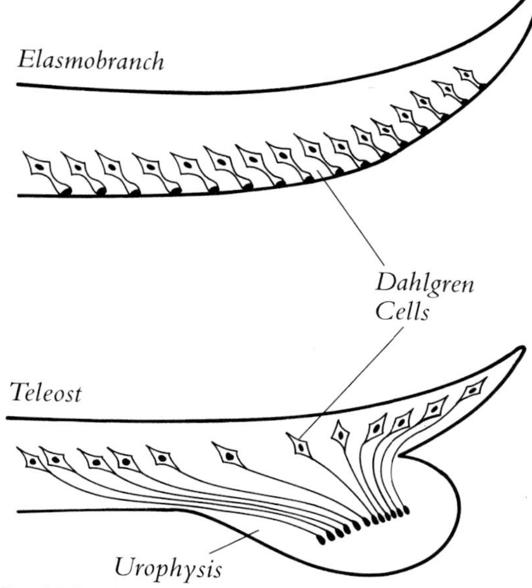

FIG. 16-6. Caudal neurosecretory system. Comparison of an elasmobranch with Dahlgren cells to a teleost with an organized urophysial neurohemal structure containing the axonal endings of the neurosecretory Dahlgren cells. (Redrawn from Bentley.[5])

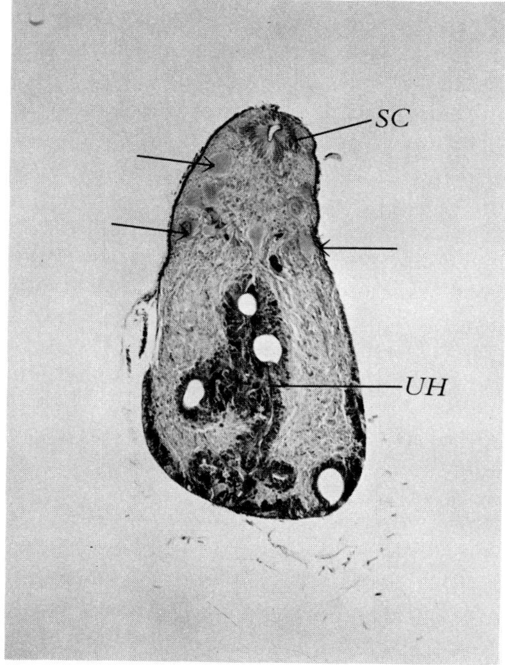

FIG. 16-7 Cross-section through the urophysial region of a teleost showing the neurosecretory cells *(arrows)* and the neurohemal urophysis *(UH)*. *SC*, spinal cord. (Courtesy Dr. Howard A. Bern and Richard Nishioka.)

the pars nervosa except that the Dahlgren secretory products will not stain with any of the NS stains commonly employed for the hypothalamo-hypophysial system. The acid violet or alcian blue procedures are employed typically to stain the NS products of the caudal NS system.

Surgical removal or ablation of this complex has proved difficult because of its rapid regenerative properties.[29] Early experiments, in fact, relied on complete removal of the tail of the fish (caudectomy), which led to the initial conclusion that this system somehow related to balance and flotation in fishes! Short-term ablation studies coupled with histological studies and quantitation of NS material in the urophysis of seawater- and freshwater-adapted fishes soon linked the system to a role in iono-osmotic regulation. The arrangement of blood vessels makes the urophysis ideally suited for storing factors that when released would travel directly to the kidneys. Venous drainage from the urophysis enters the renal portal vessels via the caudal vein and passes through the kidney prior to entering the general circulation.

Four active fractions have been prepared from urophysial extracts.[6,9,46] *Urotensin I* is a hypotensive agent assayed by monitoring a decrease in blood pressure in the rat tail artery. *Urotensin II* causes smooth-muscle contraction in the urinary bladder. The activity is usually assayed in vitro with fish urinary bladders. The urotensin II fraction also causes increased blood pressure and urine flow in eels. *Urotensin III* promotes sodium uptake across goldfish gills. This activity has not been observed in other species, however, and its general significance is questionable. *Urotensin IV* increases water transfer across the toad urinary bladder in vitro; it may be AVT.

Urotensins affect ion transport across the opercular membrane, skin, urinary bladder and intestine. Urotensin I has been characterized chemically from the white sucker, *Catostomus commersoni*.[47] It is a peptide of 41 amino acids and is structurally related to mammalian corticotropin-releasing hormone (CRH) and the amphibian peptide sauvagine. Urotensin I has CRH activity when assayed in mammals. In freshwater-adapted *Gillichthyes mirabilis* urotensin I reduces water and salt absorption by the intestine but has no effect in seawater-adapted fish.[53]

Urotensin II is a dodecapeptide chemically related to somatostatin.[64] There is no effect of urotensin II on the intestine of freshwater-adapted *Gillichthyes,* but it markedly increases water and salt absorption by the intestinal epithelium of seawater-adapted fish. Urotensin I may be important only for freshwater fishes where its action is similar to that of PRL. Urotensin II is important in marine fishes. Levels of urotensin II in the urophysis of marine *Gillichthyes* vary inversely with rainfall, implying a response to periodic dilutions of shallow coastal waters.[8]

Other Hormones

Any factors that alter the general state of the organism will undoubtedly influence iono-osmoregulatory balance. Thyroid hormones (T_3 and T_4) and growth hormone (GH) have been shown to exhibit effects on iono-osmoregulatory processes in fishes. The thyroid gland of salmonid fishes has been linked with changes in osmoregulatory processes occurring in these fishes prior to their seaward migration (see Chap. 18). Although GH has also been related to iono-osmoregulatory processes it probably does not play a direct role. Some effects attributed to GH may be due to small amounts of PRL present as a contaminant or to the similarity in structure and function of GH and PRL.

The pineal complex may also influence osmoregulation in teleosts. Pinealectomy during the spring causes a reduction in plasma cortisol levels of goldfish (*C. auratus*) that is not observed in sham-operated animals.[14] During the summer, however, pinealectomy results in higher plasma cortisol levels of fish held under long photoperiods, but it has no effect on cortisol levels of fish held under short photoperiods. Such preliminary studies suggest that a thorough examination of endocrine parameters is necessary with respect to osmoregulatory events and various environmental factors before the influence of osmoregulation in these fishes can be understood.

Salinity Preference

Migratory euryhaline teleosts exhibit changes in salinity preference at different stages in their life cycles. Salinity preference tests allow a fish to select a "preferable" salinity when presented with a choice. Thyroid hormones are implicated in salinity preference changes in salmonids and sticklebacks (see Chap. 18). Cortisol and PRL synergize in determining salinity preferences in the Gulf killifish *F. grandis.*[25] Considerable work is needed to verify these observations in other species and to demonstrate such relationships temporally with respect to natural changes in salinity preferences.

Summary of Iono-Osmotic Regulation in Freshwater Fishes

The iono-osmotic problems of freshwater fish are ion conservation and water excretion. Cortisol is the primary hormone regulating sodium balance. The gut is the major site for sodium influx, and transport of sodium from the lumen of the intestine to the blood is stimulated by cortisol. Gill transport of sodium by Keys-Wilmer cells from fresh water to the blood is also stimulated by cortisol, but this source of sodium is generally secondary to gut transport. Although kidney renin levels are higher in freshwater fish, it is not established that renin or angiotensins stimulate corticosteroid synthesis in teleosts.

Prolactin appears to be responsible for water balance with secondary influences on salt transport in freshwater-adapted or freshwater fishes. Glomerular filtration in the kidney is enhanced by effects of PRL, which reduces the glomerular-renal capsular gap, resulting in greater GFR and production of a large volume of urine. Some tubular reabsorption of sodium and other ions can occur along the kidney tubule, resulting in dilute urine that enters the bladder. Arginine vasotocin may also influence GFR by its vascular effects, being hypertensive at higher levels and possibly hypotensive at lower levels.

Another essential role of PRL occurs at the level of the gut where sodium influx is stimulated by cortisol.[38] Normally the transport of large quantities of sodium and chloride results in water uptake. Prolactin blocks the movement of water that normally would follow the transported salt. Thus PRL both increases water excretion via effects on the kidney and reduces water influx through the gut. Urotensin I may contribute to blocking ion and water absorption.

Calcium balance in freshwater-adapted and freshwater fishes may be controlled by PRL as described in Chapter 12. Prolactin may be the hypercalcemic factor controlling plasma Ca^{++} levels. Loss of Ca^{++} could contribute to the death of hypophysectomized fishes that die if retained in fresh water.

Mucous production by skin and gills is enhanced by PRL, and this mucus is presumably a hindrance to water influx and possibly salt efflux. Freshwater fishes produce more mucus than do marine or seawater-adapted animals. A characteristic of the transformation of freshwater juvenile steelhead trout (parr) to the silvery seaward migratory form (smolt) is reduction in mucous production. A mucous coating in freshwater and freshwater-adapted fishes may have other than osmoregulatory functions since it does not seem to be employed by marine fishes to reduce water losses from the skin and gills.[38]

The importance of these two major roles for PRL (that is, increased water excretion and reduction in water influx) and the stimulation of sodium transport by cortisol easily explains the inability of many freshwater euryhaline species to survive following hypophysectomy as well as the progressive changes in other species in which death does not occur. Since PRL alone can promote survival in the former group, it is assumed that these fish rely heavily on PRL for maintenance of osmotic equilibrium. Effects of PRL on calcium retention may promote survival of hypophysectomized fishes. It is interesting to note that it is those euryhaline species exhibiting one or more migrations between fresh water and sea water as a normal phase of their life history that rely less on PRL for freshwater survival. These migratory fishes possess greater flexibility in their osmo-regulating abilities than do fishes that can adapt to high or low salinities but rarely if ever must do so in nature.

Summary of Iono-Osmotic Regulation in Marine Fishes

The interrenal plays a central role in iono-osmotic regulation in marine and seawater-adapted fishes. Cortisol stimulates the Keys-Wilmer cells to transport salt but in the opposite direction of that in freshwater fishes (that is, from blood to the external medium). Transport by the gills is the major mechanism for salt excretion in marine environments, accounting for up to 90% of all salt excreted. The kidney cannot be used for salt excretion because it lacks the appropriate apparatus for concentrating urine sufficiently and its use to excrete significant quantities of salt would result in enormous water losses.

Cortisol also stimulates salt uptake by the intestinal epithelium as it did in freshwater fishes, but in marine and seawater-adapted fishes it is basically a mechanism for obtaining water and not salt. Because PRL levels are low in marine and seawater-adapted fishes, water readily follows the transported salt. Urotensin II also stimulates salt and water absorption by the intestine. The excess salt is excreted via the gills under the additional influence of cortisol. Thus, marine and seawater-adapted fishes may drink seawater, and considerable water may be taken up from the gut without concern for salt. The low levels of PRL also result in structural changes in the kidney of seawater-adapted fishes, causing decreased GFR. This mechanism is especially important in migratory species (Table 16-2). In aglomerular marine fishes, of course, glomerular filtration is not a problem.

The relative absence of PRL in marine and seawater-adapted fishes means another regulatory system is required for calcium homeostasis. Although there is ample production of calcitonin in ultimobranchial bodies of teleosts, it is apparently not functional as a hypocalcemic factor (see Chap. 12). The CS may be the source of the hypocalcemic factor (hypocalcin) that stimulates elimination of calcium.

TABLE 16-2. *Glomerular Filtration Rate in Premigratory Juvenile and Migratory Rainbow Trout* Salmo gairdneri *Maintained in Fresh Water*[36]

	ml/kg BODY WEIGHT/DAY	P
Premigratory	174.7 ± 9.6	< 0.001
Migratory	90.5 ± 7.8	–

Not only is production of PRL decreased in marine and seawater-adapted fishes but so are production and release of urotensins from the urophysis and AVT from the neurohypophysis. It would appear that radiation of freshwater fishes into the marine environment was made possible by shutting down most of the endocrine and physiological mechanisms that evolved initially to solve iono-osmotic problems in a hypo-osmotic medium. The only additional modifications required were retention of cortisol, production of urotensin II and reversal of the direction of salt transport across the gill.

References

1. Aida, K., R.S. Nishioka and H.A. Bern (1980). Changes in the corpuscles of Stannius of coho salmon (*Oncorhynchus kisutch*) during smoltification and seawater adaptation. Gen. Comp. Endocrinol. 41:663–671.
2. Ball, J.N. and D.M. Ensor (1965). Effect of prolactin on plasma sodium in the teleost, *Poecilia latipinna.* J. Endocrinol. 32:269–270.
3. Ball, J.N. and D.M. Ensor (1967). Specific action of prolactin on plasma sodium levels in hypophysectomized *Poecilia latipinna* (Teleostei). Gen. Comp. Endocrinol. 8:432–440.
4. Ball, J.N. and E.F. Hawkins (1976). Adrenocortical (interrenal) responses to hypophysectomy and adenohypophysial hormones in the teleost *Poecilia latipinna.* Gen. Comp. Endocrinol. 28:59–70.
5. Bentley, P.J. (1976). Comparative Vertebrate Endocrinology. Cambridge University Press, Chap. 8.
6. Berlind, A. (1973). Caudal neurosecretory system: A physiologist's view. Am. Zool. 13:759–770.
7. Bern, H.A. (1983). Functional evolution of prolactin and growth hormone in lower vertebrates. Am. Zool. 23:663–671.
8. Bern, H.A., S. Goldstein, R.S. Nishioka and R. Gunther (1982). Seasonal changes in the content of Urotensin II in the urophysis of the goby, *Gillichthyes mirabilis.* Acta Zool. 63:177–180.
9. Bern, H.A. and K. Lederis (1969). A reference preparation for the study of active substances in the caudal neurosecretory system of teleosts. J. Endocrinol. 45:xi–xii.
10. Butler, D.G. (1966). Effect of hypophysectomy on osmoregulation in the European eel (*Anguilla anguilla* L.). Comp. Biochem. Physiol. 18:773–781.
11. Butler, D.G., W.C. Clarke, E.M. Donaldson and R.W. Langford (1969). Surgical adrenalectomy of a teleost fish (*Anguilla rostrata* Le Seur): Effect on plasma cortisol and tissue electrolyte and carbohydrate levels. Gen. Comp. Endocrinol. 12:503–514.
12. Chan, D.K.O., I. Chester Jones, I.W. Henderson and J.C. Rankin (1967). Studies on the experimental alteration of water and electrolyte composition of the eel (*Anguilla anguilla* L.). J. Endocrinol. 37:297–317.
13. Dahlgren, U. (1914). On the electric motor nerve centers in the skates (Rajidae). Science 40:862–863.
14. Delahunty, G., C.B. Schreck and V.L. deVlaming (1977). Effect of pinealectomy, reproductive state, feeding regime and photoperiod on plasma cortisol in goldfish. Am. Zool. 17:873.
15. Dharmamba, M., N. Mayer-Goston, J. Maetz and H.A. Bern (1973). Effect of prolactin on sodium movement in *Tilapia mossambica* adapted to sea water. Gen. Comp. Endocrinol. 21:179–187.
16. Dharmamba, M. and R.S. Nishioka (1968). Response of "prolactin-secreting" cells of *Tilapia mossambica* to environmental salinity. Gen. Comp. Endocrinol. 10:409–420.
17. Donaldson, E.M., F. Yamazaki and W.C. Clare (1968). Effect of hypophysectomy on plasma osmolarity in goldfish and its reversal by ovine prolactin and a preparation of salmon pituitary "prolactin." J. Fish. Res. Board Can. 25:1497–1500.
18. Doneen, B.A. (1976). Water and ion movements in the urinary bladder of the gobiid teleost *Gillichthyes mirabilis* in response to prolactins and to cortisol. Gen. Comp. Endocrinol. 28:33–41.
19. Doneen, B.A. and H.A. Bern (1974). *In vitro* effects of prolactin and cortisol on water permeability of the urinary bladder of the teleost *Gillichthyes mirabilis.* J. Exp. Zool. 187:173–179.
20. Enami, M. (1955). Caudal neurosecretory system in the eel (*Anguilla japonica*). Gunma J. Med. Sci. 4:23–36.
21. Enami, M. (1959). The morphology and functional significance of the caudal neurosecretory system of fishes. In A. Gorbman, ed., Comparative Endocrinology. John Wiley and Sons, New York, pp. 697–724.
22. Ensor, D.M. (1982). Prolactin and osmoregulation in lower vertebrates: a phylogenetic perspective. In C.G. Scanes, M.A. Ottinger, A.D. Kenny, J. Balthazart, J. Cronshaw and I. Chester Jones, eds., Aspects of Avian Endocrinology: Practical and Theoretical Implications. Texas Tech Univ., Lubbock, Texas, pp. 329–335.
23. Ensor, D.M. and J.N. Ball (1972). Prolactin and osmoregulation in fishes. Fed. Proc. 6:1615–1623.

24. Epstein, F.H., M. Cynamon and W. McKay (1971). Endocrine control of Na-K-ATPase and seawater adaptation in *Anguilla rostrata*. Gen. Comp. Endocrinol. 16:323–328.

25. Fivizzani, A.J. and A.H. Meier (1977). Temporal synergism of cortisol and prolactin influences salinity preference of *Fundulus grandis*. Am. Zool. 17:858.

26. Fontaine, M. (1964). Corpuscles de Stannius et régulation ionique (Ca, K, Na) du milieu intérieur de l'anguille (*Anguilla anguilla* L.). C.R. Acad. Sci. 265:736–737.

27. Foskett, J.K., G.M. Hubbard, T.E. Machen and H.A. Bern (1982). Effects of epinephrine, glucagon and vasoactive intestinal polypeptide on chloride secretion by teleost opercular membrane. J. Comp. Physiol. 146:27–34.

28. Foster, R.C. (1975). Changes in urinary bladder and kidney function in the starry flounder (*Platichthys stellatus*) in response to prolactin and to freshwater transfer. Gen. Comp. Endocrinol. 27:153–161.

29. Fridberg, G., R.S. Nishioka, H.A. Bern and W.R. Fleming (1966). Regeneration of the caudal neurosecretory system in the cichlid teleost *Tilapia mossambica*. J. Exp. Zool. 162:311–336.

30. Gaitskell, R.E. and I. Chester Jones (1970). Effects of adrenalectomy and cortisol injection on the *in vitro* movement of water by the intestine of the freshwater European eel (*Anguilla anguilla* L.). Gen. Comp. Endocrinol. 15:491–493.

31. Greven, J.A.A., J.C.A. van der Meij and S.E. Wendelaar Bonga (1978). The relationship between hypocalcin and prolactin in the teleost *Gasterosteus aculeatus*. In P. Gaillard, ed., Comparative Endocrinology Proceedings, Elsevier/North Holland Biomedical Press, Amsterdam, p. 288.

32. Henderson, I.W. and I. Chester Jones (1967). Endocrine influences on the net extrarenal fluxes of sodium and potassium in the European eel (*Anguilla anguilla* L.). J. Endocrinol. 37:319–325.

33. Henderson, I.W. and N.A.M. Wales (1974). Renal diuresis and antidiuresis after injections of arginine vasotocin in the fresh-water eel (*Anguilla anguilla* L.). J. Endocrinol. 41:487–500.

34. Hirano, T. (1969). Effects of hypophysectomy and salinity change on plasma cortisol concentration in the Japanese eel, *Anguilla japonica*. Endocrinol. Jap. 16:557–560.

35. Hirano, T., D.W. Johnson, H.A. Bern and S. Utida (1973). Studies on water and ion movement in the isolated urinary bladder of selected freshwater, marine and euryhaline teleosts. Comp. Biochem. Physiol. 45A:529–540.

36. Holmes, W.N. and I.M. Stanier (1966). Studies on the renal excretion of electrolytes by the trout (*Salmo gairdneri*). J. Exp. Biol. 44:33–46.

37. Jampol, L.M. and F.H. Epstein (1970). Sodium-potassium-activated adenosine-triphosphatase and osmotic regulation by fishes. Am. J. Physiol. 218:607–611.

38. Johnson, D.W. (1973). Endocrine control of hydromineral balance in teleosts. Am. Zool. 13:799–818.

39. Johnson, D.W., H.A. Bern and T. Hirano (1972). Water and sodium movements and their hormonal control in the urinary bladder of the starry flounder, (*Platichthys stellatus*). Gen. Comp. Endocrinol. 19:115–128.

40. Jorgensen, C.B. and P. Rosenkilde (1956). On regulation and content of chloride in goldfish. Biol. Bull. 110:300–305.

41. Kamiya, M. and S. Utida (1969). Sodium-potassium-activated adenotriphosphatase activity in gills of freshwater, marine and euryhaline teleosts. Comp. Biochem. Physiol. 31:671–674.

42. Lahlou, B. and A. Giordon (1970). Le contrôle hormonal des échanges et de la balance de l'eau chez le téleostéen d'eau douce *Carassius auratus*, intact et hypophysectomisé. Gen. Comp. Endocrinol. 14:491–509.

43. Lam, T.J. (1968). Effect of prolactin on plasma electrolytes of the early-winter marine threespine stickleback, *Gasterosteus aculeatus* form *trachurus*, following transfer from sea to freshwater. Can. J. Zool. 46:1095–1097.

44. Lam. T.J. (1972). Prolactin and hydromineral regulation in fishes. Gen. Comp. Endocrinol. Suppl. 3:328–338.

45. Lam, T.J. and J.F. Leatherland (1969). Effect of prolactin on freshwater survival of the marine form (*trachurus*) of the threespine stickleback, *Gasterosteus aculeatus*, in the early winter. Gen. Comp. Endocrinol. 12:385–394.

46. Lederis, K. (1972). Recent progress in research on the urophysis. Gen. Comp. Endocrinol. Suppl. 3:339–344.

47. Lederis, K., A. Letter, D. McMaster, G. Moore and D. Schlesinger (1982). Complete amino acid sequence of urotensin I, a hypotensive and corticotropin-releasing neuropeptide from *Catostomus*. Science 218:162–164.

48. Leloup-Hatey, J. (1970). Influence de l'ablation des corpuscles de Stannius sur le fonctionmment de l'interrenal de l'anguille (*Anguilla anguilla* L.). Gen. Comp. Endocrinol. 15:388–397.

49. Loretz, C.A., and H.A. Bern (1982). Prolactin and osmoregulation in vertebrates. Neuroendocrinology 35:292–304.

50. McKeown, B.A. (1972). Effects of 2-Br-α-ergocryptine on fresh water survival in teleosts, *Xiphophorus hellerii* and *Poecilia latipinna*. Experientia 28:675–676.

51. Maetz, J., R. Motais and N. Mayer (1968). Cited by Johnson.[38]

52. Maetz, J., and E. Skadhauge (1968). Drinking rates and gill ionic turnover in relation to external salinities in the eel. Nature 217:371–373.

53. Mainoya, J.R. and H.A. Bern (1982). Effects of teleost urotensins on intestinal absorption of water and NaCl in tilapia, *Sarotherodon mossambicus,* adapted to fresh water or sea water. Gen. Comp. Endocrinol. 47:54–58.

54. Mattheiji, J.A.M., and H.W.J. Stroband (1971). The effects of osmotic experiments and prolactin on the mucous cells in the skin and ionocytes in the gills of the teleost *Cichlasoma biocellatum.* Z. Zellforsch. 121:93–101.

55. Mayer, N., J. Maetz, D.K.O. Chan, M. Forster and I. Chester Jones (1967). Cortisol, a sodium excretive factor in the eel (*Anguilla anguilla* L.) adapted to sea water. Nature 214:1118–1120.

56. Natochin, Y.V. and G.P. Gusev (1970). The coupling of magnesium secretion and sodium reabsorption in the kidney of teleosts. Comp. Biochem. Physiol. 37:107–111.

57. Nicoll, C.S., S.W. Wilson, R. Nishioka, and H.A. Bern (1981). Blood and pituitary prolactin levels in tilapia (*Sarotherodon mossambicus;* Teleostei) from different salinities as measured by a homologous radioimmunoassay. Gen. Comp. Endocrinol. 44:365–373.

58. Oduleye, S.O. (1975). The effect of hypophysectomy and prolactin therapy on water balance of the brown trout, *Salmo trutta.* J. Exp. Biol. 63:357–366.

59. Ogawa, M. (1970). Effects of prolactin on the epidermal mucous cells of the goldfish, *Carassius auratus* L. Can. J. Zool. 48:501–503.

60. Ogawa M., M. Yagasaki and F. Yamazaki (1973). The effect of prolactin on water influx in isolated gills of the goldfish, *Carassius auratus* L. Comp. Biochem. Physiol. 44A:1177–1183.

61. Olivereau, M. and A.-M. Lemoine (1968). Action de la prolactine chez l'anguille intacte. III. Effet sur la structure histologique du rein. Z. Zellforsch. 88:576–590.

62. Pang, P.K.T. and J.A. Yeel (1980). Evolution of the endocrine control of vertebrate hypercalcemic regulation. In S. Ishii, T. Hirano and M. Wada, eds., Hormones, Adaptations and Evolution. Jap. Sci. Soc. Press, Tokyo/Springer-Verlag, Berlin, pp. 103–111.

63. Parry, G. (1966). Osmotic adaptation in fishes. Biol. Rev. 41:392–444.

64. Pearson, D., J.E. Shively, B.R. Clark, I.I. Geschwind, M. Barkley, R.S. Nishioka and H.A. Bern (1980). Urotensin II: a somatostatin-like peptide in the caudal neurosecretory system of fishes. Proc. Nat'l Acad. Sci. U.S.A. 77:5021–5023.

65. Pickford, G.E., P.K.T. Pang, E. Weinstein, J. Torretti, E. Hendler and F.H. Epstein (1970). The response of the hypophysectomized Cyprinodont, *Fundulus heteroclitus,* to replacement therapy with cortisol: Effects on blood serum and sodium-potassium activated adenosine triphosphatase in the gills, kidney and intestinal mucosa. Gen. Comp. Endocrinol. 14:524–534.

66. Pickford, G.E. and J.G. Phillips (1959). Prolactin, a factor in promoting survival of hypophysectomized killifish in freshwater. Science 130:454–455.

67. Potts, W.T.W. and D.H. Evans (1966). The effects of hypophysectomy and bovine prolactin on salt fluxes in freshwater-adapted *Fundulus heteroclitus.* Biol. Bull. 131:362–368.

68. Potts, W.T.W. and G. Parry (1964). Osmotic and Ionic Regulation in Animals. Pergamon Press, Oxford.

69. Sawyer, W.H. (1972). Neurohypophysial hormones and water and sodium excretion in African lungfish. Gen. Comp. Endocrinol. Suppl. 3:345–349.

70. Schreibman, M.P. and K.D. Kallman (1969). The effect of hypophysectomy on freshwater survival in teleosts of the order Atheriniformes. Gen. Comp. Endocrinol. 13:27–38.

71. Sokabe, H., H. Oide, M. Ogawa and S. Utida (1973). Plasma renin activity in Japanese eels (*Anguilla japonica*) adapted to sea-water or in dehydration. Gen. Comp. Endocrinol. 21:160–167.

72. Specker, J.L. and C.B. Schreck (1982). Changes in plasma corticosteroids during smoltification of coho salmon, *Oncorhynchus kisutch.* Gen. Comp. Endocrinol. 46:53–58.

73. Speidel, C.C. (1919). Gland cells of internal secretion in the spinal cord of the skates. Carnegie Inst. Wash. Papers 13:1–31.

74. Speidel, C.C. (1922). Further comparative studies in other fishes of cells that are homologous to the large irregular gland cells in the spinal cord of skates. J. Comp. Neurol. 34:303–317.

75. Stanley, J.G. and W.R. Fleming (1964). Excretion of hypertonic urine by a teleost. Science 144:63–64.

76. Stanley, J.G. and W.R. Fleming (1967). Effect of prolactin and ACTH on the serum and urine sodium levels of *Fundulus kansae.* Comp. Biochem. Physiol. 20:199–208.

77. Wendelaar Bonga, S.E. and J.A.A. Greven (1975). A second cell type in Stannius bodies of two euryhaline teleost species. Cell Tissue Res. 159:287–290.

17·Endocrine Regulation of Amphibian Metamorphosis

Metamorphosis (literally a change in form or transformation) is a gradual or sudden event involving changes in body form, function and ecological niche of an animal. It occurs early in the life of most fishes and amphibians but is more dramatic in the amphibians. The amphibian larva during its short aquatic life seems to go through all of the evolutionary changes required for the first aquatic vertebrate to invade the land successfully. Detailed studies of amphibian metamorphosis in a sense allow scientists to examine the acquisition of terrestrial adaptations during the life history of a single animal. The hormones responsible for these changes and concepts related to the regulation of their secretion are discussed in this chapter.

Amphibian Life Histories

The amphibian life cycle usually is described as involving reproduction in an aquatic medium followed by embryonic development and hatching to a free-living aquatic larval form. The larva grows for a time that is characteristic for a particular species. Metamorphosis induced by thyroid hormones (see Chap. 8) occurs at the end of the larval period, and the animal enters a juvenile phase as a terrestrial or semiterrestrial creature. The juvenile possesses the general body form of the adult. Following sexual maturation, which occurs after one to several years of postmetamorphic growth, the adult returns to water to breed. Usually the adult returns more than 1 year to the same area to breed. The life cycle of a "typical" anuran is depicted in Figure 17-1.

Although primitive amphibians produced large, yolky eggs, many of the typical anurans exhibit a modified reproductive strategy often assumed to be the primitive pattern for amphibians. However, the size of the anuran egg has been markedly reduced with concomitant reduction in yolk content and an increase in the number of eggs per female. The anuran larval stage may have evolved as an intermediate feeding stage that allows for production of large numbers of offspring with several advantages to the parents.[14] The female parent with an aquatic larval feeding stage is relieved somewhat in the amount of energy (that is, yolk) that must be channelized into gamete production. Neither carnivorous parent competes for food with the larvae. In many species the larvae are herbivorous and do not assume the carnivorous habit until after metamorphosis. Urodeles that exhibit the typical amphibian life history similarly benefit from the intercalated aquatic larval feeding stage. Larvae of urodeles are all carnivorous like the adults, and separation of the adults and larvae reduces both competition for food items and the probability that adults will consume their own young for food. Among the permanently aquatic urodeles, however, there is some competition for food items, and cannibalism of young is not uncommon. Other adaptations have been emphasized in the last case, resulting in the relative success of such species.

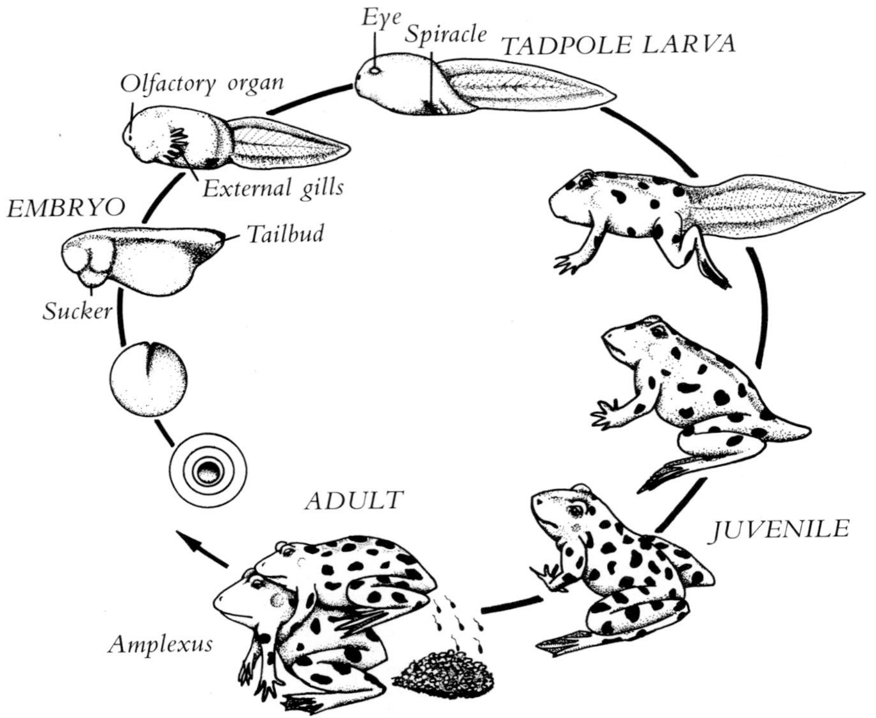

FIG. 17-1. Anuran life history. (Redrawn from Hickman et al.[48])

Some species such as the North American spadefoot toads (*Spea* spp.) have condensed the breeding season and period of larval life to only a few weeks.[6] Adult spadefoots, which live in arid habitats, spend most of their lives in underground burrows, coming out to feed and breed with the seasonal rains. In a matter of a few days they complete sexual maturation and breeding activities in temporary ponds resulting from the rain and then return to their burrows. Fertilized eggs develop into larvae, and metamorphosis into small juvenile spadefoots occurs in a few additional days. As the temporary ponds evaporate the juvenile spadefoots emerge and dig burrows in which they will "await" the next breeding season.

Not all amphibians seek water for reproduction (Fig. 17-2), and many species are permanently terrestrial and never breed in water.[62] Many anurans (for example, *Eleutherodactylus* spp., *Alytes obstetricans*), urodeles (for example, *Batracoseps,* some *Plethodon*) and some apodans deposit their eggs in moist places on land. These eggs undergo direct development, and juvenile adult forms hatch from the eggs. Most of the larval stages occur within the egg capsule. Other species (for example, *Pachymedusa dachnycolor*) attach egg masses to objects above water. When larvae hatch, they drop into the water to continue development. Still other species, such as the marsupial frog *Gastrotheca rhomboididae,* have developed specialized pouches or folds of skin in which the eggs develop to tadpoles that are then dropped into water. Viviparity occurs in a few anurans and urodeles (for example, *Nectophrynoides occidentalis, Salamandra* spp.). One salamander, *Salamandra atra,* has a gestation period in its modified oviducts of up to 4 years and gives birth to two fully metamorphosed young. Viviparity is common among apodan species, but they have not been studied extensively.[109]

Some anurans (*Pipa* spp., *Xenopus* spp., etc.) and many urodeles (*Necturus* spp., *Amphiuma* spp., *Cryptobranchus alleganiensis,* etc.) have become permanent aquatic residents. They not only breed in the water but

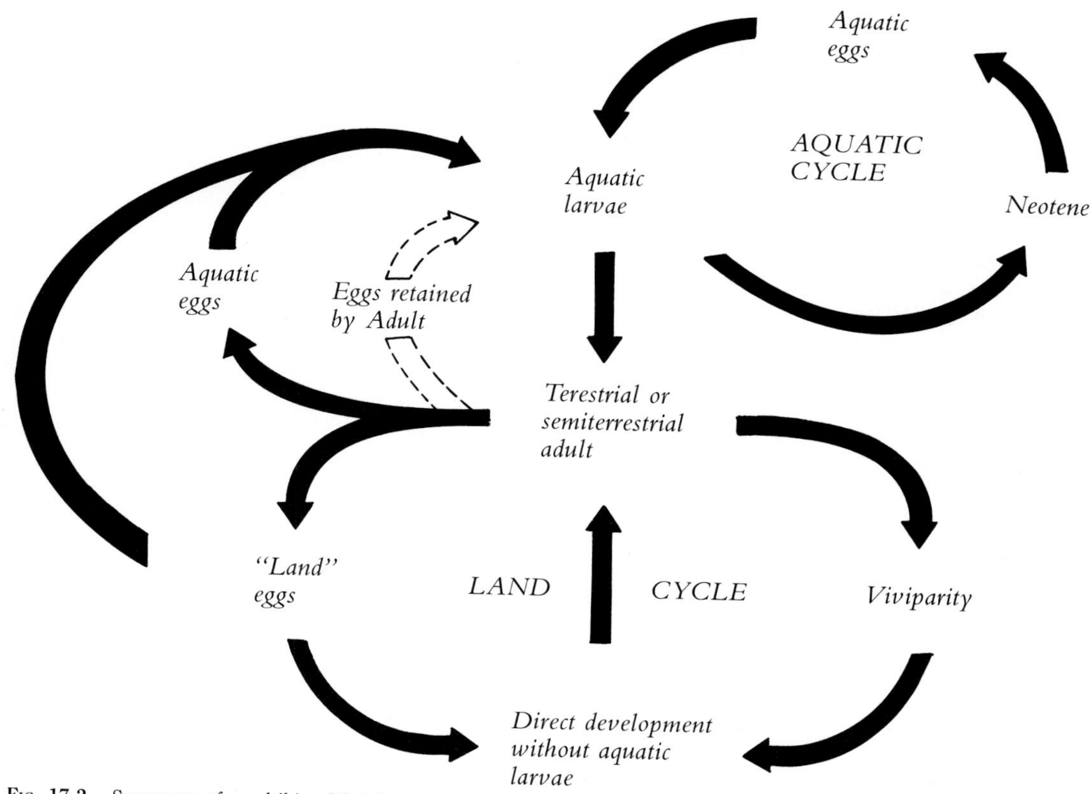

FIG. 17-2. Summary of amphibian life history patterns. Terrestrial amphibians may lay eggs in water or allow the eggs to develop on land and deposit larvae in water *(clear arrow)*. Other species may exhibit entirely aquatic life histories with or without metamorphosis. Still other species will become permanently terrestrial, either laying eggs on land or being completely viviparous.

remain aquatic throughout their entire life history. Urodeles that exhibit this behavior generally do not undergo metamorphosis or exhibit only some changes associated with the typical metamorphic event while retaining many larval features.

There are so many striking exceptions to the typical life history plan that one begins to wonder why this one pattern has been used as exemplary of the class. Probably the answer lies in the tendency for biologists to view the amphibians as the group transitional between fishes and the terrestrial amniote vertebrates. Consequently the life history pattern that most closely resembles the biochemical, physiological, morphological and behavioral alterations that might have occurred during evolution of the terrestrial vertebrates became a focal point for investigation. This pattern may not be an example of ontogeny recapitulating phylogeny, at least in the sense of progression from fish to reptile.

Metamorphosis

Metamorphosis encompasses the life history events centering around the processes whereby an aquatic amphibian larva undergoes complex changes to become a terrestrial or semiterrestrial organism.[14,71,110] Urochordates, cephalochordates, lampreys, and bony fishes exhibit comparable metamorphic changes.[56,71] Biochemical, physiological, morphological and behavioral changes occur as a consequence of endocrinological events that in turn are influenced by environmental factors. This phenomenon of metamorphosis is one of the best examples of the integration of environmental factors with endocrine events. First some morphological features of amphibian larvae and their alterations during metamorphosis will be examined. Then some of the biochemical modifications occurring during metamorphosis will be considered before the endocrinological bases for change, including an integrated mechanism controlling metamorphosis, are examined. The return of terrestrial adults to water for the purposes of breeding will be discussed under "Second Metamorphosis." Finally, there will be a discussion of the endocrine factors involved in the life histories of some amphibians that spend their entire lives in water.

Morphological Events

Anuran tadpole larvae are readily distinguishable from urodele larvae on morphological grounds (Fig. 17-3). Tadpoles lack limbs during most of their aquatic life and typically have internal gills covered with an opercular structure. Urodele larvae possess four limbs at hatching and exhibit prominent external gills. Larvae of urodeles also have prominent tail fins that regress during metamorphosis, leaving only the terrestrial-type tail. Tadpoles completely resorb the entire tail during metamorphosis. Herbivorous tadpoles exhibit shortening of the gut during metamorphosis, resulting in a shorter gut typical of carnivores. The guts of carnivorous larvae may also

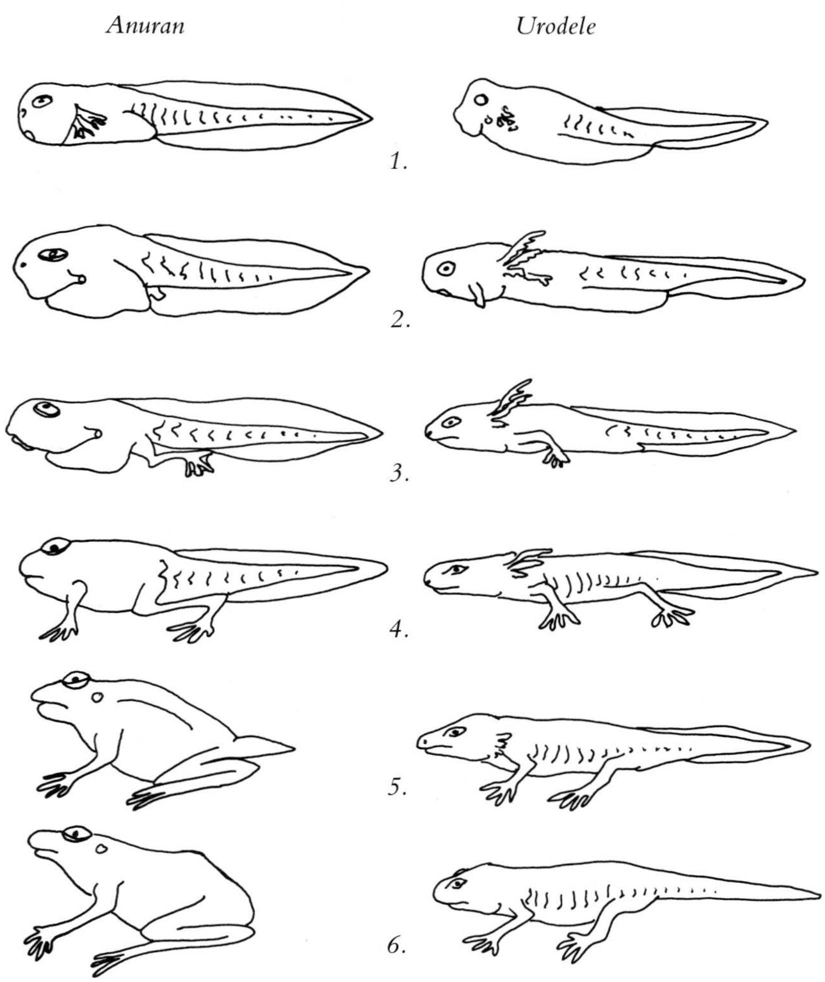

Fig. 17-3. Comparison of anuran and urodele larvae and metamorphosis.

shorten during metamorphosis, but this effect is less marked. Some of the many morphological changes that occur during metamorphosis are summarized in Table 17-1.

Growth and development of tadpoles have been studied carefully, and arbitrary stages have been established that allow investigators to compare different species or different populations of the same species. For example, this has been done for *Rana pipiens, Xenopus laevis,* and some others.[45,67,96,104]

In anurans the first obvious sign of metamorphic change is the emergence of hind limbs. Prior to this event tadpoles may be termed generally *premetamorphic.*[20] The developmental changes that occur between emergence of the hind limbs and emergence of the forelimbs comprise *prometamorphosis.* Marked elongation of the hindlimbs with respect to body length occurs during prometamorphosis. The rapid series of events following emergence of the forelimbs to achieve the definitive adult body form are designated collectively as *metamorphic climax.* The most dramatic change during climax is complete resorption of the tadpole tail. These stages of metamorphosis are summarized in Figure 17-3. Larvae may go from premetamorphosis through climax in only a few days. Large ranids, such as *Rana grylio, R. catesbeiana* and *R. clamitans,* may spend an extended period as premetamorphic or prometamorphic larvae, often not undergoing metamorphosis until the end of their second summer.

The morphological differences between urodele and tadpole larvae make it impossible to use the same terminology for staging urodeles. Metamorphosis in urodeles consists of simultaneous resorption of gills and tail fins with attendant morphological changes associated with skin, limb and head structures. There is no morphological distinction between premetamorphic and prometamorphic stages, although gill and tail fin resorption could indicate the onset of a climax stage.

Biochemical Events

Numerous biochemical changes underlying the general process of metamorphosis have been examined in considerable detail (Table 17-2). These events include: (1) a change in visual pigments in the retina, (2) production of "adult" hemoglobin in place of "larval" hemoglobin, (3) induction of a number of liver enzymes, (4) increased secretion of serum proteins by the liver, (5) induction of hydrolytic enzymes in tail tissue, (6) induction of proteolytic enzymes in the gut of herbivorous larvae and (7) thickening of the skin due to deposition of collagen fibers and keratinization.[30,49] Some of these events are described below. These biochemical changes are necessary for the transition from aquatic to terrestrial life.

Retinal Pigments. Visual pigments (rod pigments) in the retina are converted during metamorphosis from the type characteristic of freshwater fishes to that found in terrestrial amphibians and amniotes.[110] This conversion is presumably necessary for terrestrial vision and represents a fundamental change that also occurred during evolution of terrestrial vertebrates. Examination of additional amphibian species has shown that although several species do show this same change, some do not exhibit any change in visual pigments with

Table 17-1. *Life History of* Rana pipiens *at 23°C*

PERIOD	EVENTS	DURATION
Embryonic	Embryogenesis	8 days
Premetamorphic	Growth	5–6 wk
Prometamorphic	Accelerated growth of hind limbs; skin changes occur	3 wk
Metamorphic climax	Forelimbs emerge; tail resorbs; gills resorb; head and gut reconstruction; etc.	1 wk
Juvenile	Growth	–
Adult	Reproductive maturation and breeding	–

TABLE 17-2. *Summary of Some of the Biochemical Events Associated with Anuran Metamorphosis*

TISSUE	CHANGES OBSERVED
Liver	Increased RNA synthesis; induction of urea cycle enzymes (de novo); induction of serum protein synthesis
Tail	Induction of acid hydrolases and phagocytosis
Skin	Increased collagen synthesis resulting in thickening and decreased permeability; reduction in mucous secretion
Intestine & stomach	Cessation of feeding; shift from carbohydrase production to protease (pepsin) production; shortening of gut
Blood	Increase in serum proteins (from liver); change in hemoglobin from larval type to terrestrial type (increased SH groups); possible increase in hematocrit
Eye	Possible change in retinal pigments from aquatic type (porphyropsin) to terrestrial type (rhodopsin)

metamorphosis and others undergo the reverse change at metamorphosis.[12]

HEMOGLOBIN TRANSITION. A change from synthesis of larval hemoglobin to adult hemoglobin is induced by thyroid hormones.[15,16,30,55] Larval hemoglobin is adapted to extracting O_2 under aquatic conditions, (low O_2 content), and adult hemoglobin is adapted for air breathing (high O_2 content). Larval hemoglobin does not show a Bohr effect (decreasing O_2 affinity with decreasing pH), but adult hemoglobin does. This transition is similar to the change from fetal to adult hemoglobin that occurs in mammals, and it occurs during metamorphosis of anurans. In urodeles, however, this change in hemoglobin type occurs very early in life, and even certain species that never undergo metamorphosis in nature do exhibit a shift from larval to adult hemoglobin.[18,20] It is curious that this transition should occur in species that would seemingly benefit from retaining the aquatic-type hemoglobin and suggests that this change in blood pigment may not be essential for air breathing.

In the aquatic clawed frog *X. laevis,* treatment with the antithyroid drug propylthiouracil blocks all morphological changes normally associated with metamorphosis, but the transition from larval to adult hemoglobin occurs.[64] Either this event is not induced by thyroid hormones in this species, or the threshold level of thyroid hormones that induces this response is considerably less than needed for the morphological changes to occur.

NITROGEN EXCRETION: AMMONIA AND UREA. This change is reminiscent of the evolution of terrestrial vertebrates from fishes and involves induction of the ornithine-urea cycle enzymes in the tadpole liver. This does not mean de-novo induction; rather it means increased production of these enzymes, especially of carbamylphosphate synthetase and arginine synthetase.[8] Similar changes occur in at least one urodele.[94] During metamorphosis there is a gradual reduction in ammonia excretion and an increase in urea excretion (Fig. 17-4). Some

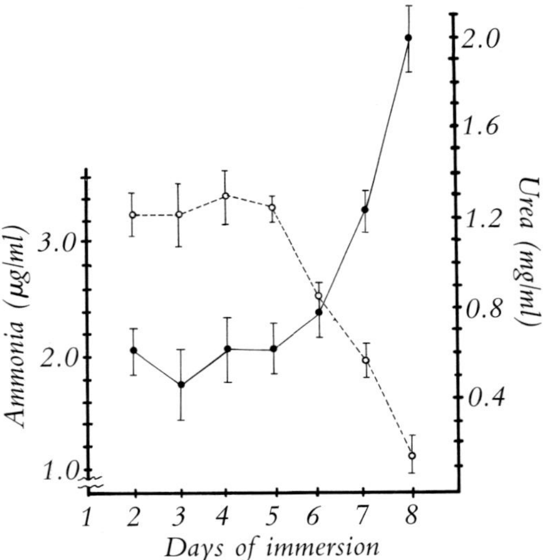

FIG. 17-4. Urea-ammonia excretion during anuran metamorphosis. Changes are shown in excretion of ammonia *(left scale; open circles)* and urea *(right scale; solid circles)* following immersion of premetamorphic *Rana catesbeiana* tadpoles in tap water containing thyroxine. (Unpublished data of C. Owen and D.O. Norris.)

additional liver enzymes stimulated by thyroid hormones include hepatic arginase, ornithine transcarbamylase and tyrosine aminotransferase.[9,51,69]

Tail Resorption. A number of investigators have reported induction by thyroid hormones of lysosomal enzymes such as acid phosphatase and collagenase in tail tissue. These enzymes are responsible for autodigestion of the tail of anurans and the tail fin of urodeles. The end products of this digestion are used for anabolic processes elsewhere in the animal. This system has been employed successfully to analyze the mechanisms whereby thyroid hormones influence gene actions and to study thyroxine-prolactin interactions. It has proved to be a useful in-vitro bioassay system.

The Endocrinological Bases for Metamorphosis

The Thyroid Axis

The importance of the thyroid gland in metamorphosis was discovered by Gudernatsch as a result of feeding horse thyroid tissue to tadpoles, causing them to undergo premature metamorphosis.[43] It was soon demonstrated convincingly that thyrotropin (TSH), triiodothyronine (T_3) and thyroxine (T_4) were effective in inducing metamorphosis in many species of anurans and urodeles. Treatment with TSH or thyroid hormones prematurely stimulates the biochemical and morphological changes associated with metamorphosis. Differences are observed, however, between events occurring during induced metamorphosis and "spontaneous" metamorphosis (Table 17-3), probably related to differences in tissue thresholds to thyroid hormones.[59,64]

Premature metamorphosis results in transformed animals that are smaller than would result from spontaneous metamorphosis that occurs after larvae have reached "normal" size for metamorphosis. Treatment with antithyroid drugs (propylthiouracil, thiourea) delays onset of metamorphosis until such treatment is terminated, and endogenous thyroid hormones or exogenous hormones bring about metamorphosis. Such treatment results in production of "giant" larvae, which if allowed to undergo metamorphosis become larger than normal transformed animals.

Most observations support a stimulatory role for the hypothalamus over TSH release from the adenohypophysis, although there have been reports of no influence over thyroid function.[42,90] Section of the infundibular stalk connecting the hypothalamus and hypophysis and insertion of an impervious barrier to prevent regeneration and transfer of materials from the hypothalamus to the hypophysis blocks metamorphosis in *A. maculatum* larvae.[29] Metamorphosis was observed only in animals that had been operated on, in which portal blood vessel regeneration had taken place. Extirpation of the preoptic nucleus of several anuran species blocks metamorphosis,[40,107,108] and removal of the posterior hypothalamus causes a specific reduction in thyroid function in *R. pipiens* tadpoles.[46]

Thyrotropin-releasing hormone (TRH) has been immunologically and biologically demonstrated in the amphibian hypothalamus as well as in other regions of the brain.[50,103]

Table 17-3. *Comparison of T_3-Induced Metamorphosis with Related Events Occurring in Spontaneous Metamorphosis*

INDUCED EVENT	SPONTANEOUS EVENT	REF.
No morphological or biochemical changes in pancreas	Biochemical and morphological changes in pancreas	2
Predominantly larval hemoglobin at TK stage[a] XXV	Larval hemoglobin almost totally replaced by adult hemoglobin at TK stage[a] XXV	55
Increase in cathepsin C only in tail tissue	Increases in cathepsin C in gill, lung, liver, kidney and tail tissues	111

[a]Refers to Taylor and Kollros stages for *Rana pipiens*.[104]

Immunoreactive TRH in the brain of *X. laevis* tadpoles increases during metamorphic climax.[58] Injections of TRH intraperitoneally or intracranially, however, have failed to induce metamorphosis in amphibian larvae.[27,36,72,102,105] However, intravenous infusion of TRH into postmetamorphic *Rana ridibunda* did activate thyroid glands.[13] Rapid destruction of TRH does not occur in amphibian plasma, but TRH is ineffective at causing TSH release from pituitaries of *R. pipiens, A. mexicanum* or *A. tigrinum* incubated in vitro.[103] It is also possible that this peptide that releases TSH in mammals may play some other role in regulating central nervous function in amphibians, such as suggested for mammals.[87] The observation that TRH can cause release of prolactin (PRL) in mammals may assume some relevance after the actions of PRL on metamorphosis are discussed in the next section.

Differentiation of cells in various regions of the amphibian brain is induced by thyroxine,[35,39,60,63,80] but thyroxine-dependent differentiation of hypothalamic cells may not necessarily be responsible for induction of later metamorphic events. The onset of metamorphosis is marked by differentiation of neurosecretory centers as evidenced by accumulation of neurosecretory material in the hypothalamus and the median eminence and by differentiation of the portal system. These events are induced by thyroid hormones and are blocked by antithyroid drugs.[23,33,38] Thyroxine treatment induces premature differentiation of catecholamine-containing cells in the hypothalamus (bordering the preoptic recess) of larval *Bufo marinus*.[63] Differentiation of these cells is not a prerequisite for metamorphosis. The catecholamine-containing cells may be involved with inhibiting TSH release after climax or in some unrelated function essential for terrestrial life.

Other Hormones Influencing Metamorphosis

Prolactin. Early studies indicated that amphibian metamorphosis could sometimes be blocked or delayed by administration of mammalian adenohypophysial or placental preparations.[7,93,98] Exogenous PRL was found to be an antimetamorphic factor.[14] Prolactin treatment blocks metamorphosis induced with either TSH or thyroid hormones and interferes with TSH at the thyroid gland and with thyroid hormones at their target tissues. However, certain liver enzymes that are normally induced by thyroid hormones are not influenced by PRL.[5,51]

Evidence that endogenous PRL plays a role in preventing or delaying amphibian metamorphosis comes from studies employing antibodies against mammalian PRL[11] and studies using ergocornine, which blocks endogenous PRL release.[17,83] The failure of mammalian TRH to induce metamorphic changes is apparently not related to stimulation of PRL release as described in mammals.[37]

Prolactin may be essential for some metamorphic events. Immunoreactive PRL has been shown to increase in bullfrog plasma during metamorphosis, reaching a peak at metamorphic climax.[112] Furthermore, the high mortality often associated with induced metamorphosis in tiger salamander larvae is eliminated if the animals also receive low doses of ovine PRL.[10] It is possible that antimetamorphic effects of mammalian PRL in amphibians are artifacts of the large doses required to block metamorphosis.

Adrenocortical Hormones. Several reports have shown that treatment of anuran larvae with corticosteroids or corticotropin (ACTH) enhances metamorphosis under some conditions.[31,47,88] There have been equivocal reports of the influence of ACTH and adrenocortical hormones on urodele larvae, ranging from enhancement to no effect to inhibition.[72,97] Do adrenocortical hormones play an essential role or are these observations related to possible permissive actions of corticosteroids such as those described in mammals (see Chap. 10)? In bullfrogs, plasma corticosterone levels increase during prometamorphosis and again during climax.[112] Circulating cortisol also increases at climax. Corticosteroids may enhance the actions of thyroid hormones during metamorphosis. These data also could be interpreted as reflecting an independent role for corticosteroids. Certainly more detailed studies are required to demonstrate a positive role for endogenous corticosteroids.

Pineal Gland. Contrasting observations have been reported on the possible relationship of the pineal complex to metamorphosis in anuran amphibians. Metamorphosis is accelerated following pinealectomy of the midwife toad *Alytes obstetricans,*[89] but an earlier study found that feeding mammalian pineal tissue to *Bufo americanus* tadpoles also accelerated metamorphosis.[1] Limited data for urodeles suggest that the pineal complex may play a stimulatory role with respect to thyroid function. Pinealectomy decreases radioiodide uptake by thyroid glands of *A. tigrinum* larvae,[34,84] although neither melatonin nor a commercial extract of bovine pineal glands has any effect on radioiodide uptake by intact larvae.[78] Circulating thyroxine and melatonin do exhibit coincident peak levels on a diurnal basis,[75] but this does not necessarily imply a cause-effect relationship. No consistent relationship has been demonstrated between pineal activity and metamorphosis, and additional studies are needed to explain these divergent observations.

A summary of some endocrine organs whose secretions may influence metamorphosis is provided in Table 17-4. Although some of these may eventually prove to be important contributory factors, the major factor will still be activation of the thyroid axis at a genetically predetermined time in the life history of each species. This activation may be influenced by environmental factors or the general endocrine state of the animal (Fig. 17-5) or by both.

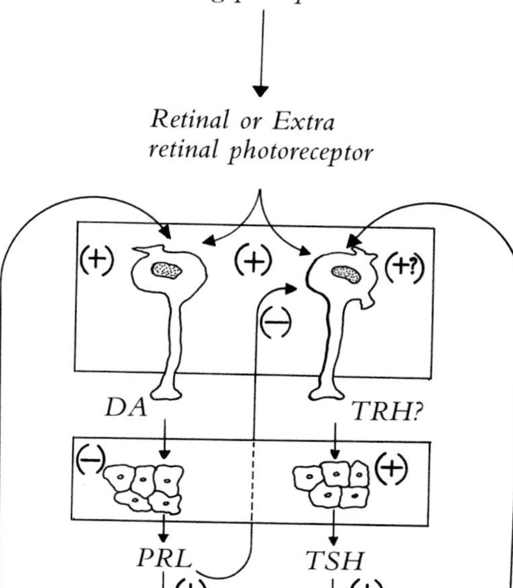

Fig. 17-5. Thyroid-prolactin interactions. A basic antagonism is present in amphibians from the nature of hypothalamic control (prolactin under inhibitory control; thyroid under stimulatory control) to interactions at the thyroid gland by prolactin *(PRL)* and thyrotropin *(TSH)* and even at some target tissues where PRL promotes larval aquatic features and thyroid hormones *(T_3/T_4)* favor metamorphosis and terrestrial life (antilarval). Length of day may be interpreted through data obtained by retinal (eye) receptors or by extraretinal receptors such as the pineal gland. DA, dopamine; TRH, thyrotropin-releasing hormone.

Table 17-4. *Hormones That Influence Amphibian Metamorphosis*

HORMONE	SOURCE	INFLUENCE
TRH	Hypothalamus	None
TSH	Adenohypophysis	Stimulatory
T_3	Thyroid	Stimulatory
T_4	Thyroid	Stimulatory
PRL	Adenohypophysis	Inhibitory, synergistic
ACTH	Adenohypophysis	Stimulatory, inhibitory
CORTICOIDS	Adrenocortical cells	Stimulatory (?)
MELATONIN	Pineal	??

Hypothesis for Endocrine Regulation of Metamorphosis

The observation that differentiation of the hypothalamic neurosecretory system in *Rana* tadpoles depended on thyroid hormones led Etkin to propose that thyroid hormones released slowly and autonomously into the circulation from the larval thyroid gland are responsible for maturation of the hypothalamic neurosecretory centers.[21,22] According to Etkin's hypothesis the maturing hypothalamus produces increasing amounts of a stimulatory factor (TRH?), which in turn elevate TSH levels. Thyrotropin accelerates production of thyroid hormones. There would follow a peak of thyroid activity responsible for metamorphic climax, including a negative feedback effect on the hypothalamus that would rapidly shut down the thyroid axis. Etkin further supposed that the immature hypothalamo-thyroid axis of Amphibia lacked any negative feedback feature and termed the proposed action of thyroid hormones on the hypothalamo-hypophysial system positive feedback. However, negative feedback has been demonstrated in larval *R. pipiens* and in *Xenopus*,[14,57] and the term positive feedback might better be replaced with the term maturational effect.[38] Etkin provided a diagram for his hypothesis depicting rising hormone levels during prometamorphosis and metamorphic climax followed by a rapid decline to premetamorphic levels (Fig. 17-6). This scheme has drawn criticism since there was originally no experimental evidence to support these conjectures and because limited experimental work suggested that timing of the thyroxine peak was incorrect. Increase in circulating thyroid hormones during late prometamorphosis and climax and subsequent decline are supported by careful measurements of plasma protein-bound iodide levels

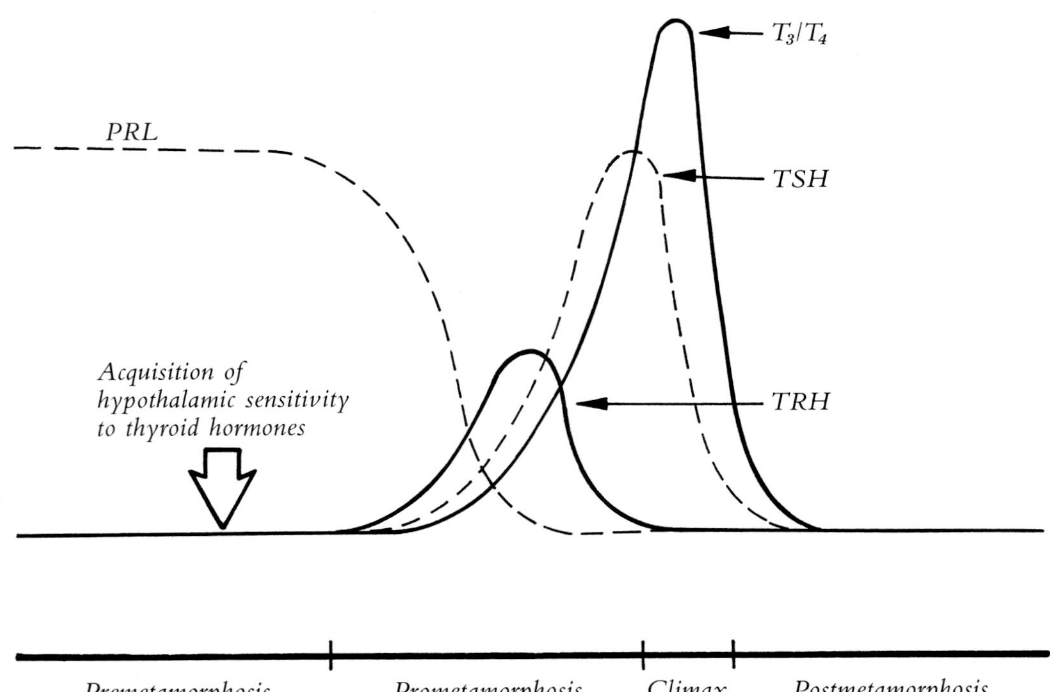

FIG. 17-6. The Etkin hypothesis. Premetamorphic anuran tadpoles at some point in development acquire a hypothalamic sensitivity to thyroxine (or T_3) resulting in hypothalamic maturation of the inhibitory prolactin center and the thyrotropic center. A rapid decrease in circulating prolactin *(PRL)* ensues, accompanied by thyroxine-induced increase in thyroid-releasing hormone (TRH) and consequent increases in thyrotropin (TSH) and thyroid hormones *(T_3/T_4)* (prometamorphosis) leading to climax. Negative feedback presumably returns the thyroid axis to a low "premetamorphic" level during the postmetamorphic period. (Based on Etkin.[23,24,28])

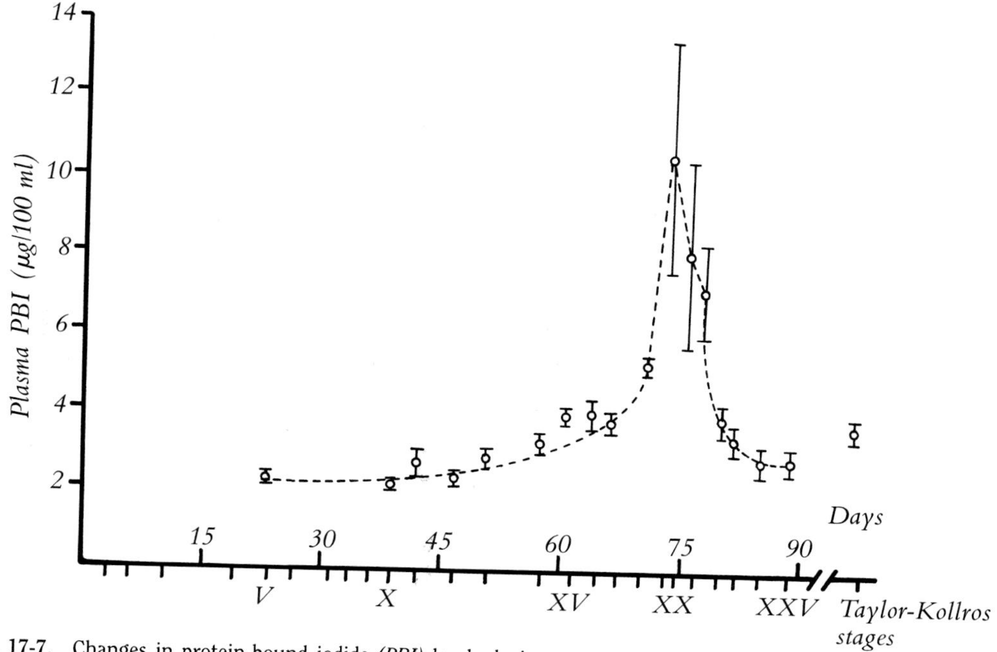

FIG. 17-7. Changes in protein-bound iodide *(PBI)* levels during anuran metamorphosis. More recent data on plasma thyroid hormone levels support this pattern for secretion and metabolism of thyroid hormones in anurans[66,112] and urodeles.[19,61] (Redrawn from Just.[54])

(Fig. 17-7) and plasma T_4 levels,[54,66,86] although the magnitude and timing of this activity do not correlate precisely with Etkin's illustration. Nevertheless, there does appear to be a sudden increase in thyroid activity correlated with differentiation of hypothalamic neurosecretory centers and the portal system that may relate to the secretory pattern of thyroid hormones following climax. Support for such a mechanism in urodeles comes from the observation that hypothalamic injections of T_4 induce metamorphosis in *A. tigrinum* larvae with a concomitant increase in thyroid gland function as measured by radioiodide uptake.[74] Similar doses of T_4 administered intraperitoneally or intramuscularly are ineffective. An intraperitoneal dose sufficient to induce metamorphosis does not activate thyroid gland function.

Demonstration of the antimetamorphic action of PRL prompted Etkin to add hypothetical PRL levels to his scheme.[24–26] Prolactin release is under inhibitory hypothalamic control in the Amphibia as it is in most vertebrates (see Chap. 4). Larvae with immature hypothalamic centers might produce excessive amounts of PRL until maturation of the PRL release-inhibiting center takes place, and PRL would prevent premature metamorphosis. Decreased tissue sensitivity to PRL could also enhance metamorphosis. The importance of PRL in preventing metamorphosis has been supported for anurans and urodeles. Treatment with antibodies prepared against mammalian PRL or with drugs that block release of PRL accelerates metamorphosis.[11,17,83] Bioassay of pituitaries of larvae and recently transformed *A. tigrinum* larvae using the pigeon crop-sac assay (see Chaps. 1 and 5) indicates a marked reduction in pituitary PRL activity following spontaneous or induced metamorphosis.[77] This may be interpreted as supportive of the modified Etkin hypothesis. Measurement of circulating PRL in bullfrogs does not support a decrease in plasma PRL during metamorphosis. Prolactin levels increase to a maximum at metamorphic climax.[112] A physiological role for PRL is supported by observations that PRL stimulates feeding and improves survival[10] of thyroxine-treated metamorphosing salamanders. The decrease in pituitary PRL of postmetamorphic tiger salamanders[77] could be interpreted as a depletion of stored hormone during metamorphosis.

"Second Metamorphosis"

There are several genera of newts, including *Notophthalmus, Triturus* and *Taricha,* that exhibit a second morphological and physiological change from a juvenile terrestrial form, sometimes termed an *eft,* to an aquatic breeding adult form (see Chap. 18).

This so-called second metamorphosis involves a limited reversal to an aquatic form, including reacquisition of a smooth, mucus-coated moist skin like that of the aquatic larvae and a return to the natal habitat.[110] Associated with these skin alterations are changes in secondary sex characters of males and occurrence of directed migration of both males and females to the breeding ponds. Prolactin treatment induces these skin changes, the migration to water (water drive), and development of the secondary sexual characters such as enhancement of the tail fin. Thyroid hormones antagonize second metamorphosis in newts, although small quantities of thyroid hormones enhance PRL effects. Thyroid hormones in newts may influence their migration to land and their preference for dry substrates (see Chap. 18).

Endocrine Factors and Life Histories of Permanently Aquatic Urodeles

Long before the role of thyroid hormones in metamorphosis was discovered, naturalists had described many species of caudate amphibians that never underwent metamorphosis but retained an essentially larval body form or at least many characteristics that were larval.[62] Some of these species never undergo metamorphosis in nature or in the laboratory (for example, *Necturus* spp.; hellbender, *C. alleganiensis;* congo eel, *Amphiuma* spp.). In other species (for example, *A. tigrinum;* red-spotted newt, *Notophthalmus viridescens;* crested newt, *Triturus cristatus;* Pacific salamander, *Dicamptodon ensatus*), some populations undergo metamorphosis, but other populations do not. Sometimes only a few individuals in a population will metamorphose, and the majority remain as larvae.

Sexual maturity occurs in a number of species of urodeles with larval type bodies but does not occur in anuran larvae although complete spermatogenesis has been reported for ranid and *Xenopus* tadpoles.[53,100] Sexual maturation may occur in larval animals by either retardation of somatic development (metamorphosis) with sexual maturation occurring at the normal time or by precocious or accelerated sexual development. The former condition has been termed *neoteny* and the latter *progenesis,* with both terms being encompassed by *paedomorphosis,* referring to retention of any larval features in a sexually reproducing form.[41] Since paedomorphosis in amphibians appears to result exclusively from delaying somatic development, the term neoteny will be used freely here.[41,81] Such individuals of a species may be referred to as *neotenes,* and the term may include extremes from reproducing larvae to those larvae exhibiting some sexual development prior to metamorphosis. Even in animals appearing to be larval in body form, some metamorphic events may have occurred, such as the hemoglobin transition[18,85] and these animals are not truly "larval" in every respect.

Species that never undergo metamorphosis and that reproduce in a larval form may be termed *obligate neotenes.* Those like *A. tigrinum* that may or may not undergo metamorphosis prior to attainment of sexual maturity are termed *facultative neotenes,* stressing their autonomy to undergo metamorphosis according to environmental and endocrine conditions. When purified thyroid hormones and TSH preparations became available it was soon discovered that obligate neotenes are of two types. Some species (inducible obligate neotenes) can be induced to undergo metamorphosis in the laboratory by treating them with thyroid or TSH preparations (for example, *Typhlomolge rathbuni, A. mexicanum*), whereas others (noninducible) are insensitive to even massive doses (*Necturus* spp., *Amphiuma* spp.).

The inducible obligate neotenes appear to have some defect in the hypothalamo-hypophysial system so that the thyroid remains quiescent.[101] The basis for neoteny in obligate neotenes is peripheral. Transplantation of skin from a species that normally responds to thyroid hormones onto the obligate neotene *Necturus maculosus* results in complete change of the graft with no metamorphic changes in the host following immersion in a solution containing T_4.[68] Obviously this obligate neotene is insensitive to thyroid hormones, and it is not simply a case of high levels of endogenous PRL or of rapid metabolism or excretion or both of thyroid hormones. Facultative neotenes and inducible obligate neotenes are sensitive to exogenous TSH or thyroid hormones, but the largest (oldest?) individuals of facultative species may not respond or may die after initiation of some metamorphic changes.[44] These observations suggest that age may be an important factor in determining the sensitivity of tissues to thyroid hormones in facultative neotenes. Reproductive maturation per se does not appear to influence the sensitivity of tissues to exogenous TSH or thyroid hormones,[74,76] although there is an inverse relationship between circulating T_4 and degree of gonadal maturation.[73,92]

Endocrine Bases for Neoteny

The hypothalamus of neotenes is not completely undifferentiated with respect to control of adenohypophysial secretion as evidenced by gonadal maturation. Furthermore, transplanted neotene pituitaries release large amounts of melanotropin as do those from other "adult" amphibians, indicating the presence of inhibitory hypothalamic control. Therefore it is reasonable to assume that some inhibitory factor is present that prevents metamorphosis.

Prolactin may be the factor important in reducing the responsiveness of tissues to thyroid hormones in neotenes.[3] Although this is probably not the case in obligate neotenes that are insensitive to thyroid hormones, PRL may be an important factor in some inducible obligate neotenes and facultative neotenes. Pituitaries from neotenic *A. tigrinum* contain larger amounts of PRL than those from immature larvae,[77] and treatment of neotenes with ergocornine (a drug that blocks PRL release) or PRL, antibodies increases their sensitivity to injected T_4.[11,17,83] Perhaps PRL retards metamorphosis in these animals by suppressing hypothalamic centers controlling TSH release.[38,83] This PRL block can be overcome by either raising T_4 levels with hormone injections into the hypothalamus or reducing PRL levels in the presence of higher endogenous levels of thyroid hormones.[11,17,74,83]

Following is an example of the possible importance of reductions in endogenous PRL: Tail height in urodeles is a PRL-dependent character,[65,83,106] and tail height can be used as a crude indicator of endogenous circulating levels of PRL. When neotenic *A. tigrinum* are brought into the laboratory, there is a reduction in tail height within 24 hours, which presumably reflects a reduction in circulating PRL. If these neotenes are held at 5°C, a temperature at which thyroid hormones are ineffective, tail regression still occurs but takes several days.[70] There is a seasonal variation in circulating thyroid hormones in these animals that correlates with the frequency of spontaneous metamorphosis in the laboratory on a seasonal basis.[73,82] The highest incidence of spontaneous metamorphosis correlates with the highest endogenous levels of T_4 (Fig. 17-8).

Environmental Factors and Metamorphosis in Facultative Neotenes

The facultative neotene *A. tigrinum* has been studied for more than 70 years in attempts to elucidate the environmental factors responsible for metamorphosis and gonadal maturation. The literature consists, however, of many misleading generalizations based upon anecdotal comments, incomplete experimental analyses and the belief that one environmental factor is responsible for blocking metamorphosis or inducing metamorphosis. Single environmental factors that have been suggested as causative agents include iodide content of the water, oxygen content of the water, drying up of the pond environment (a "do-or-die" hypothesis), altitude, temperature, photoperiod, nutrition and pH. Some of these environmental factors may be ruled out simply

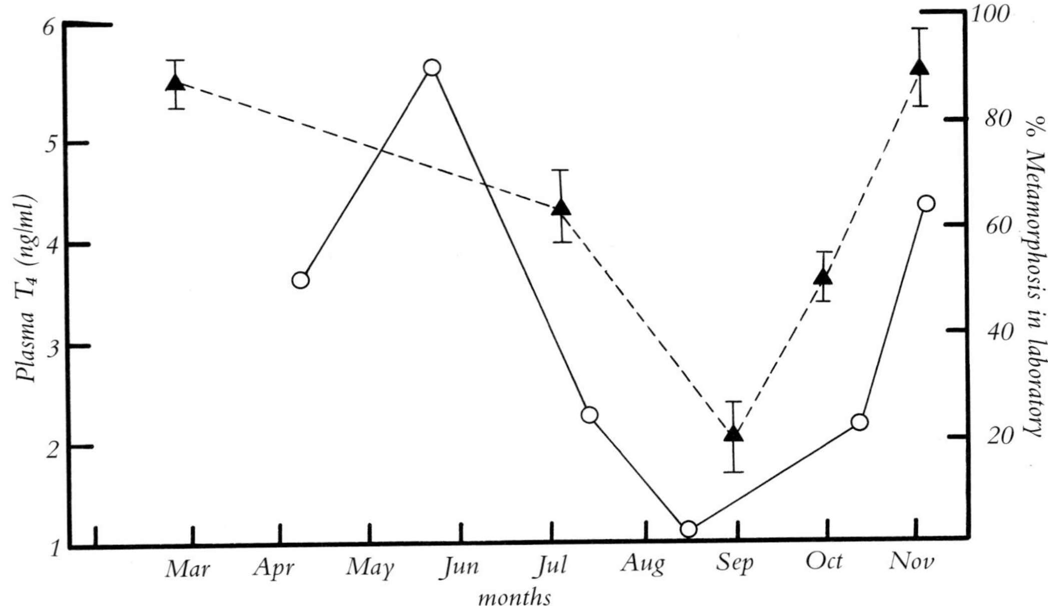

FIG. 17-8. Seasonal variations in T_4 and frequency of "spontaneous" metamorphosis. The highest occurrence of metamorphosis in field-collected neotenic tiger salamanders after they are brought into the laboratory *(open circles)* correlates with endogenous levels of T_4 *(solid triangles)*. Bringing animals into the laboratory generally further increases circulating levels,[70] pushing endogenous levels still higher and presumably causing metamorphosis. Prolactin levels decrease in captive larvae.[67]

on their inconsistency as single determinants of metamorphosis (desiccation, altitude); some because they do not explain occurrence of the facultative neotene (iodide content of the water); some because they have been shown to have no experimental basis (oxygen content or iodide content of the water), etc. Since animals in nature are constantly subjected to many environmental factors, most of which have periodic aspects to them, it would seem naive to assume that any one factor would be the causative agent sought. More likely the final word will involve interactions of multiple factors producing the endocrine state conducive to or hostile to metamorphosis. Temperature and photoperiodic fluctuations are among the most obvious factors changing in a predictable fashion in the environment, and they do influence thyroid function.[73,78] In addition pH, salinity and population density have been shown to influence thyroid function or metamorphosis or both in a number of urodele and anuran species, and these factors should not be overlooked as being cooperative agents influencing metamorphosis in facultative neotenes.

Growth rates have been implicated as regulators of metamorphosis in anurans although a number of environmental factors may directly or indirectly influence growth and development.[113] For example, temperature regimens are reported to be the primary determinants of the onset of metamorphosis in high-altitude populations of *A. tigrinum* in Colorado,[4,95] and the fastest growing individuals undergo metamorphosis earliest.[4] The rate of differentiation rather than growth appears to account for 95% of the variance in length of the larval period for anuran populations, and the major environmental factor influencing differentiation rate is temperature.[99]

Summary

Amphibian metamorphosis is controlled primarily by the activity of the thyroid axis. Many features of the endocrine regulation and of metamorphic changes themselves are similar in anurans and urodeles. The following account is somewhat hypothetical but serves as a useful generalization.

Hypothalamic and hypothalamo-hypophysial portal system differentiation is influenced by low endogenous levels of thyroid hormones. Activation of a hypothalamic TSH-releasing center and a PRL release-inhibiting center produces a sudden surge in thyroid hormone levels that brings about metamorphosis. Either an increase in thyroid hormones (typically) or possibly a decrease in PRL levels may initiate metamorphosis. The major role for endogenous PRL is delaying metamorphosis until some appropriate time, and low levels of PRL may play a role in influencing the sequence of responses to elevated thyroid hormone levels. Both PRL and thyroid hormones probably are present at all times in the circulation, and it is the relative proportions of these hormones that determine the direction development will take.

Neoteny in urodeles involves obligate or facultative suppression of metamorphosis, and the entire life history may occur in the aquatic habitat. Noninducible obligate neotenes lack tissue sensitivity to thyroid hormones. Inducible obligate neotenes appear to possess a defect with respect to the ability to release sufficient TSH to cause metamorphosis. Facultative neotenes may rely on high endogenous levels of PRL that block the sensitivity of the hypothalamus to thyroid hormones. Environmental factors in particular combinations presumably determine the endocrine state of neotenes and hence determine whether metamorphosis will precede reproductive maturation.

Metamorphosis may be influenced by the general endocrine state of amphibians, including ACTH and corticosteroids, pineal factors, gonadal state and possibly others.

The second metamorphosis or water drive involves return of terrestrial phase newts to water for purposes of breeding and is accompanied by skin changes and changes in male secondary sexual characters and gonadal maturation. Water-drive behavior, skin changes and tail height (a male secondary sexual character) are induced by PRL. Thyroid hormones may block water-drive phenomena, but small amounts enhance the responses to PRL. Similar events may take place in other urodeles and in anurans that return from a terrestrial existence to water for breeding.

References

1. Addair, J. and F.E. Chidester (1928). Pineal and metamorphosis: The influence of pineal feeding upon the rate of metamorphosis in frogs. Endocrinology 12:791–796.
2. Atkinson, B.G. and G.H. Little (1972). Growth and regression in tadpole pancreas during spontaneous and thyroid hormone-induced metamorphosis. I. Rates of macromolecular synthesis and degradation. Mech. Aging Devel. 1:299–312.
3. Berman, R.H., H.A. Bern, C.S. Nicoll and R.C. Strohman (1964). Growth promoting effects of mammalian prolactin and growth hormone in tadpoles of *Rana catesbeiana*. J. Exp. Zool. 156:353–360.
4. Bizer, J.R. (1978). Growth rates and size at metamorphosis of high elevation populations of *Ambystoma tigrinum*. Oecologia 34:175–184.
5. Blatt, L.M., K.A. Slickers and K.H. Kim (1969). Effect of prolactin on thyroxine-induced metamorphosis. Endocrinology 85:1213–1215.
6. Bragg, A.N. (1965). Gnomes of the Night. University of Pennsylvania Press, Philadelphia.
7. Brandt, W. and G. Thomas (1941). The antagonistic effect of powdered and alcoholic extracts of placenta on thyroxine in axolotls. J. Endocrinol. 2:395–398.
8. Brown, G.W. and P.P. Cohen (1958). Biosynthesis of urea in metamorphosing tadpoles. In W. McElroy and B. Glass, ed., The Chemical Basis of Development. Johns Hopkins Press, Baltimore, pp. 495–513.
9. Campantico, E., M. Olivero, A. Guardabassi, M.T. Rinaudo, C. Giunta and R. Bruno (1971). Effects of prolactin on arginase activity in the liver of *Bufo bufo* larvae under different experimental conditions. Gen. Comp. Endocrinol. 17:287–292.
10. Choun, J.L. and D.O. Norris (1974). The effects of prolactin dose on rates of TSH-induced metamorphosis, weight loss and feeding frequency in larval tiger salamanders, *Ambystoma tigrinum*. J. Colo. Wyo. Acad. Sci. 7(5):68.

11. Clemons, G.K. and C.S. Nicoll (1977). Effects of antisera to bullfrog prolactin and growth hormone on metamorphosis of *Rana catesbeiana* tadpoles. Gen. Comp. Endocrinol. 30:357–363.

12. Crim, J.W. (1975). Observations on the distribution of visual pigments in Amphibia. Comp. Biochem. Physiol. 52A:719–720.

13. Darras, V.M. and E.R. Kuhn (1982). Increased levels of thyroid hormones in a frog *Rana ridibunda* following intravenous administration of TRH. Gen. Comp. Endocrinol. 48:469–475.

14. Dodd, M.H.I. and J.M. Dodd (1976). The biology of metamorphosis. In B. Lofts, ed., Physiology of the Amphibia. Vol. 3, pp. 467–599.

15. Ducibella, T. (1974). The occurrence of biochemical metamorphic events without anatomical metamorphosis in the axolotl. Dev. Biol. 38:175–186.

16. Ducibella, T. (1974). The influence of L-thyroxine on the change in red blood cell type in the axolotl. Dev. Biol. 38:187–194.

17. Eddy, L. and H. Lipner (1975). Acceleration of thyroxine-induced metamorphosis by prolactin antiserum. Gen. Comp. Endocrinol. 25:462–466.

18. Edwards, J.A. and J.T. Justus (1969). Hemoglobins of two urodeles: Changes with metamorphosis. Proc. Soc. Exp. Biol. Med. 132:524–526.

19. Eagleston, G.W. and B.A. McKeown (1978). Changes in thyroid activity of *Ambystoma gracile* (Baird) during different larval, transforming and postmetamorphic phases. Can. J. Zool. 56:1377–1381.

20. Etkin, W. (1932). Growth and resorption phenomena in anuran metamorphosis. Physiol. Zool. 5:275–300.

21. Etkin, W. (1963). Metamorphosis-activating system of the frog. Science 139:810–814.

22. Etkin, W. (1964). Metamorphosis. In J. Moore, ed., Physiology of the Amphibia. Academic Press, New York, Vol. 1, pp. 426–468.

23. Etkin, W. (1965/1966). Hypothalamic sensitivity to thyroid feedback in the tadpole. Neuroendocrinology 1:293–302.

24. Etkin, W. (1968). Hormonal control of amphibian metamorphosis. In W. Etkin and L.I. Gilbert, eds., Metamorphosis. Appleton Century Crofts, New York, pp. 313–348.

25. Etkin, W. and A.G. Gona (1967). Antagonism between prolactin and thyroid hormone in amphibian development. J. Exp. Zool. 165:249–258.

26. Etkin, W. and A.G. Gona (1967). Antithyroid action of prolactin in the frog. Life Sci. 6:703–709.

27. Etkin, W. and A. Gona (1968). Failure of mammalian thyrotropin-releasing factor preparation to elicit metamorphic responses in tadpoles. Endocrinology 82:1067–1068.

28. Etkin, W. and A.G. Gona (1974). Evolution of thyroid function in poikilothermic vertebrates. Handbook of Physiology, Sec. 7, Endocrinology. Williams & Wilkins, Baltimore, Vol. 3, pp. 5–20.

29. Etkin, W. and W. Sussman (1961). Hypothalamo-pituitary relation in metamorphosis of Ambystoma. Gen. Comp. Endocrinol. 1:70–79.

30. Frieden, E. and J.J. Just (1970). Hormonal responses in amphibian metamorphosis. In G. Litwack, ed., Biochemical Actions of Hormones. Academic Press, New York, Vol. 1, pp. 1–52.

31. Frieden, E. and B. Naile (1955). Biochemistry of amphibian metamorphosis. I. Enhancement of induced metamorphosis by glucocorticoids. Science 121:37–39.

32. Galton, V.A. (1983). Thyroid hormone action in amphibian metamorphosis. In J.H. Oppenheimer and H.H. Samuels, eds., Molecular Basis of Thyroid Hormone Action. Academic Press, New York, pp. 445–483.

33. Gern, W.A. (1976). The effects of intrahypothalamic injection of thyroxine and hypophysial manipulation on metamorphosis of neotenic and larval tiger salamanders, *Ambystoma tigrinum*. Ph.D. thesis, University of Colorado, Boulder.

34. Gern, W.A., S.L. Nelson, P.H. Vader, K.F. DeBoer and A.G. Heath (1973). The influence of the pineal gland and melatonin on activity and behavioral circadian rhythms in neotenic tiger salamanders. J. Colo.-Wyo. Acad. Sci. 7(4):33.

35. Gona, A. (1973). Effects of thyroxine, thyrotropin, prolactin and growth hormone on the maturation of the frog cerebellum. Exp. Neurol. 38:494–501.

36. Gona, A.G. and O. Gona (1974). Failure of synthetic TRF to elicit metamorphosis in frog tadpoles or red-spotted newts. Gen. Comp. Endocrinol. 24:223–225.

37. Gona, A. and O. Gona (1974). Prolactin-releasing effects of centrally-acting drugs in the red-spotted newt, *Notophthalmus viridescens*. Neuroendocrinology 14:365–368.

38. Goos, H.J.T. (1969). Hypothalamic neurosecretion and metamorphosis in *Xenopus laevis*. IV. The effect of extirpation of the presumed TRF cells and of a subsequent PTU treatment. Z. Zellforsch. 97:449–458.

39. Goos, H.J.T., A.M. de Knect and J. de Vries (1968). Hypothalamic neurosecretion and metamorphosis in *Xenopus laevis*. I. The effect of propylthiouracil. Z. Zellforsch. 86:384–392.

40. Goos, H.J.T., H. Zwanenbeer and P. VanOordt (1969). Hypothalamic neurosecretion and metamorphosis in *Xenopus laevis*. II. The effect of thyroxine following treatment with propylthiouracil. Arch. Anat. 51:269–274.

41. Gould, S.J. (1977). Ontogeny and Phylogeny. Belknap Press, Cambridge, Mass.

42. Guardabassi, A. (1961). The hypophysis of *Xenopus laevis* Daudin larvae after removal of the anterior hypothalamus. Gen. Comp. Endocrinol. 348–363.

43. Gudernatsch, J.F. (1913). Feeding experiments on tadpoles. I. The influence of specific organs given as food on growth and differentiation. Arch. Entwick. Organ. 35:457–481.

44. Hahn, W.E. (1962). Serum protein and erythrocyte changes during metamorphosis in paedogenic *Ambystoma tigrinum mavortium.* Comp. Biochem. Physiol. 7:55–61.

45. Hamburger, V. (1960). A Manual of Experimental Embryology. University of Chicago Press.

46. Hanaoka, Y. (1967). The effects of posterior hypothalectomy upon the growth and metamorphosis of the tadpole of *Rana pipiens.* Gen. Comp. Endocrinol. 8:417–431.

47. Hanke, W. and K.H. Leist (1971). The effect of ACTH and corticosteroids on carbohydrate metabolism during the metamorphosis of *Xenopus laevis.* Gen. Comp. Endocrinol. 16:137–148.

48. Hickman, C.P., Sr., C.P. Hickman, Jr., and F.M. Hickman (1974). Integrated Principles of Zoology. C.V. Mosby Co., St. Louis, p. 505.

49. Houdry, J. and M. Dauca (1977). Cytological and cytochemical changes in the intestinal epithelium during anuran metamorphosis. Int. Rev. Cytol. Suppl. 5:337–385.

50. Jackson, I.M.D. and S. Reichlin (1974). Thyroid-releasing hormone (TRH): Distribution in hypothalamic and extra-hypothalamic brain tissue of mammalian and submammalian chordates. Endocrinology 95:854–862.

51. Jaffe, R.C. and I.I. Geschwind (1974). Influence of prolactin on thyroxine-induced changes in hepatic and tail enzymes and nitrogen metabolism in *Rana catesbeiana.* Proc. Soc. Exp. Biol. Med. 146:961–966.

52. Jaffe, R.C. and I.I. Geschwind (1974). Studies on prolactin inhibition of thyroxine-induced metamorphosis in *Rana catesbeiana* tadpoles. Gen. Comp. Endocrinol. 22:289–295.

53. Jurand, A. (1955). Zjawisko neotenii u *Xenopus laevis* Daud. Folia Biol. (Krakow) 3:315–330.

54. Just, J.J. (1972). Protein-bound iodine and protein concentration in plasma and pericardial fluid or metamorphosing anuran tadpoles. Physiol. Zool. 45:143–152.

55. Just, J.J. and B.G. Atkinson (1972). Hemoglobin transitions in the bullfrog *Rana catesbeiana,* during spontaneous and induced metamorphosis. J. Exp. Zool. 182:271–280.

56. Just, J.J., J. Kraus-Just and D.A. Check (1981). Survey of chordate metamorphosis. In L.I. Gilbert and E. Frieden, eds., Metamorphosis: A Problem in Developmental Biology. 2nd ed., Plenum Press, New York, pp. 265–326.

57. Kaye, N.W. (1961). Interrelationship of the thyroid and pituitary in embryonic and pre-metamorphic stages of the frog, *Rana pipiens.* Gen. Comp. Endocrinol. 1:1–9.

58. King, J.A. and R.P. Millar (1981). TRH, GH-RIH, and LH-RH in metamorphosing *Xenopus laevis.* Gen. Comp. Endocrinol. 44:20–27.

59. Kollros, J.J. (1961). Mechanisms of amphibian metamorphosis: Hormones. Am. Zool. 1:107–119.

60. Kollros, J.J. and V. McMurray (1956). The mesencephalic V nucleus in anurans. II. Influence of thyroid hormone on cell size and cell number. J. Exp. Zool. 131:1–26.

61. Larras-Regard, E., A. Taroug and M. Dorris (1981). Plasma T_4 and T_3 levels in *Ambystoma tigrinum* at various stages of metamorphosis. Gen. Comp. Endocrinol. 43:443–450.

62. Lynn, W.G. (1961). Types of amphibian metamorphosis. Am. Zool. 1:151–162.

63. McKenna, O.C. and J. Rosenbluth (1975). Ontogenetic studies of a catecholamine-containing nucleus of the toad hypothalamus in relation to metamorphosis. Exp. Neurol. 46:496–505.

64. Maclean, N. and S. Turner (1976). Adult hemoglobin in developmentally retarded tadpoles of *Xenopus laevis.* J. Embryol. Exp. Morphol. 35:261–266.

65. Mazzi, V., C. Vellano and M. Sacerdote (1969). Possible prolactin dependency of tail height, ambisexual character in the crested newt. Ric. Sci. 39:676–677.

66. Miyauchi, H., F.T. LaRochelle, Jr., M. Suzuki, M. Freeman and E. Frieden (1977). Studies on thyroid hormones and their binding in bullfrog-tadpole plasma during metamorphosis. Gen. Comp. Endocrinol. 33:254–266.

67. Nieuwkoop, P.D. and J. Faber (1956). Normal tables of *Xenopus laevis* (Daudin). North Holland Publishing Co., Amsterdam.

68. Noble, G.K. and L.B. Richards (1931). The criteria of metamorphosis in urodeles. Anat. Rec. 48:58.

69. Noguchi, T. (1969). Regulatory mechanism of hepatic arginase activity of anuran tadpoles during metamorphosis. J. Fac. Sci. Imp. Univ. Tokyo, Sec. 4, 11:555–577.

70. Norris, D.O. (1978). Hormonal and environmental factors involved in the determination of neoteny in urodeles. In P.J. Gaillard and H.H. Boer, eds., Comparative Endocrinology. Elsevier/North-Holland Biomedical Press, Amsterdam, pp. 109–112.

71. Norris, D.O. (1983). Evolution of endocrine regulation of metamorphosis in lower vertebrates. Am. Zool. 23:709–718.

72. Norris, D.O. Unpublished data.

73. Norris, D.O., D. Duvall, K. Greendale and W.A. Gern (1977). Thyroid function in pre- and post-spawning neotenic tiger salamanders *(Ambystoma tigrinum).* Gen. Comp. Endocrinol. 33:512–517.

74. Norris, D.O. and W.A. Gern (1976). Thyroxine-induced activation of hypothalamo-hypophysial axis in neotenic salamander larvae. Science 194:525–527.

75. Norris, D.O., W.A. Gern and K. Greendale (1981). Diurnal and seasonal variations in thyroid function of neotenic tiger salamanders *(Ambystoma tigrinum).* Gen. Comp. Endocrinol. 45:134–137.

76. Norris, D.O., R.E. Jones and D.C. Cohen (1973). Effects of mammalian gonadotropins (LH, FSH, HCG) and gonadal steroids on TSH-induced metamorphosis of *Ambystoma tigrinum* (Amphibia: Caudata). Gen. Comp. Endocrinol. 20:467–473.

77. Norris, D.O., R.E. Jones and B.B. Criley (1973). Pituitary prolactin levels in larval, neotenic and metamorphosed salamanders *(Ambystoma tigrinum).* Gen. Comp. Endocrinol. 20:437–442.

78. Norris, D.O. and J.E. Platt (1973). Effects of pituitary hormones, melatonin, and thyroidal inhibitors on radioiodide uptake by the thyroid glands of larval and adult tiger salamanders, *Ambystoma tigrinum* (Amphibia: Caudata). Gen. Comp. Endocrinol. 21:368–376.

79. Norris, D.O. and J.E. Platt (1974). T_3 and T_4 induced rates of metamorphosis in immature and sexually mature larvae of *Ambystoma tigrinum* (Amphibia: Caudata). J. Exp. Zool. 189:303–310.

80. Pesetsky, I. (1966). The role of thyroid hormones in the development of Mauthner's neuron. Z. Zellforsch. 75:138–145.

81. Pierce, B.A. and H.M. Smith (1979). Neoteny or paedogenesis? J. Herpetol. 13:119–121.

82. Platt, J.E. (1974). The role of prolactin in neoteny as found in Colorado populations of the tiger salamander *(Ambystoma tigrinum).* Ph.D. thesis, University of Colorado, Boulder.

83. Platt, J.E. (1976). The effects of ergocornine on tail height, spontaneous and T_4-induced metamorphosis and thyroidal uptake of radioiodide in neotenic *Ambystoma tigrinum.* Gen. Comp. Endocrinol. 28:71–81.

84. Platt, J.E. and D.O. Norris (1973). The effects of melatonin, bovine pineal extract and pinealectomy on spontaneous and induced metamorphosis and thyroidal uptake of ^{131}I in larval *Ambystoma tigrinum.* J. Colo.-Wyo. Acad. Sci. 7(4):40.

85. Prahlad, K.V. (1968). Induced metamorphosis: Rectification of a genetic disability by thyroid hormone in the Mexican axolotl *Siredon mexicanum.* Gen. Comp. Endocrinol. 11:21–30.

86. Regard, E., A. Taurog and T. Nakashima (1978). Plasma thyroxine and triiodothyronine levels in spontaneously metamorphosing *Rana catesbeiana* tadpoles and in adult anuran Amphibia. Endocrinology 102:674–684.

87. Reichlin, S., R. Saperstein, I.M.D. Jackson, A.E. Boyd III and Y. Patel (1976). Hypothalamic hormones. Annu. Rev. Physiol. 38:389–424.

88. Remy, C. and J.-J. Bounhiol (1971). Metamorphoses normalisees obtenues pâr l'hormone adrenocorticotrope chez des tetârds d'Alytes hypophysectomises et thyroxines. C.R. Acad. Sci. 272:455–458.

89. Remy, C. and P. Disclos (1970). Influence de l'epiphysectomie sur le developpement de la thyroide et des gonades chez les tetârds d'*Alytes obstetricans.* C.R. Soc. Biol. 164:1989–1993.

90. Rosenkilde, P. (1972). Hypothalamic control of thyroid function in Amphibia. Gen. Comp. Endocrinol. Suppl. 3:32–40.

91. Rosenkilde, P. (1979). The thyroid hormones. In E.J.W. Barrington, ed., Hormones and Evolution. Academic Press, London, Vol. 1, pp. 437–491.

92. Rosenkilde P. and I. Jorgenson (1977). Determination of serum thyroxine in two species of toads: Variation with season. Gen. Comp. Endocrinol. 33:566–573.

93. Roth, P.C.J. (1957). Influence de l'extrait placentaire humain sur la metamorphose experimentale des amphibiens. Ann. Endocrinol. 18:775–779.

94. Schultheiss, H. (1977). The hormonal regulation of urea excretion in the Mexican axolotl (*Ambystoma mexicanum* Cope). Gen. Comp. Endocrinol. 31:45–52.

95. Sexton, O.J. and J.R. Bizer (1978). Life history patterns of *Ambystoma tigrinum* in montane Colorado. Am. Midl. Nat. 99:101–118.

96. Shumway, W. (1940). Stages in the normal development of *Rana pipiens.* I. External form. Anat. Rec. 78:139–144.

97. Sluczewski, A. and P.C.J. Roth (1953). Action de la cortisone et de la corticostimuline (A.C.T.H.) associées a la thyroxine, sur la métamorphose de l'axolotl (*Ambystoma tigrinum* Green) en fonction du pH du milieu ambient. Ann. Endocrinol. 14:948–954.

98. Smith, P.E. (1926). A retardation in the rate of metamorphosis of the Colorado axolotl by injection of anterior hypophyseal fluid. Br. J. Exp. Biol. 3:239–249.

99. Smith-Gill, S.J. and K.A. Berven (1979). Predicting amphibian metamorphosis. Am. Nat. 113:563–585.

100. Swingle, W.W. (1918). The acceleration of metamorphosis in frog larvae by thyroid feeding, and the effects upon the alimentary tract and sex glands. J. Exp. Zool. 24:521–543.

101. Tassava, R.A. (1969). Survival and limb regeneration of hypophysectomized newts with pituitary xenografts from larval axolotls, *Ambystoma mexicanum.* J. Exp. Zool. 171:451–458.

102. Taurog, A. (1974). Biosynthesis of iodoamino acids. Handbook of Physiology, Sec. 7, Endocrinology. Williams & Wilkins, Baltimore, Vol. 3, pp. 101–133.

103. Taurog, A., C. Oliver, R.L. Eskat, J.C. Porter and J.M. McKenzie (1974). The role of TRH in the neoteny of the Mexican axolotl, *Ambystoma mexicanum.* Gen. Comp. Endocrinol. 24:267–279.

104. Taylor, A.C. and J.J. Kollros (1946). Stages in the normal development of *Rana pipiens* larvae. Anat. Rec. 94:7–23.

105. Vandescande, F. and M.-R. Aspeslagh (1974). Failure of thyrotropin releasing hormone to increase ^{125}I uptake by the thyroid in *Rana temporaria.* Gen. Comp. Endocrinol. 23:355–356.

106. Vellano, C. (1972). Un neuvo metado per il dosaggio biologico della prolattina. Boll. Soc. Ital. Biol. Sper. 48:360–362.

107. Voitkevich, A.A. (1962). Neurosecretory control of the amphibian metamorphosis. Gen. Comp. Endocrinol. Suppl. 1:133–147.

108. Voitkevich, A.A. (1965). Role of the neurosecretion in endocrine integration of the developmental processes. Arch. Anat. Microsc. Morphol. Exp. 54:239–260.

109. Wake, M.H. (1977). The reproductive biology of caecilians: An evolutionary perspective. In D.H. Taylor and S.I. Guttman, eds., The Reproductive Biology of Amphibians. Plenum Press, New York, pp. 73–101.

110. Wald, G. (1981). Metamorphosis: An overview. In L.I. Gilbert and E. Frieden, eds., Metamorphosis: A Problem in Developmental Biology. 2nd ed., Plenum Press, New York, pp. 1–39.

111. Wang, V.B. and E. Frieden (1973). Changes in cathepsin C activity during spontaneous and induced metamorphosis of the bullfrog. Gen. Comp. Endocrinol. 21:381–389.

112. White, B.L. and C.S. Nicoll (1981). Hormonal control of amphibian metamorphosis. In L.I. Gilbert and E. Frieden, eds., Metamorphosis: A Problem in Developmental Biology. 2nd ed., Plenum Press, New York, pp. 363–396.

113. Wilbur, H.M. and J.P. Collins (1973). Ecological aspects of amphibian metamorphosis. Science 182:1305–1314.

18·Endocrine Factors and Migratory Behavior

One of the most dramatic events in vertebrates is the predictable seasonal occurrence of massive migrations for breeding or feeding purposes. These coordinated migrations usually involve movements via the same routes between specific localities. Migratory behavior is advantageous in that it maximizes the availability of food and other resources to coordinate with breeding and rearing of the young. A species may utilize more than one location, so when resources become reduced they may move to another site. The tendency for certain individuals to migrate to particular locations (that is, *homing*) further serves to partition resources. Migration also breaks up established predator-prey relationships and parasite-host cycles. Finally, migration is an adaptive solution to what might be considered extreme environmental conditions (cold, drought, etc.). The primary disadvantages of migratory behavior are the energy costs that often contribute to the death of the migrant through exhaustion and the reduced time during which breeding and rearing of the young can occur. Obviously the advantages have outweighed the disadvantages, resulting in the evolution of this phenomenon in many species.

The initiating roles of environmental factors in migratory behavior were first recognized by Rowan who observed the photoperiodic control of migratory behavior and gonadal development in a bird, the slate-colored junco, *Junco hyemalis*.[90] The mediation of environmental changes through the endocrine system to coordinate physiology and behavior in migratory species provides an excellent topic for discussing hormonal interactions as they influence major life history events. In this chapter, environmental and endocrine factors that influence migratory behavior in salmonid fishes, urodele amphibians and birds are discussed.

Migration in Salmonid Fishes

Many species of teleostean fishes exhibit reproductive and feeding migrations during their lives in seawater, freshwater or between seawater and freshwater.[61] The species that migrate between waters of markedly different salinities have captured the imagination and interests of most scientists interested in fish migrations. Such migrations involving extensive osmoregulatory adjustments have been studied primarily in the salmonid fishes (*Salmo* spp., *Salvelinus* spp., *Oncorhynchus* spp.), the sticklebacks[2] (*Gasterosteus* spp.) and the eels (*Anguilla* spp.).

Species that migrate to freshwater for spawning and utilize the marine environment primarily as a food resource are termed *anadromous* (for example, salmonids and sticklebacks), whereas those species spending much of their lives in freshwater but that migrate to seawater for breeding purposes are termed *catadromous* (for example, eels). Anadromous species generally migrate into streams with direct access to the sea or into tributary streams of major rivers or tributary streams of lakes that drain into ocean-bound rivers. The catadromous eels are usually restricted to major rivers and their tributaries.

The Anadromous Salmonids

The family Salmonidae consists of the above-mentioned genera of primitive teleosts and exhibits a circumpolar distribution in the Northern Hemisphere. In recent years, however, salmonids have been introduced successfully in other parts of the world, including New Zealand and South America. The genus *Salmo* consists of several "trout" species. Members of the genus *Salvelinus* are known as the chars, and Pacific salmon are housed in their own genus, *Oncorhynchus.* Common names have not been restricted by scientific classification, however, and the common brook trout is *Salvelinus fontinalis,* whereas the Atlantic salmon is *Salmo salar.*

Anadromous populations are known for all three genera of salmonids although natural, nonmigratory or "lake-locked" populations occur in some species. Some Pacific salmon (for example, *O. gorbuscha,* the pink salmon) enter the estuarine environment soon after hatching and spend most of their lives at sea. The amago salmon, *O. rhodurus,* spends 4 to 5 months at sea, whereas chinook salmon, *O. tschawytscha,* spends several years. Many species can delay migration and may even develop nonmigratory freshwater populations, but they do so by sacrificing the opportunity for rapid growth and attainment of large body size with attendant greater fecundity exhibited by their anadromous cousins. Differences in timing and necessity for seaward migration and considerable variation in timing of spawning migrations and in the actual season for spawning in these fishes complicate investigations of hormonal events and related physiological environmental factors.

The development of osmoregulatory capability and the seasonal nature of migration have led to the development of the concept of *salinity preference.* Prior to seaward migration of young salmonids, their preference for water of higher salinity can be demonstrated.[5,56,66] This preference develops at different points in the life histories of the various species and may be followed by either an obligate requirement for seawater to survive or a return to preference for freshwater if access to water of higher salinity does not occur.[51,66] The abilities of sockeye (*O. nerka*), coho (*O. kisutch*) and amago salmon to develop successful "landlocked" populations is indicative of the return to freshwater preference and the retention of freshwater osmoregulatory mechanisms. Salinity preference may not play any role in directing seaward migratory behavior of young fish, but it could influence the return of adults for spawning. Returning adults are presented with waters of decreasing salinity that could serve as orientating cues. Studies of salinity preference in young salmonids are useful in determining premigratory conditions following experimental manipulations.

Salmonid Life History

The life history pattern (Fig. 18-1) described here is typical for those species spawning in the tributary streams above lakes, such as sockeye salmon, coho salmon and steelhead trout.[39,40,96] These species utilize lakes as rearing areas for the young fish prior to their migration to sea. Most of the features of this life history pattern occur in other species as well, although certain phases may be highly modified or absent.

Life of Young Fish in Fresh Water. Spawning generally occurs in the fall of the year. The eggs are laid and fertilized in a nest or *redd* prepared by the adults in the gravel stream bed. The eggs develop slowly over the winter and hatch in the following spring. Some species will spawn in the spring; development and hatching follow rapidly. Newly hatched salmonid larvae rapidly resorb their yolk sacs and become free-feeding *fry.* These fry generally are displaced passively downstream into lakes where they grow during that first summer to the *fingerling* stage (about the size of the index finger). Some species tend to form schools (for example, sockeye salmon), whereas others tend to remain solitary and territorial (steelhead trout). Fingerlings acquire dark vertical pigment bands that aid in making them less visible. These pigment bars are known as *parr marks,* and the fish are called *parr.*

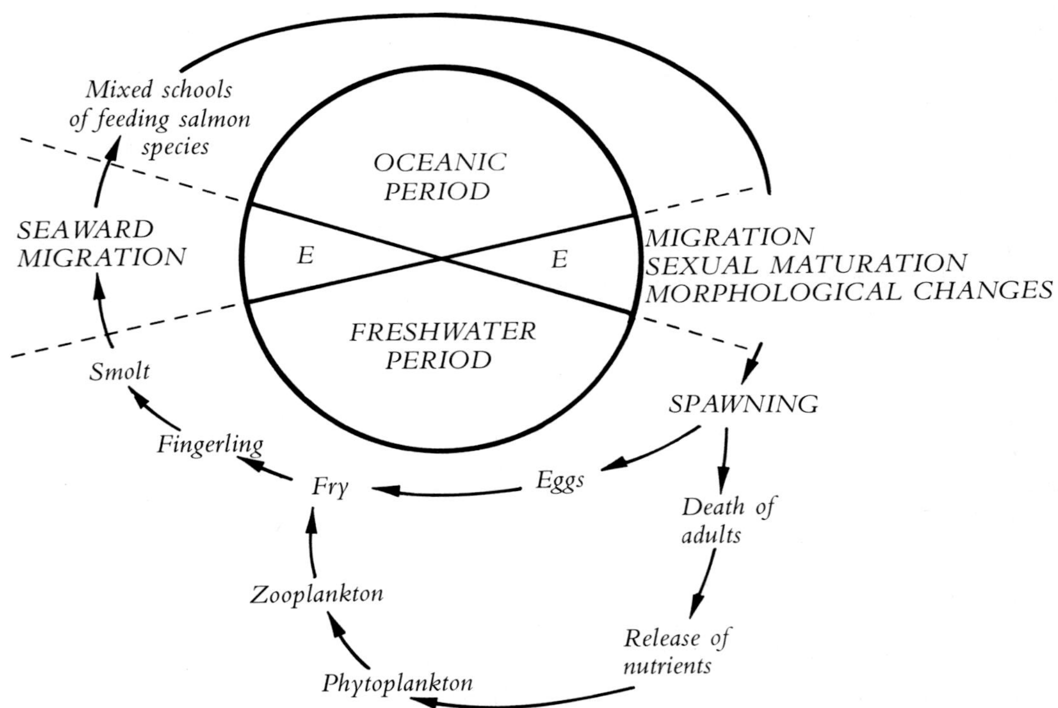

FIG. 18-1. Generalized life history for migratory salmonid fishes. *E*, estuary. See text for explanation.

Parr remain in fresh water for one to three summers, depending on the species and their rate of growth. Most parr achieve an optimal size for migration by the end of the second summer. This optimal size is probably related to energy stores, ability to swim against currents and development of osmoregulatory capacity for seawater survival. Natural selection related to observations that survival is greater for larger fish reaching the sea is probably the primary determiner of "optimal size." If the parr grows rapidly it may reach migratory size by the end of the first summer of lacustrine (lake) life. On the other hand, reduced resources, intense competition or both with other parr or other species may result in a slower growth rate so that three summers are required to reach optimal size.[23,24,41]

"SMOLTIFICATION" AND SEAWARD MIGRATION. The parr that has obtained optimal size for migration undergoes marked transformation or metamorphosis to the migratory form or *smolt.* This process typically involves silvering of the body through deposition of guanine in the scales, reduction in skin mucus, the appearance of a testable preference for water of higher salinity and the ability for osmoregulation in full seawater if challenged. There is usually a reduction in fat content that accompanies this transformation. The smolt no longer has the appearance (or the physiology) of a freshwater fish with cryptic parr marks but assumes the characteristic dark back and silver sides of a deepwater oceanic fish. These as well as some additional changes occurring during the smolt transformation of the parr are listed in Table 18-1.

Soon after the ice breaks up in the spring the smolts will begin their seaward migration during periods of peak water discharge into the effluent streams draining the lake. Premigratory behavior is characterized by a tendency to form schools and restless swimming movements around the lake (premigratory restlessness), culminating in their entering the effluent stream. Migrating coho smolts as well as pink-salmon fry exhibit positive rheotaxis (orientation to and swimming into currents) during the day, which causes them to move into the swiftest cur-

TABLE 18-1. *Behavioral, Physiological and Morphological Changes Associated with Smolt Transformation and Seaward Migration of Juvenile Salmonids*

BEHAVIOR	REF.
General restlessness and decreased territorial behavior	49, 51
Preference for water of higher salinity	3, 56, 66
Morphology	
Loss of cryptic coloration pattern (parr marks) due to guanine deposition in the scales	62
Changes in fin coloration and head shape	50, 102
Appearance of so-called chloride-secreting (Keys-Wilmer) cells in gills	50
Appearance of acidophils in proximal pars distalis of pituitary	49
Scales become less firmly attached and skin mucus is reduced	50, 61
Osmoregulation	
Increased resistance to seawater when challenged	13
Decline in renal excretory rates of water and electrolytes attributable to reduction in glomerular filtration rate	55
Changes in mineral and ionic composition of blood and other tissues	56, 69
Metabolism and Biochemistry	
Decrease in fat content and changes in fat composition as well as a reduction in the condition factor (index of fatness)	24, 50, 64
Changes in the electrophoretic patterns of hemoglobin and serum proteins	61, 109, 110
Biochemical changes leading to increased guanine deposition in the scales	101
Conversion of visual pigments from freshwater type to marine type	76
Decrease in liver glycogen	26
Changes in liver vitamins and in amino acid composition of body proteins	69
Endocrine	
Increase in interrenal activity and levels of corticosteroids	27, 82
Increase in thyroid activity	13, 22, 49

rents. A loss of visual contact during dark periods presumably reduces the intensity of the rheotaxis, and the migrants are displaced downstream.[50] Some active downstream displacement may occur also. Downstream displacement occurs primarily during the early hours of the day with the smolts holding position during most of the day by orienting upstream. This holding behavior is followed by another downstream displacement the next day. The alternating pattern of holding position and downstream displacement continues until the smolts reach the higher salinities of the estuary. The direction of migration, especially through complex freshwater systems, involves both celestial (sun-compass) and noncelestial (?) mechanisms that appear to be genetically fixed in different populations or races of salmon.[40] From the estuary the smolts will enter the ocean and begin the voracious feeding that will result in extensive growth and production of adult salmon within about 2 years.

Oceanic Existence. Relatively little is known about the life of salmonids during the 1 to 3 years they remain at sea. Extensive tagging studies by Japanese, U.S. and Canadian scientists indicate that salmon may range as far as 3500 miles from their home streams and that there is considerable mixing of North American and Asian stocks on the high seas.[78] The primary advantage of this oceanic growth period is the achievement of large size. This is essential to provide sufficient energy stores for the return migration as well as to develop a large reproductive potential. In the northern Pacific many species of salmon may be found together, but they have partitioned the food resources so that there is little interspecific competition for nutrients.[58]

Survival of each species depends upon the number and size of eggs produced. Because of the greater food supplies larger eggs provide a greater chance for survival, allowing the young to hatch at a much larger size. Similarly the advantage of producing the greatest number of offspring is to optimize the probability of maintaining the population. The largest female can produce more eggs of a larger size, and natural selection has resulted in a compromise between size and number of eggs for each species.

The Spawning Migration. Pacific salmon that have achieved a minimum size suitable for sexual maturation and making the return migration begin the most spectacular aspect of the salmonid life history: the homing migration to spawn in the same locale, indeed even the same spawning bed, from which they originated. As gonadal maturation commences in the larger individuals they tend to form separate schools and begin to move away from the immature fish toward the vicinity where their home streams enter the ocean. Once they reach the vicinity of the estuaries the migrants select the appropriate river with a high degree of accuracy and start a directed movement upstream. Observations of swimming speeds and orientation behavior by oceanic salmon strongly support their use of a sun-compass mechanism that results in their being in the appropriate region of the ocean at the correct time.[46]

Laboratory and field experiments have confirmed that salmonids utilize a keen olfactory sense to home in on the correct spawning ground. Experimental blocking of nostrils causes confusion and straying, and it has been proposed that salmonids imprint as fry on chemical cues peculiar to a given spawning ground.[46,94] The presence of these chemical cues in the effluent waters allows the salmon to choose the appropriate river to ascend. Electrophysiological studies have demonstrated dramatic increases in neural activity in the olfactory apparatus of migrating adult Pacific salmon following perfusion of the nostrils with water from their breeding site.[44,108] This response disappears if the "home water" is greatly diluted, but it establishes, at least, the ability to recognize when it has reached home. The salmon will not respond to water collected where other populations normally spawn, although weak responses were reported with water through which the fish had migrated to reach their home pond.[108] Salmon have also been shown to respond electrophysiologically to waters from downstream sources as well as to water from the breeding site.[83] This suggests that migration may involve a sequence of imprinting phenomena directing the migration as proposed by Harden Jones rather than only upon a recognition signal from the breeding site as suggested by Hasler.[45,46] The strongest support for the olfaction hypothesis is provided by the reported attraction of coho salmon to a nonhome spawning site using synthetic chemicals to which the fish had been exposed only as fry.[14,94] Coho salmon exhibit neurophysiological olfactory bulb response to the synthetic imprinting chemical several months after conditioning.[14]

The nature of the chemical signal and its source remains obscure. Nordeng proposes that smolts of the same population but of a different year class are responsible for producing a pheromone that attracts the adults.[80] Behavioral preference tests conducted on adult char, *Salmo alpinus,* suggest the fish home on bile acids produced by the smolts' liver and eliminated in their feces.[18,95] Hasler and his co-workers[47] adhere to an hypothesis that a mixture of plant chemicals and/or minerals is the signal for homing behavior. There is experimental support for both hypotheses, and the true explanation may be a combination of both. Fish may respond to an array of chemicals from various sources that characterize their spawning site.

Gonadal Maturation and Spawning. Reproductive maturation generally begins coincident with initiation of the anadromous migration, continues during upstream migration and is completed after arrival at the spawning bed. Accompanying these gonadal changes are gross changes in body form and coloration patterns, which find their most extreme expressions in the Pacific salmon. As upstream migration commenses most individuals appear as they did in the ocean, and superficially the various salmon species closely resemble one another. They cease feeding when they begin to migrate and utilize stored body fat and muscle to supply the energy for migration, production of gametes and spawning. As the time for spawning nears there is marked atrophy of the musculature that is being catabolized for energy. Deformation of the jaws and skull occurs, especially in the male salmon (Fig. 18-2). The deformation of the jaws is so extreme in Pacific salmon that it is reflected in their generic name, *Oncorhynchus,* which means "hooked nose." In addition to these changes, the skin begins to redden because of deposition of carotenoid pigments. The degree of deformation of the head and changes in skin pigmentation are diagnostic of different species and allow easy sex determination, at least by scientists. It is possible that these species-specific changes are used by the fish for species identification or sexual selection or both. The deposition of carotenoid pigments in the skin and resorption of scales have been suggested to relate to cutaneous respiration,[97] but no experimental evidence has appeared to support this hypothesis.

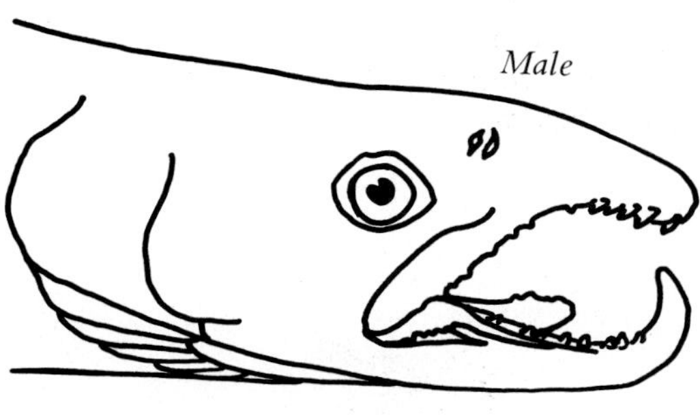

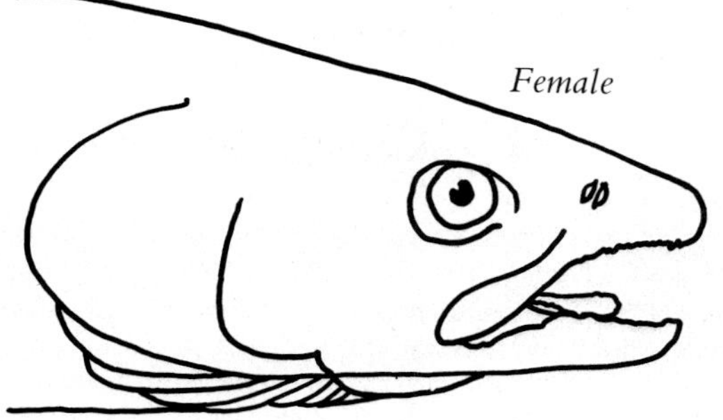

Fig. 18-2. Sexual differentiation in spawning Atlantic salmon, *Salmo salar*. Redrawn from Tchernavin[102].

The degree of morphological changes in spawning salmon, the length of the migratory journey and the energy expenditures to reach the spawning sites are also reflected in the survival rates for postspawning fish. Pacific salmon exhibit the most marked and bizarre physiological changes, frequently coupled with long migratory journeys, and all typically die after spawning (Table 18-2). Artificial attempts to prolong their lives by providing a food source have not been successful.[65] Apparently the structural and physiological changes accompanying the severe energy depletion are irreversible.

An adaptive value of the death of the spawned adults has been related to the addition of considerable nutrient supplies to the aquatic ecosystem. In general, the waters of the Pacific Northwest are nutrient poor, and a cycle of population sizes appears to be related to the numbers of dying fish. Nutrients such as phosphate provided from decaying carcasses of spawned-out salmon support algal growth, which in turn supports a large zooplankton population, the food source for the young salmon during their first few summers. Of course such a mechanism would not explain the "reason" for the death of pink salmon or chum salmon (*O. keta*), whose young are washed directly to sea after hatching.

Many individuals of other anadromous salmonids such as steelhead trout and Atlantic salmon, which have almost identical life histories, survive spawning, and the mended fish or *kelts* return to the ocean. Tagging studies have verified that such fish may return several times to spawn.

Environmental and Endocrine Factors in "Smolting" and Seaward Migration

The major environmental initiator for smolt transformation and seaward migration in parr of optimal size appears to be lengthening of the photoperiod in the spring, and it seems to be the rate of change of the daily photoperiod rather than length of day that induces smolt transformation.[12] Short photoperiod prevents the normal change in salinity preference, and long photoperiod stimulates the change.[3,22] Influx of freshwater into the lakes associated

TABLE 18-2. *Comparison of Effects of Spawning on Salmonids*

	PACIFIC SALMON (*ONCORHYNCHUS* SPP.)	MIGRATORY TROUT (*SALMO GAIRDNERI*)	NONMIGRATORY TROUT, "LAKE-LOCKED" TROUT (*SALMO GAIRDNERI*)
Relative distance of spawning migration	Great	Moderate	Short
Survival after spawning	All die	Many die	Few die
Morphological changes associated with spawning	Extreme	Moderate	Relatively slight
Hyperplasia of interrenal	Marked	Marked	Relatively slight
Interrenal degeneration	Occurs in almost all individuals	Occurs in some but less marked than in salmon	Occurs in some but less marked than in migratory rainbow trout

NOTE: These observations may also be correlated with the length of the spawning migration.

with spring runoff may alter salinity relationships and influence migratory state. Temperature is also important and may play a permissive role in downstream migration.[38,40] The capacity for osmoregulation in seawater and the change in body coloration are independent of temperature.[112] Smolt transformation may occur without seaward migration, however, if there is insufficient spring discharge from the lake.[81] Thus photoperiod operating through optic or extraoptic photoreceptors (pineal?) or both stimulates the physiological and resultant structural and behavioral changes associated with smolt transformation and a predisposition to downstream movement, but the signal to begin the actual migration may be related to the temperature, volume, or velocity of flow, or to all three, in the effluent stream.

There appears to be activation of the hypothalamo-hypophysial-thyroid axis before smolt transformation and downstream migration. William S. Hoar first described in 1939 what histologically appeared to be activated thyroid glands in migrating Atlantic salmon smolts.[49] In recent years investigators have reported increased circulatory levels of thyroid hormones in smolts of coho,[16,37,99] masou,[70] amago,[77] and chinook salmon as well as in steelhead trout.[17] Thyroid hormone levels in smolts retained in fresh water beyond the normal time for migration return to parr levels. Furthermore, examination of thyroid hormone kinetics[98] supports the interpretation that this is a surge in thyroid activity. Treatment with thyroid hormones or thyrotropin causes an increase in guanine deposition in the scales (Fig. 18-3) and a reduction in lipid reserves similar to changes associated with normal smolt transformation.[4,62,87] Furthermore, it is possible to induce a preference for water of higher salinity with mammalian thyrotropin.[3] Goitrogen treatment reverses the preference from higher to lower salinity. Thyroxine treatment also stimulates swimming

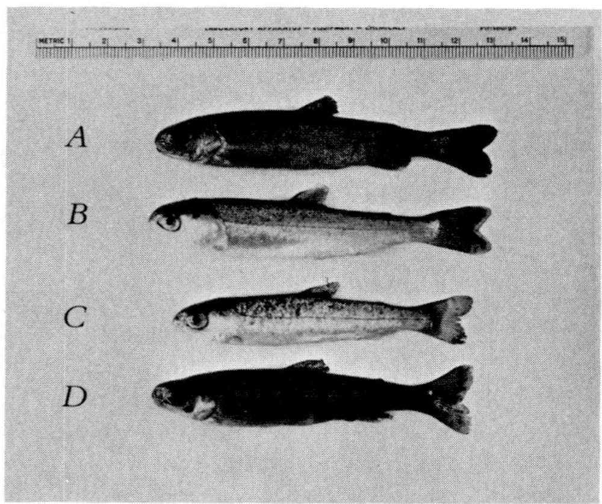

FIG. 18-3. Effects of thyroxine on guanine deposition in skin of fingerling steelhead rainbow trout. *A.* Normal fingerling. *B.* Normal fingerling immersed for 4 weeks in fresh water containing 10^{-8}M thyroxine. *C.* Radiothyroidectomized trout treated as above with thyroxine. *D.* Untreated radiothyroidectomized fish. From Norris[81].

activity in young chum, coho and sockeye salmon as well as goldfish.[53,54] Oxygen consumption is increased in smolts, [5] and it may be related to altered fat metabolism or direct effects of thyroid hormones on respiratory mechanisms or to both.

Timing of the thyroid hormone surge in smolts appears to be under lunar influence. Peak thyroid activity in coho and chinook salmon coincides with each successive new moon occurring during the migratory season.[37,38] Displacement down stream also is correlated with moon phase. Migration coincides with the appearance of the full moon.[38]

Although the surge in thyroid activity is now well documented in smolting salmonids, the significance of this surge is not understood. It does not appear until after steelhead trout have acquired the ability to osmoregulate in sea water.[13] Furthermore, the deposition of guanine in the scales has been observed in radiothyroidectomized steelhead[81] and thiourea-treated chum salmon.[52] Increased thyroid activity may be a consequence of the increased activity level of smolts rather than a causative agent for migratory behavior. On the other hand, activation of the hypothalamo-pituitary-thyroid axis may result in premigratory restlessness. Experimental studies are needed to establish a causative role for thyroid hormones in seaward migration.

Activation of the interrenal gland is evidenced by a fourfold to eightfold increase in circulating corticosteroids of *Salmo salar* smolts as compared to parr,[27,97] and the interrenal gland of smolts is hypertrophied.[82] Corticosteroids are normally involved in osmoregulatory adjustments (see Chap. 16), and interrenal hyperactivity suggests that smolts are under osmotic stress. A reduction in PRL secretion suggested by the marked reduction in mucus on the skin may also contribute to osmoregulatory stress (see Chap. 16).

Inhibition of smolt transformation by precocious sexual maturation has been hypothesized for *S. salar,*[24,25] but sexually mature smolts of *S. salar* have been reported in captivity.[92] Restless type of activity is induced by treatment of young chum, coho or sockeye salmon with testosterone.[53,54] Additional evidence against any action of gonadal hormones on salinity preference has been provided by studies of gonadectomized anadromous sticklebacks.[2] There does not appear to be any reason to implicate gonadal hormones as inhibitory to smolt transformation or migratory behavior, and, in fact, they may be positively related. However, neither testosterone nor estradiol levels increase during smoltification of amago salmon except in male exhibiting precocious testicular development.[77]

Environmental and Endocrine Factors in Spawning Migration

Circumstantial evidence implicates thyroid function in spawning migrations similar to that reported for the seaward migration. Thyroid glands of migrating Atlantic salmon and Pacific salmon show extensive cytological activity[49] (see Fig. 8-11). Upstream migrating Atlantic salmon also exhibit increased radioiodide uptake by thyroid follicles and elevated PBI levels.[28,29] Spawning salmon show reduced thyroid activity, which becomes even more depressed in mended kelts returning to sea.[29] Similar observations have been reported for cod, *Gadus morhua,* that migrate long distances in the ocean to reach their spawning grounds.[115] These observations support a general role for thyroid hormones in migratory behavior regardless whether there is any change in environmental salinity during the migration.

Intense interrenal activity has been described in migrating salmonids (Table 18-2), and extensive interrenal gland degeneration is believed to be the major causative factor in the death of Pacific salmon following spawning. It is not clear whether increased interrenal function is related to osmoregulation or metabolism or is simply a generalized response to the stressful nature of the entire migration and events of spawning. Pacific salmon in particular appear to be suffering from Cushing's syndrome, or hyperadrenocorticism,[43,88,89] and exhibit symptoms similar to those described for mammals (Chap. 10). Similar changes in interrenal function have been described for other salmonids (Table 18-2) and for cod during their marine migrations.[115]

Gonadal hormones may be implicated in initiating, continuing or ending salmonid migra-

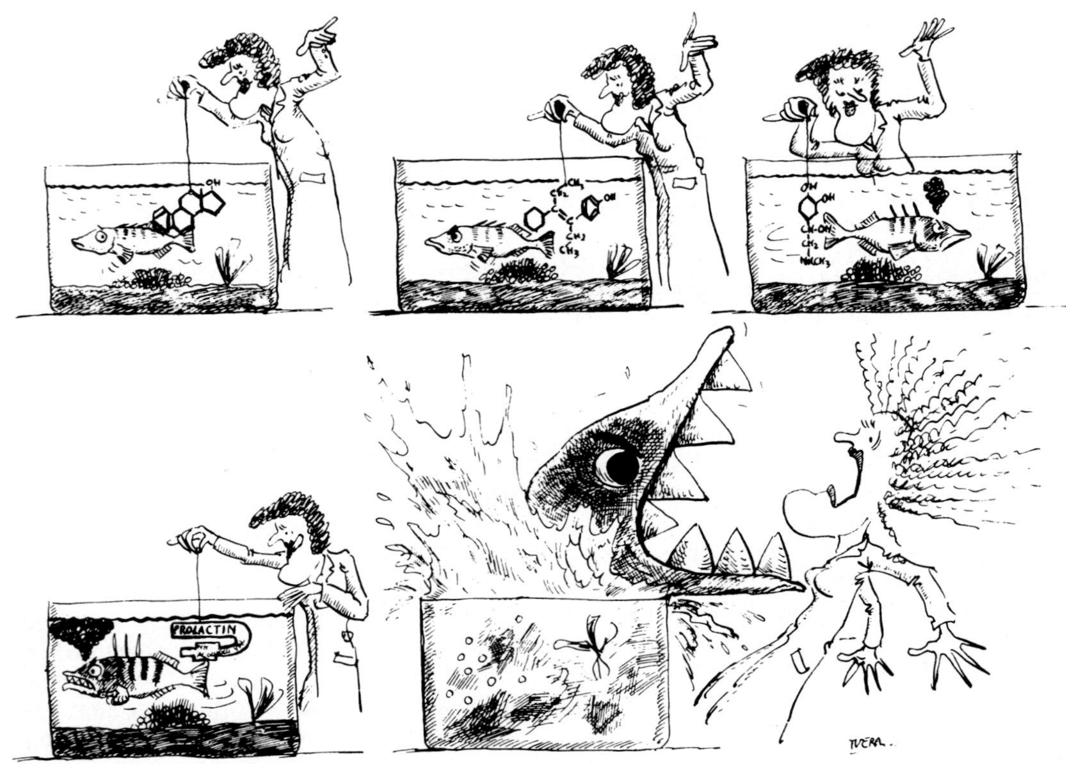

FIG. 18-4. Effects of hormones on fish behavior. (Courtesy of Mr. Frans Vera.)

tion, or they may be implicated in all three. In the ocean, gonadal maturation begins during the late spring, and the adults begin to move toward the appropriate estuaries. Extrapolation from studies with young fish suggests that gonadal hormones may affect general activity levels which would be a prerequisite for migration.[53,54] However, no cause-effect relationships have been established.

Prolactin levels as measured by a nonhomologous radioimmunoassay increase and remain elevated in sockeye salmon entering fresh water.[67] This increase is undoubtedly associated with the essential role for PRL in regulating osmo-ionic balance in fresh water (see Chap. 16). Growth hormone also increases in these same salmon, but the pattern of secretion is different and suggests a possible role in metabolism. These observations should be studied more thoroughly to confirm these results with homologous assays.

Migration in Urodele Amphibians

Migratory behavior in amphibians has not been studied extensively, although most zoologists are familiar with directed movements of anurans and urodeles associated with breeding. Seasonal migrations to water have been documented in detail for North American newts (*Taricha, Notophthalmus*) and for salamanders.[57,105,106] The water-drive behavior of *N. viridescens* was described briefly in Chapter 5 as it is employed in the red-eft bioassay for prolactin (PRL). Although most anuran and urodele migrations are either prenuptial or postbreeding events, the endocrine control of directed movements has been examined only in urodeles. In addition to the seasonal breeding and postbreeding migrations, also to be considered is the directed movement of immediate postmetamorphic juveniles away from their natal pond. Both postlarval and breeding migrations are usually associated with rainfall.[48]

Experimental studies on the migratory behavior of newts, *Taricha rivularis,* have verified that they exhibit accurate homing ability even when displaced considerable distances to strange areas.[106,107] Navigational abilities of amphibians have been reported with respect to sun-compass orientation, and the olfactory discrimination demonstrated for newts (Chap. 15) eventually may help to unravel the apparent mystery of their homing abilities.

The species to be discussed here all exhibit terrestrial juvenile forms that achieve sexual maturity and migrate back to their natal ponds for breeding purposes. Typically, individuals leave the pond following breeding and return to their terrestrial haunts until onset of the next breeding season. Eggs laid in these ponds develop into larvae that eventually undergo metamorphosis and migrate to land as juveniles.

Almost 40 years ago it was recognized that the migration of terrestrial red-spotted newts (efts)[36,85,86] and European newts[103] (*Triturus*) to water involved the pituitary hormone PRL and that water drive could be induced out of season with mammalian PRL and even by chorionic somatomammotropin.[11,32] Prolactin may induce an aquatic preference in juvenile tiger salamanders,[10] and locomotor activity is increased by PRL treatment of terrestrial-phase tiger salamanders. This induced activity may be a component of PRL-induced migratory behavior.[20] The locomotor component could be important in newts as well, since they may not remain submerged in a given pond to which they first migrate but wander in and out of several nearby ponds prior to "selecting" one in which to breed.[57] These data suggest that the migratory "water drive" involves first a type of premigratory restlessness and then induction of an aquatic preference.

The actions of exogenous PRL on water-drive behavior in newts (*N. viridescens*) depend upon when the hormone is administered.[74] The daily variation in responsiveness of the newt to PRL seems to be phased by the photoperiod operating through the production of corticosterone. The time of injecting corticosterone with respect to the time for PRL injection determines whether water-drive behavior can be induced. These results have important implications with respect to photoperiodic control of migratory behavior in urodeles, and additional studies in this direction are warranted.

Prolactin induces integumentary changes and stimulates production of mucus that is characteristic of the skin of aquatic-phase newts.[34,35] These changes are the reverse of those occurring during metamorphosis of larvae (see Chaps. 8, 17), and exogenous thyroid hormones can inhibit both the skin changes and behavioral changes attributed to PRL.[33,113] Thyroid hormones, in fact, stimulate shedding of the skin (molting) in urodeles.[60] Prolactin and androgens act synergistically in male newts to stimulate development of a number of sex accessory structures such as the nuptial pads and to cause an increase in the height of the tail,[15,111] which is employed by the male in courtship.[1,99]

Since landward migration of recently transformed urodeles is probably not controlled by PRL, the logical hormones to examine are those that are stimulatory with respect to metamorphosis, that is, thyrotropin and the thyroid hormones. Anurans invariably leave the water during or soon after metamorphosis as do many urodeles. In some urodeles, however, the metamorphosed animal may remain in the pond for an extended time. Indeed, in some populations of the tiger salamander, the metamorphosed animals may remain in the pond until ready to breed. Recently metamorphosed tiger salamanders exhibiting a preference for an aquatic medium show increased locomotor activity and eventually change to a dry-substrate preference following treatment with thyroxine (Fig. 18-5).[21] Furthermore, recently metamorphosed salamanders already exhibiting an endogenously determined dry-substrate preference have higher circulating levels of thyroxine than do others that exhibit an aquatic preference.[21] These data imply that both the movement of recently metamorphosed animals to land and the return of postbreeding animals to land involves an increase in thyroid function that induces locomotor activity and an eventual dry-substrate preference primarily through effects on the central nervous system.

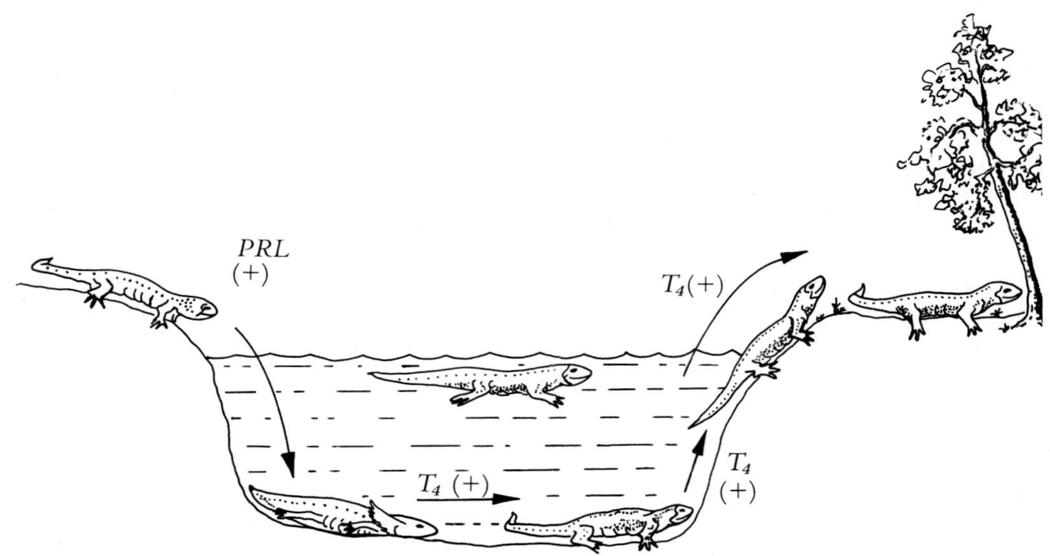

FIG. 18-5. Thyroid hormones and prolactin in the life history of urodele amphibians. Prolactin may be responsible for the migration of terrestrial adults to water for breeding, whereas thyroxine causes metamorphosis of larval offspring and may induce the landward migration of both newly metamorphosed and postbreeding salamanders. Once they are on land, thyroxine may be responsible for a long-term preference for a dry substrate.

Migration in Birds

Migration in north temperate avian species is one of the most dramatic and commonly observed animal behaviors involving precise orientation, directed movements over long distances and homing. The massive migrations that are characteristic of so many species occur twice annually and are closely timed to seasonal environmental factors. A northward migration associated with breeding occurs in the spring, and during the autumnal migration birds return to southerly wintering grounds. The reader should keep in mind that migratory behavior is extremely complex and may have evolved several times during avian phylogeny, and differences may exist in regulatory mechanisms and environmental factors directing the behavior.[6] For example, in comparison with long-distance migrants, short-distance and middle-distance migrants exhibit greater variability with respect to all aspects of migration.[7,42] Furthermore, spring migrations prior to breeding are considerably more synchronized than the fall postbreeding migrations for a given species.[84] Finally, even within a given species some populations may be migratory whereas others are sedentary.[6] A generalized accounting follows to provide a framework for discussion and to stress the common features among the species studied. This account will not include local nomadic movements that are related primarily to availability of food and water and will emphasize long-distance migrations.

Migratory Behavior

Migratory behavior can be separated into premigratory, migratory and postmigratory phases, but the discussion here centers around the premigratory phase since it is the only aspect that has been linked to endocrine phenomena. During the premigratory phase, a period of *premigratory fattening* occurs that involves selective deposition of fat into peritoneal and subcutaneous regions. These fat deposits provide energy stores to be utilized during actual migration. The duration of the fattening period and the quantity of fat deposited are correlated with the relative length of the migratory route. Associated with fattening is the appearance of premigratory restlessness or *Zugunruhe* that is most readily observed in caged birds. This behavior involves hyperactivity (hopping, fluttering) and is presumed to be evidence for a "desire" to begin the migration. At least it would increase the probability of coming in contact with other stimuli that would initiate the directed flight behavior. The relationship of premigratory fattening to Zugunruhe is not clear since some species exhibit Zugunruhe under experimental conditions without prior or coincident fattening.[6,63] In at least some species the initial phases of testicular or ovarian growth (recrudescence) in repeat migrants may take place during the spring migratory period, although the most dramatic gonadal growth occurs after the birds arrive at the breeding grounds. No gonadal development is taking place in fall migrants, however, and the gonads of these birds are in a quiescent (refractory ?) phase. Furthermore, premigratory fattening may not be obvious in fall migrants.[59] It is not clear whether Zugunruhe induces fattening in response to increased energy demands produced by the restless behavior or whether both fattening and Zugunruhe occur simultaneously in response to environmental and endocrine factors.

Environmental, Genetic and Endocrine Factors

The interest in environmental factors and endocrine mechanisms controlling avian migrations began with the classical experiments of Rowan on slate-colored juncos.[90] He demonstrated that artificially increasing the light portion (photophase) of the photoperiod induced precocious gonadal recrudescence, and the birds exhibited certain migratory behaviors out of season. Many studies have since demonstrated that long photoperiods and low light intensities induce premigratory fattening, precocious gonadal development and Zugunruhe and that low temperatures may reduce or block these responses in certain species.[6] One of the most elegant studies involved placing optical (light conducting) fibers into the brains of white-crowned sparrows.[116] It is not clear whether long photoperiods activate endocrine mechanisms or whether the length of the photophase acts as an external timing signal or *Zeitgeber* to regulate some endogenous timing mechanism that is in turn responsible for premigratory and migratory events. The annual (circannual) rhythmicity for the onset of premigratory and migratory behaviors is often difficult to tie directly with photoperiodic events, however. For example, birds may depart at precisely the same time each year from equatorial winter quarters where photic conditions exhibit little variation, and postbreeding migrants frequently depart for winter quarters long before adverse environmental conditions occur. There is, however, evidence for internal (genetically determined) factors that control migratory behavior in some species.[6] For example, a number of warbler species exhibit circannual rhythms in molting, fattening, Zugunruhe and gonadal development although maintained under constant laboratory conditions.

Long photoperiods may stimulate PRL release through stimulation of the hypothalamic center controlling PRL release. (The reader should recall that PRL release in birds is normally under stimulatory hypothalamic control; see Chap. 4.) Premigratory fattening and Zugunruhe are stimulated in migratory sparrows (*Zonotrichia* spp.) by treatment with mammalian PRL, and pituitary PRL levels are higher in migrants than in nonmigrants.[70–73,75] One possible mechanism for endocrine regulation of premigratory behavior involves the stimulation by light to release gonadotropin-releasing hormone (GnRH) from the hypothalamus, resulting in the eventual release of gonadal steroids into the blood (Fig. 18-6).[100] These steroid hormones (androgens, estrogens or both) would induce release of PRL indirectly (see Chap. 11) and indirectly cause fattening and Zugunruhe associated with the spring migration. However, the fall migration would have to occur in the absence of gonadal hormones since the avian gonads are quiescent at that time.

Prolactin and corticosteroid secretory patterns differ seasonally, and the actions of PRL on fattening can be altered by changing the phase of corticosteroids with respect to peak PRL levels.[75,96] Thus hypothalamic control of PRL and ACTH release could be the key to induction of physiological and behavioral premigratory events.

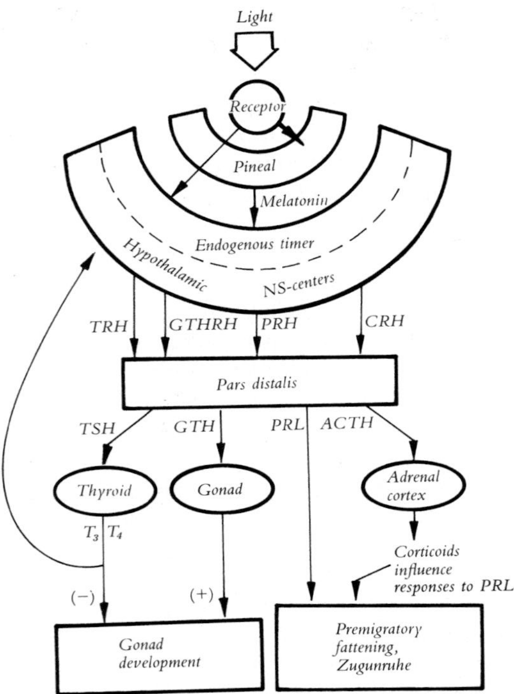

FIG. 18-6. Endocrine factors in bird migration. This diagram is an attempt to summarize the known relationships among the many endocrine glands and the influence of light on migration. See text for explanation.

Thyroid activity exhibits a positive correlation with migratory behavior in some species but not in others.[31,114] Some of the negative reports could be related to methods employed to ascertain thyroid state. Nevertheless, it seems unlikely that thyroid hormones perform any initiative roles in migratory behavior except through permissive actions such as those described in Chapter 8. Of particular importance for migratory behavior might be effects on the central nervous system that would increase the sensitivity of receptors for certain environmental cues.

Whenever an event involving hypothalamic activity and an influence of photoperiodic stimuli is considered, a possible role for the pineal complex is inevitably suggested (see Chap. 15). The pineal gland of house sparrows (*Passer domesticus*) has been demonstrated to be an essential regulator of circadian rhythms in body temperature.[30,104] Furthermore, pinealectomy inhibits testicular recrudescence in male domestic ducks and female Japanese quail.[9,93] Although the last two species are not migratory, these observations establish the pineal gland as a potential factor capable of influencing photoperiodic premigratory activities. Pinealectomy of captive white-crowned sparrows abolishes the circadian rhythmicity of Zugenruhe in both fall and spring birds, confirming a role for the pineal as a mediator of photoperiodic information at least in this species.[68]

Summary

Although there are many differences among the animals discussed in this chapter, a few generalizations may still be drawn concerning migratory behavior and its endocrine control. The seasonal appearance of premigratory events seems to be controlled by endogenous clocks that are entrained by external environmental factors (Zeitgebers), especially photoperiod. The premigratory phase is associated with deposition of energy stores (fat) and a period of increased activity (Zugunruhe). Furthermore, a general increase in the sensitivity of the nervous system may be involved here. Premigratory restlessness would seem to increase the opportunity for an individual to experience a greater range of stimuli than would a sedentary creature, and consequently a unique behavior (migration) may be initiated.

In both salmonid fishes and birds that migrate long distances some migrations are related to breeding, and most of the gonadal development occurs after they reach the breeding areas. In amphibians, however, sexual maturity and breeding conditions have been attained prior to migration. Only in the last case would it seem reasonable to ascribe a possible involvement of gonadal hormones in breeding migrations. The migration of juvenile salmonids and amphibians involves a change in body form and function (metamorphosis) in both; it is primarily related to the acquisition of new habitats. Even birds exhibit a change of dress prior to migration, although molting has not been implicated directly in migratory behavior.

The endocrine aspects of vertebrate migration are rather poorly known, and the possible role of thyroid hormones as permissive agents seems to be the only consistant relationship.

The possible actions of thyroid hormones on the nervous system may be of special importance.

Smolt transformation and seaward migration in salmonids is accompanied by increases in thyroid and interrenal (adrenocortical) activity, but if there is an initiating endocrine factor, it has not yet been identified. Rather it appears that the hormones examined only influence the responsiveness of the animal to certain environmental stimuli. Premigratory restlessness (Zugunruhe ?) is an obvious component of premigratory salmonids in freshwater. The endocrine control of the spawning runs is not well understood. The hypertrophied thyroids and interrenals of migrants attest to the demands migration places on the physiology of these fishes, and thyroid hormones may influence the acuity of olfactory receptors. Gonadal development and associated morphological changes observed in spawning animals do not occur until after these animals have entered fresh water; gonadal hormones probably do not initiate the migration. Prolactin might be involved as it is in amphibian and avian prebreeding migrations.

Recently metamorphosed salamanders exhibit increased locomotor activity (Zugunruhe ?) related to thyroid hormone treatment, and preference for a dry substrate appears to be induced by thyroid hormones. The emergence of juvenile anurans from ponds following metamorphosis may also be a response to the surge of thyroid hormones responsible for metamorphosis. The return to water in urodeles seems to involve a directed movement and preference for immersion in an aquatic substrate. Increased locomotor activity seems to be an important component as well. The water-directed migration of urodeles is stimulated by PRL, and similar hormonal relationships could be expected in anurans. Thyroid hormones may also play a permissive or enhancing role in PRL-stimulated water-drive behavior.

Avian premigratory restlessness (Zugunruhe) and fattening are induced by PRL, possibly in relation to the pattern of corticosteroid secretion. Thyroid hormones probably play permissive roles, and gonadal steroids could be important in the prebreeding migrations of some species.

References

1. Arnold, S.J. (1977). The evolution of courtship behavior in New World salamanders with some comments on Old World salamanders. In D.H. Taylor and S.I. Guttman, eds., The Reproductive Biology of Amphibians. Plenum Press, New York, pp. 141–184.

2. Baggerman, B. (1957). An experimental study on the timing and breeding and migration in the three-spined stickleback (*Gasterosteus aculeatus* L.) Arch. Neerl. Zool. 12:105–317.

3. Baggerman, B. (1963). The effect of TSH and antithyroid substances on salinity preference and thyroid activity in juvenile Pacific salmon. Can. J. Zool. 41:307–319.

4. Baraduc, M.M. (1954). Influence de la thyroxinisation de jeunes truites arc-en-ciel (*Salmo gairdneri*) sur la teneur en lipides viscéraux et periviscеraux. C. R. Acad. Sci. 238:728–730.

5. Baraduc, M.M. and M. Fontaine (1955). Etude comparée du métabolisme respiratoire de jeune saumon sédentaire (parr) et migrateur (smolt). C. R. Soc. Biol. 149:1327–1329.

6. Berthold, P. (1975). Migration: control and metabolic physiology. In D.S. Farner and J.R. King, eds., Avian Biology. Academic Press, New York, Vol. 5, pp. 77–128.

7. Berthold, P., E. Gwinner, H. Klein and P. Westrich (1972). Cited by Berthold.[6]

8. Binkley, S., E. Kluth and M. Menaker (1971). Pineal function in sparrows: Circadian rhythms and body temperature. Science 174:311–314.

9. Cardinali, D.P., A.E. Cuello, J.H. Tramezzani and J.M. Rosner (1971). Effects of pinealectomy on the testicular function of the adult male duck. Endocrinology 89:1082–1093.

10. Carl, G. (1975). Effect of prolactin on aquatic preference in the tiger salamander, *Ambystoma tigrinum.* J. Colo.-Wyo. Acad. Sci. 7:40–41.

11. Chadwick, C.S. (1941). Further observations on the water drive in *Triturus viridescens.* II. Induction of the water drive with the lactogenic hormone. J. Exp. Zool. 86:175–187.

12. Clarke, W.C. and J.E. Shelbourn (1977). Effect of temperature, photoperiod, and salinity on growth and smolting of underyearling coho salmon. Am. Zool. 17:957.

13. Conte, F.P. and H.H. Wagner (1965). Development of osmotic and ionic regulation in juvenile steelhead trout *Salmo gairdneri.* Comp. Biochem. Physiol. 14:603–620.

14. Cooper, J.C. and A.D. Hasler (1974). Evidence for retention of olfactory cues in homing coho salmon. Science 183:336–338.

15. Dent, J.N. (1975). Integumentary effects of prolactin in lower vertebrates. Am. Zool. 15:923–935.

16. Dickhoff, W.W., L.C. Folmar and A. Gorbman (1978). Changes in plasma thyroxine during smoltification of coho salmon, *Oncorhynchus kisutch.* Gen. Comp. Endocrinol. 36:229–232.

17. Dickhoff, W.W., L.C. Folmar, J.L. Mighell, and C.V.W. Mahnken (1982). Plasma thyroid hormones during smoltification of yearling and underyearling coho salmon and yearling chinook salmon and steelhead trout. Aquaculture 28:39–48.

18. Doving, K.B., R. Selset and G. Thommesen (1980). Olfactory sensitivity to bile acids in salmonid fishes. Acta. Physiol. Scand. 108:123–131.

19. Dusseau, J.W. and A.H. Meier (1971). Diurnal and seasonal variations of plasma corticosterone in the white-throated sparrow *Zonotrichia albicollis.* Gen. Comp. Endocrinol. 16:399–408.

20. Duvall, D. and D.O. Norris (1977). Prolactin and substrate stimulation of locomotor activity in adult tiger salamanders (*Ambystoma tigrinum*). J. Exp. Zool. 200:103–106.

21. Duvall, D. and D.O. Norris (1980). Stimulation of dry-substrate preference and locomotor activity in newly transformed tiger salamanders (*Ambystoma tigrinum*) by exogenous or endogenous thyroxine. Anim. Behav. 28:116–123.

22. Eales, J.G. (1965). Factors influencing seasonal changes in thyroid activity in juvenile steelhead trout, *Salmo gairdneri.* Can. J. Zool. 43:719–729.

23. Elson, P.F. (1957). The importance of size in the change from parr to smolt in Atlantic salmon. Can. Fish. Cult. 21:1–6.

24. Evropeytseva, N.V. (1959). Transformation to smolt stage and downstream migration of young salmon. Fish. Res. Board Can. Trans. Ser. No. 234, 36 pp.

25. Evropeytseva, N.V. (1960). Correlation between the processes of early gonad ripening and transformation of the seaward-migrating stage among male Baltic salmon (*Salmo salar* L.) held in ponds. Fish. Res. Board Can. Trans. Ser. No. 430, 5 pp.

26. Fontaine, M. and J. Hatey (1950). Variations de la teneur du foie en glycogène chez le jeune saumon (*Salmo salar* L.) au cours de la "smoltification." C. R. Soc. Biol. 144:953–955.

27. Fontaine, M. and J. Hatey (1954). Sur la teneur in 17-hydroxycorticostéroides du plasma de saumon (*Salmo salar* L.). C. R. Acad. Sci. 239:319–321.

28. Fontaine, M. and J. Leloup (1959). Influence de la nage a contre-courant le métabolisme de l'iode et le fonctionnement thyroïdien chez la truite arc-en-ciel (*Salmo gairdnerii* Rich.). C. R. Acad. Sci. 249:343–347.

29. Fontaine, M. and J. Leloup (1962). Le fonctionnement thyroïdien du saumon adulte (*Salmo salar* L.) a quelques etapes de son cycle migratoire. Gen. Comp. Endocrinol. 2:317–322.

30. Gaston, S. and M. Menaker (1968). Pineal function: The biological clock of the sparrow. Science 160:1125–1127.

31. George, J.C. and D.V. Naik (1964). Cyclic changes in the thyroid of the migratory starling, *Sturnus roseus* (Linnaeus), Pavo 2:37–49.

32. Gona, O. and A.G. Gona (1973). Action of human placental lactogen on second metamorphosis in the newt *Notophthalmus viridescens.* Gen. Comp. Endocrinol. 21:377–380.

33. Grant, W.C., Jr. (1961). Special aspects of the metamorphic process: second metamorphosis. Am. Zool. 1:163–171.

34. Grant, W.C. Jr. and G. Cooper IV (1964). Endocrine control of metamorphic and skin changes in *Diemictylus viridescens.* Am. Zool. 4:413–414.

35. Grant, W.C. Jr. and G. Cooper IV (1965). Behavioral and integumentary changes associated with induced metamorphosis in *Diemictylus.* Biol. Bull. 129:510–522.

36. Grant, W.C. Jr. and J.A. Grant (1956). The induction of water drive in the land stage of *Triturus viridescens* following hypophysectomy. Anat. Rec. 125:604.

37. Grau, E.G., W.W. Dickhoff, R.S. Nishioka, H.A. Bern and L.C. Folmar (1981). Lunar phasing of the thyroxine surge preparatory to seaward migration of salmonid fish. Science 211:607–609.

38. Grau, E.G., J.L. Specker, R.S. Nishioka and H.A. Bern (1982). Factors determining the occurrence of the surge in thyroid activity in salmon during smoltification. Aquaculture 28:49–57.

39. Gribanov, V.I. (1962). The coho salmon (*Oncorhynchus kisutch* Walbaum)—a biological sketch. Fish. Res. Board Can. Trans. Ser. No. 370, 83 pp.

40. Groot, C. (1965). On the orientation of young sockeye salmon (*Oncorhynchus nerka*) during their seaward migration out of lakes. Behavior Suppl. 14:198.

41. Gudjonsson, T.V. (1946). Age and body length at time of seaward migration of immature steelhead trout (*Salmo gairdneri* Richardson) in Minter Creek, Washington. M.A. thesis, University of Washington.

42. Gwinner, E. (1972). Endogenous timing factors in bird migration. In S.R. Galler, K. Schmidt-Koenig, G.J. Jacobs and R.E. Belleville, eds., Animal Orientation and Navigation. NASA, Washington, pp. 321–338.

43. Hane, S., O.H. Robertson, B.C. Wexler and M.A. Krupp (1966). Adrenocortical response to stress and ACTH in Pacific salmon (*Oncorhynchus tshawytscha*) and steelhead trout (*Salmo gairdnerii*) at successive stages in the sexual cycle. Endocrinology 78:791–800.

44. Hara, T.J., K. Ueda and A. Gorbman (1965). Electroencephalographic studies of homing salmon. Science 149:884–885.

45. Harden Jones, F.R. (1968). Fish Migration. Arnold, London.

46. Hasler, A.D. (1966). Underwater Guideposts. University of Wisconsin Press, Madison.

47. Hasler, A.D., A.T. Scholz and R.M. Horall (1978). Olfactory imprinting and homing in salmon. Am. Scient. 66:347–355.

48. Healy, W.R. (1975). Breeding and postlarval migrations of the red-spotted newt, *Notophthalmus viridescens,* in Massachusetts. Ecology 56:637–680.

49. Hoar, W.S. (1939). The thyroid gland of the Atlantic salmon. J. Morphol. 65:257–295.

50. Hoar, W.S. (1951). Hormones in fish. Publ. Ont. Fish. Res. Lab. Biol. Stud. No. 71:1–51.

51. Hoar, W.S. (1976). Smolt transformation: evolution, behavior, and physiology. J. Fish. Res. Bd. Can. 33:1233–1252.

52. Hoar, W.S. and G.M. Bell (1950). The thyroid gland in relation to seaward migration of Pacific salmon. Can. J. Res. D 28:126–136.

53. Hoar, W.S., M.H. Keeleyside and R.G. Goodall (1955). The effects of thyroxine and gonadal steroids on the activity of salmon and goldfish. Can. J. Zool. 33:428–439.

54. Hoar, W.S., D. MacKinnon and A. Redlich (1952). Effects of some hormones on the behavior of salmon fry. Can. J. Zool. 30:273–286.

55. Holmes, W.N. and I.M. Stanier (1966). Studies on the renal excretion of electrolytes by the trout (*Salmo gairdneri*). J. Exp. Biol. 44:33–46.

56. Houston, A.H. (1960). Variations in the plasma level of chloride in hatchery-reared yearling Atlantic salmon during parr-smolt transformation and following transfer into sea water Nature 185:632–633.

57. Hurlburt, S.H. (1969). The breeding migrations and interhabitat wandering of the vermillion-spotted newt *Notophthalmus viridescens* (Rafinesque). Ecol. Monogr. 39:465–488.

58. Ito, J. (1964). Food and feeding habit of Pacific salmon (Genus *Oncorhynchus*) in their oceanic life. Bull. Hokkaido Reg. Fish. Res. Lab. No. 29:85–97.

59. Johnston, D.W. (1964). Ecological aspects of lipid deposition in some postbreeding arctic birds. Ecology 45:848–852.

60. Kaltenback, J.C. (1968). Nature of hormone action in amphibian metamorphosis. In W. Etkin and L.I. Gilbert, eds., Metamorphosis. Appleton-Century-Crofts, New York, pp. 399–442.

61. Koch, H.J. (1968). Migration. In E.J.W. Barrington and C.B. Jorgenson, eds. Perspectives in Endocrinology. Academic Press, New York, pp. 305–349.

62. Landgrebe, F.W. (1941). The role of the pituitary and the thyroid in the development of teleosts. J. Exp. Biol. 18:162–169.

63. Lofts, B., R.K. Murton and A. Wolfson (1963). The experimental demonstration of premigration activity in the absence of fat deposition in birds. Ibis 105:99–105.

64. Lovern, J.A. (1934). Fat metabolism in fishes. V. The fat of the salmon in its young freshwater stages. Biochem. 28:1961–1963.

65. McBride, J.R., U.H.M. Fagerlund, M. Smith and N. Tomlinson (1965). Postspawning death of Pacific salmon: Sockeye salmon (*Oncorhynchus nerka*) maturing and spawning in captivity. J. Fish. Res. Board Can. 22:775–782.

66. Mclnerney, J.F. (1964). Salinity preference: An orientation mechanism in salmon migration. J. Fish. Res. Board Can. 21:995–1018.

67. McKeown, B.A. and A.P. van Overbeeke (1972). Prolactin and growth hormone concentrations in the serum and pituitary gland of adult migratory sockeye salmon (*Oncorhynchus nerka*). J. Fish. Res. Board Can. 29:303–309.

68. McMillan, J.P. (1972). Pinealectomy abolishes the circadian rhythm of migratory restlessness. J. Comp. Physiol. 79:105–112.

69. Malikova, E.M. (1959). Biochemical analyses of young salmon at the time of their transformation to a condition close to the smolt stage and during retention of smolts in fresh water. Fish. Res. Board Can. Trans. Ser. No. 232, 19 pp.

70. Meier, A.H., J.T. Burns and J.W. Dusseau (1969). Seasonal variations in the diurnal rhythm of pituitary prolactin content in the white-throated sparrow, *Zonotrichia albicollis.* Gen. Comp. Endocrinol. 12:282–289.

71. Meier, A.H. and K.D. David (1967). Diurnal variations of the fattening response to prolactin in the white-throated sparrow, *Zonotrichia albicollis.* Gen. Comp. Endocrinol. 8:110–114.

72. Meier, A.H. and D.S. Farner (1964). A possible endocrine basis for premigratory fattening in *Zonotrichia leucophrys gambelii.* Gen. Comp. Endocrinol. 4:584–595.

73. Meier, A.H., D.S. Farner and J.R. King (1965). A possible endocrine basis for migratory behavior in *Zonotrichia leucophrys gambelii.* Anim. Behav. 13:453–465.

74. Meier, A.H., L.E. Garcia and M.M. Joseph (1971). Corticosterone phases a circadian water-drive response to prolactin in the spotted newt, *Notophthalmus viridescens.* Biol. Bull. 141:331–336.

75. Meier, A.H. and R. MacGregor III (1972). Temporal organization in avian reproduction. Am. Zool. 12:257–271.

76. Munz, F.W. and R.T. Swanson (1965). Thyroxine-induced changes in the proportions of visual pigments. Am. Zool. 5:683.

77. Nagahama, Y., S. Adachi, F. Tashiro and E.G. Grau (1982). Some endocrine factors affecting the development of seawater tolerance during the parr-smolt transformation of the amago salmon, *Oncorhynchus rhodurus*. Aquaculture 28:81–90.

78. Neave, F. (1964). Ocean migrations of Pacific salmon. J. Fish. Res. Board Can. 21:1227–1244.

79. Nishikawa, K., T. Hiroshima, S. Suzuki and M. Suzuki (1975). Changes in circulating L-thyroxine and L-triiodothyronine of the masu salmon, *Oncorhynchus masou* accompanying the smoltification, measured by radioimmunoassay. Endocrinol. Japon. 26:731–735.

80. Nordeng, H. (1977). A pheromone hypothesis for homeward migration in anadromous salmonids. Oikos 28:155–159.

81. Norris, D.O. (1966). Radiothyroidectomy in the salmonid fishes *Salmo gairdnerii* Richardson and *Oncorhynchus tshawytscha* Walbaum. Ph.D. thesis, University of Washington.

82. Olivereau, M. (1962). Modifications de l'interrenal du smolt (*Salmo salar* L.) au cours du passage d'eau douce en eau de mer. Gen. Comp. Endocrinol 2:565–573.

83. Oshima, K., A. Gorbman and H. Shimada (1969). Memory-blocking agents: Effects on olfactory discrimination in homing salmon. Science 165:86–88.

84. Preston, F.W. (1966). The mathematical representation of migration. Ecology 47:375–392.

85. Reinke, E.E. and C.S. Chadwick (1939). Inducing land stage of *Triturus viridescens* to assume water habitat by pituitary implants. Proc. Soc. Exp. Biol. Med. 40:691–693.

86. Reinke, E.E. and C.S. Chadwick (1940). The origin of the water drive in *Triturus viridescens*. Induction of water drive in the thyroidectomized and gonadectomized land phases by pituitary implantations. J. Exp. Zool. 83:223–233.

87. Robertson, O.H. (1949). Production of the silvery smolt stage in rainbow trout by intramuscular injection of mammalian thyroid extract and by thyrotropic hormone. J. Exp. Zool. 110:337–355.

88. Robertson, O.H., M.A. Krupp, C.B. Favour, S. Hane and S.F. Thomas (1961). Physiological changes occurring in the blood of Pacific salmon (*Oncorhynchus tshawytscha*) accompanying sexual maturation and spawning. Endocrinology 68:733–746.

89. Robertson, O.H. and B.C. Wexler (1959). Hyperplasia of adrenal cortical tissue in Pacific salmon (genus *Oncorhynchus*) and rainbow trout (*Salmo gairdneri*) accompanying sexual maturation and spawning. Endocrinology 65:225–238.

90. Rowan, W. (1925). Relation of light to bird migration and developmental change. Nature 115:494–495.

91. Salthe, S.N. and J.S. Mecham (1974). Reproductive and courtship patterns. In B. Lofts, ed., Physiology of the Amphibia. Academic Press, New York, Vol. 2, pp. 310–522.

92. Saunders, R.L. and E.B. Henderson (1965). Precocious sexual development in male post-smolt Atlantic salmon reared in the laboratory. J. Fish. Res. Board Can. 22:1567–1570.

93. Sayler, A. and A. Wolfson (1967). Avian pineal gland: Progonadotropic response in the Japanese quail. Science 158:1478–1479.

94. Scholz, A.T., R.M. Horrall, J.C. Cooper and A.D. Hasler (1976). Imprinting to chemical cues: The basis for home stream selection in salmon. Science 192:1247–1249.

95. Selset R. and K.B. Doving (1980). Behavior of mature anadromous char (*Salmo alpinus* L.) towards odorants produced by smolts of their own population. Acta. Physiol. Scand. 108:113–122.

96. Shapovalov, L. and A.C. Taft (1954). The life histories of the steelhead trout (*Salmo gairdneri gairdneri*) and silver salmon (*Oncorhynchus kisutch*) with special reference to Waddell Creek, California and recommendations regarding their management. State of Calif. Fish. Bull. 98.

97. Smirnov, A.I. (1959). Functional significance of the prespawning changes in the integument of the salmon (with particular reference to the genus *Oncorhynchus*). Zool. Zh. No. 5. Cited by Nikolsky, G.V., The Ecology of Fishes, Academic Press, New York, p. 166.

98. Specker, J.L., J.J. DiStefano III, E.G. Grau, R. Nishioka and H.A. Bern (1984). Development-associated changes in throxine kinetics in juvenile salmon. Endocrinology, in press.

99. Specker, J.L. and C.B. Schreck (1982). Changes in plasma corticosteroids during smoltification of coho salmon, *Oncorhynchus kisutch*. Gen. Comp. Endocrinol. 46:53–58.

100. Stetson, M. and J.E. Erickson (1972). Hormonal control of photoperiodically induced fat deposition in white-crowned sparrows. Gen. Comp. Endocrinol. 19:355–362.

101. Svard, P.O. (1958). Acid-soluble nucleotides from the blood of metamorphosing salmon. Nature 182:1448–1449.

102. Tchernavin, V.C. (1943). The breeding characters of salmon in relation to their size. Proc. Zool. Soc. Lond. B113:206–232.

103. Tuchmann-Duplessis, H. (1949). Action de l'hormone gonadotrope et lactogene sur le comportment and les caracteres seuels secondaires du Triton nor-

mal et castre. Arch. Anat. Microsc. Morphol. Exp. 38:302–317.

104. Turek, F.W., J.P. McMillan and M. Menaker (1976). Melatonin: Effects of the circadian locomotor rhythm of sparrows. Science 194:1441–1443.

105. Twitty, V.C. (1941). Data on the life history of *Ambystoma tigrinum californiense* Gray. Copeia 1941:1–3.

106. Twitty, V., D. Grant and O. Anderson (1966). Course and timing of the homing migration in the newt *Taricha rivularis.* Proc. Natl. Acad. Sci. 56:864–871.

107. Twitty, V., D. Grant and O. Anderson (1967). Home range in relation to homing in the newt *Taricha rivularis* (Amphibia: Caudata). Copeia 1967:649–653.

108. Ueda, K., T.J. Hara and A. Gorbman (1967). Electroencephalographic studies on olfactory discrimination in adult spawning salmon. Comp. Biochem. Physiol. 21:133–143.

109. Vanstone, W.E. and F.C.-W. Ho (1960). Plasma proteins of coho salmon, *Oncorhynchus kitsutch,* as separated by zone electrophoresis. J. Fish. Res. Board Can. 18:393–399.

110. Vanstone, W.E., E. Roberts and H. Tsuyaki (1964). Changes in the multiple hemoglobin patterns of some Pacific salmon, Genus *Oncorhynchus,* during the parr-smolt transformation. Can. J. Physiol. Pharmacol. 42:697–704.

111. Vellano, C. (1972). Un nuovo metado per il dosaggio biologico della prolattina. Boll. Soc. Ital. Biol. Sper. 48:360–362.

112. Wagner, H.H. (1974). Photoperiod and temperature regulation of smolting in steelhead trout (*Salmo gairdneri*). Can. J. Zool. 52:219–234.

113. Wald, G. (1981). Metamorphosis: an overview. In L.I. Gilbert and E. Frieden (eds.), Metamorphosis: A Problem in Developmental Biology, 2nd ed. Plenum Press, New York, pp. 1–39.

114. Wilson, A.C. and D.S. Farner (1960). The annual cycle of thyroid activity in white-crowned sparrows of eastern Washington. Condor 62:414–425.

115. Woodhead, A.C. and P.M.J. Woodhead (1965). Seasonal changes in the physiology of the Barents Sea cod, *Gadus morhua* L., in relation to its environment. I. Endocrine changes particularly affecting migration and maturation. ICNAF Spec. Publ. 6:692–715.

116. Yokoyama, K. and D.S. Farner (1978). Induction of *Zugenruhe* by photostimulation of encephalic receptors in white-crowned sparrows. Science 201:76–79.

19·Endocrine Regulation of Metabolism in Mammals

Metabolism is the total of enzyme catalyzed chemical reactions that are involved in maintaining the structure and functions of an organism. Complex molecules can be constructed from simple building blocks: simple sugars, amino acids, fatty acids and nucleotides. Conversely, complex molecules (proteins, triglycerides, polysaccharides) can be degraded to provide building blocks for synthesis of other complex molecules. The ultimate energy source for all activities of any organism is that stored in chemical bonds. Simple sugars can be degraded to carbon dioxide and water, releasing energy that can be used to drive other processes.

It should not be surprising to learn that essential interconversions of carbohydrates, lipids and proteins as well as the consumption of simple sugars for energy are regulated by hormones. Abnormal metabolism is responsible for the overt symptoms of many endocrine disorders, and by far the most common disorder, diabetes mellitus, is caused by a deficiency in a metabolic hormone, insulin.

Maintenance of any organism involves utilization of energy derived from hydrolysis of chemical bonds. Carbohydrates represent the most immediate energy source for synthesis of adenosine triphosphate (ATP) or other high-energy reserves (such as guanosine triphosphate (GTP) or creatine phosphate). In mammals as in other vertebrates, glucose is the primary carbohydrate energy source. All of the cell's machinery for energy production (oxidative metabolism) relies on hydrolysis of chemical bonds in glucose and glucose metabolites. Glucose and its intermediates may be utilized as precursors in the synthesis of many other essential molecules, including lipids of all sorts, proteins and nucleic acids. It is possible to convert other molecules (amino acids, glycerol, lactate) to glucose, which can be used in the synthesis of ATP or other compounds as needed. Production of glucose from amino acids, glycerol or lactate is termed *gluconeogenesis.*

The major tissues involved in oxidative metabolism in mammals are liver, muscle, fat, nervous and kidney cortex. In addition, red blood cells, the kidney medulla and the testes have low oxidative capacities and produce lactate through anaerobic respiration. Lactate is released into the blood and must be metabolized by other tissues (primarily liver and kidney cortex). Each tissue performs highly specialized functions, and the generalized metabolic schemes for metabolism are modified for the special requirements of each tissue.

Many differences exist in the oxidative and synthetic processes that occur in different tissues, and it is important to understand these differences before discussing endocrine regulatory mechanisms that operate in the intact organism. The homeostasis of energy metabolism can only be appreciated fully when one is aware of the roles played by these tissues as they are influenced by diet, starvation and muscular work. The principal ways in which muscle, liver, adipose tissue and brain metabolism relate to carbohydrate, lipid and protein stores will be examined, as will their regulation under different physiological conditions.

Dietary differences determine to a considerable extent the endogenous mechanisms for metabolic homeostasis. Carnivores eat other organisms that consist primarily of protein and absorb principally amino acids from the gut as well as lesser amounts of fatty acids, glycerol and monosaccharides. Herbivores such as the ruminants have a bacterial flora in their guts that digests cellulose to glucose. The bacteria metabolize glucose and produce a variety of compounds for their own use as well as by-products such as short-chain fatty acids. Fatty acids and amino acids constitute the major oxidative substrates absorbed by the ruminant. Omnivores, such as ourselves, obtain a greater proportion of carbohydrates in their diets than do either carnivores or ruminants. The proportions of carbohydrates, proteins and lipids vary from meal to meal in human diets. The composition of metabolites in hepatic portal blood of animals with these varied diets places different demands on the regulatory mechanisms that must be employed in utilization, conversion, excretion and storage processes.

In this chapter general aspects of hormonal influence on carbohydrate, lipid and protein metabolism under differing physiological conditions are considered.

Intermediary Metabolism

The complete pathway for carbohydrate-based energy metabolism is the oxidation of glucose to CO_2 and water, yielding a net increase in ATP. Complete oxidation of glucose involves *glycolysis,* the *tricarboxylic acid* (TCA) or *citric acid cycle* and the *electron transport chain.* Generally glycolysis involves stepwise conversion in the cytosol of the six-carbon glucose molecule to two three-carbon intermediates known as pyruvate (Fig. 19-2). A small quantity of ATP is produced by oxidation of glucose to pyruvate. An alternative pathway by which glucose may be oxidized is the *pentose phosphate pathway* (Fig. 19-3), which is

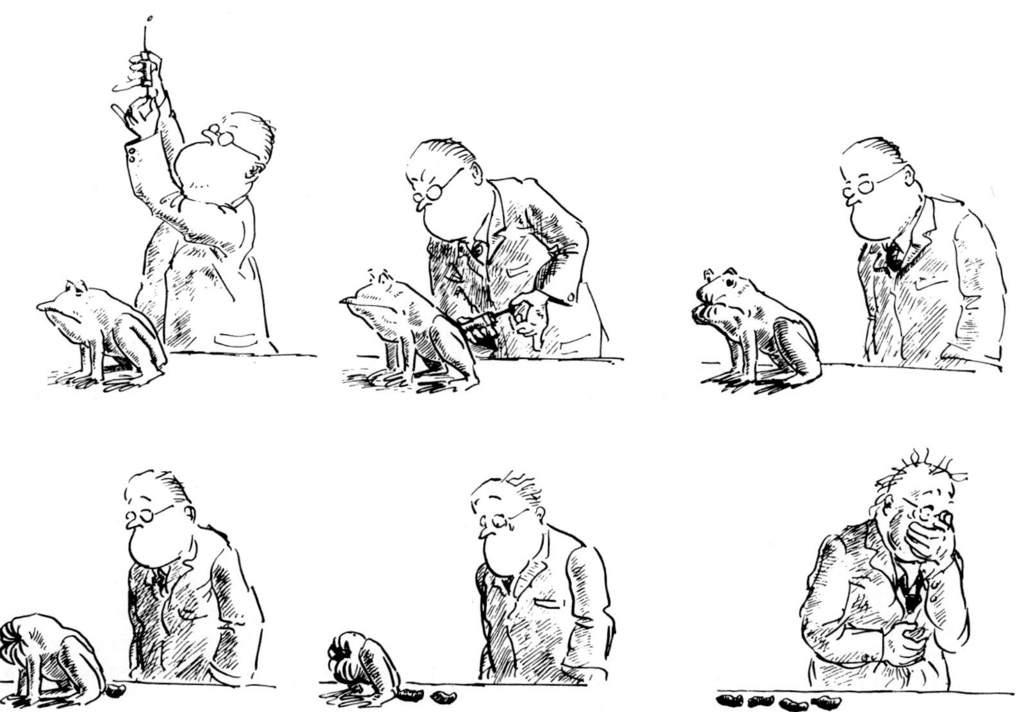

Fɪɢ. 19-1. Endocrine control of metabolism. (Courtesy of Mr. Frans Vera.)

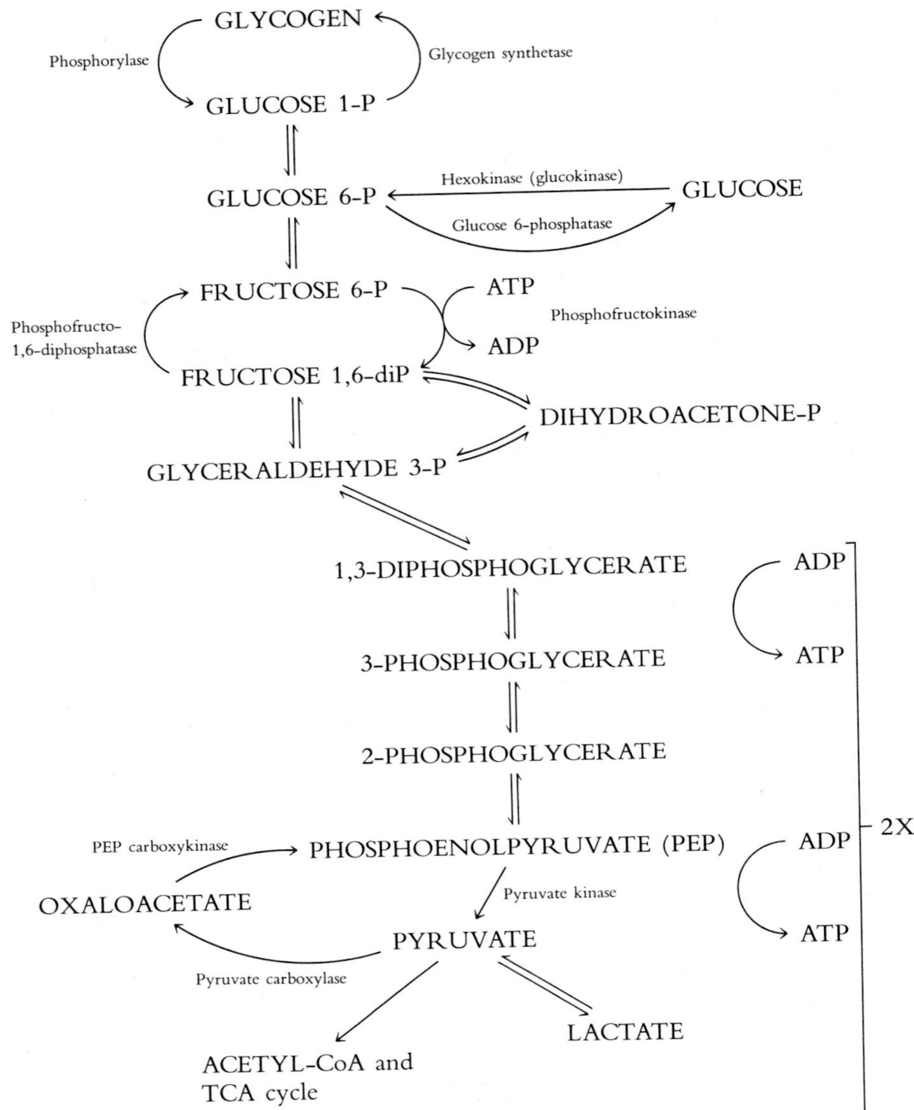

FIG. 19-2. Glycolysis. This scheme summarizes the steps in glucose oxidation through the Embden-Meyerhof pathway. Only those enzymes responsible for regulatory steps are indicated. *P*, phosphate.

closely linked to lipid synthesis. This pathway metabolizes about 30% of the glucose oxidized in the liver cell and provides reduced compounds (NADPH) necessary for fatty acid synthesis, for inactivation of steroids (see Chap. 9) and for drug detoxification. Some of the pentose sugar produced may be utilized for ribose and deoxyribose synthesis and in formation of nucleotides for later incorporation into nucleic acids. In the TCA cycle (Fig. 19-4), pyruvate enters the mitochondrion where it is oxidized to CO_2 and acetate in the form of acetylcoenzyme A (acetyl-CoA). Acetyl-CoA is further oxidized to yield more CO_2 and a quantity of special reduced compounds (such as NADH). Electrons are transferred from these reduced compounds sequentially through a chain of electron acceptor-donor molecules

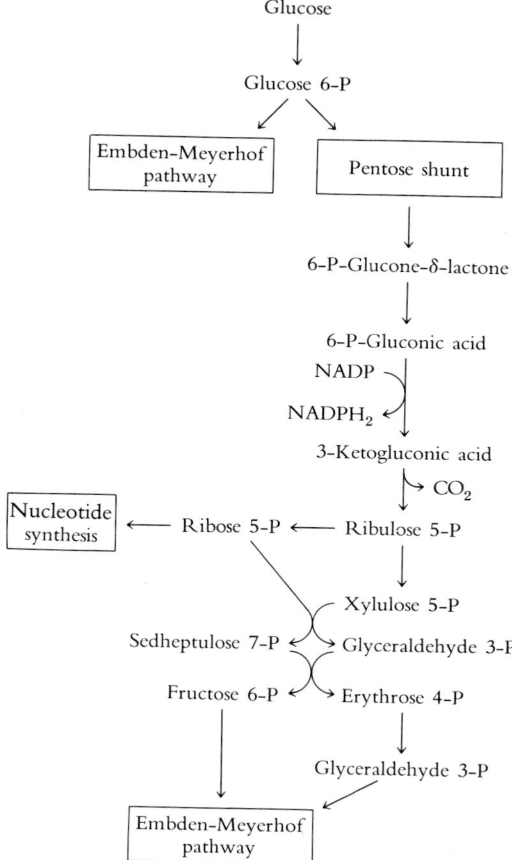

FIG. 19-3. Major steps in the pentose shunt. This is an alternate pathway for glucose oxidation resulting in a return to the Embden-Meyerhof pathway via glyceraldehyde 3-P and fructose 6-P. The pentose shunt generates sugars for nucleotide synthesis and reduced hydrogen donors ($NADPH_2$) for lipogenesis.

Glycolysis

There are three limiting steps in glycolysis (Fig. 19-2), each of which is catalyzed by a unidirectional enzyme (that is, the reaction may be catalyzed only in one direction because of thermodynamic considerations). Free glucose enters a cell by facilitated diffusion but cannot be utilized by that cell until it has been phosphorylated. This step is catalyzed by a unidirectional enzyme, *hexokinase* (most tissues) or *glucokinase* (liver). Phosphorylated glucose may be polymerized and stored as glycogen *(glycogenesis),* which constitutes a temporary reserve of glucose within the cell, or it may undergo glycolysis (including the pentose phosphate pathway). Hydrolysis of glycogen *(glycogenolysis)* is accomplished by the enzyme complex known as the *phosphorylase* system. The events in glycogenesis and glycogenolysis are summarized in Figure 19-6.

The second limiting step in glucose metabolism involves the unidirectional enzyme *phosphorylase fructokinase* (PFK), which is responsible for converting fructose 6-phosphate (derived directly from glucose 6-phosphate) to fructose 1,6-diphosphate. This step is essentially irreversible and commits the cell to oxidize glucose to pyruvate. The presence of substrate (fructose 6-phosphate) activates PFK, and this reaction is considered to be the major rate-limiting step in glycolysis.

The final limiting step in glycolysis is the irreversible conversion of phosphoenol pyruvate (PEP) to pyruvate by the enzyme *pyruvate kinase.* Sufficient energy is released upon hydrolysis of PEP to synthesize ATP directly.

known as the electron transport chain (Fig. 19-5). At each transfer, an electron drops to a lower energy state while releasing a small quantity of energy, some of which can be trapped in the synthesis of ATP. The final electron acceptor is oxygen (O_2), which, when reduced by acceptance of electrons, forms water. If oxygen is not available (i.e., under anaerobic conditions), this sequence is altered by conversion of pyruvate to lactate (Fig. 19-2). Neither the TCA cycle nor the electron transport chain of the mitochondrion functions under anaerobic conditions.

The Tricarboxylic Acid Cycle and Electron Transport

The TCA cycle is regulated primarily through the availability of acetate for combining with coenzyme A to yield acetyl-CoA. Either glycolysis through pyruvate or oxidation of fatty acids (see below) provides acetyl-CoA for TCA-cycle metabolism. The availability of certain TCA-cycle intermediates such as oxaloacetate may also influence operation of the TCA cycle. Such intermediates may be synthesized from amino acids (see gluconeogenesis). Utilization of the reduced compounds (for ex-

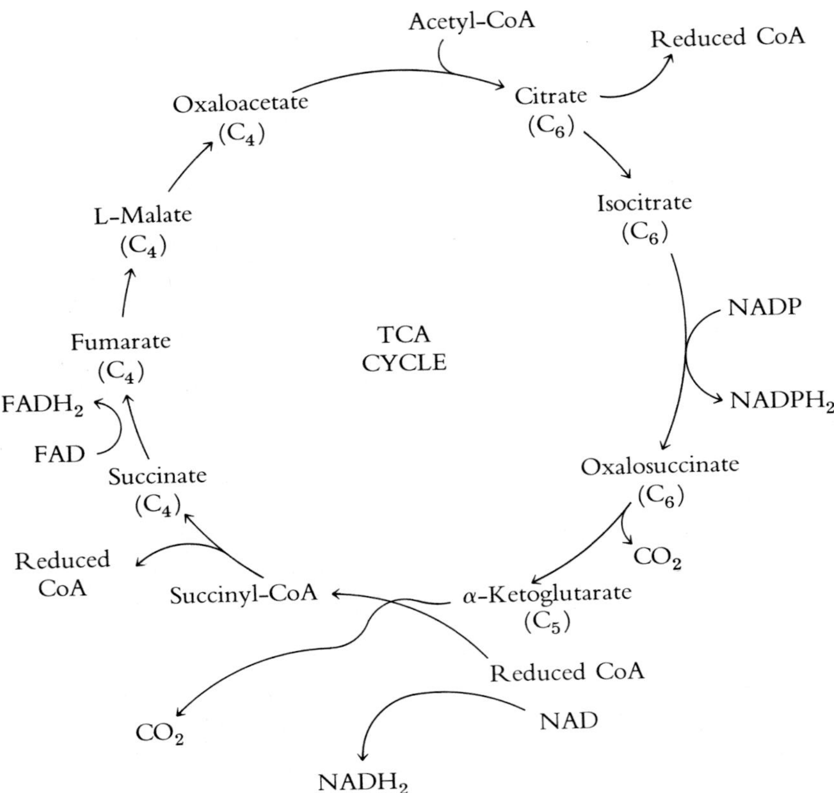

Fig. 19-4. The tricarboxylic acid *(TCA)* cycle. Acetyl-CoA formed from pyruvate is further oxidized here to CO_2 and hydrogens with accompanying electrons that are transferred to receptors of the electron transport chain (Fig. 19-5). The TCA cycle is also known as the Krebs citric acid cycle.

ample, NADH) generated by the TCA cycle also determine its continued operation. For example, the unavailability of oxygen as the final electron acceptor will not allow utilization of reduced compounds produced by the TCA cycle, causing the system to halt with an accumulation of pyruvate. Increase in this substrate determines the conversion of pyruvate to lactate by lactate dehydrogenase (an enzyme that catalyzes this reaction in either direction)

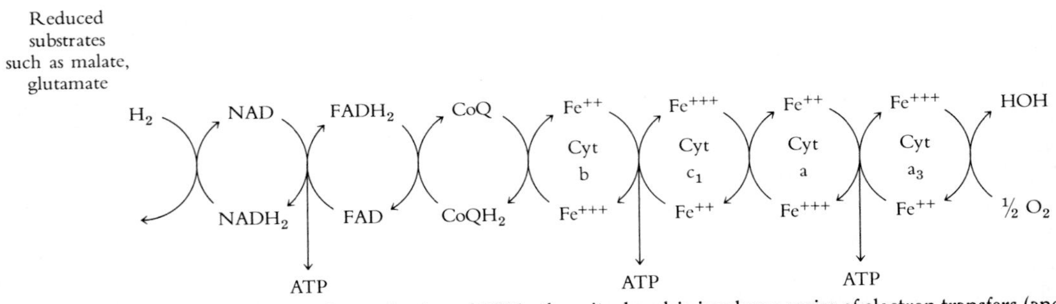

Reduced substrates such as malate, glutamate

H_2 NAD $FADH_2$ CoQ Fe^{++} Fe^{+++} Fe^{++} Fe^{+++} HOH

Cyt b Cyt c_1 Cyt a Cyt a_3

$NADH_2$ FAD $CoQH_2$ Fe^{+++} Fe^{++} Fe^{+++} Fe^{++} ½ O_2

ATP ATP ATP

Fig. 19-5. The cytochrome system. The production of ATP in the mitochondria involves a series of electron transfers (and hydrogen ions) with the final electron acceptor being oxygen and resulting in the production of water. The molecules involved include nicotinamide-adenine dinucleotide (NAD → $NADH_2$), flavin-adenine dinucleotide (FAD → $FADH_2$), and a series of iron-containing (Fe) pigments known as the cytochromes (b, c, a, a_3).

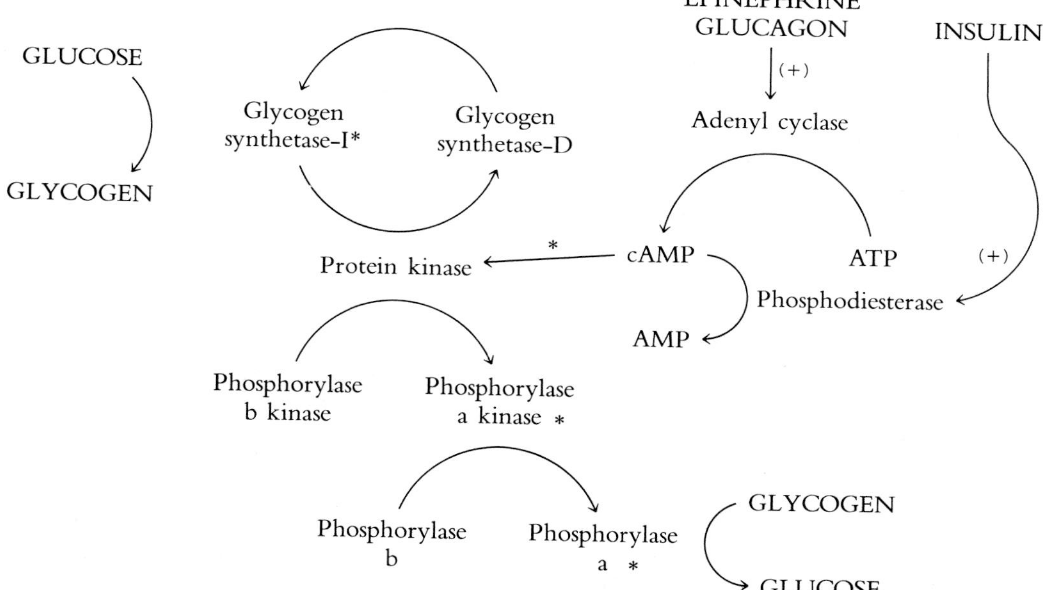

Fig. 19-6. Glycogenolysis and glycogenesis. The control of phosphorylase and glycogen synthetase activities by cAMP-dependent protein kinase. The a form of phosphorylase and the I form of glycogen synthetase are the active (*) enzymes. (See also Fig. 1-5.)

depending upon relative availability of substrates.

Lipogenesis and Lipolysis

Synthesis of fatty acids is accomplished essentially by combining units of acetyl-CoA to form fatty acyl-CoA molecules. This synthesis requires NADPH produced in part through efforts of the pentose phosphate pathway. Esterification of fatty acids (linkage to glycerol via ester bonds) involves coupling of three long-chain fatty-acyl-CoA units one at a time to glycerol phosphate to form monoglycerides, diglycerides and finally triglycerides (neutral fats). Triglycerides may be stored or, as in the case of the liver, be coated with lipoprotein and secreted as droplets into the blood. Fatty acid and triglyceride synthesis is shown in Figure 19-7. Cholesterol synthesis (see Chap. 9) also involves acetyl-CoA as a precursor and is accomplished in the liver.

Lipids are transported in the blood in several ways. Small fatty acids are released directly into the blood where they are referred to as free fatty acids or *nonesterified fatty acids* (NEFA). The latter name is more suitable than "free" because NEFAs have low solubility in aqueous medium and must form a complex with serum albumin for transport. Larger fatty acids are transported as triglycerides (esterified: attached by ester bonds to glycerol). The liver packages triglycerides and releases them in small protein-coated droplets called *very low density lipoproteins* (VLDL). A small amount of cholesterol is also present in VLDLs. Hydrolysis of VLDLs including the triglycerides occurs in capillary beds of adipose and certain other tissues by the activity of *lipoprotein lipase.* Fatty acids and glycerol are released and can diffuse into the adjacent cells.

Larger transport droplets called *low density lipoproteins* (LDL) contain about 60% of the cholesterol that occurs in human blood. These LDLs are about 2 nm in diameter and consist of about 1500 cholesterol esters surrounded by a phospholipid-cholesterol layer and coated with about 20 molecules of apoprotein B and some minor apoproteins. The apoprotein acts as a binding protein for receptors located in pits on the surface of various cellular types. The nature of the apoproteins determines to

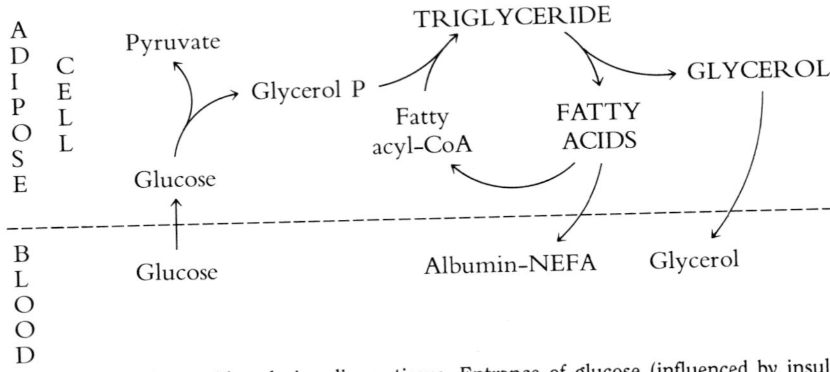

FIG. 19-7. The triglyceride-fatty acid cycle in adipose tissue. Entrance of glucose (influenced by insulin) stimulates glycolysis and production of glycerol P, which is involved in esterification with three fatty acyl-Co A molecules (lipogenesis). Triglycerides may be hydrolyzed (lipolysis) to fatty acids and glycerol that may enter the blood. Fatty acids are transported in the blood in association with albumin and are referred to as free or nonesterified fatty acids (NEFA). P, phosphate.

what cellular type a lipoprotein droplet can bind. The LDL is internalized to complete the transfer of cholesterol from the liver. Steroidogenic tissues utilize LDLs as an important source of cholesterol for synthesizing androgens, estrogens, progesterone, corticosteroids and vitamin D_3.

High density lipoprotein (HDL) droplets transport cholesterol from tissues to the liver where it is metabolized and excreted. About 30% of the blood cholesterol in humans is found in HDLs, and HDLs may provide some cholesterol for steroidogenesis. In rats, HDLs transport most of the cholesterol. There appears to be a relationship between HDLs (especially one type known as HDL_2) and the risk of heart attack. Normal HDL levels are 45 and 55 mg/dl in blood of men and women, respectively. Higher risk of heart attack is correlated with lower levels of HDLs. A great deal is yet to be learned about HDL levels, metabolism and health before we can draw firm conclusions from these observations. For example, what is the meaning of the high HDL levels reported for runners or higher levels (80–100 mg/dl) observed in alcoholics?

Fatty acid mobilization (Fig. 19-7) involves hydrolysis of triglycerides by the enzyme *triglyceride lipase* releasing a fatty acyl-CoA and diglyceride. The diglyceride is hydrolyzed by diglyceride lipase to yield another fatty acid plus monoglyceride. Monoglyceride lipase hydrolyzes the latter to yield glycerol and fatty acids. Fatty acids may be metabolized through the β-oxidation process (Fig. 19-8) to acetyl-CoA, which can be used to synthesize ATP, or

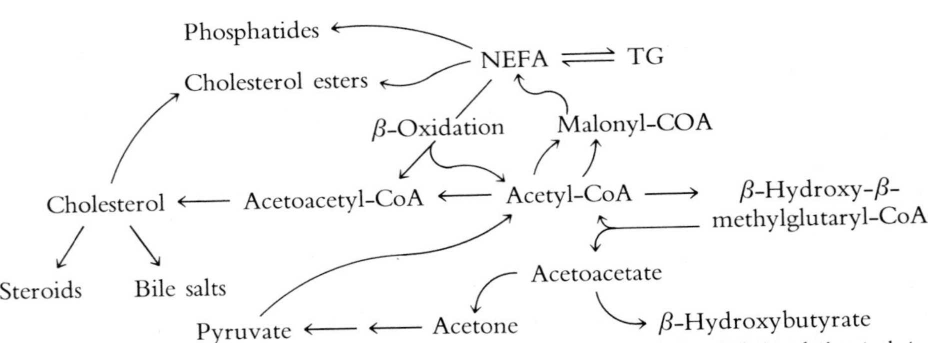

FIG. 19-8. β-Oxidation of fatty acids. Oxidation of nonesterified fatty acids *(NEFA)* and their relation to ketone body formation. *TG,* triglycerides; acetone, acetoacetate and β-hydroxybutyrate are collectively termed ketone bodies.

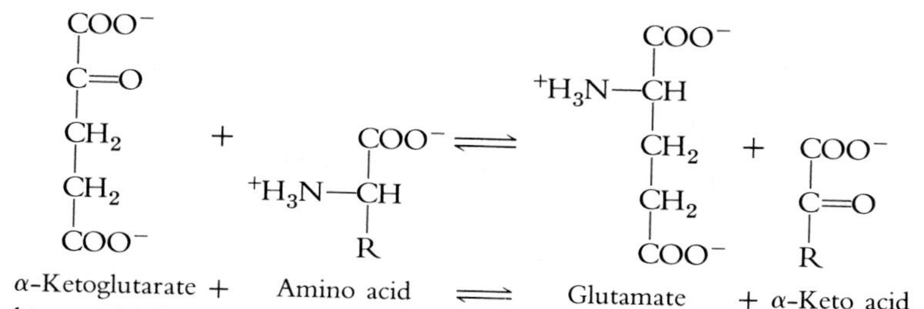

$$\begin{array}{c}COO^-\\ |\\ C{=}O\\ |\\ CH_2\\ |\\ CH_2\\ |\\ COO^-\end{array} + \begin{array}{c}COO^-\\ |\\ {}^+H_3N{-}CH\\ |\\ R\end{array} \rightleftharpoons \begin{array}{c}COO^-\\ |\\ {}^+H_3N{-}CH\\ |\\ CH_2\\ |\\ CH_2\\ |\\ COO^-\end{array} + \begin{array}{c}COO^-\\ |\\ C{=}O\\ |\\ R\end{array}$$

α-Ketoglutarate + Amino acid ⇌ Glutamate + α-Keto acid

FIG. 19-9. General transamination reaction. The amino acid reacts with α-ketoglutarate to form glutamate and an α-keto acid. The α-ketoglutarate is regenerated from glutamate by a separate reaction involving glutamate dehydrogenase and NAD.

they may be secreted directly into the blood through which they travel to another tissue for oxidation or use in resynthesis of fat. Glycerol similarly may be converted to glycerol phosphate in the same tissue or released into the blood. Glycerol phosphate may contribute to resynthesis of glucose (gluconeogenesis) or may again participate in fat synthesis.

Gluconeogenesis

Gluconeogenesis occurs primarily from amino acids, but glycerol or lactate may also provide gluconeogenic substrates. Dietary or tissue proteins must first be hydrolyzed to amino acids, which may in turn be deaminated via transaminase reactions to yield glucose intermediates (ketoacids) plus ammonia (see Fig. 19-9). The ammonia is generally combined with CO_2 via the urea cycle to form urea for excretion. This process is extremely important in carnivores, which assimilate large quantities of amino acids from their diets and relatively little carbohydrate.

The process of gluconeogenesis is essentially a reversal of glycolysis but must utilize different pathways because of the unidirectional nature of hexokinase (glucokinase), PFK and pyruvate kinase. Alanine, for example, may be converted directly to pyruvate through transamination (Fig. 19-10). Pyruvate may then be converted to oxaloacetate by a unidirectional enzyme, *pyruvate carboxylase* and ATP (Fig. 19-11). Other amino acids (except for leucine) may be transaminated to various glucose intermediates (Table 19-1) and find their way through pyruvate or oxaloacetate, or both, to glucose. The conversion of aspartate directly to oxaloacetate is depicted in Figure 19-10. It should be noted that transamination reactions require an ammonia acceptor; in this case, as for alanine, the acceptor is α-ketoglutarate. In liver mitochondria the resulting glutamate can be readily deaminated back to α-ketoglutarate by *glutamic acid dehydrogenase* with the ammonia being transferred directly into the urea cycle.

Oxaloacetate is converted to PEP by another unidirectional enzyme, *PEP carboxykinase,* and GTP. Increased levels of PEP influence resynthesis of fructose 1,6-diphosphate, which is directed to glucose 6-phosphate by a third unidirectional step catalyzed by *fructose 1,6-diphosphatase.* Finally, the last unidirectional enzyme in the gluconeogenic scheme, *glucose*

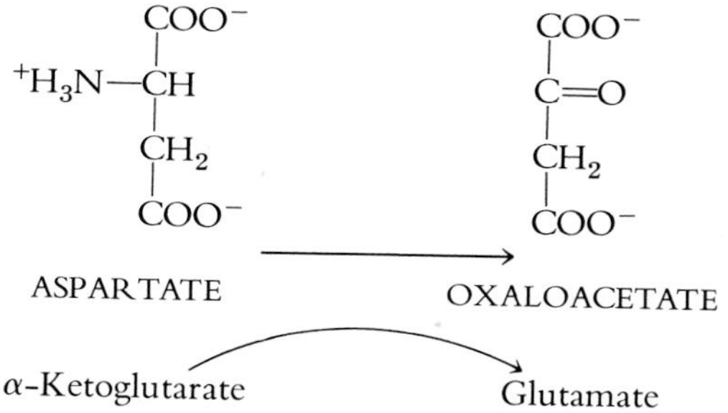

$$\begin{array}{c}COO^-\\ |\\ {}^+H_3N{-}C\\ |\\ CH_3\end{array} \xrightarrow{\text{Glutamate-pyruvate transaminase}} \begin{array}{c}COO^-\\ |\\ C{=}O\\ |\\ CH_3\end{array}$$

ALANINE → PYRUVATE

α-Ketoglutarate → Glutamate

$$\begin{array}{c}COO^-\\ |\\ {}^+H_3N{-}CH\\ |\\ CH_2\\ |\\ COO^-\end{array} \longrightarrow \begin{array}{c}COO^-\\ |\\ C{=}O\\ |\\ CH_2\\ |\\ COO^-\end{array}$$

ASPARTATE → OXALOACETATE

α-Ketoglutarate → Glutamate

FIG. 19-10. Transamination of alanine to pyruvate and of aspartate to oxaloacetate. Both of these reactions are reversible.

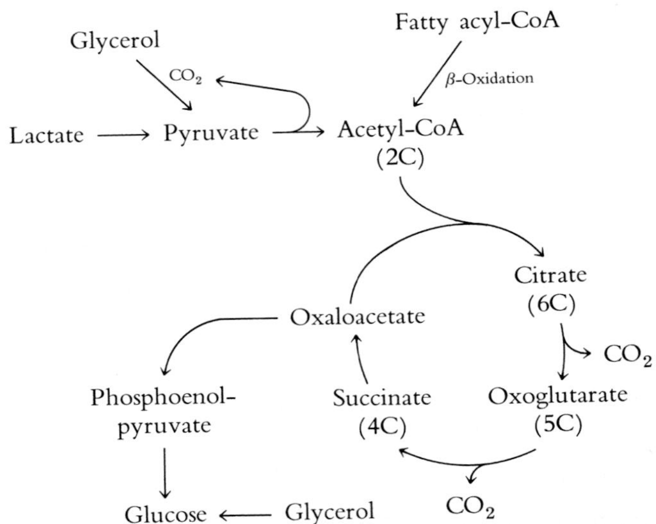

FIG. 19-11. Metabolism of pyruvate or acetyl-CoA via the TCA cycle. The carbons lost as CO_2 in formation of oxaloacetate are such that the carbons of acetyl-CoA are the ones lost and the glucose produced from oxaloacetate would not contain the carbons found in the pyruvate or acetate. Hence, gluconeogenesis technically does not occur in this manner (see text).

6-phosphatase, produces free glucose that can diffuse from the cell into the blood. However, this final step does not occur in most tissues and is unique to those tissues that participate in regulating circulating glucose levels, that is, liver and kidney cortex.

Production of glucose from amino acids, like the complete oxidation of glucose, involves both cytosol and mitochondrial events. Pyruvate produced in the cytosol via glycolysis may enter the mitochondrion or may be converted by pyruvate carboxylase to oxaloacetate while still in the cytosol. Mitochondrial membranes are not permeable to oxaloacetate, but mitochondrial oxaloacetate produced in the TCA cycle or through transamination of amino acids may be converted first to other intermediates, such as malate, which may diffuse into the cytosol and may be reconverted to oxaloacetate. This mitochondrial shuttle was proposed to account for observations in the rat and some other species in which PEP carboxykinase was found only in the cytosol, yet transamination to oxaloacetate occurred within the mitochondrion. In rabbits, however, PEP carboxykinase is present in mitochondria, whereas in the guinea pig the enzyme is found in both compartments. These observations emphasize that caution must be used in generalizing about cytological localization of specific metabolic events in gluconeogenesis when considering different species.

TABLE 19-1. *Some Amino Acid Precursors for Certain Gluconeogenic Substrates Formed by Deamination or Transamination of Amino Acids*

GLUCONEOGENIC SUBSTRATE	POTENTIAL AMINO ACID SOURCE
Pyruvate	Ala, Ser, Gly
α-Ketoglutarate	Arg, Lys, His
Propionate	Val, Thr, Ile

After Newsholme and Start.[8]

Lipids may contribute to gluconeogenesis following hydrolysis of triglycerides to fatty acids and glycerol. Glycerol may be phosphorylated to glycerol phosphate and converted to a three-carbon intermediate in glycolysis (Fig. 19-2). Glycerol phosphate can be oxidized to acetyl-CoA or can be a source of glucose via the gluconeogenic pathway. Since fatty acids inhibit glycolysis, it is more likely that glycerol metabolism will follow the gluconeogenic pathway. Fatty acids through oxidation to acetyl-CoA do not constitute any net synthesis of glucose intermediates. Although oxaloacetate can be synthesized in the TCA cycle, the two carbons of acetyl-CoA will be lost as CO_2 and cannot end up in the glucose molecule (Fig. 19-11). An accumulation of acetyl-CoA in liver results in formation of ketone bodies (Fig. 19-8), which enter the blood and are metabolized by other tissues or excreted.

Lactate under aerobic conditions is converted to pyruvate by lactate dehydrogenase and can be directed toward glucose synthesis through the gluconeogenic pathway. However, no new net synthesis of glucose occurs in this manner since glucose probably was the original source of the lactate. Muscles may release lactate following vigorous contraction when sufficient oxygen is not available. Several other tissues, for example, red blood cells, normally respire anaerobically and contribute lactate for gluconeogenesis. The liver and kidney cortex metabolize lactate that has entered the blood from other tissues.

Metabolic Events of Particular Tissues

Liver

The mammalian liver is capable completely of (1) removing from or releasing glucose to the blood, (2) storing of glucose as glycogen, (3) metabolizing glucose to CO_2 and water with attendant production of ATP, (4) synthesizing triglycerides from fatty acids and glycerol for storage or transport as lipoprotein droplets to other tissues, (5) hydrolyzing triglycerides to fatty acids that may be released or further oxidized to acetyl-CoA for ATP production, (6) synthesizing other lipids or ketone bodies and (7) performing gluconeogenesis from amino acids, glycerol or lactate precursors. In addition, there are myriads of other synthetic activities performed by the liver, including synthesis of a wide range of proteins (renin substrate, somatomedins, serum albumin, etc.), phospholipids and urea, as well as conjugation of steroids and detoxification of many drugs, including alcohol.

In omnivores and in carnivores the major dietary carbohydrate is glucose. Ruminants take in little carbohydrate through their diets. The most important metabolic role for the liver of omnivores, ruminants and carnivores is to provide adequate circulating oxidative fuels during periods of acute or prolonged fasting and to process and direct excessive fuels to adipose tissue for storage as fat. The role differs in relation to the sources of energy in the diet. The liver is anatomically situated ideally for this role since about 70% of its blood supply comes directly through the portal vein, which drains the gut and contains the absorbed products of digestion as well as insulin from the endocrine pancreas. In humans the liver rapidly removes excess glucose by a facilitated diffusion mechanism that is augmented by the enzyme glucokinase, which has a high affinity for glucose and converts it to glucose 6-phosphate. Unlike the hexokinase that phosphorylates glucose in other tissues, hepatic glucokinase is not inhibited by accumulation of product (glucose 6-phosphate), and uptake of glucose is maximized. Cell membranes are impermeable to phosphorylated forms of glucose, and only four metabolic avenues are open to it. Glucose 6-phosphate may be converted to glucose 1-phosphate, formed into a complex with uridine and added to a glycogen polymer by glycogen synthetase (uridine-diphosphoglucose-glycosyl transferase), or it may be oxidized to pyruvate via the glycolytic pathway and, depending on oxygen availability, be converted to lactate or completely oxidized in the mitochondria to CO_2 and water. An alternative route for glucose 6-phosphate is the pentose phosphate pathway whereby reduced NADPH is produced. Reduced NADP ($NADPH_2$) is utilized for fatty acid synthesis. About 30% of the glucose oxidized by the liver will pass through the pentose phosphate pathway. Finally, glucose 6-phosphate may be dephosphorylated by glucose 6-phosphatase to free glucose, which can diffuse back into the blood. The direction of glucose 6-phosphate metabolism is determined by the overall metabolic requirements of the organism at any moment and its dietary state. Metabolism is then altered accordingly by the endocrine environment.

The major lipids of importance in liver metabolism occur as triglycerides, long-chain fatty acids, short-chain fatty acids, cholesterol and cholesterol esters. For the moment the first two groups will be considered. Fatty acids and glycerol are absorbed from the gut following enzymatic hydrolysis of triglycerides and are reconverted to triglycerides in the intestinal epithelial cells. Large droplets of triglycerides as well as some cholesterol and cholesterol esters are coated with lipoprotein and released into the intercellular spaces around the epithelial cell. These droplets or *chylomicrons* enter lacteals, the blind capillaries of the lymphatic system, and eventually enter the blood vascular system via the thoracic ducts. Chylomicrons are similar to the VLDLs produced by the liver except they do not contain cholesterol. The coating of chylomicrons and the triglycerides are hydrolyzed by lipoprotein lipase localized in the endothelial cells of capillaries in adipose and, to a lesser extent, muscle tissues, and released fatty acids and glycerol are directly absorbed by these tissues. The high local concentrations of these substances allow them to readily diffuse into adipose or muscle cells.

Nonesterified fatty acids and glycerol released from hydrolysis of triglycerides in the gut may diffuse directly into intestinal capillaries, bind to albumin and travel to the liver via the portal vein. Uptake of NEFA and glycerol is simply a function of concentration, and since intracellular NEFA and glycerol are essentially nonexistent because of their rapid metabolism, a considerable quantity may be removed from the blood with ease. Although 99.9% of the plasma NEFAs form a complex with albumin, the total capacity for NEFA transport is rather low. Consequently most long-chain fatty acids enter the system as triglycerides in chylomicrons.

Nonesterified fatty acids and glycerol accumulated by the liver cell may be used for energy through β-oxidation, for glucose synthesis (glycerol only) or for long chain fatty acid and triglyceride synthesis. Liver cells of mammals are capable of storing relatively small amounts of triglycerides.

Liver cells oxidize NEFAs to acetyl-CoA when conditions dictate mobilization of fatty acids and gluconeogenesis. Much of the acetyl-CoA is converted to ketone bodies as previously described. Since liver cells lack the necessary enzymes to metabolize ketone bodies further, they are released into the blood. Other tissues especially muscle and brain, remove these ketone bodies, reconvert them to acetyl-CoA and synthesize ATP. As in the case of NEFA oxidation, ketone bodies do not provide net sources of glucose because of the production of CO_2 from acetate in the TCA cycle.

If glycogen and glucose are limited as a consequence of lowered blood glucose, amino acids may be deaminated (transamination) to provide gluconeogenic substrates. Under conditions of glycogen depletion the liver must maintain sufficient circulating glucose through gluconeogenic processes to provide adequate energy sources for the brain and other obligate users of glucose (for example, red blood cells). Note that the cortical portion of the kidney is capable of carrying out gluconeogenesis as well as limited oxidation of glucose or storage as glycogen, and it aids the liver in maintaining sufficient levels of glucose during periods of food deprivation or low dietary intake of carbohydrates.

Excessive levels of amino acids stimulate gluconeogenesis in liver cells. If glycogen stores are adequate, the carbohydrate produced is converted to fatty acids and glycerol. Triglycerides are synthesized and exported as VLDLs destined for storage in adipose tissue.

Adipose Tissue

Adipose tissue functions primarily as a storage reservoir for respiratory fuel. Nonesterified fatty acids, long chain fatty acids and glycerol obtained from hydrolysis of chylomicrons or VLDL in the capillary beds of adipose tissue are readily accumulated by adipose cells, and the fatty acids are esterified with glycerol to triglycerides. Neutral fats are an excellent storage form because 1 g of fat when hydrolyzed produces nine times more energy per gram than does an equivalent weight of glucose stored as glycogen. Consequently much more stored fat fuel can be packed into a limited space. If migratory birds, such as the ruby-throated hummingbird that migrates hundreds of miles nonstop over ocean, were to rely solely on stored glycogen, they would be too heavy to fly!

Triglycerides can be hydrolyzed on demand by a lipase complex consisting of triglyceride lipase, diglyceride lipase and monoglyceride lipase to yield longchain fatty acids and glycerol. Triglyceride lipase appears to be the rate-limiting enzyme in this pathway and the one that is regulated by hormones. Longchain fatty acids are hydrolyzed to smaller fatty acids (NEFAs). Glycerol and NEFAs enter the blood where the latter form a complex with serum albumin and are transported to other tissues such as muscle or liver where they can be utilized as energy sources.

Glycolysis is regulated in adipose cells primarily by the availability of glucose. Therefore the rate of entrance of glucose into the cell determines the rate of glycolysis. Increased levels of glucose 6-phosphate augment formation of NADPH via the pentose phosphate pathway and synthesis of glycerol phosphate, both of which enhance lipogenesis. A decrease in glucose 6-phosphate similarly enhances lipolysis. This relationship between glycolysis and lipid metabolism is the basis for the *glucose-fatty acid cycle* (Fig. 19-7), which theoretically can regulate fatty acid mobilization simply by the availability of glucose. When glucose becomes scarce this mechanism would favor conservation of available glucose and would provide additional substrates for energy metabolism (NEFA) and gluconeogenesis (glycerol).

Muscle

Muscle cells are specialized for oxidizing glucose to produce the ATP needed for sustaining contraction. Red muscle is especially rich in mitochondria, TCA enzymes and electron transport molecules for complete oxidation of glucose to CO_2 and water. In contrast, white muscles (such as the pectoral muscles of domestic chickens) are specialized for anaerobic oxidation of glucose to lactate and have few mitochondria. The account here deals only with red muscle. Because of the high rate of glycolysis and aerobic oxidation of glucose in muscle as compared to liver, most of the detailed knowledge of these biochemical pathways has been generated from studies of muscle. Liver does not carry on as much oxidative phosphorylation as does muscle, and the components in this system are more difficult to study in liver because of the low rates of reaction.

Uptake and oxidative metabolism of glucose by muscle cells is very similar to events occurring in liver, with only a few important differences. Glucose is accumulated by facilitated transport, but the enzyme, hexokinase, responsible for phosphorylation of glucose has a lower affinity for substrate than liver glucokinase and is inhibited by accumulation of product. Only two routes are readily available to glucose 6-phosphate in muscle. Synthesis of glycogen is accomplished by the glycogen synthetase system, and the musculature may store more total glycogen than does the liver. For example, in humans the liver stores about 70 g of glucose as glycogen, whereas the musculature stores about 120 g. However, muscle glycogen is not available to provide glucose for export from the muscle cell because, unlike liver cells, muscle cells lack glucose 6-phosphatase and cannot hydrolyze glucose 6-phosphate to free glucose that could diffuse into the blood.

The second pathway for metabolism of glucose 6-phosphate in muscle is glycolysis. When muscle is performing only moderate work, the blood can supply glucose to maintain sufficient ATP levels. Greater work loads will draw upon glycogen reserves, and if demand exceeds the ability of blood to supply sufficient O_2, muscular activity may be maintained for a limited time by rapid anaerobic metabolism of glucose to lactate. The pentose phosphate pathway for glucose metabolism is not very important in muscle.

Muscle cells may also utilize NEFAs directly as an energy source and can utilize VLDL synthesized by the liver as a source of NEFAs because, like adipose tissue, some muscle capillary beds have cells that produce lipoprotein lipase. However, the extent of the contribution of exogenous NEFA to overall muscle metabolism has not been determined. Ketone bodies when present in the blood are also a ready source of energy for muscle cells, which can resynthesize acetyl-CoA and under aerobic conditions synthesize ATP. Muscle cells may synthesize and store triglycerides, which can also be hydrolyzed to provide fatty acids for energy production. The ability for muscle to metabolize endogenous or exogenous lipids for energy becomes extremely important under conditions of fasting.

Brain

The brain and rest of the nervous system have a high specific requirement for glucose as the principle energy source. Nervous tissue has lost the ability to store glycogen, does not store triglycerides and must therefore rely exclusively on blood for its source of glucose. Deprivation of glucose for only a matter of minutes can produce cell death and irreparable damage to the brain. Red blood cells and cells of the kidney medulla and the testes have similar high glucose requirements, but these cells utilize glucose only anaerobically, whereas brain also has a high O_2 requirement for glucose oxidation. Since muscle glycogen cannot be released it is the liver, and to a limited extent the kidney cortex, that must provide glucose for these tissues through glycogenolysis and gluconeogenesis. Under conditions of starvation, alternative energy sources provide some glucose (Table 19-2), and other substrates must be utilized by the brain for energy.

Hormones Regulating Metabolism

Metabolism is influenced by many hormones that affect the availability of substrates and the activity of key enzymes in glycolysis, gluconeogenesis, glycogenolysis, lipogenesis and lipolysis. These hormones include *insulin* and *glucagon* from the endocrine pancreas (Chap. 13), *epinephrine* from the adrenal medulla (Chap. 10), *glucocorticoids* from the adrenal cortex (Chap. 10), *growth hormone* (GH) and *β-lipotropin* (LPH) from the adenohypophysis (Chap. 5), *thyroid hormones* (Chap. 8) and *gonadal steroids* (Chap. 11). In addition, the *cyclic nucleotides* (cAMP, cGMP) or the *prostaglandins* or both (see Chaps. 1, 15) may be important mediators of the action of one or more of the above hormones. Insulin-like growth factors (somatomedins, IGF-I, etc.) also influence metabolism (Chap. 15). Metabolism may be affected by drugs such as caffeine that alter the activity of cyclic nucleotide-degrading enzymes (phosphodiesterases).

These metabolic hormones may be classified according to their general effects on metabolism of carbohydrates, fats or protein (Table 19-3). Because of the existence of such interrelationships between these classes of compounds, many metabolic hormones influence all of them. Hormones may be considered glycolytic (insulin), glycogenolytic (epinephrine, glucagon, thyroid hormones) or gluconeogenic (epinephrine, GH, glucocorticoids). They may be lipogenic (insulin) or lipolytic (epinephrine, thyroid hormones, GH, LPH) with respect to mobilization of fatty acids. Some of these hormones are protein anabolic, that is, they increase the general synthesis of proteins and favor nitrogen retention (insulin, GH, thyroid hormones, androgens) or protein

TABLE 19-2. *Sources for Blood Glucose Utilized by Brain During Starvation*

	GLUCOSE PRODUCED (G/DAY)	
	3–4 DAYS OF STARVATION	SEVERAL WEEKS OF STARVATION
Total required by brain	120	120
Glucose precursors		
Glycerol	19	19
Lactate/Pyruvate	39	39
Amino acids	41	16
Total	99	74
Remainder from ketone bodies	21	46

After Newsholme and Start.[8]

NOTE: Presumably the additional energy comes from utilization of ketone bodies.

TABLE 19-3. *Generalized Actions of Hormones with Respect to Protein, Carbohydrate and Lipid Metabolism*

HORMONE	PROTEIN	CARBOHYDRATE	LIPID
Insulin	Anabolic	Hypoglycemic, glycogenic, antiglycogenolytic	Lipogenic, antilipolytic
Epinephrine		Glycogenolytic, hypergly- cemic, gluconeogenic	Lipolytic
Glucagon		Hyperglycemic, glycogeno- lytic	
Growth hormone	Anabolic	Hyperglycemic, gluconeo- genic	Lipolytic
Glucocorticoids	Antianabolic	Hyperglycemic, gluconeo- genic, inhibits periperal utilization	
Thyroxine	Anabolic or catabolic	Hyperglycemic, glycogeno- lytic	Lipolytic
Androgens	Anabolic		

catabolic (glucocorticoids, thyroid hormones). Increased levels of circulating glucose (hyperglycemia) are caused by epinephrine, glucagon, thyroid hormones, GH, glucocorticoids and estrogens, whereas only insulin is hypoglycemic.

The following accounts of metabolism under differing physiological conditions emphasize the importance of insulin, glucagon, epinephrine, GH, and glucocorticoids as the major metabolic regulators, with glucocorticoids and thyroid hormones exhibiting permissive actions with respect to GH. The extent of involvement by LPH is not yet clear. The hormones that predominate under three conditions will be examined: regulation following digestion of a meal (postabsorptive), responses to acute stress and responses to chronic stress (starvation).

Endocrine Regulation Following Feeding

Insulin is the major hormone responsible for regulating carbohydrate, amino acid and lipid levels in omnivores and carnivores in the immediate postabsorptive state. The factors that regulate insulin release were discussed in Chapter 13. Insulin increases the rate of transport of glucose into liver, muscle and adipose cells. In liver, this stimulates glycogenesis and production of VLDLs and LDLs. Glucose entry into muscle cells stimulates glycogenesis and glycolysis. This increase observed in muscle glycolysis appears to be due simply to an increase in substrates. In adipose tissues, glucose entry favors fatty acid synthesis and esterification, mainly by substrate effects.

Entry of amino acids into muscles stimulated by insulin enhances protein synthesis. In the liver and to some extent the kidney cortex, excess amino acids are deaminated (transaminated), and if sufficient glucose and glycogen are present, these molecules will contribute to lipogenesis for export as lipids to adipose tissue for storage. Insulin depresses gluconeogenesis in liver cells by favoring incorporation of amino acids into protein and also in adipose cells, although the latter have not been extensively studied.

In addition to effects of insulin on the cell membrane and transport of glucose and amino acids, insulin alters lipid and carbohydrate metabolism through effects on enzymes. In muscle and probably in liver, insulin interferes with the enzyme protein kinase by increasing the proportion of the enzyme that is inactive. Protein kinase is responsible for two important enzymatic interconversions. The first involves conversion of inactive phosphorylase-b-kinase to an active form, which in turn catalyzes phosphorylation of another enzyme, phosphorylase-b, to an active form, phosphorylase-a (Fig. 19-6). Phosphorylase-a is responsible for cleaving a glucose 1-phosphate residue from glycogen. Conversion of glucose 1-phosphate to glucose 6-phosphate is determined by substrate levels. At the same time, protein kinase catalyzes inactivation of glycogen synthetase also through phosphorylation. Thus, phosphorylation via protein kinase activates glycogenolysis (phosphorylase-a) and inhibits glycogenesis (glycogen synthetase), resulting in an increase in intracellular glucose 6-phosphate. Insulin favors glycogen synthesis by inhibiting protein kinase activity. This effect may be caused by an insulin-induced reduction in cAMP related to an insulin-induced increase in cGMP (see Chap. 1).

Insulin also increases the amount of glucokinase in liver cells and reduces the amount of glucose 6-phosphatase. These changes seem to reflect alterations in rates of synthesis of these enzymes and would increase glycolysis. There are no apparent effects on these enzyme levels in either muscle or adipose tissue.

NEFA synthesis and triglyceride synthesis are increased in liver by insulin. In adipose tissue, insulin increases synthesis of lipoprotein lipase, which enhances lipogenesis. Insulin also stimulates triglyceride synthesis in adipose tissue from either glucose or acetyl-CoA, but the mechanism of this effect is not fully understood. Lipolysis is inhibited by insulin in adipose cells by a reduction in activity of triglyceride lipase that is correlated with a reduction in cAMP levels. Thus, insulin in adipose tissue is both lipogenic, largely through effects on substrate availability, and antilipolytic, through an effect on cAMP levels. Although the effects of insulin on lipid metabolism in liver and adipose tissue are marked, there seems to be no influence of insulin on lipid metabolism in muscle.

Immediately following a high protein meal, then, insulin may be considered the most important single hormone since it directs excess fuels obtained from the diet into storage. Somewhat later, GH and insulin work cooperatively in that GH stimulates some lipolysis, which provides utilization of fatty acids for meeting energy requirements of protein anabolic processes that are being stimulated by GH. Such cooperative action also conserves glucose for those tissues that have specific requirements for glucose (for example, the brain) while encouraging others (muscle) to use an alternative fuel.

Herbivore metabolism differs markedly from that of carnivores. Most studies have been done with ruminants. Digestion in these large herbivores is accomplished by bacterial flora that reside in a special region of the gut known as the rumen. The bacteria digest cellulose to release glucose. This glucose is utilized by the bacteria and is not available for absorption into the ruminant. Instead, the ruminant absorbs fatty acids and amino acids resulting from metabolism and death of bacteria. Glucagon is the main hormone released after feeding, and it stimulates gluconeogenesis from amino acids. Studies of cattle and sheep indicate that insulin increases incorporation of lipids into adipose tissue. Growth hormone directs energy to skeletal muscle. During periods between feedings, the glucocorticoids are responsible for maintaining gluconeogenesis.

Effects of Acute Stress on Metabolism

Acute stress such as the "flight-or-fight" response and exercise produces profound alterations in energy metabolism that are mediated primarily by epinephrine released from the adrenal medulla and to some extent by glucagon from the endocrine pancreas. Hyperglycemia can occur following release of epinephrine due to a direct inhibition of insulin release (see Chap. 13).

In muscle, epinephrine activates adenyl cyclase and increases cAMP with resultant activation of protein kinase, as discussed previously. Increased activity of protein kinase accelerates glycogenolysis and inhibits glycogen synthesis in muscle even when insulin levels are high during the immediate postabsorptive state. Since muscle lacks glucose 6-phosphatase, the released glucose is utilized within the muscle cell for oxidative phosphorylation as is glucose taken up from the blood. Although epinephrine has been shown experimentally to activate glycogenolysis in liver, large (pharmacological) doses are required, and it is probably glucagon that is responsible for effects on glycogenolysis observed under physiological conditions. Reduced blood sugar levels due to increased glucose utilization would be sufficient to induce glucagon release, which through the same cAMP mechanism would stimulate glycogenolysis in liver.

Epinephrine also stimulates cAMP production in adipose tissue where it increases activity of triglyceride lipase, resulting in an increase in blood NEFAs and glycerol. A similar effect may occur in those muscles where triglyceride stores have been produced. The release of fatty acids and their use for fuel during prolonged exercise such as marathon running protects liver glycogen stores from metabolism by muscle and makes them available for tissues with high glucose requirements such as brain.

The increase in plasma NEFAs and their uptake by liver tends to inhibit glycolytic enzymes and increase acetyl-CoA for ATP synthesis or ketone body formation. Accumulation of acetyl-CoA favors conversion of pyruvate obtained from lactate to oxaloacetate and resynthesis of glucose via the gluconeogenic pathway. Thus, increases in fatty acids can influence glucose availability in association with the glucose-fatty acid cycle.

Effects of Chronic Stress (Starvation) on Metabolism

During fasting or early starvation in humans there is an elevation in GH levels as well as in glucagon levels. The liver is capable of storing glucose in the form of glycogen sufficient for only about 12 to 24 hours of fasting, during which time all of the stored liver glucose is depleted. Fatty acid mobilization and oxidation become the major source of energy for ATP synthesis in muscle, and gluconeogenesis from amino acids in the liver and kidney cortex becomes the primary source for blood glucose. Growth hormone and possibly LPH stimulate lipolysis in adipose tissue and provide the required fatty acids. Glycerol also produced from triglyceride hydrolysis can be used as a gluconeogenic precursor. The action of GH on adipose tissue requires the presence of glucocorticoids. Furthermore, glucocorticoids inhibit peripheral utilization of amino acids for protein synthesis and increase levels of transaminases in liver, which are necessary for converting amino acids to ketoacids for gluconeogenesis. The latter effect may be a secondary action of glucocorticoids but nevertheless contributes significantly to the altered metabolism of starvation.

Glucagon normally stimulates glycogenolysis in liver and enhances entry of amino acids into the gluconeogenic pathway. The resultant increase in blood glucose under nonemergency conditions enhances glucose uptake by adipose tissue and stimulates lipogenesis. However, in the fasting animal, glucose levels cannot be maximally elevated by glucagon because of lack of stored glycogen reserves. Instead, glucagon stimulates lipolysis by a cAMP-dependent activation of triglyceride lipase. These effects of glucagon and GH on adipose tissue become even more important during later stages of starvation when there is a greater emphasis on consumption of lipid fuels than on using amino acids via gluconeogenesis.

Oxidation of fatty acids by liver produces large amounts of acetyl-CoA, of which a considerable proportion under starvation conditions is converted to ketone bodies and secreted into the blood. Ketone bodies are removed from the blood by muscle, which reconverts them to acetyl-CoA for ATP synthesis. Thus an increase in ketone body production reduces glucose requirements by the musculature and the need for catabolism of amino acids. Ketone bodies, like fatty acids, depress glycolysis and favor their own utilization as energy sources. The brain, which normally has a high requirement for glucose (almost 100% of its energy demands are met by blood glucose), switches to predominant use of ketone bodies and drastically reduces its requirement for glucose. This lessened demand for glucose further reduces reliance on protein and amino acids for energy while at the same time encouraging use of triglyceride stores. In humans this switch by the brain from glucose to ketone bodies occurs after about 3 to 10 days of starvation, but the mechanism responsible for this switch is not known. If this switch did not occur, however, protein would be preferentially degraded over fat for energy, resulting in serious protein deficiencies, and would reduce significantly the survival time during total starvation. It has been calculated that if this change from amino acid emphasis and attendant nitrogen loss via urea production and excretion did not occur, death would ensue within about 21 days. However, it is well known that obese people tolerate starvation for as long as 240 days without ill effects largely because of this reduction in reliance on glucose by the nervous system and other tissues. Eventually the fat reserves will be depleted, and the body must again rely on proteins and gluconeogenesis, with rapid appearance of protein deficiencies that, if not alleviated, will lead to death. Under conditions of semistarvation (insufficient caloric intake such that some body reserves must be consumed daily to meet energy requirements of the organism), the switch over to ketone body utilization and fat depletion does not occur, and protein deficiencies become prevalent very early. Under total starvation protein deficiencies do not appear until much later, when lipid reserves have been depleted.

The Role of Protein Anabolic Steroids in Metabolism

Many hormones have been shown to produce nitrogen retention (reduction in nitrogen excretion as urea due mainly to increased protein synthesis) including GH, thyroid hormones, estrogens and insulin. Kochakian and co-workers in the mid 1930s demonstrated that androgens also produced nitrogen retention, but the mechanism of their action was very different from the above hormones. Growth hormone, for example, stimulates new protein synthesis primarily in tissues other than muscle, whereas androgens produce their most marked effects in the musculature. Estrogens produce their protein anabolic effects only on selected tissues (uterus, mammary gland, female genital tract, skin, skeleton) and have rather little effect on overall nitrogen balance. Progesterone, which is clearly protein anabolic with respect to certain target tissues such as the uterus, actually produces a negative effect on nitrogen balance (increases total nitrogen excretion) and cannot be considered protein anabolic with respect to overall metabolism. Thyroid hormones are protein anabolic in thyroidectomized but not hypophysectomized animals, suggesting that this effect is mediated through GH release.

The first claim for rejuvenating (protein anabolic) effects of androgens stems from the experiments of Brown-Séquard in 1889, who reported effects of extracts prepared from animal testes on himself. Since these unsubstantiated claims, testosterone and other androgenic steroids have been shown to cause stimulation of protein synthesis, which is supported by glycogen reserves and influenced by availability of protein in the diet. The observation that it is not possible to dissociate the protein anabolic effect (nitrogen retention) from the androgenic effect has resulted in formulation of the descriptive title *anabolic-androgenic steroid* for such compounds. Androgens do not apparently influence amino acid transport but increase activity of amino acid activating enzymes. The effect of anabolic-androgenic steroids wears off with continued treatment, however, and nitrogen metabolism returns to normal.

The potential effect of anabolic-androgenic steroids on strength and endurance has resulted in their use for athletic training programs. Few adequately controlled and properly designed studies have been published. Results are divided between claims of improved performance and no effect. Treatment with synthetic testosterone analogues depresses secretion of gonadotropins and testosterone and decreases spermatogenesis. Furthermore, liver disfunction was reported in 80% of persons examined who had taken C_{17}-alkylated derivatives of testosterone. There are numerous reports of hepatitis, liver failure and fatal liver cancer related to use of protein anabolic-androgenic steroids. These physiological effects and their implications on the health of the user must be weighed against the short-term questionable benefits.

Readings on Endocrine Regulation of Metabolism

1. Goldsworthy, G.J. and P. Cheeseman (1978). Comparative aspects of the endocrine control of energy metabolism. In P.J. Gaillard and H.H. Boers, eds., Comparative Endocrinology. Elsevier/North-Holland Biomedical Press, Amsterdam, pp. 423–436.
2. Gwynne, J.T. and J.F. Strauss III (1982). The role of lipoproteins in steroidogenesis and cholesterol metabolism in steroidogenic glands. Endocr. Revs. 3:299–329.

3. Klachko, D.M., R.R. Anderson and M. Heimberg (1978). Hormones and Energy Metabolism. Plenum Publ. Co., New York.

4. Kochakian, C.D. (1976). Anabolic-Androgenic Steroids. Springer-Verlag, Berlin, 725 pp. Handbuch der experimentellen Pharmakologie, Vol. 43.

5. McKerns, K.W. (1969). Steroid Hormones and Metabolism. Appleton-Century-Crofts, New York.

6. Meister, A. (1965). Biochemistry of the Amino Acids, Vol. I and II. Academic Press, New York.

7. Miller, A.T. (1968). Energy Metabolism. F.A. Davis Co., Philadelphia.

8. Newsholme, E.A. and C. Start (1973). Regulation in Metabolism. John Wiley and Sons, New York.

9. Orskov, E.R. (1982). Protein Nutrition in Ruminants. Academic Press, New York.

10. Ryan, A.J. (1981). Anabolic steroids are fool's gold. Fed. Proc. 40:2682–2688.

11. Trenkle, A. (1981). Endocrine regulation of energy metabolism in ruminants. Fed. Proc. 40:2536–2541.

I·Introduction to Vertebrate Tissues

During embryonic development the process of gastrulation defines the three primary germ layers: *ectoderm, mesoderm* and *endoderm.* The ectoderm gives rise to the nervous system, including the neural crest and its derivatives, the epidermis, the lining of the oral cavity and parts of certain sense organs. The endoderm gives rise to the mucosal lining of the gut and a number of derivatives of the gut, including the lungs, thyroid gland, liver and pancreas. Mesoderm is the source of muscle, dermis, linings of the coelomic cavity (peritoneum, pleura, pericardium) and blood vessels (endothelium), and special organs such as the kidneys, adrenal cortex and the gonads.

The primary germ layers give rise to four primary tissues: *epithelium, connective tissues, muscle* and *nervous tissue.* Ectoderm gives rise to nervous tissue and certain epithelia. Endoderm gives rise to both covering epithelia and glandular epithelia. Mesoderm gives rise to special epithelia (mesothelia, endothelia), in addition to glandular epithelia, the elements of the various connective tissues and all muscle. The origin of primordial germ cells that eventually reside in the gonads in at least some vertebrates has been traced to endoderm, although it is possible that mesoderm may be involved in some species.

In response to various stimuli a given tissue may exhibit no morphologically observable response, degeneration (*atrophy, resorption*) or growth. The last response may be due simply to an increase in cell size (*hypertrophy*) or to increased cellular divisions with an actual increase in cell numbers (*hyperplasia*) or both. *Tumors* (neoplasms) are abnormal proliferations of tissues (*neoplasia*) having no normal physiological function. Such growths may be classified as either benign (harmless) or malignant (very harmful or likely to cause death; i.e., a cancer). The term *adenoma* refers to a benign tumor of glandular origin that may or may not synthesize and release abnormal amounts of hormones. Connective tissue tumors are called *sarcomas,* whereas a lymphatic tumor is a *lymphoma.* Malignant growths of any epithelial tissue, including glandular epithelia, are termed *carcinomas.* Some carcinomas also produce excessive quantities of hormones or hormone-like substances, as in the production of gastrin (stimulates HCl acid secretion in the stomach) by a pancreatic carcinoma.

Epithelium

Epithelia consist of closely associated cells organized into sheets that develop into coverings of both outer and inner surfaces or are modified into glandular structures. Little intracellular material is found between the cells of epithelia. They are typically associated with a distinct basement membrane. These cells may also occur as tubes (ducts, cords) or spheres (follicles, acini). Individual cell shape may differ markedly, and some cells may exhibit specialized adornments such as cilia or microvilli (brush border). Cilia are often sensory structures. Cilia may be responsible for producing currents to aid the flow of materials through a duct or other passageway as a result of coordinated rhythmic beating. Microvilli greatly increase the total surface area of cells. Presence of microvilli is a clue to an epithelium involved in transport of molecules between the cells and extracellular fluids. Epithelia may consist of a single layer or sheet of cells (simple) or several layers of one (stratified) or several (compound) types of simple epithelia. Some examples of epithelia are listed below.

Simple squamous epithelium: thin, flat cells organized in sheets such as the peritoneum

Simple cuboidal epithelium: cube-shaped cells comprising the lining of certain ducts such as portions of the nephron

Simple columnar epithelium: tall, rectangular cells that may also be found lining certain ducts

Stratified squamous epithelium; epidermis

Glandular epithelium: cords of cells as in the adrenal cortex, acini (solid balls of cells with a central duct) as found in the exocrine pancreas, follicles or hollow balls of cells as those comprising the thyroid gland

Connective Tissue

The cells of connective tissue are generally separated from one another by extensive intracellular material (matrix) that they have secreted. Mesenchyme derived from mesoderm gives rise to four basic kinds of connective tissue: *blood and lymph-forming tissues, connective tissue proper, cartilage* and *bone.*

Blood-Forming Tissues

The blood-forming elements give rise to circulating *erythrocytes* or red blood cells (RBCs) and *leukocytes* or white blood cells (WBCs) in adult vertebrates. The RBCs of mammals are unique among the vertebrates in that the mature circulating cell lacks a nucleus. The WBCs are further subdivided into cells with granular cytoplasm, the granulocytes (*eosinophils, basophils, neutrophils*) and agranulocytes (*lymphocytes, monocytes, plasma cells*). Circulating eosinphils are identical to those associated with many organs such as the uterus and the lung. Basophils may be identical to tissue mast cells.

Connective Tissue Proper

A large number of tissue types are lumped under the title of connective tissue proper, including *loose fibrous connective tissue, dense fibrous connective tissue* (e.g., tendons), *elastic* and *reticular connective tissue,* and *adipose tissue.* The fibrous components are proteins (collagen, elastin, reticular fibers) and are found in the different connective tissue types to various extents.

Adipose tissue consists of cells that contain large amounts of fat restricted to a central vacuole which confines the cytoplasm to a thin rim adjacent to the plasmalemma. In rodents there are two readily distinguishable types of adipose tissue termed *white* and *brown fat.* White adipose tissue shows regular variations in the amount of stored fat with nutritional state. Brown fat is found in particular locations and does not vary with nutritional state. It has been correlated with hibernating behavior. In most mammals it is not possible to differentiate brown and white types of adipose tissue.

Cartilage

Cartilage cells (*chondrocytes*) secrete a matrix consisting of a glycoprotein, chondromucoid, that contains the sulfonated polysaccharide chondroitin sulfate. The extensive matrix between the chondrocytes may have few fibrous components (*hyaline cartilage*) or may contain collagen (*fibrocartilage*) or elastin fibers (*elastic cartilage*). Cartilage may also be strengthened by addition of calcium salts.

Bone

Bone is the strongest connective tissue and the most dense. The extensive matrix of bone is comprised of crystalline calcium salts, primarily calcium phosphate, and very little water. Bone occurs in a uniformly dense, compact form (*compact bone*) and in a less dense, more easily modified form (*cancellous or spongy bone*). The bone-forming cells are known as *osteoblasts* and are rich in phosphatase. Osteoblasts that have become embedded within the bone matrix are termed *osteocytes.* Giant multinucleated cells, the *osteoclasts,* containing hydrolytic enzymes are responsible for bone destruction (*resorption*). The osteoblasts and osteoclasts are responsible for bone forming, resorption and re-forming in accordance with physical stresses placed on bone and with physiological demands and sources of calcium and phosphate.

Muscle

Mesoderm gives rise to three basic muscle types: smooth, striated and cardiac. *Smooth muscle* is frequently termed involuntary muscle since it is under control of the autonomic nervous system. Primarily it is associated with internal organs and is found in such places as the gut wall, blood vessels, various ducts and the wall of the uterus. Individual muscle cells are smaller than striated cells and the contractile elements (myofibrils) are not highly organized within the cell. Smooth muscle is characterized by slow, rhythmic contractions.

Striated or *skeletal muscle* is the so-called voluntary muscle tissue that is under conscious control, although it may also be influenced by the autonomic system. Striated muscle cells are large cells with myofibrils so highly organized as to produce regular bands or striations when the cells are viewed with the aid of a microscope. Movements of the skeleton are controlled by striated muscles that are attached to the bone by dense fibrous connective tissue. In addition, a few sphincter muscles are also of this type and hence are under conscious control (e.g., the urinary bladder sphincter).

Cardiac muscle possesses properties of both skeletal muscle (striations due to highly organized myofibrils) and smooth muscle (rhythmic contractions that are innate properties of cardiac muscle cells). Instead of inserting on bones, the cardiac cells connect directly to one another through specialized tendinous attachments known as intercalated disks.

Nervous Tissue

Nervous tissue is specialized for integrative functions and conduction of information throughout the body. *Neurons* are specialized cells for conducting electrochemical neural impulses to coordinate body processes. *Neurosecretory neurons* produce neurohormones that are secreted into the blood vascular system and constitute a second type of control mechanism. The central nervous system also contains *glial cells* (neuroglia) whose functions are not entirely understood. *Schwann cells* secrete the myelin sheath characteristic of certain peripheral neurons.

II·Adrenergic Receptors

Two types of adrenergic receptors for epinephrine and norepinephrine are known: *alpha* and *beta* receptors. Alpha adrenergic receptors bind in order of decreasing affinities epinephrine, norepinephrine and the sympathomimetic drugs (that is, drugs that mimic sympathetic catecholamines) phenylephrine and isoproteronol. Ergot alkaloids (for example, ergocryptine, ergocornine) and other so-called alpha blockers, such as phentolamine and dibenamine, antagonize binding to alpha receptors without instigating adrenergic-type responses in target cells. Alpha receptors are associated with smooth muscles involved in responses such as vasoconstriction, uterine contractions and relaxation of intestinal muscles. Beta adrenergic receptors exhibit highest affinity for isoproteronol followed by epinephrine, norepinephrine and phenylephrine. Activation of beta receptors is associated with responses characteristic for epinephrine, including vasodilation, relaxation of uterine muscles and cardiac acceleration.

Norepinephrine operates primarily by binding to alpha receptors, whereas epinephrine usually binds readily to both alpha and beta receptors. Thus norepinephrine will cause vasoconstriction as will epinephrine. However, in the presence of an alpha blocker, epinephrine will cause vasodilation. The relative absence of alpha receptors in cardiac muscle explains the insensitivity of the heart to circulating norepinephrine.

Many cells that are not innervated by either sympathetic or parasympathetic fibers may possess alpha or beta receptors or both. Ergot alkaloids, which directly inhibit release of prolactin and MSH from the adenohypophysis (see Chap. 5), probably bind to alpha receptors on these cells. Noninnervated melanophores in the skin of certain amphibians and reptiles possess alpha or beta receptors or both and respond in vitro to exogenous catecholamines with melanin dispersion. Propranolol inhibits the binding of epinephrine to rat liver cell membranes demonstrating the presence of beta receptors in these cell membranes.

III·Additional Readings in Endocrinology

This appendix consists of a listing of selected reviews and books relating specifically to the material covered in this textbook. In addition, a listing of some of the more important journals and serials is provided so that the interested reader may obtain a better knowledge of trends in endocrine research and update the material provided here.

Selected Sources

General and Comparative Endocrinology

ADLER, N.T. (1981). Neuroendocrinology of Reproduction. Plenum Publ., New York.

BARRINGTON, E.J.W. (1979/80). Hormones and Evolution. Vol. 1 and 2, Academic Press, London.

BENTLEY, P.J. (1982). Comparative Vertebrate Endocrinology, 2nd ed. Cambridge University Press, London.

DEGROOT, L.J., G.F. CAHILL, JR., L. MARTINI, D.H. NELSON, W.D. O'DELL, J.T. POTTS, JR., E. STEINBERGER and A.I. WINEGRAD (1979). Endocrinology, 3 vol. Grune and Stratton, New York.

DUNN, M.J. (1983). Renal Endocrinology. Williams & Wilkins, Baltimore.

GORBMAN, A., W.W. DICKHOFF, S.R. VIGNA, N.B. CLARK and C.L. RALPH (1983). Comparative Endocrinology. John Wiley and Sons, New York.

GRAY, C.H. and V.H.T. JAMES. (1979–). Hormones in Blood. Academic Press, New York.

HADLEY, M.E. (1984). Endocrinology. Prentice-Hall, Englewood Cliffs, New Jersey.

HELLER, H. (1974). Molecular aspects in comparative endocrinology. Gen. Comp. Endocrinol. 22:315–332.

HERSHMAN, J.M. (1977). Endocrine Pathophysiology: A Patient Oriented Approach. Lea & Febiger, Philadelphia.

HERSHMAN, J.M. (1980). Management of Endocrine Disorders. Lea & Febiger, Philadelphia.

ISHII, S., T. HIRANO and M. WADA (1980). Hormones, Adaptations and Evolution. Japan. Sci. Soc., Tokyo/Springer-Verlag, Berlin.

JAFFE, B.M. and H.R. BEHRMAN (1974). Methods of Hormone Radioimmunoassay. Academic Press, New York.

JONES, T.C., U. MOHR and R.D. HUNT (1983). Endocrine System. Monographs on Pathology of Laboratory Animals. Springer-Verlag, Berlin.

KRIEGER, D.T. and J.C. HUGHES (1980). Neuroendocrinology. Sinaur Associates, Sunderland, MA.

MCCANN, S.M. (1974, 1977). Endocrine Physiology I, II. University Park Press, Baltimore.

MARTIN, C.R. (1976). Textbook of Endocrine Physiology. Williams & Wilkins, Baltimore.

NOVY, M.J. and J.A. RESKO (1981). Fetal Endocrinology. Academic Press, New York.

PANG, P.K.T. and A. EPPLE (1980). Evolution of Vertebrate Endocrine Systems. Texas Tech University, Lubbock, TX.

SHIRE, J.G.M. (1976). The forms, uses and significance of genetic variation in endocrine systems. Biol. Rev. 51:105–141.

TRIBE, M.A. and M.R. ERAUT (1978). Hormones, Book II. Cambridge University Press, London.

TURNER, C.D. and J.T. BAGNARA (1976). General Endocrinology, 6th ed. W.B. Saunders Co., Philadelphia.

VILLEE, D.S. (1975). Human Endocrinology, A Developmental Approach. W.B. Saunders Co., Philadelphia.

WEITZMAN, E.D. (1976). Circadian rhythms and episodic hormone secretion in man. Annu. Rev. Med. 27:225–243.

WILLIAMS, R.H. (1981). Textbook of Endocrinology. W.B. Saunders Co., Philadelphia.

General Endocrinology of Nonmammalian Groups

FARNER, D.S. and J.R. KING (1971–). Avian Biology. Academic Press, New York, continuing series.

GANS, C. (1969–). Biology of the Reptilia, Academic Press, New York, continuing series.

HARDISTY, M.W. and I.C. POTTER (1971–). The Biology of Lampreys. Academic Press, New York, 3 Vol.

HOAR, W.S. and D.J. RANDALL (1969–). Fish Physiology. Academic Press, New York, continuing series.

LOFTS, B. (1974, 1976). Physiology of the Amphibia. Academic Press, New York, Vol. 2, 3.

PLETHES, G., P. PECZELY and R. RUDAS (1981). Recent Advances of Avian Endocrinology. Plenum Publ., New York.

SCANES, C.G., M.A. OTTINGER, A.D. KENNY, J. BALTHAZART, J. CRONSHAW and I. CHESTER JONES (1982). Aspects of Avian Endocrinology. Practical and Theoretical Implications. Texas Tech University, Lubbock, TX.

Mechanisms of Hormone Action

BRADSHAW, R.A. and G.N. GILL (1983). Evolution of Hormone-Receptor Systems, A.R. Liss, New York.

CATT, K.J. and M.L. DUFAU (1977). Peptide hormone receptors. Annu. Rev. Physiol. 39:529–549.

FELDMAN, D. (1975). The role of hormone receptors in the action of adrenal steroids. Annu. Rev. Med. 26:83–90.

GOLDBERGER, R.F. and K.R. YAMAMOTO (1982). Biological Regulation and Development, Vol. 3A, Hormone Action. Plenum Publ., New York.

LAMBLE, J.W. (1981). Towards Understanding Receptors. Elsevier/North Holland Biomedical Press, Amsterdam.

LOWENSTEIN, W.R. (1978). Epithelia as Hormone and Drug Receptors. Springer-Verlag, New York.

MALKINSON, A.M. (1975). Hormone Action. Outline Studies in Biology. Chapman and Hall, London.

MAINWARING, W.I.P. (1975). Steroid hormone receptors: A survey. Vitam. Horm. 33:223–246.

MAINWARING, W.I.P. (1976). The Mechanism of Action of Androgens. Monogr. in Endocrinol., Springer-Verlag, New York.

PEPEU, G., M.J. KUHAR, and S.J. ENNA (1980). Receptors for Neurotransmitters and Peptide Hormones. Raven Press, New York.

PITOT, H.C. and M.B. YATVIN (1973). Interrelationships of mammalian hormones and enzyme levels *in vivo*. Physiol. Rev. 53:228–325.

Hypothalamo-Hypophysial System

BAGNARA, J.T. and M.E. HADLEY (1973). Chromatophores and Color Change: The Comparative Physiology of Animal Pigmentation. Prentice-Hall, Englewood Cliffs, N.J.

BALL, J.N. (1981). Hypothalamic control of the pars distalis in fishes, amphibians and reptiles. Gen. Comp. Endocrinol. 44:135–170.

BEERS, R.F. and E.G. BASSETT (1980). Polypeptide Hormones. Raven Press, New York.

BERN, H.A. (1983). Functional evolution of prolactin and growth hormone in lower vertebrates. Am Zool. 23:663–671.

BESSER, G.M. and L. MARTINI (1978/82). Clinical Neuroendocrinology. Academic Press, New York.

BLACKWELL, R.E. and R. GUILLEMIN (1973). Hypothalamic control of adenohypophysial secretions. Annu. Rev. Physiol. 35:357–390.

BUCKINGHAM, J.C. (1977). The endocrine function of the hypothalamus. J. Pharm. Pharmacol. 29:649–656.

FONTAINE, M. and M. OLIVEREAU (1975). Aspects of the organization and evolution of the vertebrate pituitary. Am. Zool. 15, Suppl. 1:61–80.

GIVENS, J.R., J.T. ROBERTSON and A.E. KITABCHI (1983). The Hypothalamus. Year Book Medical Publ., Chicago.

GRIFFITHS, E.C. and G.W. BENNETT (1983). Thyrotropin-releasing Hormone. Raven Press, New York.

GUILLEMIN, R. and J.E. GERICH (1976). Somatostatin: Physiological and clinical significance. Annu. Rev. Med. 27:379–388.

HOLMES, R.L. and J.N. BALL (1974). The Pituitary Gland, A Comparative Account. Cambridge University Press, London.

HUGHES, J. (1983). Opioid peptides. Br. Med. Bull. 39:1–100.

JACKSON, I.M.D. and W.W. VALE (1981). Extrapituitary functions of hypothalamic hormones. Fed. Proc. 40:2543–2569.

JUTISZ, M. and K.W. MCKERNS (1980). Synthesis and Release of Adenohypophyseal Hormones. Plenum Publ., New York.

KNOBIL, E. (1974). On the control of gonadotropin secretion in the Rhesus monkey. Recent Prog. Horm. Res. 30:1–35.

KRIEGER, D.T. (1983). Brain peptides: What, where and why? Science 222:975–985.

MACLEOD, R.M. and U. SCAPAGNINI (1980). Central and Peripheral Regulation of Prolactin Function. Raven Press, New York.

MARTIN, J.B., S. REICHLIN and K.L. BICK (1981). Neurosecretion and Brain Peptides. Adv. Biochem. Psychopharmacol. 28:1–708.

OKSCHE, A. (1976). The neuroanatomical basis of comparative neuroendocrinology. Gen. Comp. Endocrinol. 29:225–239.

PANG, P.K.T., P.B. FURSPAN, and W.H. SAWYER (1983). Evolution of neurohypophysial hormone actions in vertebrates. Am. Zool. 23:655–662.

REICHLIN, S. (1984). The Neurohypophysis. Plenum Publ., New York.

SAWYER, C.H. (1978). History of the neurovascular concept of hypothalamo-hypophysial control. Biol. Reprod. 18:325–328.

TIXIER-VIDAL, A. and M.G. FARQUHAR, eds. (1975). The Anterior Pituitary. Academic Press, New York.

Thyroid

DEVISSCHER, M. (1980). Thyroid Gland, Comprehensive Endocrinology. Raven Press, New York.

DICKHOFF, W.W. and D.S. DARLING (1983). Evolution of thyroid function and its control in lower vertebrates. Am. Zool. 23:697–708.

HARLAND, W.A. and J.S. ORR (1975). Thyroid Hormone Metabolism. Academic Press, New York.

OPPENHEIMER, J.H. and H.H. SAMUELS (1983). Molecular basis of thyroid hormone action. Academic Press, New York.

STERLING, K. and J.H. LAZARUS (1977). The thyroid and its control. Annu. Rev. Physiol. 39:349–372.

WERNER, S.C. and S.H. INGBAR (1982). The Thyroid. Hoeber-Harper, New York.

Calcium and Phosphate Metabolism

CLARK, N.B. (1983). Evolution of calcium regulation in lower verebrates. Am. Zool. 23:719–728.

COPP, D.H. and S.W.Y. MA (1978). Endocrine control of calcium metabolism in vertebrates. In P.J. Gaillard and

H.H. Boer, eds., Comparative Endocrinology. Elsevier/North-Holland Biomedical Press, Amsterdam, pp. 243–254.

Dacke, C.G. (1979). Calcium Regulation in Sub-Mammalian Vertebrates. Academic Press, London.

Katz, A.I. and M.D. Lindheimer (1977). Actions of hormones on the kidney. Annu. Rev. Physiol. 39:97–134.

Massry, S.G. and H. Fleisch (1980). Renal Handling of Phosphate. Plenum Medical Book Co., New York.

Norman, A.W. (1979). Vitamin D: The Calcium Homeostatic Steroid Hormone. Academic Press, New York.

Pancreas

Andreani, D., P.J. Lefebvre and V. Marks (1980). Current Views on Hypoglycemia and Glucagon. Academic Press, London

Creutzfeldt, W. (1980). Gut feelings about the endocrine pancreas. The entero-insular axis. Frontiers of Hormone Res. 7:1–310.

Drouin, P., L. Mejean, and G. Derby (1979). Artificial Pancreas Clinical Applications. W.B. Saunders Co., Philadelphia.

Erlandsen, S.L. (1980). Types of pancreatic islet-cells and their immunocytohemical identification. In, P.J. Fitzgerald and A.B. Mornson, eds., Pancreas. Williams & Wilkins, Baltimore.

Falkmer, S. and S.O. Emdin (1981). Insulin evolution. In Dodson et al., eds., Structural Studies on Molecules of Biological Interest., Oxford University Press, London.

Grillo, T.A.I., L. Leibson, and A. Epple (1976). The Evolution of Pancreatic Islets. Pergamon, Oxford.

Skyler, J.S. and G.F. Cahill (1981). Diabetes Mellitus. Yorke Medical Books.

Unger, R.H. and R.E. Dobbs (1978). Insulin, glucagon, and somatostatin secretion in the regulation of metabolism. Annu. Rev. Physiol. 40:307–343.

Gastrointestinal Peptides

Barrington, E.J.W. (1982). Evolutionary and comparative aspects of gut and brain peptides. Br. Med. Bull. 38:227–232.

Brown, J.C., J.R. Dryburgh, S.A. Ross and J. Dupré (1975). Identification and actions of gastric inhibitory polypeptide. Recent Prog. Horm. Res. 31:487–532.

Mutt, V. (1982). Chemistry of the gastrointestinal hormones and hormone-like peptides and a sketch of their physiology and pharmacology. Vit. Horm. 39:231–427.

Polak, J.M. and S.R. Bloom (1982). Localization of regulatory peptides in the gut. Br. Med. Bull. 38:303–307.

Rehfeld, J.F. and E. Amdrup (1979). Gastrins and the Vagus. Academic Press, New York.

Sernka, T.J. and E.D. Jacobson (1979). Gastrointestinal Physiology. The Essentials. Williams & Wilkins, Baltimore.

Adrenocortical Hormones

Andrews, R.V. (1979). The physiology of crowding. Comp. Biochem. Physiol. 63A:1–6.

Chester Jones, I. and I.W. Henderson (1976–1980). General, Comparative, and Clinical Endocrinology of the Adrenal Cortex. Academic Press, New York, Vols. 1, 2, 3.

Davis, J.O. and R.H. Freeman (1976). Mechanisms regulating renin release. Physiol. Rev. 56:1–56.

Delrio, G. and J. Brachet (1980). Steroids and their Mechanism of Action in Nonmammalian Verebrates. Raven Press, New York.

Idler, D.R. (1972). Steroids in Nonmammalian Vertebrates. Academic Press, New York.

Idler, D.R. and B. Truscott (1980). Phylogeny of vertebrate adrenal corticosteroids. In P.K.T. Pang and A. Epple, eds., Evolution of Vertebrate Endocrine Systems. Texas Tech University, Lubbock, TX, pp. 357–372.

James, V.H.T. (1979). Adrenal Gland, Comprehensive Endocrinology. Raven Press, New York.

Jones, M.T., B. Gillham, M.F. Dallman and S. Chattopadhyay (1979). Interaction within the Brain-Pituitary-Adrenocortical System. Academic Press, New York.

Leung, K. and A. Munck (1975). Peripheral actions of glucocorticoids. Annu. Rev. Physiol. 37:245–272.

Pickering, A.D. (1981). Stress and Fish. Academic Press, New York.

Selye, H. (1976). The Stress of Life. McGraw-Hill, New York.

Adrenal Medulla

Axelrod, J. (1975). Relationship between catecholamines and other hormones. Recent Prog. Horm. Res. 31:1–26.

Coupland, R.E. (1979). Catecholamines. In E.J.W. Barrington, ed., Hormones and Evolution. Academic Press, London, Vol. 1, pp. 309–340.

Coupland, R.E. and T. Fujita (1976). Chromaffin, Enterochromaffin and Related Cells. Elsevier Scientific Publ. Co., Amsterdam.

Reproductive Endocrinology

Austin, C.R. and R.V. Short (1972–). Reproduction in Mammals. Cambridge University Press, London, 7 vol.

Breeder, C.M. and D.E. Rosen (1966). Modes of Reproduction in Fishes. Am. Mus. Nat. History, Nat. History Press, Garden City, N.Y.

Brenner, R.M. and N.B. West (1975). Hormonal regulation of the reproductive tract in female mammals. Annu. Rev. Physiol. 37:273–302.

Channing, C.C. and S.J. Segal (1982). Intraovarian control Mechanisms. Plenum Publ, New York.

Cole, H.H. and P.T. Cupps (1977). Reproduction in Domestic Animals, 3rd ed. Academic Press, New York.

De Brux, J., R. Mortel and J.P. Gautray (1981). The Endometrium, Hormonal Impacts. Plenum Publ., New York.

Eskin, B.A. (1980). Menopause, Comprehensive Management. Masson Publ., New York.

Flamigni, C. and J.R. Givens (1982). The Gonadotropins. Academic Press, New York.

Greenwald, G.S. and P.F. Terranova (1983). Factors Regulating Ovarian Function. Raven Press, New York.

Holmes, R.L. and C.A. Fox (1979). Control of Human Reproduction. Academic Press, New York.

Johnson, A.D. and C.W. Foley (1974). The Oviduct and Its Functions. Academic Press, New York.

Jones, R.E. (1978). The Vertebrate Ovary. Plenum Publ., New York.

NATHANIELSZ, P.W. (1978). Endocrine mechanisms of parturition. Annu. Rev. Physiol. 40:411–445.

PEAKER, M. (1978). Comparative Aspects of Lactation. Symp. Zool. Soc. Lond., No. 41. Academic Press, New York.

PERRY, J.S. (1972). The Ovarian Cycle of Mammals. Hafner Publishing Co., New York.

PERRY, J.S. and I.W. ROWLANDS (1969). Biology of Reproduction in Mammals. Blackwell Scientific Publications, Oxford. J. Reprod. Fertil. Suppl. 6.

REITER, R.J. and B.K. FOLLETT (1980). Seasonal Reproduction in Higher Vertebrates. Prog. in Reprod. Biol. 5:1–221.

SCHWARTZ, N.B. and M. HUNZICKER-DUNN (1981). Dynamics of Ovarian Function. Raven Press, New York.

STEINBERGER, A. and E. STEINBERGER (1980) Testicular Development, Structure and Function. Raven Press, New York.

STEINETZ, B.G., C. SCHWABE and G. WEISS (1982). Relaxin: Structure, Function and Evolution. Ann. N.Y. Acad. Sci. 380:1–244.

TAYLOR, D.H. and S.I. GUTTMAN (1977). The Reproductive Biology of Amphibians. Plenum Publ., New York.

TOVERUD, S.U. and A. BOASS (1979). Hormonal control of calcium metabolism in lactation. Vit. Horm. 37:303–347.

VAN TIENHOVEN, A. (1983). Reproductive Physiology of Vertebrates. 2nd ed. Cornell University Press, Ithaca, N.Y.

ZUCKERMAN, L. and B.J. WEIR, eds. (1977). The Ovary. Academic Press, New York, 3 vol.

Miscellaneous

ERYTHROPOEITIN

GORDON, A.S. (1973). Erythropoietin. Vit. Horm. 31:106–174.

KININS

GROSS, F. and H.G. VOGEL (1980). Enzymatic Release of Vasoactive Peptides. Raven Press, New York.

SANDER, G.E. and C.G. HUGGINS (1972). Vasoactive peptides. Annu. Rev. Pharmacol. 12:227–264.

SEMIOCHEMICALS

BIRCH, M.C. (1974). Pheromones. North-Holland Publishing Company, Amsterdam.

MULLER-SCHWARZE, D. and R.M. SILVERSTEIN (1980). Chemical Signals, Vertebrates and Aquatic Inverebrates. Plenum Publ., New York.

SHOREY, H.H. (1976). Animal Communication by Pheromones. Academic Press, New York.

VANDENBERGH, J.G. (1983). Pheromones and Reproduction in Mammals. Academic Press, New York.

PINEAL

AXELROD, J., F. FRASCHINI and G.P. VELO (1982). The Pineal Gland and Its Endocrine Role. Plenum Publ., New York.

KAPPERS, J.A. and P. PEVET (1979). Pineal Gland of Vertebrates Including Man. Prog. Brain Res. 52:1–562.

MINNEMAN, K.P. and R.J. WURTMAN (1976). The pharmacology of the pineal gland. Annu. Rev. Pharmacol. Toxicol. 16:33–52.

RALPH, C.L. (1983). Evolution of pineal control of endocrine function in lower vertebrates. Am. Zool. 23:597–606.

RELKIN, R. (1983). The Pineal Gland. Elsevier Biomedical, New York.

WURTMAN, R.J. (1975). The effects of light on man and other mammals. Annu. Rev. Physiol. 37:467–484.

PROSTAGLANDINS

COLQUHOUN, D. (1975). Physiological and pharmacological roles of prostaglandins. Annu. Rev. Pharmacol. 15:285–306.

HORTON, E.W. (1972). Prostaglandins. Monogr. in Endocrinol. Springer-Verlag, New York.

PHARRISS, B.B. and J.E. SHAW (1974). Prostaglandins in reproduction. Annu. Rev. Physiol. 36:391–412.

RAMWELL, P.W. (1973). The Prostaglandins. Plenum, New York.

SOMATOMEDIN

VAN WYK, J.J. and L.E. UNDERWOOD (1975). Relation between growth hormone and somatomedin. Annu. Rev. Med. 26:427–441.

VAN WYK, J.J. and L.E. UNDERWOOD, R.L. HINTZ, D.R. CLEMMONS, S.J. VOINA and R.P. WEAVER (1974). The somatomedins: A family of insulinlike hormones under growth hormone control. Recent Prog. Horm. Res. 30:259–294.

THYMUS

BACH, J.F. (1977). Thymic hormones: Biochemistry and biological and clinical activities. Annu. Rev. Pharmacol. Toxicol. 17:281–292.

LUCKEY, T.D. (1973). Thymic Hormones. University Park Press, Baltimore.

Serials

Advances in Cyclic Nucleotide Research
Advances in Prostaglandin and Thromboxane Research
Annual Review of Biochemistry
Annual Review of Medicine
Annual Review of Pharmacology and Toxicology
Annual Review of Physiology
Annual Research Reviews: Endocrinology and Medicine
- Anti-Diuretic Hormone
- Hypothalamic Releasing Factors
- Oxytocin
- Peripheral Metabolism and Action of Thyroid Hormones
- The Pineal
- Prolactin
- Renin
- Thyroid

Chemical Zoology
Pharmacological Reviews
Recent Advances in Steroid Biochemistry
Recent Progress in Hormone Research
Vitamins and Hormones
Yearbook of Endocrinology

Journals

Acta Endocrinologica
American Zoologist
Annales d'Endocrinologie
Biology of Reproduction
Cell and Tissue Research
Comparative Biochemistry and Physiology
Endocrine Reviews
Endocrinologica Japonica
Endocrinology
General and Comparative Endocrinology
Journal of Clinical Endocrinology and Metabolism
Journal of Endocrinology
Hormones and Behavior
Hormones and Metabolic Research
Molecular and Cellular Endocrinology
Neuroendocrinology
Peptides

IV·Glossary of Abbreviations

This glossary is included as an aid to the student in dealing with the bewildering jargon of endocrinology that necessitates inclusion of more than 130 abbreviations in this textbook. The glossary is separated into two parts. The first is an alphabetical listing of hormones, paracrines, neurotransmitters, growth factors, enzymes and miscellaneous substances plus a few hormone-related terms. The second part is a listing of anatomical abbreviations. Each abbreviation is followed by an explanation of what it represents and any synonyms. Use the index to locate these terms in the text.

Abbreviations for Hormones, Neurotransmitters and Related Substances or Processes

A_I = angiotensin I (A_{II} = angiotensin II, A_{III} = angiotensin III).
AAAD = adrenal ascorbic acid depletion
ABP = androgen-binding protein
ACh = acetylcholine
ACTH = corticotropin = adrenocorticotropin, adrenocorticotropic hormone
ADH = antidiuretic hormone = AVP in mammals
APUD = amine precursor uptake and decarboxylation
AR = aromatase
AST = aspargtocin = AT
AVP = arginine vasopressin = ADH
B = corticosterone
BEI = butanol-extractable iodide
cAMP = cyclic adenosine monophosphate
CBG = corticosteroid-binding globulin
cGMP = cyclic guanosine monophosphate
CCK-PZ = see PZ-CCK
COH = compensatory ovarian hypertrophy
COMT = catechol-O-methyltransferase
CRH = corticotropin-releasing hormone = ACTH-RH
CG = chorionic gonadotropin
CS = chorionic somatomammotropin (human = hCS) = PL
CT = calcitonin, thyrocalcitonin
DA = dopamine
DES = diethylstilbestrol
DHC = 1,25-dihydroxycholecalciferol = 1,25-DHC
DHEA = dehydroepiandrosterone
DHEAS = dehydoepiandrosterone sulfate
DHT = dihydrotestosterone
DIT = diiodotyrosine
DOPA = dihydroxyphenylalanine
E = epinephrine = adrenaline
E_2 = estradiol
EGF = epidermal growth factor
END = endorphin
ENK = enkephalin
ERY = erythropoietin
F = cortisol
FFA = free fatty acids = NEFA

FSH = follicle-stimulating hormone = follitropin
FSH-RH = see GnRH
GH = growth hormone = somatotropin, STH
GH-RH = growth hormone-releasing hormone = GRH, STH-RH
GH-RIH = growth hormone release-inhibiting hormone = somatostatin
GIP = glucose-dependent insulinotropic peptide (formerly gastric inhibitory peptide)
GLT = glumitocin = GT
GnRH = gonadotropin-releasing hormone = LHRH, FSH-RH
GRH = see GH-RH
GRP = gastrin-releasing peptide
GTH = gonadotropin = LH and/or FSH
HDL = high density lipoprotein
HIOMT = hydroxyindole-O-methyltransferase
HSD = hydroxysteroid dehydrogenase = 3βHSD
HT = 5-hydroxytryptamine, serotonin = 5-HT
ICSH = interstitial cell-stimulating hormone; see LH
IGF = insulinlike growth factor
IST = isotocin, ichthyotocin = IT
LATS = long-acting thyroid stimulator
LDL = low density lipoprotein
LH = luteinizing hormone = lutropin, ICSH
LH-RH = see GTH-RH
LPH = lipotropin
LSH = lymphocyte stimulating hormone
LT = leukotrienes (LTA = A series, etc.)
LTH = luteotropin, luteotropic hormone, lactogen = prolactin (PRL)
LVP = lysine vasopressin
LVT = lysine vasotocin
MAO = monoamine oxidase
MIS = mullerian inhibiting substance
MIT = monoiodotyrosine
MSA = multiplication stimulating activity
MSH = melanotropin = melanophore-stimulating hormone, melanocyte-stimulating hormone, intermedin
MSH-RIH = MSH release-inhibiting hormone
MST = mesotocin = MT
NAT = N-acetyltransferase
NE = norepinephrine = noradrenaline
NEFA = nonesterified fatty acids = FFA
NGF = nerve growth factor
NSAID = nonsteroid anti-inflammatory drugs
NSILA-S = nonsuppressible insulinlike activity soluble peptide
OAAD = ovarian ascorbic acid depletion
OXY = oxytocin = OT
PAG = pineal antigonadotropic peptides
PBI = protein-bound iodide
PG = prostaglandins (PGE = E series, etc.)
PHI = porcine histidine isoleucine peptide
PL = placental lactogen, see CS
PMSG = pregnant mare serum gonadotropin
PNMT = phenylethanolamine N-methyltransferase
PP = pancreatic polypeptide
PRIH = prolactin release-inhibiting hormone = PRL-RIH
PRL = prolactin = LTH
PROG = progesterone = P
PTH = parathyroid hormone
PVP = phenypressin
PZ-CCK = pancreozymin-cholecystokinin
rT_3 = reverse T_3 (3,3′,5-triiodothyronine)
SBG = steroid-binding globulin
STH = see GH
STH-RH = see GH-RH
T = testosterone
T_3 = triiodothyronine, (3,5,3′-triiodothyronine) = liothyronine
T_4 = thyroxine = tetraiodothyronine (3,5,3′,5′-tetraiodothyronine)
TBG = thyroxine-binding globulin
Tgb = thyroglobulin
TRF = see TRH
TRH = thyrotropin-releasing hormone = TRF
TSH = thyrotropin = thyroid-stimulating hormone
TYR = tyrosine
VAT = valitocin = VT

VIP = vasoactive intestinal peptide, vasoactive intestinal polypeptide
VLDL = very low density lipoprotein

Some Anatomical Abbreviations

CL = corpus luteum
HHA = hypothalamo-hypophysial axis
HHPS = hypothalamo-hypophysial portal system
IFN = infundibular nucleus
MAH = modified adenohypophysial tissue (Agnatha)
ME = median eminence
NH = neurohypophysis
NIL = neurointermediate lobe (fishes)
NLT = nucleus lateralis tuberis
NS = neurosecretory
NSM = neurosecretory material
NSN = neurosecretory neuron
PD = pars distalis
PI = pars intermedia
PN = pars nervosa
PON = preoptic nucleus = NPO
ppd = proximal pars distalis (fishes)
PT = pars tuberalis (tetrapods)
PV = pars ventralis = VL (elasmobranchs)
PVN = paraventricular nucleus
rpd = rostral pars distalis (fishes)
SCO = subcommissural organ
SON = supraoptic nucleus (anamniotes)
SV = saccus vasculosus (fishes)
UH = urohypophysis (bony fishes)
VL = ventral lobe = PV (elasmobranchs)

Index

Page numbers in *italics* indicate figures; numbers followed by "t" indicate tables.